CAPNOGRAPHY: CLINICAL ASPECTS

Nancy,

Best wishes,

[illegible] 8/20/08

CAPNOGRAPHY: CLINICAL ASPECTS
CARBON DIOXIDE OVER TIME AND VOLUME

Edited by

J.S. Gravenstein MD Drhc
Graduate Research Professor, Emeritus, Department of Anesthesiology
University of Florida College of Medicine
Gainesville, Florida, USA

Michael B. Jaffe PhD
Advanced Technology Projects Manager, Respironics-Novametrix, LLC
Wallingford, Connecticut, USA

David A. Paulus MD
Professor of Anesthesiology, Department of Anesthesiology and Mechanical Engineering
University of Florida College of Medicine and Engineering
Gainesville, Florida, USA

CAMBRIDGE
UNIVERSITY PRESS

PUBLISHED BY THE PRESS SYNDICATE OF THE UNIVERSITY OF CAMBRIDGE
The Pitt Building, Trumpington Street, Cambridge, United Kingdom

CAMBRIDGE UNIVERSITY PRESS
The Edinburgh Building, Cambridge CB2 2RU, UK
40 West 20th Street, New York, NY 10011-4211, USA
477 Williamstown Road, Port Melbourne, VIC 3207, Australia
Ruiz de Alarcón 13, 28014 Madrid, Spain
Dock House, The Waterfront, Cape Town 8001, South Africa

http://www.cambridge.org

First published 2004

Printed in the United Kingdom at the University Press, Cambridge

Typeface: Ehrhardt 10/11pt System: QuarkXpress®

A catalog record for this book is available from the British Library

Library of Congress Cataloging in Publication data

ISBN 0 521 54034 8

CONTENTS

CONTRIBUTORS

Ozan Akça MD
Assistant Director, Outcomes Research Institute
Assistant Professor, Department of Anesthesiology
Neuroscience and Anesthesia ICU
University of Louisville
Louisville, Kentucky, USA

John T. Anderson MD FACS
Assistant Professor of Surgery
Department of Surgery
Trauma Surgery and Surgical Critical Care
University of California, Davis Health System
Sacramento, California, USA

Michael Banner PhD
Professor
Anesthesiology and Physiology
University of Florida College of Medicine
Gainesville, Florida, USA

Prasad Betadpur MD
Fellow, Pulmonary and Critical Care Medicine
University of Virginia Health Systems
Charlottesville, Virginia, USA

Francesca Bernabè MD
Medical Doctor in Anesthesia and Intensive Care
Department of Perioperative Medicine
Intensive Care and Emergency Medicine
Trieste University School of Medicine
Trieste, Italy

David G. Bjoraker MD
Associate Professor of Anesthesiology
University of Florida College of Medicine
Gainesville, Florida, USA

Lluis Blanch Torra MD
Critical Care Center
Hospital de Sabadell
Corporacio Parc Tauli
Sabadell, Spain

Edwin A. Bowe MD
Professor and Chair
Department of Anesthesiology
University of Kentucky
Lexington, Kentucky, USA

Philip G. Boysen MD FACP FCCP FCCM
Professor of Anesthesiolgy and Medicine
Chair, Department of Anesthesiology
University of North Carolina School of Medicine
Chapel Hill, North Carolina, USA
UNC-Chapel Hill
Chairman, Department of Anesthesiology
Chapel Hill, North Carolina, USA

Justin C. Cahill MD
Resident
Section of Emergency Medicine
Yale-New Haven Hospital
New Haven, Connecticut, USA

Brian Carmack MD
Department of Emergency Medicine
Orlando Regional Medical Center
Orlando, Florida, USA

Ira M. Cheifetz MD FCCM FAARC
Associate Professor of Pediatrics
Division Chief, Pediatric Critical Care Medicine
Medical Director, Pediatric Intensive Care Unit and
Pediatric Respiratory Care
Duke Children's Hospital
Durham, North Carolina, USA

David C. Cone MD
Associate Professor of Emergency Medicine and
Public Health
Chief, Division of EMS
Section of Emergency Medicine
Yale University School of Medicine
New Haven, Connecticut, USA

Nancy Craig RRT
Supervisor Respiratory Care
Children's Hospital of Boston
Boston, Massachusetts, USA

Bernhard Dahme PhD
Professor of Clinical Psychology
Psychological Institute III
Respiratory Psychophysiology Laboratory
University of Hamburg
Hamburg, Germany

Daniel P. Davis MD FACEP
Associate Professor of Clinical Medicine
Division of Emergency Medicine
University of California
San Diego, California, USA

Ronald Dueck MD
Clinical Professor
Department of Anesthesiology
University of California
San Diego, California, USA
Veterans Affairs Hospital
San Diego, California, USA

Jay L Falk MD
Clinical Professor of Medicine and
Emergency Medicine
University of Florida College of Medicine
Chief Academic Medical Officer
Orlando Regional Healthcare
Academic Chairman
Department of Emergency Medicine
Orlando Regional Medical Center
Orlando, Florida, USA

Roger Fletcher MD FRCA
Formerly Honorary Lecturer
Department of Anaesthesia
University Hospital, Lund, Sweden
Formerly at the Department of Anaesthesia
Manchester Royal Infirmary
Manchester, England

Michael Frakes BSN CFRN CCRN EMTP FP-C
Flight Nurse
LIFE STAR/Hartford Hospital
Hartford, Connecticut, USA

Andrea Gabrielli MD
Associate Professor of Anesthesiology and Surgery
Division of Critical Care Medicine
Medical Director Respiratory Care Services
Medical Director Hyperbaric Medicine
Shands Hospital at the University of Florida
Gainesville, Florida, USA

Thomas J. Gallagher MD
Professor of Anesthesiology and Surgery
University of Florida College of Medicine
Gainesville, Florida, USA

Julian M. Goldman MD
Harvard Medical School
Departments of Anesthesia and Biomedical
Engineering
Massachusetts General Hospital
Boston, Massachusetts, USA
Adjoint Associate Professor
University of Colorado School of Medicine
Denver, Colorado, USA

J.S. Gravenstein MD Drhc
Graduate Research Professor, Emeritus
Department of Anesthesiology
University of Florida College of Medicine
Gainesville, Florida, USA

Loren Greenway PhD FCCP
Administrative Director Pulmonary Medicine
Intermountain Healthcare
LDS Hospital
Salt Lake City, Utah, USA

Antonino Gullo MD
Full Professor in Intensive Care
Head, Department of Perioperative Medicine
Intensive Care and Emergency
Department of Perioperative Medicine
Intensive Care and Emergency Medicine
Trieste University, School of Medicine
Trieste, Italy

Adrian Karl Hamburger MD
Resident in Anesthesia
Department of Anesthesia and Critical Care
Massachusetts General Hospital
Boston, Massachusetts, USA

Donna S. Hamel RRT RCP FAARC
Research Coordinator
Duke Children's Hospital
Durham, North Carolina, USA

Amy V. Isenberg MD MPH
Fellow, Departments of Anesthesiology and
Preventive Medicine
University of North Carolina, School of Medicine
Chapel Hill, North Carolina, USA

Michael B. Jaffe PhD
Advanced Technology Projects Manager
Respironics-Novametrix, LLC
Wallingford, Connecticut, USA

Robert R. Kirby MD
Professor of Anesthesiology
Chief, Anesthesiology Service
Malcom Randall Veterans Affairs Medical Center
Gainesville, Florida, USA

E.F. Klein Jr MD FCCM
Professor of Anesthesiology
Division of Pediatric Anesthesiology
University of Arkansas for Medical Sciences
Little Rock, Arkansas, USA

A. Joseph Layon MD
Professor, Departments of Anesthesiology, Surgery, and Medicine
University of Florida College of Medicine
Gainesville, Florida, USA
Medical Director/Division Chief, Division of Critical Care Medicine
Shands Hospital at the University of Florida
Gainesville, Florida, USA

Emilio B. Lobato MD
Associate Professor of Anesthesiology
University of Florida College of Medicine
Assistant Chief, Anesthesiology Service
Medical Director, Operating Room Services
Chief, Cardiac Anesthesia
Malcom Randall VA Medical Center, NF/SG VHS
Gainesville, Florida, USA

Umberto Lucangelo MD
Assistant Professor in Anesthesia and Intensive Care
Department of Perioperative Medicine
Intensive Care and Emergency Medicine
Trieste University School of Medicine
Trieste, Italy

Paul E. Marik MD FCCP FCCM
Professor, University of Pittsburgh
University of Pittsburgh Medical Center
Pittsburgh, Pennsylvania, USA

Alicia E. Meuret PhD
Director, Psychophysiology Program
Center for Anxiety and Related Disorders
Boston University
Boston, MA, USA

Timothy E. Morey MD
Associate Professor
Department of Anesthesiology
University of Florida
Gainesville, Florida, USA

Joseph Orr PhD
Research Assistant Professor
Department of Anesthesiology
University of Utah
Salt Lake City, Utah, USA

Mehmet S. Ozcan MD
Fellow, Division of Critical Care Medicine
Department of Anesthesiology
University of Florida College of Medicine
Shands Hospital at the University of Florida
Gainesvilles, Florida, USA

David A. Paulus MD
Professor of Anesthesiology
Department of Anesthesiology and Mechanical Engineering
University of Florida College of Medicine and Engineering
Gainesville, Florida, USA

George A. Ralls MD
Department of Emergency Medicine
Orlando Regional Medical Center
Orlando, Florida, USA

Thomas Ritz PhD
Senior Research Scholar and Lecturer
Psychological Institute III
Respiratory Psychophysiology Laboratory
University of Hamburg
Hamburg, Germany

Walton T. Roth MD
Professor of Psychiatry
Department of Psychiatry and Behavioral Sciences
Stanford University
Palo Alto, California, USA

Thorsten Schäfer, Priv-Doz Drmed
Ruhr-Universität Bochum
Institut für Physiologie
Bochum, Germany

Peter W. Scherer MD PhD
Professor of Bioengineering
Department of Bioengineering
University of Pennsylvania
Philadelphia, Pennsylvania, USA

Gerd Schmalisch Priv-Doz Drscnat
Clinic of Neonatology (Charité Campus Mitte)
Humboldt-University
Berlin, Germany

Salvatore Silvestri MD FACEP
Medical Director
Orange County EMS System
Orange County, Florida, USA
Faculty Attending and Director/Division of EMS
Department of Emergency Medicine
Orlando Regional Medical Center
Orlando, Florida, USA
Clinical Assistant Professor
Department of Emergency Medicine
University of Florida College of Medicine
Gainesville, Florida, USA

Bob Smalhout MD PhD
Formerly Founder and Head
Institute of Anaesthesiology
University Hospital
Utrecht, The Netherlands

Daniel E. Supkis MD
Covenor of IEC/ISO Joint Working Group for Respiratory Gas Monitors and
Associate Professor of Anesthesiology
MD Anderson Cancer Center
Houston, Texas, USA

Robert Joseph Thomas MD MMSc
Instructor in Medicine
Harvard Medical School
Division of Pulmonary, Critical Care and Sleep Medicine
Beth Israel Deaconess Medical Center
Boston, Massachusetts, USA

John E. Thompson RRT
Director of Clinical Technology
Children's Hospital of Boston
Associate in Anesthesia
Harvard Medical School
Boston, Massachusetts, USA

Jonathon Dean Truwit MD
E. Cato Drash Professor
Senior Associate Dean, Clinical Affairs
Chief, Pulmonary and Critical Care Medicine
University of Virginia Health Systems
Charlottesville, Virginia, USA

Joseph Varon MD FACP FCCP FCCM
Professor, The University of Texas Health Science Center
St. Luke's Episcopal Hospital
Houston, Texas, USA

Kevin R. Ward MD
Associate Professor and Director of Research
Department of Emergency Medicine
Associate Director
VCU Reanimation Engineering Shock Center (VCURES)
Virginia Commonwealth University
Richmond, Virginia, USA

Marvin A. Wayne MD FACEP FAAEM
Associate Clinical Professor
University of Washington School of Medicine
Assistant Clinical Professor
Section of Emergency Medicine Yale University
Emergency Medical Services Medical Director
Bellingham/Whatcom County
Bellingham, Washington, USA

Charles Weissman MD
Professor and Chair
Department of Anesthesiology and Critical Care Medicine
Hebrew University – Hadassah School of Medicine
Jerusalem, Israel

Daphne Willner MD
Resident
Department of Anesthesiology and Critical Care Medicine
Hadassah–Hebrew University Medical Center
Jerusalem, Israel

Kai Zhao PhD
Department of Bioengineering
University of Pennsylvania
Philadelphia, Pennsylvania, USA

PREFACE

This work explores carbon dioxide from physiology to clinical application of capnography. Included are discussions of physiological concepts and traditional uses of intra-operative and non-operative capnography. We have considered both applications where capnography has gained a foothold and is fast becoming a standard of care as well as the newer emerging applications. This calls for expertise in diverse fields. We persuaded over 40 specialists to give account of their findings and applications in essays that could stand as independent reports. As a consequence, this book is in some respects more of a symposium than a textbook while it covers a comprehensive range of topics relating to the application of capnography in health care. For the readers' comfort we have accepted some overlap and repetition. We have also allowed for differences in perspectives inherent in the background of the author. We are particularly pleased with the historical section of the book, which comprises unique contributions from some of the pioneers of capnography.

J.S. Gravenstein
M.B. Jaffe
D.A. Paulus

COMMONLY USED ABBREVIATIONS

Abbreviation: Subscripts

A, alv	alveolar
a	arterial
aw	airway
B, b	barometric
d, ds	dead space
E, exp	expiratory
I, insp	inspiratory
Fx,i	fractional concentration of component i in medium x
Px,i	partial pressure of component i in medium x
V	gas volume
ATP	ambient temperature and barometric pressure
ATPD	ambient temperature and barometric pressure, dry
ATPS	ambient temperature and barometric pressure, saturated with water vapor under these conditions
BTPS	body temperature, barometric pressure and saturation with water vapor under these conditions

Examples

P_aCO_2	partial pressure of carbon dioxide in arterial blood
$P_{et}CO_2$	partial pressure of carbon dioxide at end-tidal
P_ACO_2	partial pressure of carbon dioxide in alveolar gas
F_ECO_2	fractional concentration of carbon dioxide in expired gas

Reference

Quanjer, P.H., Sly, P.D. & Stocks, J. (1995). Respiratory function measurements in infants: symbols, abbreviations and units. *Eur. Respir. J.*, **8(6)**: 1039–1056.

INTRODUCTION

The American Society of Anesthesiologists (ASA) says in its standards for basic anesthetic monitoring:

> *To ensure adequate ventilation of the patient during all anesthetics ... every patient receiving general anesthesia shall have the adequacy of ventilation continually evaluated ... Continual monitoring for the presence of expired carbon dioxide shall be performed unless invalidated by the nature of the patient, procedure or equipment. Quantitative monitoring of the volume of expired gas is strongly encouraged. When an endotracheal tube or laryngeal mask is inserted, its correct positioning must be verified by clinical assessment and by identification of carbon dioxide in the expired gas. Continual end-tidal carbon dioxide analysis, in use from the time of endotracheal tube/laryngeal mask placement, until extubation/removal or initiating transfer to a postoperative care location, shall be performed using a quantitative method, such as capnography, capnometry, or mass spectroscopy*[1].

This ringing endorsement and requirement of capnography by the ASA as well as other medical societies focuses our attention on the successful ventilation of the lungs, as documented by the appearance of carbon dioxide (CO_2) with every exhalation. However, the traditional time-based capnography says nothing about the volumes of gas that delivered the CO_2. Volumetric capnography, which provides a volume-based view of ventilation, as such brings us wonderful additional intelligence.

The current spotlight on and the growing recognition of the clinical value of time- and volume-based capnography are well deserved. Too many patients have died because of ventilation-related problems. But capnography has much more to offer. For example, a readily available sign of a severe pulmonary embolism is the decrease in end-tidal CO_2 at constant tidal volume and minute ventilation. This directs our attention to the delivery of CO_2 to the alveoli and thus to pulmonary blood flow. In consequence, capnography tells a story not only about ventilation but it can also provide crucial information on circulation, specifically pulmonary blood flow.

And that is not all. In malignant hyperthermia oxygen consumption and CO_2 production go into overdrive. Long before the fever sets in, CO_2 production is racing ahead and its concentration in the expired gas rises dramatically, best seen when we can combine the measurements of volume and CO_2 so that we can calculate the volume of CO_2. Thus, capnography generates early warning signs of a rare but treacherous complication of metabolism. This is but one example of how capnography can alert us to the unexpected appearance of CO_2 in the body, or to its decrease.

When we take stock of capnography, we recognize that these measurements can provide important insight and crucial information on ventilation *and* on circulation *and* on metabolism. How these three factors interact will be an important aspect of the book before you.

In a patient who has suffered trauma to the brain or who undergoes an intracranial operation or who has a mass occupying lesion in the brain, the arterial CO_2 levels must be carefully controlled in order to avoid a devastating rise in intracranial pressure or damaging hyperventilation. While we want to monitor arterial CO_2 tension in such patients, the management of ventilation will be greatly assisted by capnography, exemplifying another value of capnography.

To recapitulate: The data provided by capnography must be interpreted with a keen awareness that ventilation *and* circulation *and* metabolism can affect end-tidal values. Interpretation of the data is greatly aided by volumetric capnography. Furthermore, the effects of CO_2 on organs such as the brain make control of ventilation and consequently of arterial CO_2 tension an essential component of good clinical management.

In view of these four perspectives on capnography, we have decided to collate much of the leading *clinical section* of this book in four subsections that concentrate on ventilation, circulation, metabolism and organ effects. In each of these subsections you will find clinical examples and much practical information. We follow the *clinical section* with a look at the basic physiology of CO_2, a history of CO_2 measurements with perspectives from the fathers of time and volumetric capnography and end it with a detailed examination of the technology that makes all of this possible.

---

[1] www.asahq.org/publicationsAndServices/standards/02.pdf

CLINICAL PERSPECTIVES

PART 1

CLINICAL PERSPECTIVES 1

J.S. Gravenstein & D.A. Paulus

Who should be monitored?

Unless you are on cardiopulmonary bypass or in deep hypothermia, you must breathe, that is, you must ventilate your lungs to pick up oxygen and deliver carbon dioxide (CO_2) from the lungs to the outside. Detecting – breath after breath – appropriate volumes of gas and concentrations of CO_2 in the exhaled gas (it is no longer air!) proves in one stroke several important facts:

1 CO_2 is being generated by metabolic processes during which the body utilizes oxygen.
2 Venous blood brings the CO_2 from the periphery to the heart.
3 The heart pumps blood through the lungs.
4 Ventilation of the lungs – spontaneous or manual or mechanical – conveys the CO_2 and other gases to the outside. As long as no contrivance, such as a ventilator, is attached to the patient, the journey of CO_2 ends here, as far as we are concerned. This adds up to an enormous amount of important information should we suspect a problem with CO_2 production, its transport to the heart and to the lungs and its elimination in the exhaled gas.

Subsequent chapters in this book will deal in considerable detail with specific issues of CO_2 production, transport, and analysis. Here we will examine different time- and volume-based capnograms and invite the reader to analyze them with a clinical eye with a special focus on problems related to ventilation, by far the most common clinical application of capnography.

Before presenting different capnographic patterns a word of caution. A capnogram, whether time or volume based, presents a snapshot. Even a trend plot running over several minutes represents but a brief episode in a phase of a patient's disease. More often than not, capnography is recruited to help with the diagnosis and interpretation of an acute process (intubation, embolism, bronchospasm, adjustment of ventilation, bicarbonate infusion, etc.). We must remember that the body has uncounted mechanisms to compensate for disturbances. These mechanisms can affect cardiac output, pulmonary blood flow, ventilation, acid–base balance, and renal physiology. In short, every acute change in ventilation and circulation with effects on CO_2 homeostasis will induce changes. When we observe capnographic data during such unsteady states, we must be aware of the fact that capnography can tell only a small part of the story and that the data in front of us are likely to change until a new steady state has been reached. Clinicians toil to help the body to make this new steady state as physiologic as possible.

The normal time-based capnogram

For many years the only widely available capnographic display plotted CO_2 along a time axis. The phases were labeled in different ways, for example as shown diagrammatically in Figure 1.1.

Time-based capnography can use either an on-airway (or "mainstream") method, which uses a cuvette containing a cell in which the concentration of CO_2 is assessed or a side-stream system, which relies on aspirating gas close to the patient's face and bringing it via a long capillary tube to the gas analyzer.

Difficulties arise when we try to determine when in the respiratory cycle the phases were recorded. Figure 1.2 shows tracings obtained during mechanical ventilation of an anesthetized patient. The time plots represent from top to bottom flow, mainstream capnogram, side-stream capnogram, and airway pressure.

Observe that the mainstream capnogram precedes the side-stream capnogram by the transport time of gas in the capillary connecting the sampling port (usually on the "Y" of the breathing circuit close to the patient's mouth) to the gas analyzer. At the end of inspiration the dead-space of the patient will be filled with air. Thus, the first exhaled gas (about 150 ml for the average adult) of anatomic dead-space without CO_2 will not be recognized by the capnograph. Phase I (without CO_2) of the capnogram, therefore, contains a little exhaled gas. Finally, a respiratory pause at the end of expiration will leave stagnant gas in the cuvette of the mainstream analyzer or under the sampling port of the side-stream analyzer. Thus, time-based capnograms show the end of exhalation only when end-tidal values are abruptly interrupted by a breath that washes away the CO_2. If phase III of a time-based capnogram is horizontal, we cannot separate the end-expiratory portion that may represent a respiratory pause from an ongoing exhalation delivering a steady level of CO_2. Indeed, should the patient be in respiratory arrest, the plateau would eventually slowly decay as the gas-aspirating side-stream analyzer begins to aspirate air (or gas from the breathing circuit). Despite these limitations, time-based capnography has been widely adopted and has greatly enhanced the safety of patients at risk of inadequate ventilation.

Before interpreting the capnogram, we must ascertain that artifacts have not distorted the tracing. Two sources of distortions can be recognized as detailed below.

Mechanical

Here we include improper calibration of the gas analyzer as discussed in Chapter 39. A leak in the sampling tube of a side-stream gas analyzer can allow

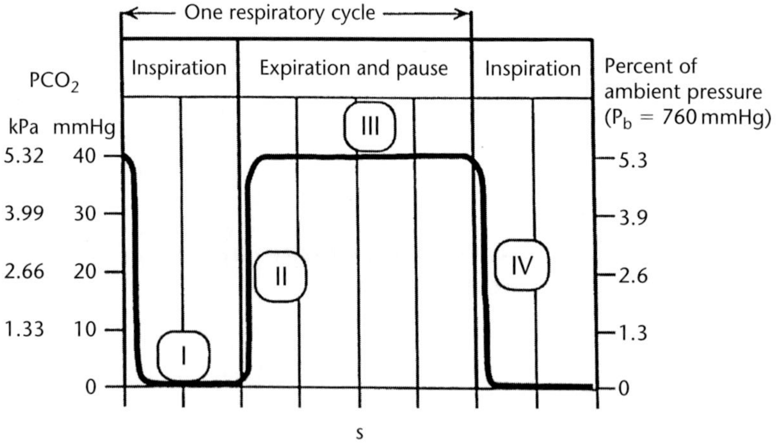

Figure 1.1 The capnogram has four phases: I: inspiration; II: the appearance of CO_2 during early expiration; III: the plateau phase, with or without a respiratory pause; and IV: the descending slope of the inspiratory phase. With a respiratory rate of 10 breaths/min, one respiratory cycle would last 6 s. The ratio of inspiration to expiration is assumed to be 1:2. Gases assumes to be dry; barometric pressure (P_b) is 760 mmHg.

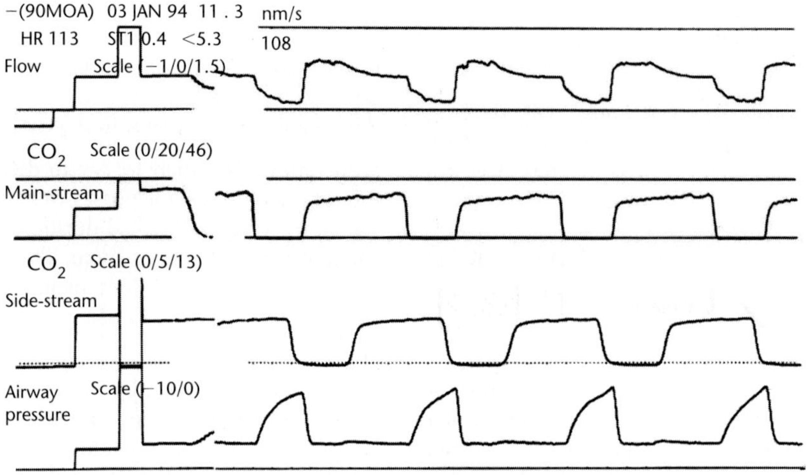

Figure 1.2 Tracing from a patient during controlled ventilation using a circle breathing system. Tracings from top to bottom are flow, mainstream capnogram, side-stream capnogram, and airway pressure. Observe that flow and pressure show relatively short fluctuations with inspiration and expiration and the side-stream capnogram is out of phase. With side-stream analyzers the gas has to be carried from the patient to the analyzer through a capillary. Inspiration and expiration on the pressure and flow recording are not simultaneous with inspiration and expiration on the capnogram. The plateaus of the capnograms extend into the respiratory pause and last until the next inspiration arrives.

air to be aspirated and thus dilute the sampled CO_2. One special circumstance can lead to the "steepled" capnogram discussed in Chapter 6 (Capnography during anesthesia). Obstruction of the sampling catheter would cause the capnogram to be dampened, slurring up- and down-slopes of the capnogram and causing falsely high inspired and falsely low end-expired CO_2 values.

Observe that the side-stream capnograms are a little more rounded than the on-airway capnograms (Figure 1.2). Thus, the side-stream capnographic signals have undergone some damping brought about when the front of the gas column traveling in the long capillary tube undergoes some mixing with adjoining gas. This damping problem becomes more troublesome with rapid respiration as shown in Figure 1.3. With rapid ventilation as encountered in pediatric anesthesia, the system might not have sufficient time to reach 100% of the required response, thus displaying higher than actual inspired and lower than actual expired CO_2 values. The response time of capnographs are discussed in Chapter 39.

A water trap with a large internal volume (Figure 1.4) can also introduce artifacts when high airway pressures during inspiration compress gas in the trap. This gas expands during expiration and enters the gas

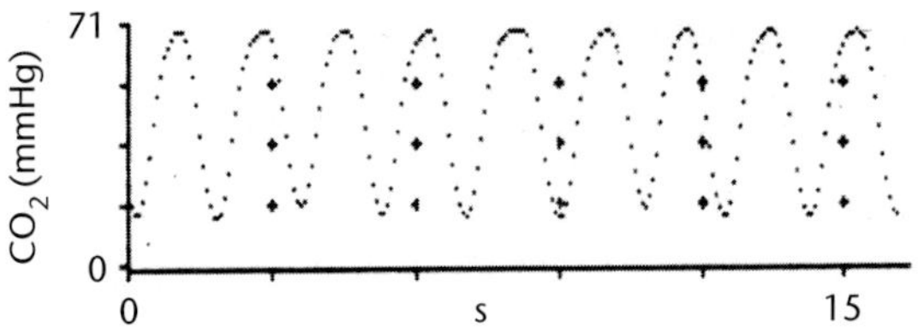

Figure 1.3 A capnogram without a well-defined plateau does not enable end-tidal partial pressure of CO_2 ($P_{et}CO_2$) to be deduced. End-tidal values are reported to be 70.5 mmHg; however, they are likely to be much higher in this tachypneic child. Observe that the inspired values show a PCO_2 of 14.9 even though there was no rebreathing. The respiratory rate exceeded the capnograph's power of resolution. A capnogram without a plateau in phase III may not give meaningful end-tidal values for any other gas exhaled by the patient. Inspect the capnogram before accepting as valid data presented by the instrument.

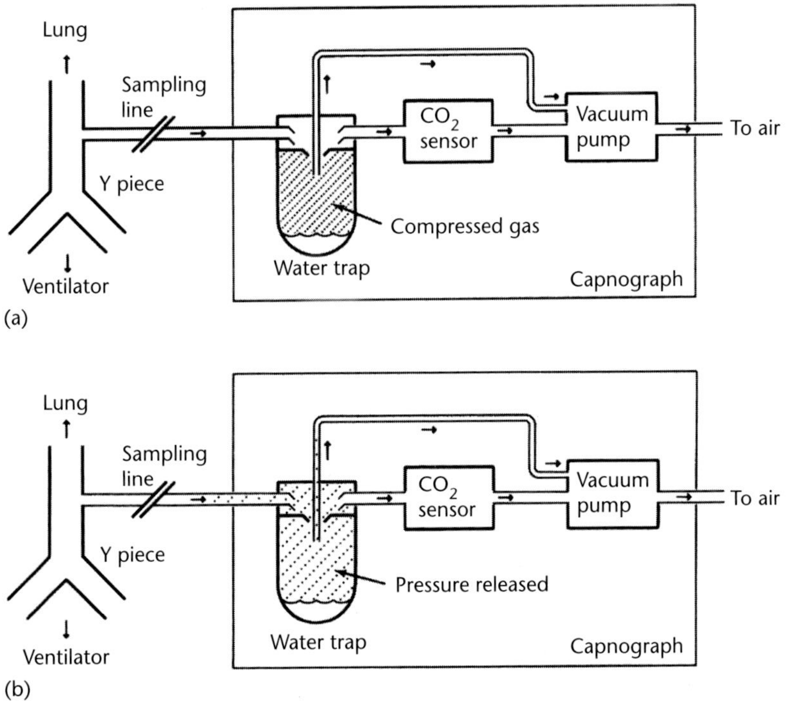

Figure 1.4 Capnograms artifact and water traps. Large water traps (>10 ml) produce artifact, which has its origin in the phase of respiration and whose appearance depends on respiratory rate. (a): At the end of inspiration, the system is pressurized at peak airway pressure (P_{aw}) and filled with fresh gas, except for the lower part of the water trap, which holds a gas mixture containing CO_2 (shaded). (b): At the beginning of expiration, P_{aw} decreases to baseline. The pressurized gas mixture in the lower part of the water trap expands and some flows into the sampling tube, the CO_2 content of which is eventually detected by the capnograph. Its appearance on the capnograph depends on what part of an earlier breath is moving through the water trap when the P_{aw} drops to baseline. With constant sampling flow and tube length, it depends on respiratory rate.

stream to be analyzed, thus introducing an artifact (van Genderingen & Gravenstein, 1987). Modern side-stream capnographs use small water traps and/or filters.

Clinical artifacts

The smooth outline of the capnogram might be dented by the patient taking a breath while undergoing mechanical ventilation. Figure 1.5 shows an example. This pattern has been baptized a "curare cleft", an unfortunate appellation. Calling it a curare cleft implies that not enough muscle relaxant drugs had been given so that the patient was capable of initiating a breath. Instead of focusing on incomplete relaxation, the clinician should ask why the patient attempts to breathe while being mechanically ventilated. The answer might be that the patient's partial pressure of CO_2 in arterial blood (P_aCO_2) exceeds physiological limits and that in the face of partial paralysis a troubled respiratory center attempts to correct hypercarbia. Increasing minute ventilation would be a better measure than deepening the muscle relaxation. An alternative explanation might be that the patient, unable to signal pain because of almost complete paralysis, gasps in desperation. Rather than blocking the response with deeper muscle paralysis, the patient should be better anesthetized. Finally, a "curare cleft" can be generated by pushing on the patient's chest, as might well happen when the surgeon leans on the chest during an operation. Only if the clinician is persuaded that none of these explanations apply and that a hiccup must be held responsible for the "curare cleft" and the brief inspiratory efforts interfere with the surgical procedure should the degree of muscle relaxation be increased.

Finally, cardiogenic oscillations might ripple the down-slope of the capnogram (Figure 1.6). These interesting, heart rate synchronous, small inspirations

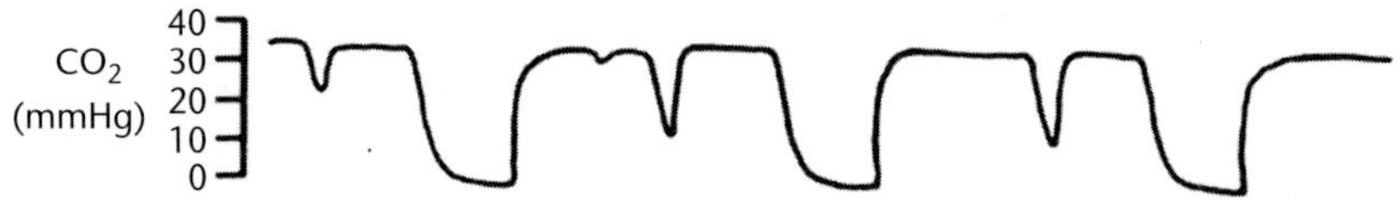

Figure 1.5 Capnogram showing a breathlet in the plateau (phase III). This capnogram shows a patient making inspiratory efforts during mechanical ventilation, but the capnogram cannot reveal the circumstances of the inspiratory effort. Only examination of the patient and analysis of all clinical factors can guide the clinician in deciding to adjust the ventilator, give drugs, or initiate other maneuvers. The patient's minute ventilation, level of anesthesia, degree of muscle relaxation, and metabolic state and the impact of external stimuli require consideration.

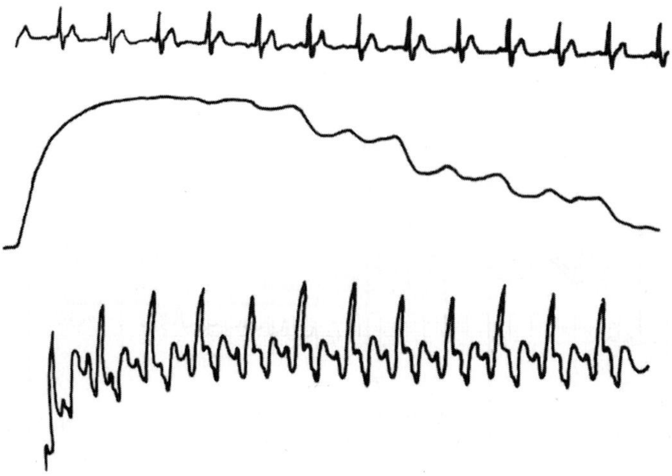

Figure 1.6 Simultaneous electrocardiogram (ECG) and capnogram with cardiogenic oscillations and pneumotachogram. Cardiogenic oscillations in the capnogram (middle) were generated from a healthy volunteer who breathed into a mouthpiece, to which a pneumotachograph (set at high sensitivity) and side-stream capnograph sampling connector was attached. An ECG (top) was recorded simultaneously. Oscillations appeared on the capnogram only on the down-slope (phase IV). The oscillation occurred at the same rate as the heartbeat, but they were not synchronous because of the delayed response of the side-stream capnograph, 2–3 s after the pneumotachogram. In order to generate a pneumotachogram, the subject kept his glottis open after an exhalation was completed.

and expirations give evidence that cardiac contractions and relaxations in the chest cause fluctuations of the lung volume with tidal volumes of about 10 ml, the recording of which generates a pneumocardiogram (Bijaoui *et al.*, 2001). Evidence of these cardiogenic tidal volumes can also be seen in the movement of inspiratory and expiratory valves of the breathing system. During the respiratory pause in mechanical ventilation the valves can be seen to flutter synchronously with the heartbeat.

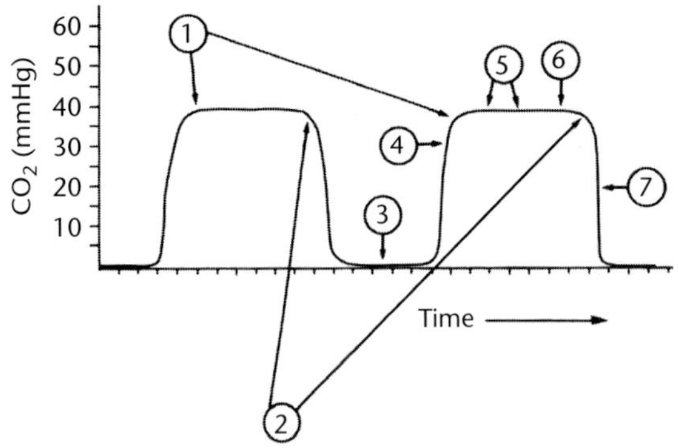

Figure 1.7 (1) *Plateau/onset* – Is there a pattern giving evidence of ventilation? (2) *Plateau/end* – Are peak values appropriate? Are the ventilator settings and the patient's respiratory pattern consistent with the capnogram and capnographic findings? (3) *Baseline* – Is the inspired CO_2 tension zero (normal baseline) or is there evidence for rebreathing (elevated baseline)? (4) *Upstroke* – Is there evidence for slow exhalation (slanted upstroke)? (5) *Plateau/horizontal* – Is there evidence of uneven emptying of lungs? (6) *Plateau/smooth* – Is expiration interrupted by inspiratory efforts? (7) *Downstroke* – Is the downstroke steep or is there evidence of slow inspiration or partial rebreathing?

In summary, a capnogram should have well-defined four phases. Figure 1.7 lists points to be considered when deciding whether or not to accept a capnogram of a quality sufficient for clinical interpretation.

Interpreting an artifact-free time-based capnogram

Cardio-vascular issues

The presence of a capnogram signifies that the patient's lungs are perfused. In cardiac arrest the lungs will not be perfused but with successful resuscitation CO_2 will appear in the exhaled gas, as discussed in greater detail in Chapter 20. In general, the capnogram will give evidence of acutely reduced pulmonary perfusion coincident with a drop in cardiac output. Figure 1.8 shows an example of momentary-induced ventricular fibrillation as practiced during implantation of a pacemaker/defibrillator. This will produce a typical pattern of decreasing capnographic tracings (Figure 1.8). During the first seconds of arrest without pulmonary perfusion, the lung yields quickly decreasing amounts of CO_2 either from the stagnant blood or from lung tissue. With successful defibrillation and re-establishment of pulmonary perfusion CO_2 once again appears in the exhaled breath. Of course, with continued cessation of pulmonary blood flow and continued ventilation, the capnogram will eventually show zero. If ventilation is stopped during cardiac arrest, a time side-stream capnogram will gradually reach zero values as the

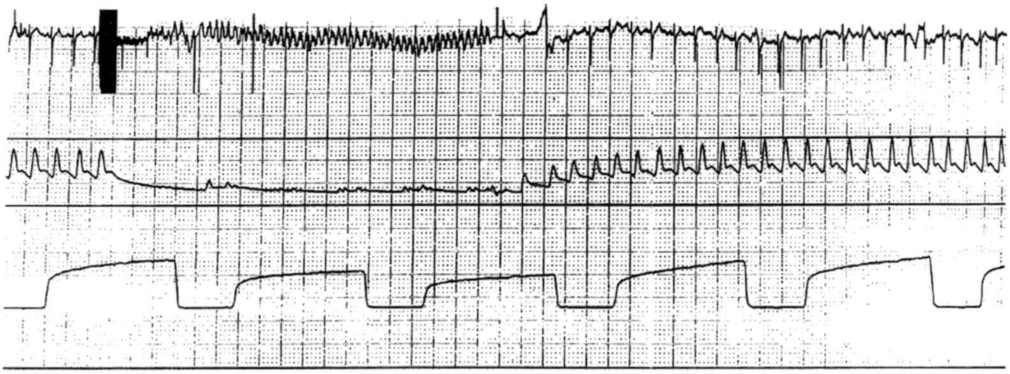

Figure 1.8 A patient undergoing the implantation of an automatic internal cardiac defibrillator was monitored with electrocardiogram (ECG) (top), radial arterial pressure (middle), and mainstream capnography (bottom). Induced ventricular fibrillation (black areas in ECG) and defibrillation are apparent in the ECG tracing. Observe decay of arterial pressure. During absent pulmonary blood flow the patient's lungs were ventilated and with two breaths the $P_{et}CO_2$ fell from 35 mmHg before fibrillation to 22 mmHg before defibrillation.

system continues to aspirate gas (about 200 ml/min), thus eventually aspirating room air. An on-airway (mainstream) system might show steady values (high or low) if the gas in the cuvette of the system remained stationary.

Some changes in end-tidal values develop slowly and are thus more readily recognized in trend-plots. For example, showers of air emboli can produce areas of alveolar dead-space (ventilated but not perfused alveoli) perhaps associated with a decrease of cardiac output. Soon the air bubbles either pass through the lungs or make it into the alveoli to be exhaled. This process causes the telltale transient dip in end-tidal CO_2 values as shown in Figure 1.9. This capnogram comes from a patient undergoing a posterior fossa operation in the sitting position and suffering from a typical shower of air emboli. Such ventilation/perfusion ($\dot{V}/\dot{Q}$) abnormalities are discussed in greater detail in Chapter 30.

Pulmonary issues

The most important use of capnography in the field, in the intensive care unit, and in the operating room comes with the establishment of an artificial airway. Intubation of the esophagus instead of the trachea still kills people who depend on a tracheal tube for ventilation. Capnography tells whether or not the tube is in the esophagus. Details of this essential application of capnography in different settings are discussed in considerable detail in several subsequent chapters.

In an artifact-free capnogram, normal end-tidal CO_2 values (between 35 and 45 mmHg) suggest normal ventilation. However, because a $\dot{V}/\dot{Q}$ mismatch (see Chapter 30) can cause the end-tidal values to appear normal while arterial values are high, the clinician will consider other evidence confirming adequate ventilation. First the clinician will need to assess the minute volume in the light of the patient's age, and weight. We are reassured if the patient's end-tidal CO_2 values are within the normal range and his tidal volume and minute ventilation fall within the ranges given in Table 1.1. But observe that the adult range of minute ventilation covers a wide span. In general, recumbent patients under anesthesia requiring mechanical ventilation need larger tidal volumes to maintain normal blood gas values than spontaneously breathing patients sitting upright. Selection of the optimal minute ventilation must also take into account dead-space ventilation. Every tidal volume ventilates dead-space as well as the alveoli. If we wish to double minute ventilation we might double the respiratory rate. However, as we increase the respiratory rate without changing tidal volume, we increase dead-space ventilation in parallel with alveolar ventilation. Doubling tidal volume instead of changing respiratory rate would greatly improve alveolar ventilation without increasing dead-space ventilation.

During anesthesia and with mechanical ventilation typically we use relatively low respiratory rates (8–10 breaths/min) and large tidal volumes (10–12 ml/kg).

Figure 1.10 shows a capnogram from a patient with chronic obstructive lung disease. The reported end-tidal CO_2 pressure of 42 mmHg is likely to be distinctly lower than the P_aCO_2 of this patient, as the patient does not show a plateau of phase III and the still rising values were interrupted by the next inspiration.

If the plateau of the capnogram (phase III) does not become almost horizontal before the next breath brings

Figure 1.9 The capnogram shows a trend of slow decrease in peak expiratory CO_2 from about 34 to a low of 22 mmHg, and then an increase to 35 mmHg. Inspiratory values remained normal. This trend is compatible with a brief shower of air emboli in a patient undergoing a posterior fossa craniectomy in the sitting position.

Table 1.1 Average respiratory values for resting, healthy patients

Parameter	Adult range	Neonatal range
Respiratory rate	10–15 breaths/min	30–40 breaths/min
Tidal volume	7–10 ml/kg	5–7 ml/kg
Minute ventilation	5–10 l/min	200–300 ml/kg/min

the transition to phase IV we must wonder how long the CO_2 levels would have continued to rise had an inspiration not interrupted exhalation. Patients with obstructive lung disease, such as asthma, will often show such a sloping phase III (Figure 1.10). The end-tidal partial pressure of CO_2 ($P_{et}CO_2$) will then fail faithfully to represent P_aCO_2. $\dot{V}/\dot{Q}$ mismatch is discussed in Chapter 30. Asthmatic patients exhibiting such sloping phase III of the capnogram often respond to the inhalation of bronchodilators (or general anesthesia with a halogenated agent) with an improvement of their capnogram and rising $P_{et}CO_2$ until the improved gas exchange has corrected the problem.

Small tidal volumes will represent relatively low effective alveolar ventilation, that is, with shallow breathing dead-space will make up more than the usual 30% of tidal volume. In such circumstances the end-tidal CO_2 values might appear normal and the capnogram can look quite unremarkable. Yet, an interposed large tidal volume can reveal a $P_{et}CO_2$ much higher than expected.

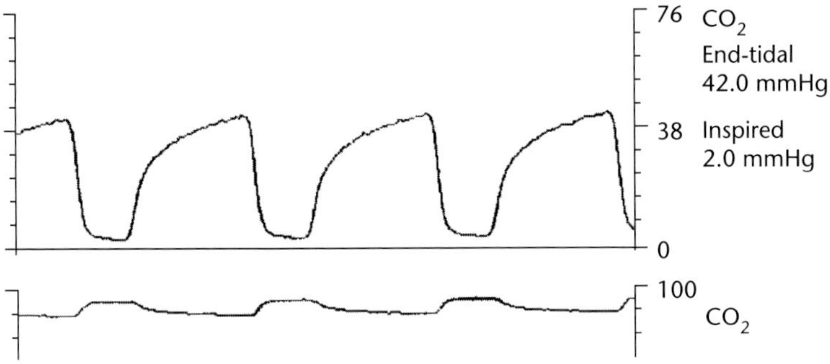

Figure 1.10 Capnogram with sloping phases II and III. The patient has chronic obstructive pulmonary disease. Every mechanical breath interrupts the patient's slow expiration so that the capnogram cannot develop end-tidal CO_2 tensions representative of alveolar arterial gas.

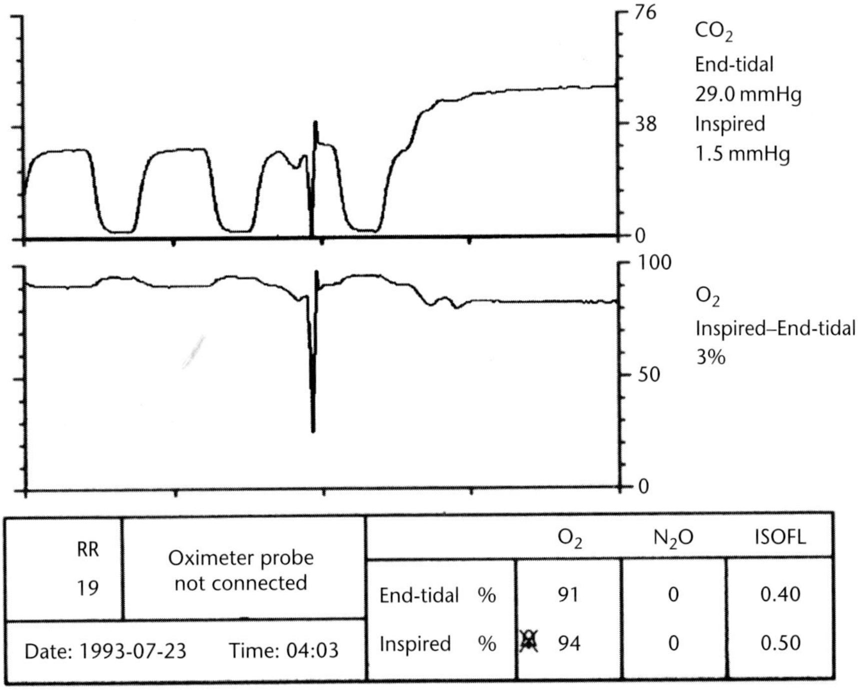

Figure 1.11 A patient undergoing thoracotomy was intubated with an endotracheal tube that enables the blocking of one mainstem bronchus while collecting gas from the blocked as well as the ventilated lung. The left part of the capnogram comes from the ventilated lung showing a $P_{et}CO_2$ of 29 mmHg. The P_aCO_2 was 46 mmHg. The right part of the capnogram represents gas sampled distal to the blocker in the right lung showing a PCO_2 of 48 mmHg. The PCO_2 of the mixed venous blood sampling through a pulmonary arterial catheter was 49 mmHg.

Intubation of a mainstem bronchus will result in relative hyperventilation of the intubated lung, producing low $P_{et}CO_2$ values. Once both lungs are ventilated without changing the tidal volume, the end-tidal values will normalize. In the unventilated airways CO_2 will equilibrate with venous blood as seen in Figure 1.11.

In the discussion of time-based capnography the question of the adequacy of ventilation, that is the adequacy of CO_2 elimination and dead-space ventilation pops up repeatedly. Thus, it would be nice to be able to look at dead-space ventilation as it relates to tidal volume. Enter volume-based capnography (see also Chapters 30 and 31).

The normal volume-based capnogram

An individual tracing of the time-based capnogram left a number of questions unanswered, which the single breath volume-based capnogram provides. In Figure 1.12 the solid line denotes the expiratory portion and the inspiratory portion (not always shown) is denoted by a dashed line. In general, the data offered by the volume-based capnogram refine the information offered by time-based capnography. Again, we ask for an artifact-free tracing and we think about ventilation and circulation. We can then scan the phases of the capnogram for detailed information. The questions to be raised for each phase are numbered and enumerated in Figure 1.12. Our first and most important question is: do we have evidence for ventilation of the lungs? If not, is the endotracheal tube in the esophagus or is the patient in cardiac arrest? Once we are reassured about that, we proceed to examine details. The inspired CO_2 tension should be zero. If not, there is evidence of rebreathed carbon dioxide as discussed in Chapter 6. We usually assume a normal dead-space to occupy about 1 ml/pound (0.5 ml/kg) or for the average adult about 150 ml or approximately one-third of the tidal volume. The volume-based capnogram provides a convenient opportunity to confirm this fact. A larger than normal dead-space points either to an equipment dead-space (see Chapter 6), exhausted CO_2 absorber, or ventilation of unperfused lung segments (see Chapter 30). Ideally, the transition from phase I to II should be abrupt. It is usually isn't because as alveolar gas passes through the dead-space it first mixes with the dead-space gas and then rapidly displaces it. This process should result in a steep rise of the capnogram in phase II. If the alveoli empty grossly unevenly, as in severe emphysematous or obstructive lung disease,

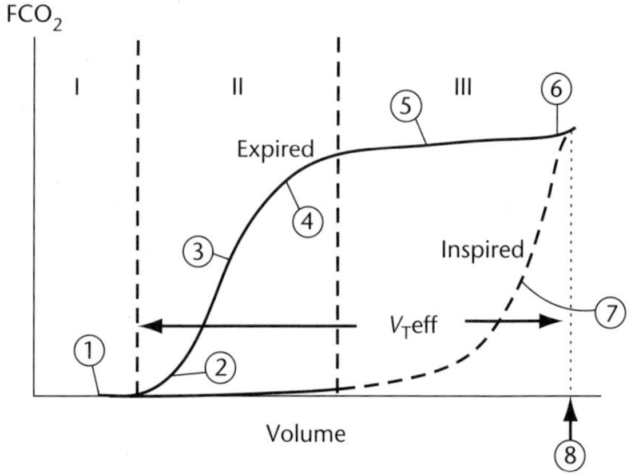

Figure 1.12 A solid line denotes the expiratory portion; the inspiratory portion, if shown, is denoted by a dashed line. The three phases are 'denoted' by I, II, and III. (Numbers 1–8 represent the checklist and comments below.) (1) *Phase I*: Is the inspired CO_2 tension zero (normal baseline) or is there evidence for rebreathing (elevated baseline)? Does the volume of phase I reasonably reflect the anatomical and apparatus dead-space? (Plus possibly compressed volume if the program does not subtract this) Please note that the vertical interrupted line for phase I does not intersect the abscissa at the dead-space volume. (2) *Angle between phases I and II*: Is the transition clearly defined? (3) *Slope of phase II*: Is there evidence for slow exhalation (slanted up-slope)? When the transition to phase III is slurred, think of obstructive pulmonary disease. (4) *Angle between phases II and III*: Is the transition clearly defined? (5) *Slope of phase III*: Is the slope almost level (children and young adults) or is there a clear gradient (i.e. evidence of uneven emptying in patients with lung disease)? (6) *End of phase III*: What is the final value? Is expiration interrupted by inspiratory efforts? Are peak values appropriate? The area under the expiratory limb represents the volume of expired CO_2. (7) *Down-slope (if inspiratory limb shown)*: Is the down-slope steep or is there evidence of partial rebreathing? The area under inspiratory limb represents the volume of inspired CO_2; the area between the curves represents the volume of CO_2 eliminated. (8) *Exhaled volume and exhaled CO_2 volume*: Are the values consistent with the expected value and ventilator setting?

the slope will be slanted. The angle between the up-slope and the plateau indicates that the addition of CO_2 from the alveoli is now beginning to become homogeneous. A lazy up-slope and a slurred transition again indicate a troubled lung that empties its CO_2 unevenly. A horizontal (or nearly so) plateau shows a lung that fairly prodigiously adds CO_2 to every milliliter of exhaled gas. Healthy children and young adults often show nearly horizontal plateaus. Cardiogenic oscillations, as described above, can put a heartbeat synchronous ripples on the plateau. At the end of the plateau we hope to read the true end-tidal value for CO_2. As already mentioned, it should be between 35 and 45 mmHg:

- If the inspiratory limb is inscribed, we would expect a steep fall of CO_2 in the inspired gas, soon reaching zero, unless the patient is rebreathing CO_2 – as discussed above. The area under the inspiratory limb is the volume of inspired CO_2; and the area between the curves represents the volume of CO_2 eliminated.
- Since we have plotted the tidal volume on the abscissa, we can check the exhaled volume and compare it with the expected value for the patient. Remember that inspired and expired volumes are often not identical either because of a respiratory quotient of less than one (more oxygen consumed than CO_2 exhaled) or because the uptake or elimination of anesthetic gases cause a discrepancy. Nitrous oxide here is the culprit because we often give it in relatively high concentrations (up to 70%). Its solubility co-efficient of 0.47 for blood at body temperature predicts that many liters will go into solution in the body and will eventually again appears in the exhaled gas.

The gas last inhaled will fill the patient's dead-space. It will be the gas first exhaled and should be free of CO_2. If it is not, the patient is rebreathing exhaled CO_2 – linked to the type of equipment in use or an equipment malfunction – or CO_2 is being added to the inspired gas. For example, at the end of anesthesia some anesthetists like to add CO_2 so as to allow hyperventilation for the elimination of anesthetic gases without causing the patient to develop a respiratory alkalosis.

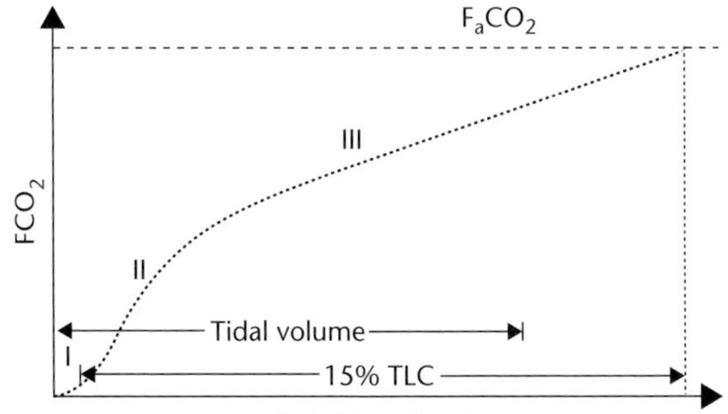

Figure 1.13 Volume-based capnogram from a patient with chronic obstructive pulmonary disease. TLC is the total lung capacity. Observe that the transition from phase II to the plateau phase III is difficult to discern. (Reproduced with permission from Anderson, J.T., Owings, J.T. & Goodnight, J.E. (1999). Bedside noninvasive detection of acute pulmonary embolism in critically ill surgical patients. *Arch. Surg.*, **134**: 869–874).

Figure 1.13 comes from an asthmatic patient. The slanted up-slope indicates the tardy entry of CO_2 into the exhaled gas as is typical in patients with obstructive pulmonary disease. Conditions that increase dead-space ventilation (ventilated but not perfused alveoli), such as emboli (tumor, gas, clot) or right to left shunts will stand out clearly in the volume-based capnogram that shows the large dead-space (Figure 1.14). With a decrease in cardiac output the volume of CO_2 delivered to the lungs will also decrease. As the volume-based capnogram enables the calculation of the exhaled CO_2, we can quantify the

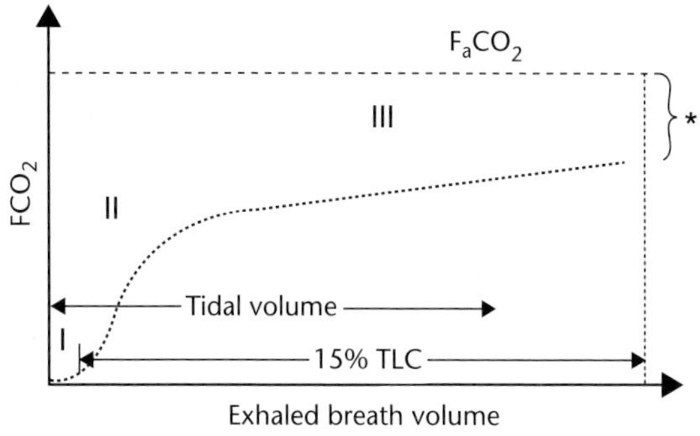

Figure 1.14 Volume-based capnogram from a patient with pulmonary embolism. Observe the large difference between end-tidal and arterial CO_2 tension. The asterisk shows the size of the alveolar dead-space at end-expiration. (Reproduced with permission from Anderson, J.T., Owings, J.T. & Goodnight, J.E. (1999). Bedside noninvasive detection of acute pulmonary embolism in critically ill surgical patients. *Arch. Surg.*, **134**: 869–874).

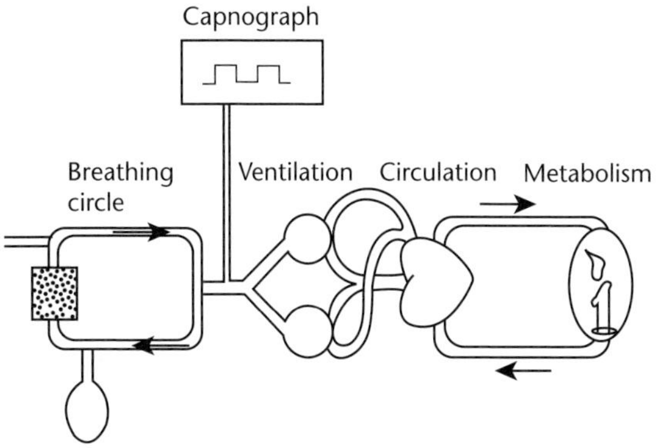

Figure 1.15 End-tidal values can be affected by a number of mechanisms, starting with the generation of CO_2 in the cell (candle), the transport of venous blood to the heart (cardiac output), the pulmonary blood flow (part of which may be shunted past ventilated alveoli), ventilation (part of which may be blocked from perfused alveoli), the breathing system (which may cause rebreathing, hyperventilation, or hypoventilation), and ending with the capnograph (which may fail because of artifacts or incorrect calibration).

change better than with the time-based capnography that allows us only to report the end-tidal values.

Summary

Whether using time- or volume-based capnography, many questions will confront the clinician when abnormal capnographic data call for an analysis. Figure 1.15 recapitulates the fact that many components of the system can cause trouble – starting with cellular metabolism (remember malignant hyperthermia) to mechanical problems related to the airway, ventilation, and monitors. These topics, buttressed by exhaustive references, will be discussed in detail in subsequent chapters.

References

Bijaoui, E., Baconnier, P.F. & Bates, J.H.T. (2001). Mechanical output impedance of the lung determined from cardiogenic oscillations. *J. Appl. Physiol.*, **91**: 859–865.

van Genderingen, H.R. & Gravenstein, N. (1987). Capnogram artifact during high airway pressures caused by a water trap. *Anesth. Analg.*, **66**: 185–187.

VENTILATION: ADEQUACY OF BREATHING ASSESSMENT

SECTION **1a**

CAPNOGRAPHY AND RESPIRATORY ASSESSMENT OUTSIDE OF THE OPERATING ROOM

2

E.B. Lobato & R.R. Kirby

Introduction

Since gas exchange is a primordial function of the lungs and the conductive airways, evaluation of respiratory function is of paramount importance. Although the respiratory system contributes to functions other than gas exchange, the traditional assessment evaluates the mechanical efficiency of the airway, lungs, and thoracic cavity to provide gas exchange through analysis of the forces generated to move air to and from the alveoli.

Clinicians evaluate this function by visual observation of chest expansion, depth and rate of respirations, use of respiratory muscles, and the quality and quantity of breath sounds. Quantitative information is obtained by measuring thoracic/pulmonary compliance (change of volume related to change in pressure) and calculating airways resistance. Additional, more complex techniques involve measurement of lung volumes and capacities with spirometry, which also evaluates airway patency, and lung/thorax expansion. Factors that affect these measurements include pain, fatigue, and poor understanding by the patient (and perhaps the clinician) of how the test is to be carried out. As a result, assessment of airway obstruction or lung restriction is reliable only insofar as the ability of the patient to optimally perform the tests is unimpaired. They are effort dependent, and the inability or unwillingness of the patient to expend the requisite effort renders them useless.

Perhaps the ultimate test for adequate ventilation is the invasive determination of arterial carbon dioxide (CO_2) partial pressure (P_aCO_2). In general, an elevation in P_aCO_2 (hypercapnia) represents decreased respiratory rate (RR), depth, or both; inefficient alveolar ventilation (ventilation/perfusion ($\dot{V}/\dot{Q}$) inequalities); or production of CO_2 in excess of the patient's ability to excrete it. A reduction in P_aCO_2 (hypocapnia) results from excessive alveolar ventilation in relation to CO_2 production. Measurement of P_aCO_2, although a true reflection of ventilatory efficiency, is far from ideal since it is invasive and intermittent.

Capnography has been utilized in surgical patients for almost two decades to confirm tracheal intubation and to assess the efficiency of ventilation. Measurement of exhaled CO_2, and particularly the end-tidal PCO_2 ($P_{et}CO_2$), is an established standard of care in patient monitoring (American Society of Anesthesiologists, 2004). In conjunction with P_aCO_2, capnography provides a semiquantitative assessment of $\dot{V}/\dot{Q}$ mismatch by changes in the P_aCO_2–$P_{et}CO_2$ difference (normal <5 mmHg). Capnograms consist of two types: (1) the concentration of CO_2 is plotted against expired volume, otherwise known as single breath time concentration CO_2 curve (Romero *et al.*, 2000); (2) the concentration of CO_2 is plotted against time during a respiratory cycle.

The latter technique has been in use for several decades and requires less elaborate equipment than is required to generate instantaneous CO_2 concentration as related to expiratory volume.

Although capnography has been utilized for years as a standard in the operating room to assist in airway and ventilatory management, it is also increasingly employed outside of the operating room as a non-invasive, continuous trend monitor of P_aCO_2 and airway dynamics. The value of capnography to assess the efficacy of cardiopulmonary resuscitation during low perfusion states or cardiac arrest has been established, and it is now considered as standard of care to determine endotracheal tube position by the American Heart Association (2000). Colorimetric capnometry is fast, convenient, and useful to verify tracheal intubation in a non-operating room setting. However, it can present problems as reported by Puntervoll *et al.* (2002). They compared colorimetric methodology with mainstream capnography and found that in emergency situations in which CO_2-containing air may be present in the esophagus, capnography should be the preferred method of verifying tracheal, and not esophageal, intubation. The tested colorimetric CO_2 indicator was very sensitive to low CO_2 values and thus may falsely indicate correct tracheal intubation, even when the tube is in the esophagus.

In respiratory care, capnography is utilized to determine lung volumes, provide assessment of the mechanical efficiency of the respiratory system, evaluate patients in respiratory distress, and monitor the treatment of patients with reactive airways disease. Potential advantages include its non-invasive nature, lack of the need for patients to exert maximal effort, and the ability to provide continuous values, thus making trend assessments feasible.

Capnography and lung volumes

The traditional determination of lung volumes and ventilation is by analysis of the expired concentration of a trace gas, such as nitrogen or helium, during a single breath (*washout*) against exhaled volume. Nitrogen washout provides an estimate of functional residual capacity, total lung volume, dead-space volume, and alveolar volume. If CO_2 is substituted for nitrogen or helium, a similar washout curve is generated (Romero *et al.*, 2000). This technique is known as single breath capnography ($SBTCO_2$) (Figure 2.1), which is divided into three phases. Phase I consists of anatomical dead-space, which contains little to no CO_2. This phase is followed by a steep increase in CO_2 concentration as gas from the conductive airways is mixed with alveolar gas (phase II). A plateau follows (phase III) in which there is no change in exhaled CO_2 concentration. Phase III represents alveolar emptying. Occasionally, a terminal upswing is seen (phase IV), particularly in obese or pregnant individuals. Factors such as uneven or delayed alveolar emptying (from slow compartments) contribute to this aberration.

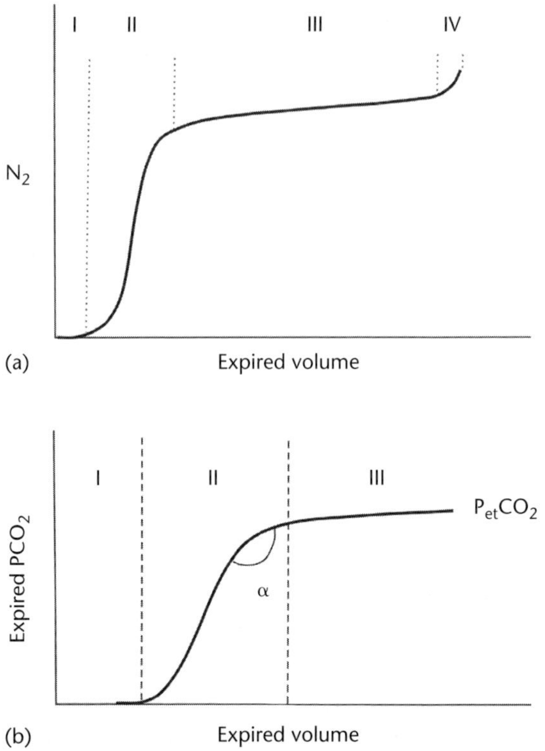

Figure 2.1 Curves of exhaled nitrogen (a) and CO_2 (b) concentration versus expired volume during a single breath "washout" test. Both show the traditional division into phases I–IV (for full explanation, see text). N_2: nitrogen.

Uses of time capnography

As was mentioned previously, since $SBTCO_2$ requires sophisticated software and equipment, clinicians typically utilize exhaled CO_2 concentration against time during a respiratory cycle. A number of applications are available.

Trend monitor of alveolar ventilation

Capnography can be used as a continuous monitor of alveolar ventilation in patients with lung disease or hemodynamic instability. Although such use does not replace arterial blood gas analysis, it may decrease the required frequency (Tobias *et al.*, 1994). In stable patients with body temperature that remains constant, the P_aCO_2 and $P_{et}CO_2$ can be used as surrogates, since their difference is 1–5 mmHg in normal individuals (Liu *et al.*, 1992; Frieson & Alswang, 1996). When changes in temperature, cardiovascular function, and CO_2 production occur, capnography used to trend P_aCO_2 can be misleading. The primary reason capnography has not replaced arterial blood gas analysis to determine P_aCO_2 is related to variability in the three physiological parameters that determine $P_{et}CO_2$: (1) production of CO_2; (2) delivery of CO_2 via pulmonary blood flow; and (3) elimination of CO_2.

Trend monitoring of dead-space ventilation

Components of a time capnogram are similar to those of an $SBTCO_2$ capnogram (Figure 2.2) (Bhavani-Shankar *et al.*, 1995; Schmmitz & Shapiro, 1995) and consist of a square wave in which phase I represents the CO_2-free gas from the airways (anatomical and physiology of the dead space). Phase II consists of a rapid S-shaped upswing on the tracing which is due to mixture of dead-space gas with alveolar gas. Phase III, the alveolar plateau (CO_2-rich gas from the alveoli). Unlike $SBTCO_2$, a descending limb results from the inspiratory phase during which the fraction of inspired CO_2 decreases to zero.

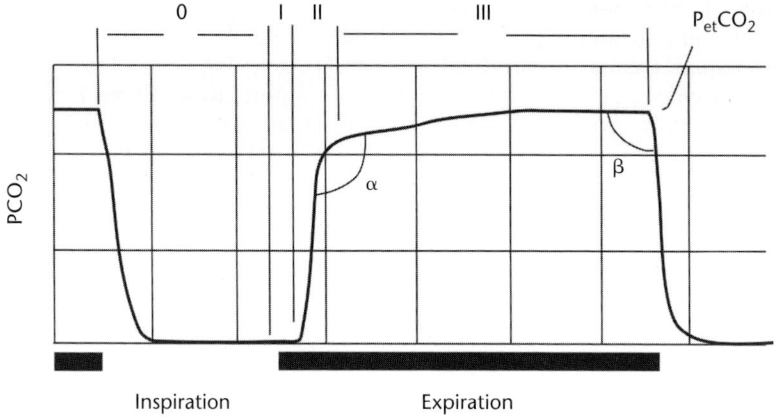

Figure 2.2 Time capnogram showing exhaled PCO_2 versus time. All three phases are shown. Alpha (α) angle: angle between phases II and III; beta (β) angle: angle between phase III and inspiratory limb (phase 0). (Reproduced with permission from Bhavani-Shankar, K., Kumar, A.Y., Moseley, H.S.L. & Ahyee-Hallsworth, R. (1995). Terminology and the current limitations of time capnography: a brief review. *J. Clin. Monit.*, **11**: 175–182.)

The capnograph also exhibits two angles (Bhavani-Shankar *et al.*, 1995): (1) the α angle, between phases II and III, and (2) the β angle between the end of phase III and the beginning of inspiration. The α angle is about 110°. It increases as the slope of phase III increases. The slope of phase III is dependent on $\dot{V}/\dot{Q}$ relationships within the lungs. Alpha angle values are important in assessing airway obstruction. Other factors that can produce changes in the α angle include equipment-related characteristics, capnometer response time, and the patient's respiratory cycle time. The β angle can be used to assess the extent of rebreathing. During rebreathing of CO_2, an increase in the angle from the normal 90° occurs, since the descending slope becomes less vertical in the presence of inspired CO_2.

Assessment and monitoring of patients with airway obstruction

Capnography may represent a useful alternative to spirometry in the evaluation of patients with asthma or chronic obstructive lung disease. The normal rectangular shape of the capnograph is affected by various degrees of airway obstruction (Figure 2.3) (You *et al.*, 1994; Yaron *et al.*, 1996; Strömberg & Gustafsson, 2000). Parameters used to assess airway obstruction include: (1) slope of the alveolar plateau, which can be related to end-tidal CO_2 ($ETCO_2$); (2) radius of minimal curvature of the α angle; (3) time necessary to pass from 25% to 75% of the $P_{et}CO_2$; and (4) β angle. Several studies have shown significant correlation between these capnographic indices and spirometric measures in stable patients. You *et al.* (1994) found a good correlation in asthmatic patients between the end-tidal slope (phase III) obtained by the capnograph and the forced expiratory volume in 1 s.

Capnography in patients with reactive airway disease does not require the patient's cooperation or

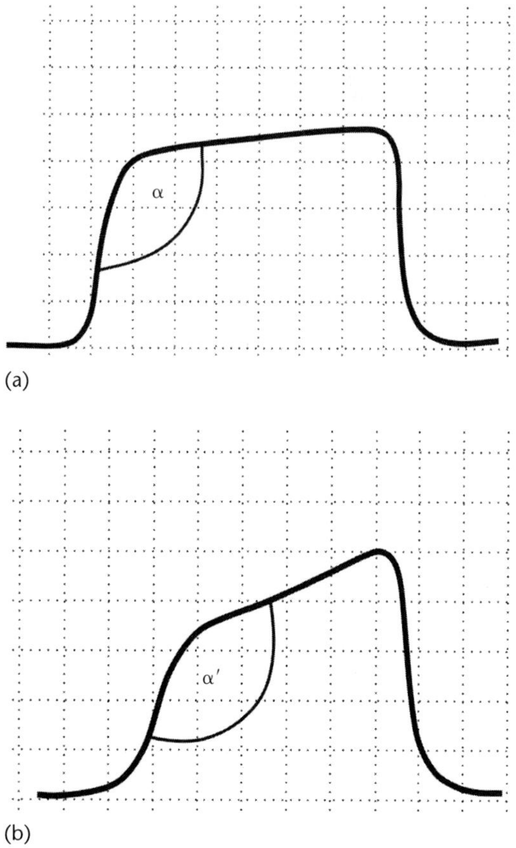

Figure 2.3 (a) Normal capnogram showing alpha (α) angle of 105°. (b) Capnogram during acute bronchospasm showing an alpha (α′) angle of 140°.

wakefulness. Therefore, it can be used continuously in a number of clinical situations. Limitations result from several factors, particularly the analyzer's dynamic characteristics; expiratory flow rate; duration of the expiratory phase; and artifacts derived from the upper airway, such as nasal obstruction and pulsatile waves of carotid origin. These factors require criteria for adequate use, interpretation, and assessment of airway patency.

Evaluation of non-intubated patients with and without respiratory distress

Capnography has been utilized in emergency departments to evaluate patients in respiratory distress. Plewa *et al.* (1995) evaluated 29 patients with symptoms of dyspnea and an RR >16/min in a level 1 trauma center/community hospital emergency department. Their primary goal was to assess the ability of $P_{et}CO_2$ to predict P_aCO_2. Although there was a significant correlation with P_aCO_2, they found that within two standard deviations, $P_{et}CO_2$ underestimated P_aCO_2 by as much as 16 mmHg and overestimated it by up to 5 mmHg. Values of $P_{et}CO_2$ correlated reasonably well with P_aCO_2 only in patients who were able to provide a forced expiratory volume. It was less accurate in patients who could only breathe at tidal volume levels or had pulmonary disease.

By contrast, in patients without respiratory failure who were seen in the emergency room for a variety of conditions, capnography correlates reasonably with P_aCO_2. Barton and Wang (1994) studied 76 patients and found a close relationship between $P_{et}CO_2$ and P_aCO_2, even when the values were compared during respiratory and non-respiratory acidosis ($r^2 = 0.899$). Mainstream capnometry appears to provide more accurate $P_{et}CO_2$ than conventional sidestream capnometry during spontaneous breathing in non-intubated patients (Casati *et al.*, 2001).

In a later prospective observational study conducted in an urban county hospital of adult patients undergoing procedural sedation, patients were monitored for vital signs, depth of sedation per the physician by the Observer's Assessment of Alertness/Sedation scale (OAA/S), pulse oximetry, and nasal-sample $P_{et}CO_2$ (Miner *et al.*, 2002). There was no correlation between $P_{et}CO_2$ and the OAA/S score. Using the criteria of a $P_{et}CO_2 > 50$ mmHg, an absolute change > 10 mmHg, or an absent waveform, the authors suggested the $P_{et}CO_2$ may add to the safety of procedural sedation not readily assessed by other means in the emergency department by quickly detecting hypoventilation.

Finally, Takano *et al.* (2003) determined the utility of portable capnometry in general wards and in in-home care in 41 spontaneously breathing patients. The mean difference between P_aCO_2 and vital capacity $P_{et}CO_2$ (VC-$ETCO_2$) was 0.5 mmHg, and was not statistically significant. Regression analysis showed a close correlation between VC-$ETCO_2$ and P_aCO_2 ($r = 0.91$, $P < 0.0001$). Thus, VC-$ETCO_2$ was highly correlated with P_aCO_2, a finding similar to that of Plewa *et al.* (1995). In contrast, tidal volume, $ETCO_2$, and P_aCO_2 differed by an average of 9 mmHg. The investigators concluded that VC-$ETCO_2$ measured by portable capnometry gives a reliable point estimate of P_aCO_2 and can be useful to evaluate the respiratory condition of spontaneously breathing patients in general wards and in-home care.

Detection of occult hyperventilation in syncope and chronic fatigue syndrome

Capnography also has been utilized as a part of diagnostic maneuvers in the evaluation of syncope in children and adolescents (Naschitz *et al.*, 1998; Martinon-Torres *et al.*, 2001). Spontaneous hyperventilation is thought to play a relevant role in the pathophysiology of pediatric neurocardiogenic syncope, and it could characterize a specific subtype of response to orthostatic stress in susceptible patients. Inclusion of capnography in tilt-test protocols may improve the assessment of syncope in children. The capnography head-up tilt test (CHUTT) was found to be predictive of associated psychogenic hyperventilation, as one of the main reasons for syncope in 6% of cases (Figure 2.4).

Similar findings were reported in the chronic fatigue syndrome (CFS) (Naschitz *et al.*, 2000). Thirty-two consecutive patients with CFS and 32 healthy volunteers were evaluated with the aid of the CHUTT. The main outcome measures were blood pressure (BP), heart rate (HR), RR, and $P_{et}CO_2$ recorded during recumbence and tilt. Patients with CFS developed significantly lower systolic and diastolic BP, and $P_{et}CO_2$, in addition to a significant rise in HR and RR ($P < 0.01$) during tilt. The postural tachycardia syndrome occurred in 44%, vasodepressor reaction in 41%, cardio-inhibitory reaction in 13%, and hyperventilation in 31% of cases in CFS patients. One or more end points of the CHUTT were reached in 78% of patients with CFS but in none of the controls.

Capnometry monitoring for respiratory status during pediatric seizures

To determine the reliability and clinical value of $P_{et}CO_2$ by oral/nasal capnometry for monitoring pediatric patients presenting post-ictal or with active seizures, investigators studied 166 patients (105 patients with active seizures, 61 post-ictal patients) (Abramo *et al.*, 1997). The $ETCO_2$ was measured by oral/nasal sidestream capnometry, together with RR, SpO_2, and HR every 5 min until 60 min had elapsed.

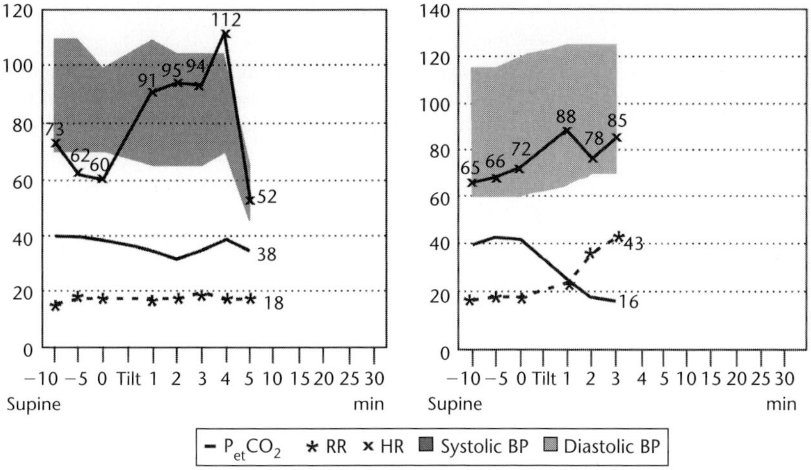

Figure 2.4 Values of BP, HR, RR, and $P_{et}CO_2$ during a CHUTT test in a patient with the diagnosis of syncope. Hyperventilation occurred immediately after tilt and continued until the patient lost consciousness. (Reproduced with permission from Naschitz, J.E., Hardoff, D., Bystritzki, I., Yeshurun, D., Gaitini, L., Tamir, A. & Jaffe, M. (1998). The role of the capnography head-up tilt test in the diagnosis of syncope in children and adolescents. *Pediatrics*, **101**: 1–6.)

The correlation between $P_{et}CO_2$ and capillary PCO_2 was significant ($r^2 = 0.97$; $P < 0.0001$). The investigators concluded that dependable $P_{et}CO_2$ values could be obtained in pediatric seizure patients using an oral/nasal cannula capnometry circuit and that continuous $P_{et}CO_2$ monitoring provided a reliable assessment of pulmonary status to assist with decisions to provide ventilatory support.

Capnometry during endoscopy procedures

Outpatient endoscopy procedures often require significant sedation, and unrecognized respiratory depression is a constant risk. Apnea or disordered respiration occurs commonly during therapeutic upper endoscopy and frequently precedes the development of hypoxemia, with disastrous outcomes reported. Forty-nine patients undergoing therapeutic upper endoscopy were monitored with pulse oximetry, automated BP measurement, and visual assessment (Vargo *et al.*, 2002). Graphic assessment of respiratory activity with sidestream capnography was performed in all patients. Episodes of apnea or disordered breathing detected by capnography were documented and compared with the occurrence of hypoxemia, hypercapnia, hypotension, and abnormal respiratory activity recognized by endoscopy personnel.

Simultaneous RR measurements obtained by capnography and by auscultation with a pre-tracheal stethoscope verified that capnography was an excellent indicator of RR when compared with auscultation ($r = 0.97$, $P < 0.001$). Fifty-four episodes of apnea or disordered respiration occurred in 28 patients (mean duration 70.8 s). Only 50% of apnea or disordered respiration episodes were eventually detected by pulse oximetry, and none were detected by visual assessment. Potentially important abnormalities in respiratory activity are undetected with pulse oximetry and visual assessment.

Conclusions

Capnography has potential applications as a tool for evaluation of the respiratory system outside of the operating room. Uses include the evaluation and monitoring of patients who present with a variety of conditions in the emergency department, including respiratory failure and reactive airways disease, and in a variety of outpatient or diagnostic settings (pediatric syncope, CFS). Current evidence suggests that capnography generally correlates well with $P_{et}CO_2$, but is less reliable in patients with significant $\dot{V}/\dot{Q}$ mismatch or in those who are unable to produce forced exhalations.

References

Abramo, T.J., Wiebe, R.A., Scott, S., Goto, C.S. & McIntire, D.D. (1997). Noninvasive capnometry monitoring for respiratory status during pediatric seizures. *Crit. Care Med.*, **25**: 1242–1246.

American Heart Association (2000). International Guidelines 2000 for CPR and ECC. **102(suppl. I)**: 1-370.

American Society of Anesthesiologists (2004). Standards for Basic Anesthetic Monitoring. Approved by the House of Delegates 21 October 1986 and last amended on 15 October 2003.

Barton, C.W. & Wang, E.S.J. (1994). Correlation of end-tidal CO_2 measurements to arterial P_aCO_2 in nonintubated patients. *Ann. Emer. Med.*, **23**: 560–563.

Bhavani-Shankar, K., Kumar, A.Y., Moseley, H.S.L. & Ahyee-Hallsworth, R. (1995). Terminology and the current limitations of time capnography: a brief review. *J. Clin. Monit.*, **11**: 175–182.

Casati, A., Gallioli, R., Passaretta, R., Scandroglio, M., Bignami, E. & Torri, G. (2001). End tidal carbon dioxide monitoring in spontaneously breathing, nonintubated patients. *Minerva Anesthesiol.*, **67**: 161–164.

Frieson, R.H. & Alswang, M. (1996). End-tidal PCO_2 monitoring via nasal cannulae in pediatric patients: accuracy and sources of error. *J. Clin. Monit.*, **12**: 155–159.

Liu, S.Y., Lee, T.S. & Bongard, F. (1992). Accuracy of capnography in nonintubated surgical patients. *Chest*, **102**: 1512–1515.

Martinon-Torres, F., Rodriguez-Nunez, A., Fernandez-Cebrian, S., Eiris-Punal, J., Perez-Munuzuri, A. & Martinon-Sanchez, J.M. (2001). The relation between hyperventilation and pediatric syncope. *J. Pediatr.*, **138**: 894–897.

Miner, J.R., Heegaard, W. & Plummer, D. (2002). End-tidal carbon dioxide monitoring during procedural sedation. *Acad. Emerg. Med.*, **9**: 275–280.

Naschitz, J.E., Hardoff, D., Bystritzki, I., Yeshurun, D., Gaitini, L., Tamir, A. & Jaffe, M. (1998). The role of the capnography head-up tilt test in the diagnosis of syncope in children and adolescents. *Pediatrics*, **101**: 1–6.

Naschitz, J.E., Rosner, I., Rozenbaum, M., *et al.* (2000). The capnography head-up tilt test for evaluation of chronic fatigue syndrome. *Semin. Arthritis Rheu.*, **30**: 79–86.

Plewa, M.C., Sikora, S., Engoren, M., Tome, D., Thomas, J. & Deuster, A. (1995). Evaluation of capnography in nonintubated emergency department patients with respiratory distress. *Acad. Emerg. Med.*, **2**: 901–908.

Puntervoll, S.A., Soreide, E., Jacewicz, W. & Bjelland, E. (2002). Rapid detection of oesophageal intubation: take care when using colorimetric capnometry. *Acta Anaesthesiol. Scand.*,**46**: 455–457.

Romero, P.V., Lucangelo, U., Lopez Aguilar, J., Fernandez, R. & Blanch, L. (2000). Physiologically based indices of volumetric capnography in patients receiving mechanical ventilation. *Eur. Respir. J.*, **10**: 232–233.

Schmmitz, B.D. & Shapiro, B. (1995). Capnography. *Resp. Care Clin. N. Am.*, **1**: 107–117.

Strömberg, N.O.T. & Gustafsson, P.M. (2000). Ventilation inhomogeneity assessed by nitrogen washout and ventilation–perfusion mismatch by capnography in stable and induced airway obstruction. *Pediatr. Pulm.*, **29**: 94–102.

Takano, Y., Sakamoto, O., Kiyofuji, C. & Ito, K. (2003). A comparison of the end-tidal CO_2 measured by portable capnometer and the arterial PCO_2 in spontaneously breathing patients. *Respir. Med.*, **97**: 476–481.

Tobias, J.D., Flanagan, J.F.K., Wheeler, T.J. & Garrett, J.S. (1994). Noninvasive monitoring of end-tidal CO_2 via nasal cannulas in spontaneously breathing children during the perioperative period. *Crit. Care Med.*, **22**: 1805–1808.

Vargo, J.J., Zuccaro Jr, G., Dumot, J.A., Conwell, D.L., Morrow, J.B. & Shay, S.S. (2002). Automated graphic assessment of respiratory activity is superior to pulse oximetry and visual assessment for the detection of early respiratory depression during therapeutic upper endoscopy. *Gastrointest. Endosc.*, **55**: 826–831.

Yaron, M., Padyk, P., Hutsinpiller, M. & Cairns, C.B. (1996). Utility of the expiratory capnogram in the assessment of bronchospasm. *Ann. Emerg. Med.*, **28**: 403–407.

You, B., Peslin, R., Duvivier, C. & Vu, V.D. (1994). Expiratory capnography in asthma: evaluation of various shape indices. *Eur. Respir. J.*, **7**: 318–323.

VENTILATION: AIRWAY MANAGEMENT

SECTION **1b**

AIRWAY MANAGEMENT: PREHOSPITAL SETTING

3

B. Carmack, S. Silvestri, G.A. Ralls & J.L. Falk

Airway management is among the most critical and challenging aspects of prehospital practice. Maintaining the integrity of the airway and oxygenation of the brain is critical to successful outcomes. Toward this end, a wide array of airway devices are available to EMS personnel and several complementary methods are available to verify proper airway placement. Devices to facilitate airway management include the BVM, esophageal–tracheal combitube, LMA, and the ETT. The BVM has been in existence since the implementation of early prehospital advanced life support systems. Devices such as the EOA and esophageal gastric tube airway (EGTA), which were once utilized as alternative airway techniques, have been replaced by the esophageal–tracheal combitube. Currently, the combitube and the LMA are the two most popular alternative airway devices. While each of these devices has a role to play, endotracheal intubation has remained the preferred technique. When properly placed, ETTs afford the best chance for adequate oxygenation, ventilation, and airway protection. Maintaining oxygenation and ventilation using adjuncts such as the pocket mask or BVM remains the first priority following simple airway opening maneuvers. For providers not trained in endotracheal intubation, and for patients in whom endotracheal intubation cannot be accomplished, devices utilized in modern prehospital systems include the esophageal–tracheal combitube and the LMA. Table 3.1 reviews some of the advantages and disadvantages of the LMA and combitube.

Endotracheal intubation remains the most definitive means of airway control and is consistently thought of as the "gold standard" (Pennant & Walker, 1992; Clinton & McGill, 1998; Nolan, 2001; Wayne *et al.*, 2001). The indications for endotracheal intubation in the prehospital setting are similar to those in other clinical settings and include a patient's inability to oxygenate, ventilate, or to protect his/her airway. The American Heart Association (AHA, 2000) considers endotracheal intubation the ventilatory adjunct of choice in cardiac arrest because it maintains airway patency, facilitates suctioning of secretions, permits delivery of concentrated oxygen mixtures, provides a route of administration of certain medications, allows delivery of a selected tidal volume, and protects the trachea from aspiration. Unfortunately for all parties involved, it also is the most technically difficult skill for the clinicians to master and extensive training is required for competence to be achieved. A study of anesthesia residents performing intubation in the operating room (OR) under attending supervision showed that a mean of 57 intubations were necessary to achieve a 90% success rate, and over 90 intubations were needed for a success rate >95% to be achieved (Konrad *et al.*, 1998). Most paramedics are simply not afforded comparable intubation volume on live patients. Indeed, the bulk of paramedic airway training is performed on manikins. Additionally, as opposed to the controlled setting of the OR, in paramedic practice this procedure takes place under a multitude of adverse circumstances. Some of the difficulties the paramedic will

Table 3.1 Advantages and disadvantages of LMA and combitube

Advantages	Disadvantages
LMA	
Ease of insertion	Stability during patient movement
Ease of cuff insufflation	Unsecured airway
Faster insertion time	
Less gastric insufflation	
Quicker learning curve	
Better skill retention	
Availability of live patient training	
Pediatric use indicated	
Effective advanced airway device	
Combitube	
Secure airway	Live patient training unavailable
Effective advanced airway device	Slow insertion time
	More difficult skill retention
	No pediatric use

have to face in carrying out this action are a loud, noisy environment, poor patient positioning, cervical spine immobilization, lack of ancillary personnel to assist in the procedure, lack of neuromuscular blocking agents, intoxicated and combative patients, and blood and vomitus in the airway. It is a procedure that requires comprehensive training and a structured program of continuing education to maintain the acquired skills.

Given that it is a difficult but necessary procedure performed in the prehospital setting, it is not unexpected that complications might arise. Complications during intubation attempts in the prehospital setting include oropharyngeal and dental trauma, laryngeal and vocal cord injury, esophageal intubation, mainstem bronchus intubation, lack of oxygenation and ventilation for unacceptable periods of time during repeated intubation attempts, delayed chest compressions in arrest patients, and failure to recognize misplaced tubes (Falk & Sayre, 1999; AHA, 2000). While these are the immediate complications of intubation, many of these can lead to the long-term sequelae of anoxic brain injury and death. Unrecognized esophageal intubation represents a great danger in prehospital airway management. In the OR, unrecognized esophageal intubation accounts for 15% of all catastrophic injuries to patients including brain damage and death, making it the single-most critical anesthetic incident associated with injuries of this type (Cheney *et al.*, 1989; Goldberg *et al.*, 1990; MacLeod *et al.*, 1991).

The true incidence of unrecognized misplaced intubations (UMI) in the prehospital setting has been a subject of investigation in recent years. Initial reports indicated UMI rates in the range of 1–5% (Stewart *et al.*, 1984; Shea *et al.*, 1985; Pointer, 1988; Jenkins *et al.*, 1994; Bozeman *et al.*, 1996; Sayre *et al.*, 1998; Falk & Sayre, 1999). While these early studies reported UMI rates, their methodologies did not include determination of the incidence of UMI as a primary outcome measure. In general, these studies reported UMI rates incidental to the primary study objectives. Katz and Falk (2001) were the first to combine determination of the incidence of UMI rate in a prehospital system as a primary outcome measure with a standardized, physician emergency department (ED) confirmation process for all prehospital placed ETTs. The position of the ETTs upon arrival at the ED is a more relevant issue. Tubes can migrate. Simple flexion or extension of the neck can change the position of the tube by up to 5 cm (Birmingham *et al.*, 1986). Irrespective of whether the patient is esophageally intubated initially or correctly intubated in the field with the tube migrating out of the trachea during transport, the catastrophic result to the patient is the same.

In the Katz and Falk study (2001), 108 consecutive prehospital intubated patients were evaluated to determine ETT position upon arrival at the ED. The overall UMI rate was an alarming 25%. Two-thirds of the misplaced tubes were in the esophagus and one-third was in the hypopharynx. This study was conducted in a regional prehospital system in which expired carbon dioxide (CO_2) monitoring was inconsistently utilized. Recent studies using a similar methodology reported the incidence of UMI, in three different prehospital systems, to be in the range of 7.0–10% (Silvestri *et al.*, 2003; Jemmett *et al.*, 2003; Jones *et al.*, 2003). These data confirm the fact that UMI represents a significant national problem. Accordingly, systematic efforts to better equip our paramedics to continuously monitor tube position both at the time of initial insertion and throughout the prehospital phase of treatment are indicated.

For decades direct visualization of the ETT passing through the cords during intubation has been considered the "gold standard" for confirming intubation. Indeed, if the clinician sees the tube pass through the vocal cords, he/she should feel reasonably confidant that the tube is in the correct position. However ideal, it is not always possible to achieve direct visualization, particularly in the prehospital setting where airways are often contaminated with blood or vomitus. Additionally, despite accurate direct visualization during placement, the tube may become dislodged in transport such that ongoing monitoring is required. Even in the case of direct visualization, the American College of Emergency Physicians (ACEP) currently recommends verification of ETT placement with secondary confirmatory techniques such as end-tidal CO_2 ($ETCO_2$) detection or use of an esophageal detector device (EDD) (ACEP, 2002).

Clinical signs such as observing chest rise with ventilation, auscultation of the chest and epigastrium, and condensation of the ETT had long been used and taught as sound indicators of tube location. It is now understood that these techniques are not foolproof, and additional techniques of confirmation are needed (Birmingham *et al.*, 1986). Lack of clearly observed chest rise may occur in patients with obesity, obstructive or restrictive lung disease, and women with large breasts who are correctly intubated (Birmingham *et al.*, 1986). Even more concerning, observation of chest rise and fall has been witnessed in esophageally intubated patients as the stomach distends with ventilation causing upward movement of the chest. Gas then escapes up the esophagus causing the chest wall to fall (Birmingham *et al.*, 1986). Auscultation of breath sounds also can be misleading and is made ever more difficult in the loud prehospital setting (Birmingham *et al.*, 1986). In one study, auscultation of the axillae alone failed to identify 15% of esophageal intubations (Andersen & Hald, 1989). Auscultation of the epigastrium fairs no better. In thin patients, tracheal breath sounds may be transmitted to the epigastric area simulating gastric insufflation (Birmingham *et al.*, 1986). In esophageal intubations, abdominal distention does not always occur, and examiners judged movements of the epigastrium normal in 90% of esophageal intubation in one study (Birmingham *et al.*, 1986; Andersen & Hald, 1989). While reservoir bag compliance is often discussed in the setting of the OR, this is unreliable in the prehospital setting where paramedics utilize stiff self-inflating bags on patients with varying lung compliance (Birmingham *et al.*, 1986). Studies in both dogs and humans reveal that condensation in the ETT occurs in approximately 85% of esophageal intubations (Andersen & Hald, 1989; Kelly *et al.*, 1998). Clinical assessment of the intubated patient is not without use, but rather simply requires more dependable secondary confirmatory techniques to reliably determine and monitor the location of the ETTs.

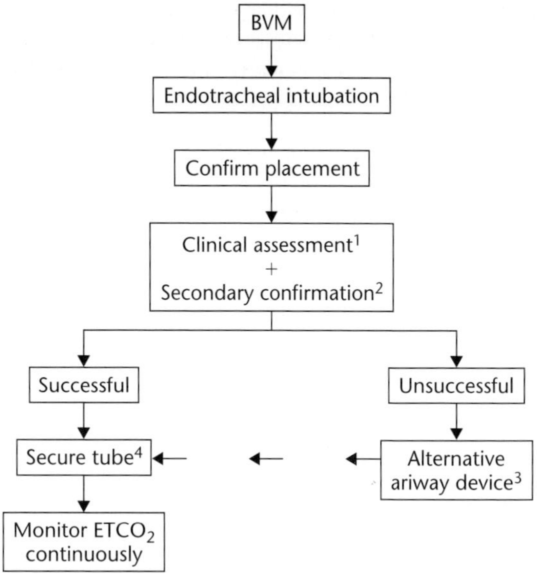

Figure 3.1 Suggested prehospital airway management algorithm. [1]Assessment variables: chest/epigastric sounds, chest rise and fall, tube condensation, patient skin/mucous membrane color (i.e. pink versus cyanotic), tube marker at corner of mouth. [2]Devices: EDD, $ETCO_2$ detector, or capnography. [3]BVM, LMA, or combitube. [4]Adjuncts that help stabilize the tubes: ETT holders, rigid cervical collar/spinal immobilization.

Given the inadequacies of clinical assessment, investigators turned to technological devices in an effort to improve results. Pulse oximetry is one such device. It may take several minutes for oxygen desaturation to occur in patients with misplaced ETTs, especially in cases of adequate preoxygenation (Birmingham *et al.*, 1986; Guggenberger *et al.*, 1989). At the time of desaturation, the deleterious consequences of hypoxia to the brain and heart may already be manifest. In contradistinction, expired CO_2 monitoring can identify the problem before critical hypoxemia becomes manifest, giving clinicians an opportunity to rectify the problem before the patient suffers any adverse consequences (Vaghadia *et al.*, 1989). The multiple variables involved in the process of endotracheal intubation are depicted in a suggested prehospital airway management algorithm in Figure 3.1.

The EDD is an apparatus that greatly improved upon the other methods available to detect ETT position. It consists of either a self-inflating bulb or a syringe that is attached to the ETT, and it exploits the differences in anatomy and physical properties of the esophagus and trachea to distinguish between the two (Bozeman *et al.*, 1996; AHA, 2000). By using either a bulb or syringe, suction is applied to the ETT. If the tube is in the esophagus, the suction will cause the floppy esophageal walls to collapse and prevent free aspiration of air through the device (Bozeman *et al.*, 1996; AHA, 2000). If the tube is placed in the trachea, however, the rigid cartilaginous rings will prevent collapse of the airway and permit aspiration of into the device (Bozeman *et al.*, 1996; AHA, 2000). The EDD has a good performance record in the OR and in the ED with reported sensitivities and specificities in the 95%+ range (Bozeman *et al.*, 1996; Pelucio *et al.*, 1997; Kasper & Deem, 1998; O'Connor & Swor, 1999). The device does have some limitations. Inaccurate results in patients with morbid obesity, pulmonary edema, bronchospastic disease, or ETT obstruction as in the case of an airway contaminated with blood or vomitus have been reported (Lang *et al.*, 1996; Coontz & Gratton, 2002). Specifically in obese patients with a body mass index (BMI) >35, the device has a false negative rate of 11–30% (Lang *et al.*, 1996). Furthermore, an EDD cannot provide continuous, breath-to-breath monitoring of ETT position. Additionally, it is contraindicated in pregnant patients and children under 5 years old (Coontz & Gratton, 2002). Despite its apparent efficacy within the hospital, Pelucio *et al.* (1997) showed that the EDD performed poorly in the hands of paramedics. In 168 intubations, it only detected 50% of esophageal intubations (5/10) in the field. This even excluded the 11 cases in which the paramedic was unable to interpret the result. In a direct comparison study, the EDD was shown to be inferior to capnography (Knapp *et al.*, 1999). The most consistently accepted use for the EDD in confirming airway placement is in the cardiac arrest patient when capnographic waveform analysis is unavailable or semiquantitative colorimetric capnometry fails to register expired CO_2 (AHA, 2000; Coontz & Gratton, 2002).

Capnography has emerged as the technology best able to assess the location of an ETT. While this technology had been available for many years within the hospital, it was not until the late 1980s and early 1990s that it was being used with any regularity in the prehospital setting.

Semiquantitative colorimetric devices are the most basic capnometer, and consist of a clear dome overlying a piece of litmus paper that changes color when CO_2 is detected (Krauss, 2003). A typical device would have the capacity to produce one of three readings, an A reading (purple): $PCO_2 \leq 2.28$ mmHg ($\leq$0.3%); a B reading (beige): PCO_2 of 3.8–7.6 mmHg (0.5–1.0%); and a C reading (yellow): $PCO_2 > 15.2$ mmHg (>2.0%) (Wayne *et al.*, 1999). Quantitative devices typically utilize infrared absorption spectroscopy, since of the exhaled gases only CO_2 and H_2O absorb infrared light (Sanders, 1989). In the sensor unit water vapor is removed, and all wavelengths of light are filtered except those which correspond with CO_2 (Sanders, 1989).

The efficacy of $ETCO_2$ in detecting ETT location has been the subject of much research in the last two decades and is best approached analyzing its use in two situations, patients in cardiac arrest and those not in cardiac arrest. Of the two, the non-arrest situation is by far the clearer. The semiquantitative colorimetric device performed extremely well in non-arrest patients in all major settings. In the prehospital setting, Ornato *et al.* (1992) showed that colorimetric $ETCO_2$ has a sensitivity of 100% with a specificity of 93%, in the non-arrest patient cohort, respectively. Additionally, the study would have had a specificity of 100% had it not been for provider error in using the device. The single false positive reading occurred in a spontaneously breathing patient who had been esophageally intubated. The provider recorded an $ETCO_2$ reading as positive prior to inflation of the cuff of the ETT. Once the cuff was inflated, the colorimetric device indicated an esophageal intubation, which was confirmed by physical exam, and the patient was reintubated tracheally with appropriate color change on the $ETCO_2$ device. MacLeod *et al.* (1991) reported nearly identical data for colorimetric $ETCO_2$ on non-arrest patients intubated in the prehospital and ED setting. A similar study on patients undergoing intubation in the OR revealed that a disposable colorimetric $ETCO_2$ device correctly identified all tracheal and esophageal intubations (Goldberg *et al.*, 1990). The efficacy of the colorimetric device has also been substantiated in non-arrest infants and children with 100% sensitivity and specificity (Bhende *et al.*, 1992). The indisputable data supporting the use of capnometry in non-arrest patients has led to the widespread prehospital use of economic, disposable devices in the US.

Use of colorimetric devices in patients in cardiac arrest has some limitations. For patients in cardiac arrest, Ornato *et al.* (1992) and MacLeod *et al.* (1991) studies yielded sensitivities and specificities of 69–72% and 100%, respectively. While all esophageal intubations were correctly identified by the device remaining purple (low $ETCO_2$), additional patients, who were tracheally intubated, had no color change on the indicator. This could have prompted paramedics to remove a correctly placed ETT. In cardiac arrest patients the low $ETCO_2$ may result from markedly diminished pulmonary blood flow despite endotracheal placement of the tube. In this case, it is the low cardiac output that results in very low delivery of CO_2 to the lungs for excretion that causes a low $ETCO_2$. These low CO_2 values may be insufficient to cause a color change in colorimetric devices.

However, in a study by Hayden *et al.* (1995) on patients undergoing out-of-hospital cardiac arrest, a sensitivity of 95.6% was demonstrated with the colorimetric $ETCO_2$ device. In this study, a large number of the positive results were in the intermediate (beige) range on the detector. Even in cardiac arrest, colorimetric $ETCO_2$ devices can provide useful information. When a positive result is obtained, the clinician can be assured that the ETT has been placed correctly. When a negative result is obtained, the situation is more complex and several things must be considered. Failure to obtain a color change during cardiac arrest can be an indicator of prolonged arrest time with poor pulmonary perfusion (low cardiac output), severe ventilation–perfusion mismatch as in a massive pulmonary embolus, or a misplaced ETT (Ornato *et al.*, 1992). If a negative result is obtained with a colorimetric device during cardiac arrest, a second method of detection is recommended such as the EDD or repeat direct visualization (Falk & Sayre, 1999; AHA, 2000). Furthermore, some information regarding the prognosis of the patient may be obtained from the $ETCO_2$ device in these patients. A purple reading on the detector in a tracheally intubated cardiac arrest patient is associated with a low incidence of return of spontaneous circulation, and in one study carried a 0% survival to hospital discharge (Ornato *et al.*, 1992; Hayden *et al.*, 1995). When patients do experience a return of spontaneous circulation it is accompanied by an immediate increase in $ETCO_2$ concentration that often precedes other clinical signs of the patients improvement. This should prompt cessation of chest compressions to check for a pulse (Garnett *et al.*, 1987; Ornato *et al.*, 1992; Idris *et al.*, 1994). The data illustrating the limitations of the colorimetric device in cardiac arrest patients is certainly not sufficient to dissuade the clinician from using the device in these situations. Rather, the clinician must be aware of the possible reasons for a negative result in this circumstance.

Recently continuous capnography has become available to prehospital systems. Along with the advance in technology comes improved reliability, particularly with respect to utilization on patients in cardiac arrest. The threshold for detection of exhaled CO_2 is significantly lower in capnography as opposed to colorimetric capnometry (O'Connor & Swor, 1999). Additionally, the tracing produced during measurement of partial pressure of CO_2 at end-tidal ($P_{et}CO_2$) from a properly placed ETT is characteristic. The reliability of the capnographic waveform during cardiac arrest and resuscitation has been verified in both animal and human models (Falk *et al.*, 1988; Sayah *et al.*, 1990). If this waveform is present, regardless of its amplitude, the tube can be confidently judged to be correctly placed (Falk & Sayre, 1999; Grmec, 2002). Every major study either evaluating the efficacy of capnography in arrest and non-arrest patients or comparing it to other methods of detection have demonstrated the superiority of continuous capnography in this setting. Knapp *et al.* (1999) revealed capnography to have a 0% error rate in a study on non-arrest intensive care unit (ICU) patients, clearly performing better than auscultation, a self-inflating EDD, and a lighted stylet. A recent study by Singh *et al.* (2003) showed capnography to be superior to the semiquantitative colorimetric device in a prehospital setting in both arrest and non-arrest patients. This was further verified in a very convincing study by Grmec (2002) of 345 prehospital intubations in which capnography had a 100% sensitivity and specificity in both arrest and non-arrest patients compared to capnometry which had 88% sensitivity and 100% specificity in the arrest population. The fact that digital capnography offers the most advantages to confirming ETT position in both arrest and non-arrest patients clearly makes it the technology of choice in the prehospital setting.

Table 3.2 summarizes a comparative analysis of the EDD, capnometry, and capnography. The most significant advantages of capnography include 100% sensitivity and specificity in determining ETT location, with or without cardiac arrest, and the ability to monitor ETT location continuously.

Besides overcoming the limitations of capnometry in detecting ETT location in arrest patients, capnography also solves several other problems. Theoretical concern had been expressed regarding false positives in patients who had ingested carbonated beverages shortly prior to intubation. Esophageal intubation in these patients may reveal $P_{et}CO_2$ consistent with tracheal placement of the tube. The morphology of the waveform is strikingly different and the $P_{et}CO_2$ rapidly falls to zero within 10–15 s of ventilation (Garnett *et al.*, 1989). In this instance, the operator would be alerted very quickly that the tube was incorrectly placed, prompting repeat intubation. This scenario illustrates the continuous monitoring advantage of capnography. Colorimetric devices may provide ongoing assessment, but fail when the litmus paper in the device gets wet. Capnographic devices may be equipped with an alarm indicating unacceptably low CO_2 concentration while giving an easily visible ongoing breath-to-breath waveform. Given that ETTs do not infrequently become dislodged in transport, this aspect is especially important in the prehospital setting.

Evidence supporting the use of $P_{et}CO_2$ for intubation confirmation produced in the last 15 years has led to the formulation of position statements by several major organizations. The American Society of Anesthesiologists (ASA) was the first organization to

Table 3.2 Comparison of EDD, colorimetric $ETCO_2$ detection (capnometry), and capnography*

Conditions	EDD	Capnometry	Capnography
Use in patients with adequate perfusion	3+	4+	4+
Use in patients with cardiac arrest (static evaluation)	3+	2–3+	4+
Ability to monitor continuously	1+	2–3+	4+
Use in pediatric patients (<5 years old)	1+	2–3+	4+
Use in pregnancy	0	2–3+	4+

0: contraindicated.

* Scale: 0–4 (0: least useful; 4+: most useful).

make $P_{et}CO_2$ monitoring a standard for basic anesthetic monitoring in 1990 (ASA, 2003). In 1998, these standards were extended to include all patients receiving anesthesia care regardless of their geographic location (ASA, 2003). By 1999, the National Association of EMS Physicians had produced a position paper that cited the use of $P_{et}CO_2$ monitoring in all patients with perfusing rhythms, and recommended a combination of techniques to assess tube location in the cardiac arrest patient. The updated Advanced Cardiac Life Support Guidelines 2000 of the AHA, included a recommendation for the use of secondary confirmatory devices, such as $ETCO_2$ detectors for ETT confirmation even with accurate direct visualization and gave this action a IIa classification (acceptable, probably helpful) (AHA, 2000). The American College of Emergency Physicians (ACEP) initially addressed this issue in 1994 indicating that $P_{et}CO_2$ monitoring of tracheal intubation was "desirable", but "not mandatory". The 2002 ACEP policy statement now fully supports $P_{et}CO_2$ measurement during emergency intubation.

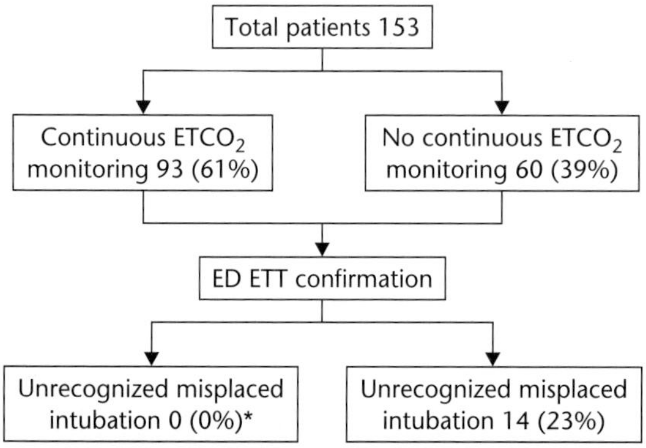

Figure 3.2 Prehospital ETT placement and $ETCO_2$ use. *Misplaced intubation rate greater for no $ETCO_2$ monitoring group versus $ETCO_2$ monitoring group by 23.3% (95% confidence interval: [13.4%, 36.0%]).

Perhaps the most compelling association between continuous $P_{et}CO_2$ monitoring and unrecognized misplaced intubation (UMI) comes from the study by Silvestri *et al.* (2004). This was a follow-up study conducted in the same regional EMS system that experienced a misplaced endotracheal intubation rate of 25% (Katz & Falk, 2001). In the intervening interval a protocol requirement for continuous $P_{et}CO_2$ monitoring was implemented within the EMS system. Of the 153 patients who received prehospital endotracheal intubation, continuous $P_{et}CO_2$ monitoring was used in 93 (61%) after intubation and in 60 (39%), continuous $P_{et}CO_2$ monitoring was not used after intubation. The overall incidence of UMI was 9%. In the group in which continuous $P_{et}CO_2$ monitoring was utilized,

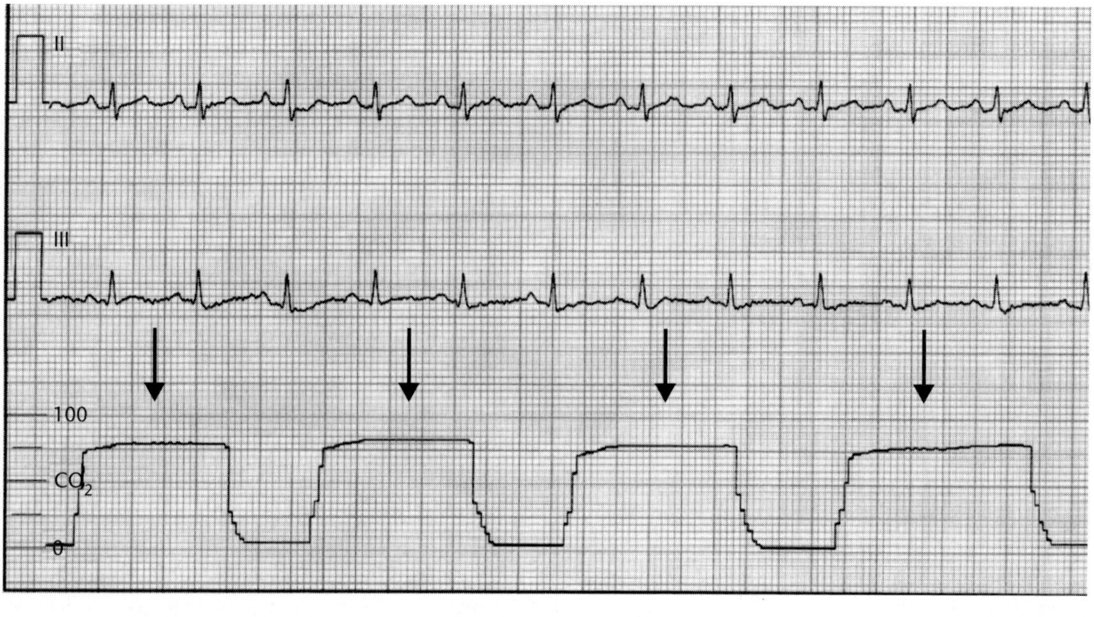

Figure 3.3 Prehospital (LifePak-12®) tracing of characteristic waveforms (arrows) in an intubated patient being ventilated via a BVM after successful resuscitation.

there were no UMI. In the group in which continuous $P_{et}CO_2$ monitoring was not utilized, there were 14 (23%) UMI (Figure 3.2) (Silvestri *et al.*, 2004). The 9% UMI rate was similar to results obtained in other recent studies yielding rates of 7.0–10% (Jemmett *et al.*, 2003; Jones *et al.*, 2003).

Without a doubt, $P_{et}CO_2$ measurement has revolutionized the way in which prehospital providers can assess ETT placement. It has the potential, when used appropriately, to eliminate the most disastrous airway complication, unrecognized esophageal intubation. Figures 3.3 and 3.4 depict characteristic capnographic waveforms with and without adequate perfusion, respectively. Supported by several major medical organizations, $ETCO_2$ detection has emerged as the standard of care in airway confirmation. Medical personnel are not the only ones to recognize this fact; representatives from the legal world have also made their voice clear on this issue. William H. Ginsburg, a lawyer from Los Angeles, in an article published in the *Annals of Emergency Medicine* stated,

> from a legal point of view, a physician, EMT, or paramedic who does not use a disposable $ETCO_2$ detector in the process of intubation, in the absence of electronic capnography, is not acting as the average reasonable reputable physician, EMT or paramedic would under the same or similar circumstances, in the same or similar location and therefore may be said to have breached his or her duty to exercise reasonable care.
>
> Ginsburg (1993)

Based on the evidence presented, a suggested algorithm for the paramedic to follow is represented in Figure 3.5.

One final consideration of prehospital airway management is prehospital rapid sequence intubation (RSI). Despite reported complications of prehospital RSI (Mizelle *et al.*, 2002; Dunford *et al.*, 2003), this procedure is gaining field acceptance. With the practice of pharmacologically facilitated (i.e. paralytic or sedative) intubation, the problem of UMI is magnified. National organizations are currently developing a prehospital RSI position statement. Components of this position paper include considerations for use of alternative advanced airway devices (e.g. an LMA or combitube), minimum standards for initial and ongoing training, continuous monitoring of airway location (e.g. capnography), and close medical oversight.

In summary, an optimal prehospital approach to airway management maximizes the patient's oxygenation and ventilation, while minimizing hypoxic intervals. Alternative airway devices play key adjunctive roles in facilitating effective ventilation. While endotracheal intubation remains the gold standard for the prehospital management of respiratory failure, the ability to continuously monitor ETT location is essential. Capnography has been shown to be the most useful modality for determining tube location both with and without cardiac arrest. Implementation of continuous capnography for prehospital airway management is an effective EMS system risk management strategy.

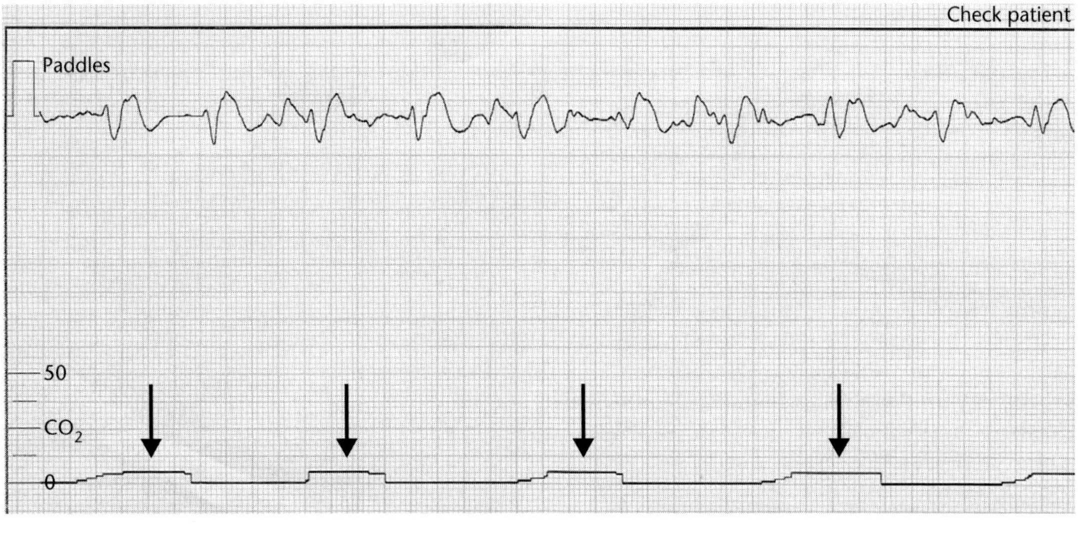

Figure 3.4 Prehospital (LifePak-12®) tracing of waveforms (arrows) in a prehospital asystolic patient, undergoing cardiopulmonary resuscitation (CPR) and attempted resuscitation. Note that although the amplitude of the waveform is low (corresponding to an $ETCO_2 < 10$ mmHg), the characteristic waveform is still present and indicative of endotracheal location of the tube.

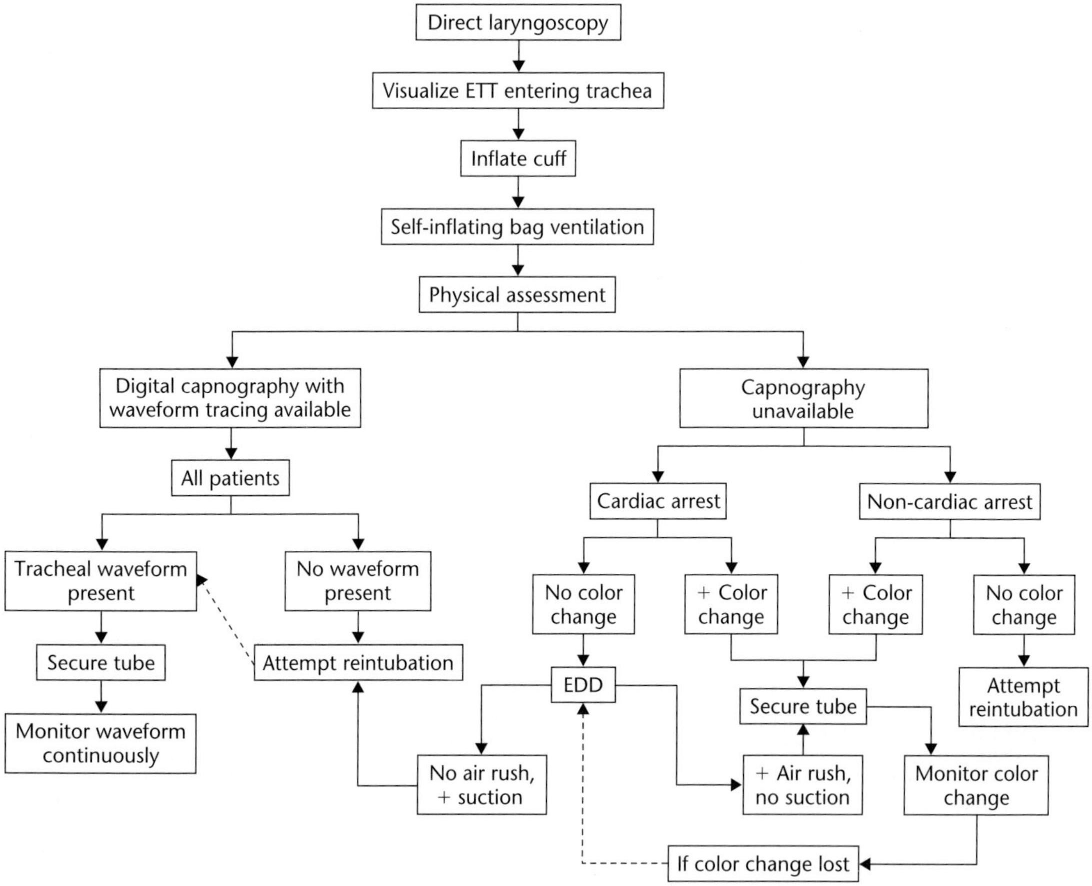

Figure 3.5 Prehospital airway algorithm of secondary confirmatory processes of ETT location determination.

References

American College of Emergency Physicians. Board of Directors (1995). Policy statements: expired carbon dioxide monitoring. *Ann. Emerg. Med.*, **25**: 441.

American College of Emergency Physicians. Clinical Policies Committee (2002). Verification of endotracheal tube placement. *Ann. Emerg. Med.*, **40**: 551–552.

American Heart Association (2000). Guidelines 2000 for cardiopulmonary resuscitation and emergency cardiovascular care. *Circulation*, **102(suppl. 8)**: 186–189.

American Society of Anesthesiologists (2003). Standards for Basic Anesthetic Monitoring. Available at www.asahq.org.

Andersen, K.H. & Hald, A. (1989). Assessing the position of the tracheal tube: the reliability of different methods. *Anaesthesia*, **44**: 984–985.

Bhende, M.S., Thompson, A.E., Cook, D.R. & Saville, A.L. (1992). Validity of a disposable end-tidal CO_2 detector in verifying endotracheal tube placement in infants and children. *Ann. Emerg. Med.*, **21**: 142–145.

Birmingham, P.K., Cheney, F.W. & Ward, R.J. (1986). Esophageal intubation: a review of detection techniques. *Anesth. Analg.*, **65**: 886–891.

Bozeman, W.P., Hexter, D., Liang, H.K. & Kelen, G.D. (1996). Esophageal detector device versus detection of end-tidal carbon dioxide level in emergency intubation. *Ann. Emerg. Med.*, **27**: 595–599.

Cheney, F.W., Posner, K., Caplan, R.A. & Ward, R.J. (1989). Standard of care and anesthesia liability. *J. Am. Med. Assoc.*, **261**: 1599–1633.

Clinton, J.E. & McGill, J.W. (1998). Basic airway management and decision-making. In: Roberts, J.R. & Hedges, J.R. (eds) *Clinical Procedures in Emergency Medicine*, 3rd edition. WB Saunders Company, Philadelphia.

Coontz, D.A. & Gratton, M. (2002). Rules of engagement: how to reduce the incidence of unrecognized esophageal intubations. *J. Emerg. Med. Serv.*, **27**:(June) 44–59.

Dunford, J.V., Davis, D.P., Ochs, M., Doney, M. & Hoyt, D.B. (2003). Incidence of transient hypoxia and pulse rate reactivity during paramedic rapid sequence intubation. *Ann. Emerg. Med.*, **42**: 721–728.

Falk, J.L. & Sayre, M.R. (1999). Confirmation of airway placement. *Prehosp. Emerg. Care*, **3**: 273–278.

Falk, J.L., Rackow, E.C. & Weil, M.H. (1988). End-tidal carbon dioxide concentration during cardiopulmonary resuscitation. *New Eng. J. Med.*, **318**: 607–611.

Garnett, A.R., Ornato, J.P., Gonzalez, E.R. & Johnson, E.B. (1987). End-tidal carbon dioxide during cardiopulmonary resuscitation. *J. Am. Med. Assoc.*, **257**: 512–515.

Garnett, A.R., Gervin, C.A. & Gervin, A.S. (1989). Capnographic waveforms in esophageal intubation: effect of carbonated beverages. *Ann. Emerg. Med.*, **18**: 387.

Ginsburg, W.H. (1993). When does a guideline become a standard? The new American Society of Anesthesiologists guidelines give us a clue. *Ann. Emerg. Med.*, **22**: 1891–1896.

Goldberg, J.S., Rawle, P.R., Zehnder, J.L. & Sladen, R.N. (1990). Colorimetric end-tidal carbon dioxide monitoring for tracheal intubation. *Anesth. Analg.*, **70**: 191–194.

Grmec, S. (2002). Comparison of three different methods to confirm tracheal tube placement in emergency intubation. *Intens. Care Med.*, **28**: 701–704.

Guggenberger, H., Lenz, G. & Federle, R. (1989). Early detection of inadvertent oesophageal intubation: pulse-oximetry vs. capnography. *Acta Anaesth. Scand.*, **33**: 112–115.

Hayden, S.R., Sciammarella, J., Viccello, P., Thode, H. & Delagi, R. (1995). Colorimetric end-tidal CO_2 detection for verification of endotracheal tube placement in out-of-hospital cardiac arrest. *Acad. Emerg. Med.*, **2**: 499–502.

Idris, A.H., Staples, E.D., O'Brien, D.J., Melker, R.J., Rush, W.J., Del Duca, K.D. & Falk, J.L. (1994). End-tidal carbon dioxide during extremely low cardiac output. *Ann. Emerg. Med.*, **23**: 568–572.

Jemmett, M.E., Kendall, K.M., Fourre, M.W. & Burton, J.H. (2003). Unrecognized misplaced endotracheal tubes in a mixed urban to rural setting. *Acad. Emerg. Med.*, **10**: 961–965.

Jenkins, W.A., Verdile, V.P. & Paris, P.M. (1994). The syringe aspiration technique to verify endotracheal tube position. *Ann. Emerg. Med.*, **12**: 413–416.

Jones, J.H., Murphy, M.P., Dickson, R.L. & Somerville, G.G. (2003). Emergency physician verified prehospital intubation, missed rates by ground paramedics. *Acad. Emerg. Med.*, **10**: 448–449 [abstract].

Kasper, C.L. & Deem, S. (1998). The self-inflating bulb to detect esophageal intubation during emergency airway management. *Anesthesiology*, **88**: 898–902.

Katz, S.H. & Falk, J.L. (2001). Misplaced endotracheal tubes by paramedics in an urban emergency medical services system. *Ann. Emerg. Med.*, **37**: 32–37.

Kelly, J.J., Eynon, C.A., Kaplan, J.L., de Garavilla, L. & Dalsey, W.C. (1998). Use of tube condensation as an indicator of endotracheal tube placement. *Ann. Emerg. Med.*, **31**: 575–578.

Knapp, S., Kofler, J., Stoiser, B., Thalhammer, F., Burgmann, H., Posch, M., Hofbauer, R., Stanzel, M. & Frass, M. (1999). The assessment of four different methods to verify tracheal tube placement in the critical care setting. *Anesth. Analg.*, **88**: 766–770.

Konrad, C., Schüpfer, G., Wietlisbach, M. & Gerber, H. (1998). Learning manual skills in anesthesiology: is there a recommended number of cases for anesthetic procedures? *Anesth. Analg.*, **86**: 635–639.

Krauss, B. (2003). Capnography in EMS: a powerful way to objectively monitor ventilatory status. *J. Emerg. Med. Serv.*, **28**:(January) 29–41.

Lang, D.J., Wafai, Y., Salem, M.R., Czinn, E.A., Halim, A.A. & Baraka, A. (1996). Efficacy of self-inflating bulb in confirming tracheal intubation in the morbidly obese. *Anesthesiology*, **85**: 246–253.

MacLeod, B.A., Heller, M.B., Gerard, J., Yealy, D.M. & Menegazzi, J.J. (1991). Verification of endotracheal tube placement with colorimetric end-tidal CO_2 detection. *Ann. Emerg. Med.*, **20**: 267–270.

Mizelle, H.L., Rothrock, S.G., Silvestri, S. & Pagane, J. (2002). Preventable morbidity and mortality from prehospital paralytic assisted intubation: can we expect outcomes comparable to hospital-based practice? *Prehosp. Emerg. Care*, **6**: 472–475.

Nolan, J.D. (2001). Prehospital and resuscitative airway care: should the gold standard be reassessed? *Curr. Opin. Crit. Care*, **7**: 413–421.

O'Connor, R.E. & Swor, R.A. (1999). Verification of endotracheal tube placement following intubation. National Association of EMS Physicians Standards and Clinical Practices Committee. *Prehosp. Emerg. Care*, **3**: 248–250.

Ornato, J.P., Shipley, J.B., Racht, E.M., Slovis, C.M., Wrenn, K.D., Pepe, P.E., Almeida, S.L., Ginger, V.F. & Fotre, T.V. (1992). Multicenter study of a portable, hand-size, colorimetric end-tidal carbon dioxide detection device. *Ann. Emerg. Med.*, **21**: 518–523.

Pelucio, M., Halligan, L. & Dhindsa, H. (1997). Out-of-hospital experience with the syringe esophageal detector device. *Acad. Emerg. Med.*, **4**: 563–568.

Pennant, J.H. & Walker, M.B. (1992). Comparison of the endotracheal tube and laryngeal mask airway management by paramedic personnel. *Anesth. Analg.*, **74**: 531–534.

Pointer, J.E. (1988). Clinical characteristics of paramedics' performance of endotracheal intubation. *J. Emerg. Med.*, **6**: 505–509.

Sanders, A.B. (1989). Capnometry in emergency medicine. *Ann. Emerg. Med.*, **18**: 1287–1290.

Sayah, A.J., Peacock, W.F. & Overton, D.T. (1990). End-tidal CO_2 measurement in the detection of esophageal intubation during cardiac arrest. *Ann. Emerg. Med.*, **19**: 857–860.

Sayre, M.R., Sackles, J.C., Mistler, A.F., Evans, J.L., Kramer, A.T. & Pancioli, A.M. (1998). Field trial of endotracheal intubation by basic EMTs. *Ann. Emerg. Med.*, **31**: 228–233.

Shea, S.R., MacDonald, J.R. & Gruzinski, G. (1985). Prehospital endotracheal tube airway or esophageal gastric tube airway: a critical comparison. *Ann. Emerg. Med.*, **14**: 102–112.

Silvestri, S., Ralls, G., Carter, E., Senn, A., Rothrock, S., Giordano, P. & Falk, J. (2003). Improvement in misplaced endotracheal tube recognition within a regional emergency medical services system. *Acad. Emerg. Med.*, **10**: 445 [abstract].

Silvestri, S., Ralls, G., Krauss, B., Thundiyil, J., Rothrock, S., Senn, A., Carter, E. & Falk, J. (2004). The effectiveness of prehospital use of continuous end-tidal carbon dioxide monitoring on the rate of unrecognized misplaced intubation within a regional emergency medical services systems. [submitted]

Singh, A., Megargel, R.E., Schnyder, M.R. & O'Connor, R.E. (2003). Comparing the ability of colorimetric and waveform end tidal capnography to verify endotracheal tube placement in the prehospital setting. *Acad. Emerg. Med.*, **10**: 466–467 [abstract].

Stewart, R.D., Paris, P.M., Winter, P.M., Pelton, G.H. & Cannon, G.M. (1984). Field endotracheal intubation by paramedical personnel. *Chest*, **85**: 341–345.

Vaghadia, H., Jenkins, L. & Ford, R. (1989). Comparison of end-tidal carbon dioxide, oxygen saturation, and clinical signs for detection of oesophageal intubation. *Can. J. Anaesth.*, **36**: 560–564.

Wayne, M.A., Slovis, C.M. & Pirrallo, R.G. (1999). Management of difficult airways in the field. *Prehosp. Emerg. Care*, **3**: 290–296.

Wayne, M.A., Delbridge, T.R., Ornato, J.P., Swor, R.A. & Blackwell, T. (2001). Concepts and application of prehospital ventilation. *Prehosp. Emerg. Care*, **5**: 73–78.

CAPNOGRAPHY: AIRWAY MANAGEMENT IN THE INTENSIVE CARE UNIT SETTING 4

P.N. Betadpur & J.D. Truwit

Capnography has become an invaluable tool in airway management in the critically ill patient. Specifically, capnography has become our standard to confirm airway cannulation of the endotracheal tube or proper seating of a laryngeal mask airway. Conversely, capnography has proven to be a useful adjunct during placement of gastric tubes as it readily detects errant airway cannulation. In this chapter we focus on the use of capnography in airway management and its adjunctive role in enteric tube placement in the intensive care unit (ICU) setting.

Airway cannulation with an endotracheal tube

While the decision to intubate in our institution is made on a case-by-case basis, the indications for intubation include hypoxia ($S_PO_2 < 70\%$), altered mental status with inability to protect airway, severe acidosis, profound respiratory failure rate and known major overdose. For placement of an emergent airway, the patient is placed in the supine position, and shifted closer to head of the bed. We use midazolam, fentanyl and/or etomidate for sedation, and succinylcholine for paralyzing the patients. A carbon dioxide (CO_2) monitor is attached to the endotracheal tube adapter (see Figure 4.2). After suctioning of oral secretions, the patient's trachea is intubated. The passage of the tube through the vocal cords is confirmed by the presence of CO_2 as visualized by the capnogram or by a change in color of the capnographic detector placed at the end of the tube. The proper placement of the tube is further confirmed by auscultation for equal breath sounds on both sides of the chest. In addition, capnography can be used to guide blind nasal intubation, for example in patients with facial trauma. During this procedure, the capnographic waveform is observed and the tube continues to be slowly advanced into the trachea provided the mainstream capnographic waveform remains displayed.

In our difficult intubations and in patients who lose a secure airway due to agitation or transport, a short acting paralytic such as succinylcholine (10 mg, half-life of <2 min) is often employed to facilitate securing the airway. In such instances, the capnographic confirmation of the airway placement is an invaluable tool in the assessment of the airway. Frequently, it is the only confirmation of tube location until a chest radiograph can be obtained. This is especially true in patients in whom auscultatory confirmation is difficult. If unable to intubate via the trachea, the patient is pre-oxygenated and an emergency tracheostomy is performed. Should the tracheostomy fail, a cricothyroidotomy may be performed.

The absence of CO_2 typically signifies esophageal intubation. However, the clinician needs to remain aware of circumstances that can introduce CO_2 into the esophagus and stomach. If bag mask ventilation precedes intubation, this can lead to mixing of exhaled gas in the pharynx. Continued bag mask ventilation can force this CO_2 contaminated gas into the esophagus and stomach leading to the measurement of CO_2 for possibly several breaths even if the endotracheal tube cannulates the esophagus (Sum-Ping *et al.*, 1989, 1991).

Capnographic recordings, if not properly interpreted, can mislead the clinician to believe that the endotracheal tube is not within the trachea. These false-negative capnography recordings can be detected in the event that the endotracheal tube is obstructed. This could result from plugging the tip of endotracheal tube with mucus or blood, or when the endotracheal tube abuts the tracheal wall and thus impedes or prevents exhalation. Apnea and severe bronchospasm lead to dramatically reduced exhalation and thus lead to flat-line capnograms that too would falsely suggest the endotracheal tube does not rest within the trachea.

Unintended bronchial intubation is difficult to detect, with time-capnography alone because the capnogram is generally typical in shape and shows normal end-tidal values. Gandhi *et al.* (1991) described an atypical case of the migration of an endotracheal tube into the right main bronchus that was identified when the end-tidal CO_2 ($P_{et}CO_2$) suddenly decreased by 6 mmHg. A prospective Australian study (Szekely *et al.*,

1993; McCoy *et al.*, 1997) found that endobronchial intubation was the most common cause of arterial desaturation. It has been suggested that signs of bronchial intubation may include changes in peak inspiratory pressure and arterial oxygen saturation (Szekely *et al.*, 1993).

Despite the concerns noted above capnography appears to be a reliable means of monitoring airway cannulation and has been considered to be a "front-line" monitor for intubation, disconnection and obstruction (Szekely *et al.*, 1993).

Maintenance of a secure airway

Continuous use of capnography allows for the detection of an airway leak or dislodged endotracheal tube. An agitated or confused patient may dislodge an endotracheal tube. Significant endotracheal movement can occur with flexion and extension of the neck (Conrardy *et al.*, 1976). Disconnection of the patient from the ventilator will be discovered quickly by a capnogram that suddenly shows a flat line. Disconnect alarms given by the ventilator will underscore the capnographic alarm. Changes in S_pO_2, heart rate and blood pressure follow later should the disconnection not be detected and corrected. Dislodgment of the endotracheal tube is always a concern during transportation of patients to and from the ICU. While the capnogram will reflect a reduced partial pressure of CO_2 in arterial blood, the measurement of both flow and CO_2 enhances monitoring (Sum-Ping *et al.*, 1989). Capnography provides continuous monitoring for early detection of such an untoward event. In support of this claim, a recent Sentinel Event report by the Joint Commission on Accreditation of Healthcare Organizations (JCAHO) reviewed 23 ventilator-associated deaths and injuries. The review of these cases found that 65% of deaths or injuries were related to malfunction or misuse of the alarm, 52% were related to ventilator tubing disconnect and that 26% were related to a disconnected tracheal or endotracheal tube. The use of capnography as an additional tool to alert caregivers to early loss of airway or ventilator circuit disconnection contributes importantly to patient safety (JCAHO, 2002). Guidelines from major critical care societies throughout the world vary. None have yet mandated $P_{et}CO_2$ for confirmation of endotracheal tube placement although some have strongly suggested using it and most have classified as desirable, especially during transport. For example, the latest American Heart Association guidelines (2000) endorse secondary confirmation of tube placement in all patients by $P_{et}CO_2$ monitoring immediately after intubation and during transport. Like any other tool, capnography is not a substitute for vigilance. The use of capnography as an additional tool to alert caregivers to early loss of airway disconnection is an asset for patient safety when combined with adequate and appropriate nursing supervision.

Assessment of enteric tube placement

Over 4.3 million small bore feeding tubes and 7 million Salem sump tubes are sold in the US per year.[1] Recently, the incidence of airway cannulation and placement into the trachea of feeding tubes as detected by bedside radiography has been documented at 2% (Rassias *et al.*, 1998). Inadvertent tracheal placement of feeding tubes and their use can result in complications such as pneumothorax, feeding pneumonitis, hydropneumothorax, bronchopleural fistula, empyema and pulmonary hemorrhage with the associated increased mortality, morbidity, length of stay and cost (Wendell *et al.*, 1991; Tornero *et al.*, 1992).

Current practice after feeding tube placement is to obtain an abdominal X-ray to ensure that the tube is in the stomach or small bowel prior to initiating tube feeds or administering medications. Unfortunately, complications may have occurred by the time a radiograph is obtained. Feeding tubes placed via oral or nasal routes are normally passed to a depth of 50–80 cm from the nares or lips in adult patients in order to reach the desired gastric and small bowel location. Should a feeding tube be placed into the respiratory system and advanced to the same depth, a pneumothorax could result (Wendell *et al.*, 1991) given that in adults, the trachea ranges 9–15 cm in length.

Other techniques to determine if the tube tip is in the lung stomach or small bowel include pH testing, visual inspection of the tube aspirates, insufflation of air via the tube while auscultating over the epigastrium, listening for air movement at the tube's proximal end and utilizing pressure manometry attached to the tube (Araujo-Preza *et al.*, 2002). All have proven fallible, with tubes detected in the lungs on X-ray evaluation. Furthermore, these tests do not detect in real-time inadvertent placement into the trachea. More definitive techniques to prevent inadvertent placement include fluoroscopy, endoscopy and direct visualization of the tube passing into the esophagus. However, these techniques are labor intensive, expensive and add extra discomfort or radiation to the patient.

[1] Verbal communication, John Bonner, Kendall Healthcare.

A two-step radiographic approach (Roubenoff & Ravich, 1989) has also been clinically used, whereby the feeding tube is placed 30 cm into the esophagus and a chest radiograph obtained. If the film demonstrates esophageal placement then it is advanced and final confirmation is obtained by an abdominal X-ray. This process is expensive and time consuming.

A study from the Queen's University Teaching Hospitals (Kindopp *et al.*, 2001) evaluated the use of capnography to eliminate the need of a two-step radiographic approach. Eligible patients were those 18 years or older and designated as needing a feeding tube by the ICU physician. Two-step radiography was used in each feeding tube placement. Capnography was performed at the midway position, which was defined as tube distance of 30 or 35 cm for oral or nasal approach, respectively. Prior to recording a syringe was used to push air through the tube to clear any secretions, which may have interfered with gas aspiration, by the capnograph. The results were recorded as: normal, abnormal, or purge warning, or no capnogram. A chest radiograph was obtained and feeding tube was interpreted as being intra-esophageal, tracheobronchial or indeterminate, or not visible. Based on the results of the radiograph, the procedure was then completed if the feeding tube was localized to the esophagus otherwise it was abandoned. For those procedures where the tubes were advanced to the completion distance, a confirmatory radiograph was obtained to determine the final tube position to use.

One hundred feeding tubes placement attempts were included in the study. Eleven were placed into the airways as diagnosed by radiography, for an incidence of 11%. Nine of these were found in the right main stem bronchus and two in the left main stem bronchus. For each of these 11 placements the capnograph displayed a capnogram comparable to that of endotracheal tube monitoring. There were 89 placements where the tube was not placed in the lung; 86 were in the esophagus and the capnograph read "purging" in all 86. In this small study, capnography was therefore 100% sensitive and 100% specific. A normal respiratory capnogram indicated tracheal placement and the lack of a normal trace indicated either esophageal or intra-oral placement. ICU patients are considered at high of complications associated with feeding tube placement.

The authors of this study still recommend obtaining and reviewing one radiograph after tube placement to ascertain final position prior to use. Eliminating at least one radiograph per feeding tube placement compared to the two-step radiography method translates to less patient positioning for radiographs, less radiation exposure and less time. The main limitations of the study were the small sample size with only 11 tracheal placements.

A prospective study of patients from the medical ICU (MICU) at the University of Virginia (Truwit *et al.*, 2002) showed that airway cannulation occurred in 22 of 217 patients studied, with an incidence rate of 10%. This is consistent with the findings of Kindopp *et al.* (2001). This study also provided an accompanying survey of bedside clinicians which indicated that airway cannulation was believed more likely with small bore feeding tubes, using a nasal approach and in sedated patients (nasal in awake). The study found that airway cannulation was indeed more common with a nasal approach but contrary to the survey results, airway cannulation was more likely in an awake patient and did not vary with enteric tube diameter. Furthermore, the *a priori* presence of the endotracheal tube was associated with reduced airway cannulation. This study confirmed the findings of Kindopp *et al.* and others (D'Souza *et al.*, 1994; Asai, 1994; 1998; 2002) provided insight into common misconceptions of clinicians. Furthermore, this technique provides continuous monitoring during feeding tube insertion (Figure 4.1). Continuous monitoring has been useful with the nasogastric tubes, but on occasion the smaller diameter feeding tubes can have ports obstructed by lubricant jelly. The indwelling wire does not interfere with CO_2 signal detection.

Our standing policy in the MICU is for the placement of all nasogastric and orogastric tubes with capnographic assessment, usually done by the critical care

1 Connect the capnograph to the gastric tube/$P_{et}CO_2$ adapter.

2 Connect the adapter to the proximal port of the feeding tube.

3 Insert the gastric tube and observe the $P_{et}CO_2$ waveform throughout insertion.

4 If a capnogram appears, stop the insertion and determine the CO_2 level. If it is 15 mmHg or greater the immediately withdraw tube and attempt to replace.

5 If the level of CO_2 is 15 mmHg or lower, wait 3 breaths to determine if the CO_2 will dissipate. If the levels do not dissipate or if the waveform persists (versus a flat CO_2 line), remove the tube and attempt reinsertion.

6 Obtain an abdominal film for confirmation of placement of small bore feeding tubes and confirm placement of the Salem sump tube by auscultation and aspiration of stomach contents.

Figure 4.1 Protocol for using $P_{et}CO_2$ device during gastric tube insertion. (Reproduced with permission from Burns, S.M., Carpenter, R. & Truwit, J.D. (2001). Report on the development of a procedure to prevent placement of feeding tubes into the lungs using end-tidal CO_2 measurements. *Crit. Care Med.*, **29**: 936–939.)

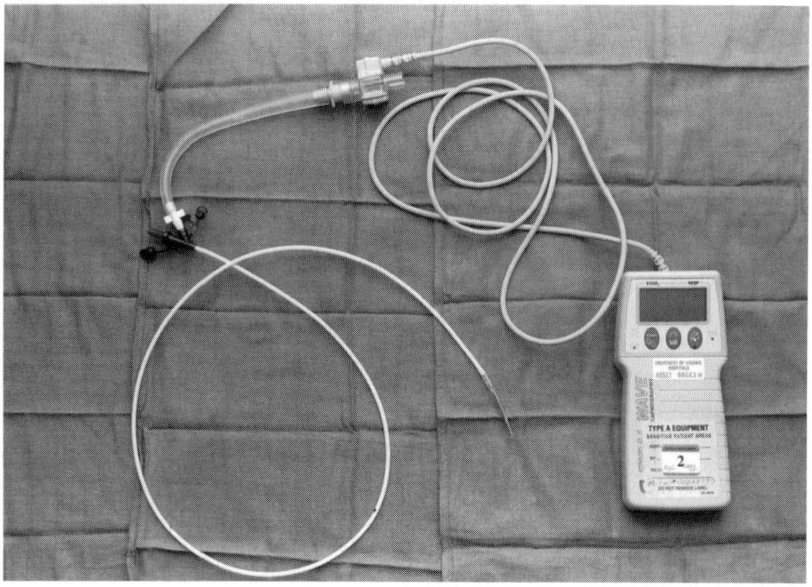

Figure 4.2 Feeding tube $ETCO_2$ placement device: connection to soft bore feeding tube. The feeding tube connection device consists of an endotracheal tube adapter (which is connected to the capnograph), a 10-cm length of tubing and a respiratory "christmas tree" adapter. The respiratory "christmas tree" adapter is connected to the proximal port of the soft bore feeding tube. Either the feeding port (with stylet in place) or the side "medication" port may be used. The $P_{et}CO_2$ is monitored during tube insertion. (Reproduced with permission from Burns, S.M., Carpenter, R. & Truwit, J.D. (2001). Report on the development of a procedure to prevent placement of feeding tubes into the lungs using end-tidal CO_2 measurements. *Crit. Care Med.*, **29**: 936–939.)

nurses in the unit.[2] In the past two trained nurses were required for the placement of the tubes, however this no longer applies. With an upgraded CO_2 monitor, there is no longer a need for placing adapters for or additional tubing for connection to the capnographs (Figure 4.2). As always, small bore feeding tube (i.e. Dobhoff) placement requires an abdominal X-ray to verify the placement of the tube prior to use, even in spite of capnographic assessment for the placement of the same. It has been our observation over the course of the 2 years that our complication rate in nasogastric and orogastric tube placement has decreased, especially the rate of inadvertent placement to tubes in the lungs and subsequent pneumothorax. This is mainly attributed to the mandatory use of the capnograph for all tube placements.

Large bore feeding tubes such as Salem sump tubes can be used for medication administration and tube feeding without X-ray verification if initial verification is done with capnograph. Placement verification with air bolus must be documented every 8 h on the nursing assessment. In patients with endotracheal tubes, gastric tube placement should generally be oral rather than nasal. These procedural guidelines are applicable to our MICU alone, and are not implemented hospital wide. At the time of writing this article, comparative data on the complication rate with and without the use of capnography is not available.

[2] University of Virginia, MICU policy statement 226, gastric tubes.

Conclusion

Capnography is a valuable adjunct in providing safe care to the critically ill patient and as a diagnostic tool. In this chapter we reviewed its value in airway management (insertion and maintenance) and for providing safer passage of feeding tubes. The added safety that capnography provides is so compelling that we have instituted the use of capnography as routine care for all patients during insertion of endotracheal tubes and gastric tubes.

References

Ahrens, T. & Sona, C. (2003). Capnography – application in acute and critical care. *AACN Clin. Issue.*, **14**: 123–132.

American Heart Association (2000). Guidelines 2000 for cardiopulmonary resuscitation and emergency cardiovascular care. *Circulation*, **102**: I86–I89.

Araujo-Preza, C.E., Melhado, M.E., Gutierrez, F.J., Maniatis, T. & Castellano, M.A. (2002). Use of capnometry to verify feeding tube placement. *Crit. Care Med.*, **30**: 2255–2259.

Asai, T. (1998). Use of a tracheal tube and capnograph for insertion of a feeding tube. *Anaesthesia*, **53**: 93.

Asai, T. (2002). Use of a capnograph during feeding tube insertion. *Crit. Care Med.*, **30**: 1674.

Asai, T. & Stacey, M. (1994). Confirmation of feeding tube position: how about capnography? *Anaesthesia*, **49**: 451.

Burns, S.M., Carpenter, R. & Truwit, J.D. (2001). Report on the development of a procedure to prevent placement of feeding tubes into the lungs using end-tidal CO_2 measurements. *Crit. Care Med.*, **29**: 936–939.

Chan, M.F. (1996). Complications of upper gastrointestinal endoscopy. *Gastrointest. Endosc. Clin. North Am.*, **6**: 287–303.

Conrardy, P.A., Goodman, L.R., Lainge, F. & Singer, M.M. (1976). Alteration of endotracheal tube position. Flexion and extension of the neck. *Crit. Care Med.*, **4**: 7–12.

D'Souza, C.R., Kilam, S.A., D'Souza, U., Janzen, E.P. & Sipos, R.A. (1994). Pulmonary complications of feeding tubes: a new technique of insertion and monitoring malposition. *Can. J. Surg.*, **37**: 404–408.

Gandhi, S.K., Munshi, C.A., Coon, R. & Bardeen-Henschel, A. (1991). Capnography for detection of endobronchial migration of an endotracheal tube. *J. Clin. Monit.*, **7**: 35–38.

Holland, R., Webb, R.K. & Runciman, W.B. (1993). The Australian Incident Monitoring Study. Esophageal intubation: an analysis of 2000 incident reports. *Anaesth. Intens. Care*, **21**: 608–610.

Joint Commission on Accreditation of Healthcare Organizations, *Sentinel Event Alert*. Issue 25, February 26, 2002.

Kindopp, A.S., Drover, J.W. & Heyland, D.K. (2001). Capnography confirms correct feeding tube placement in intensive care unit patients. *Can. J. Anaesth.*, **48**: 705–710.

McArthur, C.D. (2003). AARC clinical practice guideline. Capnography/capnometry during mechanical ventilation – 2003 revision and update. *Respir. Care*, **48**: 534–539.

McCoy, E.P., Russell, W.J. & Webb, R.K. (1997). Accidental bronchial intubation. An analysis of AIMS incident reports from 1988 to 1994 inclusive. *Anaesthesia*, **52**: 24–31.

Rassias, A.J., Ball, P.A. & Corwin, H.L. (1998). A prospective study of tracheopulmonary complications associated with the placement of narrow-bore enteral feeding tubes. *Crit. Care*, **2**: 25–28.

Roubenoff, R. & Ravich, W.J. (1989). Pneumothorax due to nasogastric feeding tubes. Report of four cases, review of the literature, and recommendations for prevention. *Arch. Intern. Med.*, **149**: 184–188.

Sum-Ping, S.T., Mehta, M.P. & Anderton, J.M. (1989). A comparative study of methods of detection of esophageal intubation. *Anesth. Analg.*, **69**: 627–632.

Sum-Ping, S.T., Mehta, M.P. & Symreng, T. (1991). Reliability of capnography in identifying esophageal intubation with carbonated beverage or antacid in the stomach. *Anesth. Analg.*, **73**: 333–337.

Szekely, S.M., Webb, R.K., Williamson, J.A. & Russell, W.J. (1993). The Australian Incident Monitoring Study. Problems related to the endotracheal tube: an analysis of 2000 incident reports. *Anaesth. Intens. Care*, **21**: 611–616.

Tornero, C., Herrejon, A. & Salcedo, M. (1992). Pneumothorax, atelectasis, and pleural effusion secondary to the placement of an enteral feeding tube. *Rev. Clin. Esp.*, **191**: 286–287.

Truwit, J.D., Marshall, M., Matsumura, W., Fuerst, C., Carperter, R. & Burns, S. (2002). Assessing the frequency of gastric tube placement into the airway in the critically ill patient. *Am. J. Respir. Crit. Care Med.*, **165**: A791.

Vargo, J.J., Zuccaro Jr, G., Dumont, J.A., Conwell, D.L., Morrow, J.B. & Shay, S.S. (2002). Automated graphic assessment of respiratory activity is superior to pulse oximetry and visual assessment for the detection of early respiratory depression during therapeutic upper endoscopy. *Gastrointest. Endosc.*, **55**: 826–831.

Wendell, G.D., Lenchner, G.S. & Promisloff, R.A. (1991). Pneumothorax complicating small bore feeding tubes. *Arch. Intern. Med.*, **151**: 599–602.

AIRWAY MANAGEMENT IN THE OPERATING ROOM

5

D.G. Bjoraker

Respiratory events constitute the largest class of injury in the American Society of Anesthesiology Closed Claims Study (522 of 1541 cases; 34%). (Caplan *et al.*, 1990). Death or brain damage occurred in 85% of the cases and most outcomes (72%) were considered to be preventable with better monitoring. Three-fourths of the adverse respiratory events were due to inadequate ventilation (196 cases; 38%), esophageal intubation (94 cases; 18%) and difficult tracheal intubation (87 cases; 17%) (Caplan *et al.*, 1990). In 48% of the esophageal intubations, auscultation of breath sounds was claimed and documented. In the pediatric age group (age 15 years or younger), respiratory events were more common than for adults (43%) (Morray *et al.*, 1993). Pediatric claims for inadequate ventilation resulted in death (70%) or brain damage (30%). Reviewers judged that 89% of the pediatric inadequate ventilation claims could have been prevented with pulse oximetry and/or capnography (Morray *et al.*, 1993).

Unrecognized esophageal intubation was identified as an important cause of cardiac arrest attributed solely to anesthesia at one institution (Keenan & Boyan, 1985). Over 15 years four of the 27 cardiac arrests among 163,240 anesthetic cases were attributed to esophageal intubation. In a study of malpractice claims brought against Washington State anesthesiologists from 1971 to 1982 esophageal intubation was a significant cause of cardiac arrest, brain damage, and death (Solazzi & Ward, 1984). Seven of the 192 claims were brought for esophageal intubation; several cases documented successful chest auscultation. In an American Society of Anesthesiologists' Committee on Professional Liability survey 18 of 29 cases of unrecognized esophageal intubation that caused injury included documentation of auscultation of the chest (Birmingham *et al.*, 1986).

Confirmation of tracheal intubation with capnography

The usually more controlled circumstances of airway management in the operating room (OR) often provide better conditions, better monitoring, and the availability of more experienced personnel, particularly when a problem occurs, than is available in other critical care environments or the emergency department. The apparent reliability of direct visualization of the placement of an endotracheal tube into the trachea would seem to make it the "gold standard" of successful intubation. However direct visualization is often either not possible or the observations made may be incorrectly interpreted. Also, the misplacement of the tube during or prior to securing it or during changes in the patient's position may result in esophageal intubation subsequent to correct initial placement. Radiographic examination of head and neck flexion and extension demonstrate tube movement by as much as 5 cm which could result in extubation (Conrady *et al.*, 1976). In infants and neonates, the problem of accidental extubation by changing head position is even more critical because of the small dimensions involved (Bosman & Foster, 1977).

The ideal method of confirming endotracheal intubation has become an enduring search since the first reports of tracheal tube placement nearly a century ago. Although the pathologist may claim to be the final judge of endotracheal tube location, even his observation is disqualified by its protracted delay, long after the clinical necessity of deciding whether the airway has been properly secured. Knapp *et al.* (1999) in a critical care setting of non-cardiac arrest patients found capnography to be the most reliable method for rapid evaluation of endotracheal tube position with no failures in 152 examinations. Murray and Modell (1983) demonstrated in dogs that disconnection, obstruction, removal, and esophageal placement of the endotracheal tube was evident in a single respiratory cycle. Partial extubation of the trachea and intermittent kinking or obstruction of the endotracheal tube created a recognizable, erratic capnogram pattern, although not greatly changing the maximum expired carbon dioxide (CO_2) concentration. Tobias and Higgins (1995) found capnography to be a useful adjunct when performing cricothyrotomy puncture both for transtracheal jet ventilation and for anesthetic injection. Although airway management in the OR may be more controlled than in the emergency department, Salem and Wafai's list

(1997) of false positives and false negatives for the use of capnography to confirm intubation is still applicable (Table 5.1). Their list concentrates on the generally used technique of time-based capnography with side-stream expiratory gas sampling.

While the detection of CO_2 by capnography after apparent completion of a difficult intubation procedure may suggest success, it may more precisely indicate only that the tube tip is somewhere in the respiratory path, perhaps not where the intubationist desires. Deluty and Turndorf (1993) described the blind nasal placement of an Endotrol® tube that resulted in a normal time-capnogram and partial pressure of CO_2 at end-tidal ($P_{et}CO_2$), but was associated with high inspiratory pressure, a large cuff inflation volume, and the inability to pass a fiberscope into the trachea through the Endotrol® tube. Subsequently, the tube was found to be at a 90° angle to the glottic opening with the tip imbedded in pharyngeal mucosa. The Murphy eye was located over vocal cords, thus accounting for the normal capnogram. Deluty and Turndorf's successful recognition of this malpositioned endotracheal tube was based on vigilance in recognizing unexpected clinical features and their persistence in seeking an explanation; valuable principles in management of the airway. Other methods of confirming intubation that may have been helpful have been extensively reviewed elsewhere (Salem, 2001; DeBoer *et al.*, 2003).

Table 5.1 Capnography confirmation of endotracheal intubation

False-negative results
Gas sampling problems
Disconnection
Apnea
Equipment failure
Kinked or obstructed tracheal tube
Unintentional PEEP to a loosely fitted or uncuffed tube
Dilution of proximal sampling by fresh gas flow in Mapleson D systems or Dryden absorber
Low sampling flow rates
Gas sampling line leaks
Patient problems
Severe upper- or lower-airway obstruction
Very large alveolar dead-space
Low cardiac output, severe hypotension
Obstruction of pulmonary circulation
Embolism, pulmonary atresia, or stenosis; surgical interruption
Severe lung disease
Cardiac arrest
False-positive results
Bag-and-mask ventilation before intubation
After ingestion of antacids or carbonated beverages (e.g. Coke, 7-Up, carbonated mineral water)
Tube in pharynx

Reproduced with permission from Salem, M.R. & Wafai, Y. (1997). Practical confirmation of endotracheal intubation in the trauma patient. *Anesthesiol. News*, **23(1)**: 4, 9–11, 12, 30–33.
PEEP: positive end-expiratory pressure.

Esophageal CO_2 detection

As the management of the difficult airway in the OR is usually not associated with the non-production of CO_2 (e.g. cardiac arrest, severe hypotension), the assumption that CO_2 will be detected in the respiratory tract is usually valid. The converse, namely that respiratory levels of CO_2 will *not* be detected in the esophagus is also usually valid, but not always. Sum-Ping *et al.* (1989) found esophageal $P_{et}CO_2$ levels of 0.6 ± 0.6% compared with tracheal levels of 4.9 ± 0.7%. Seven of their 21 patients had capnograms similar to tracheal waveforms, but greatly reduced in amplitude. One patient had an end-expired esophageal CO_2 level of 2.0%. Volumetric capnography rather than time capnography would have further amplified the notable differences between the tracheal and esophageal CO_2 levels that Sum-Ping *et al.* detected.

When mask ventilation is difficult over a prolonged period, partial pressure of CO_2 in arterial blood (P_aCO_2) may rise substantially and the CO_2 tension of exhaled gas entering the hypopharynx will also be increased. A subsequent ventilation effort may return this ventilatory dead-space gas not just to the trachea, but also to the esophagus and stomach (Sum-Ping, 1987). Not surprisingly, later esophageal intubation would yield CO_2. The clinical scenario becomes more complicated if the gastro-esophageal sphincter is particularly incompetent and to–fro gastric ventilation is as easily or more easily achieved than pulmonary ventilation. If esophageal intubation then occurs, initial breaths may contain substantial CO_2, potentially exceeding 5% if prolonged hypercarbia has occurred. A capnography pattern indicating declining CO_2 in each subsequent breath over several breaths will help identify esophageal intubation (Sum-Ping, 1987).

Prior ingestion of carbonated beverages or antacids may cause intragastric release of large amounts of CO_2 perhaps greater than 20% (Sum-Ping *et al.*, 1991). In an experiment in swine, Sum-Ping *et al.* (1991) demonstrated that esophageal capnography could detect $P_{et}CO_2$ levels as high as 5.3% after intragastric administration of a carbonated beverage. It is an oversimplification to assume that the decline of esophageal CO_2 with each subsequent breath will behave as a classic single compartment washout curve. Variables affecting the CO_2 decay will include the quantity of material ingested, the volume of liquid within the stomach, the release of CO_2 from the ingested solution, the excretion of CO_2 via mucosal absorption, the volume of gas within the stomach, the mixing of gastric ventilation with gas in the stomach, and the volume of gastric ventilation entering and the volume exiting the stomach. The volumes of gastric inspired and expired gas may change as intragastric volumes and pressures, and esophageal pressures change with each ventilation.

Endobronchial tube placement recognition

If ventilation is initiated through an endotracheal tube inadvertently placed into an endobronchial position, no substantially unusual capnography or ventilatory parameters may be immediately evident. However, if a properly positioned endotracheal tube migrates into an endobronchial position and the ventilator settings are unchanged, then several observations may alert the anesthesiologist to the tube malposition. The $P_{et}CO_2$ concentration will decrease and the peak inspiratory pressure will increase (Figure 5.1) (Gandhi *et al.*, 1991). Alveolar ventilation and P_aCO_2 are inversely related. When the endotracheal tube slips into a bronchial position, the entire ventilation is delivered to that lung, approximately doubling the ventilation/perfusion ($\dot{V}/\dot{Q}$) ratio and reducing the alveolar CO_2 tension in the ventilated lung (Gandhi *et al.*, 1986). Since capnography reflects only the CO_2 tension of the ventilated lung, a sudden decrease in $P_{et}CO_2$ is observed. If the endobronchial position persists, over time the arterial blood gases will indicate a decreased pH and oxygen tension and an increase in CO_2 tension. If the resistance to ventilation through the malpositioned tube becomes extremely high and the delivery of the prior alveolar ventilation is prevented then the under-ventilation could result in an unchanged or increased observed $P_{et}CO_2$ (Riley & Marcy, 1985; Gandhi *et al.*, 1986; Riley *et al.*, 1986).

Ezri *et al.* (2003) noted frequent endobronchial migration of the tube tip in morbidly obese patients undergoing laparoscopy gastroplasty. Oxygenation was not impaired and the $P_{et}CO_2$ did not change in any of the affected patients; direct optical examination was the single indicator of malposition. These observations are not necessarily in conflict with the circumstances discussed above where the $P_{et}CO_2$ concentration decreases and the peak inspiratory pressure increases. Anatomical tube tip migration beyond the carina does not always mean that the tube is sealed in the bronchus, essentially initiating one-lung ventilation.

In the Australian Incident Monitoring Study (AIMS) of the first 3947 cases reported, 154 were for accidental bronchial intubations (McCoy *et al.*, 1997). Of these 154 cases, the capnogram remained normal or unremarkable approximately 90% of the time with the remaining cases split between decreasing and increasing $P_{et}CO_2$ (Table 5.2). In only one case was endobronchial intubation suspected based only on capnography; in an

Table 5.2 Response of $P_{et}CO_2$ concentration during accidental bronchial intubation

$P_{et}CO_2$ response	Number of cases (n = 154)	Total (%)
Normal	23	14.9
Decreased	9	5.8
Increased	7	4.6
Not known	115	74.7

Reproduced with permission from McCoy, E.P., Russell, W.J. & Webb, R.K. (1997). Accidental bronchial intubation: an analysis of AIMS incident reports from 1988 to 1994 inclusive. *Anaesthesia*, **52**: 24–31.

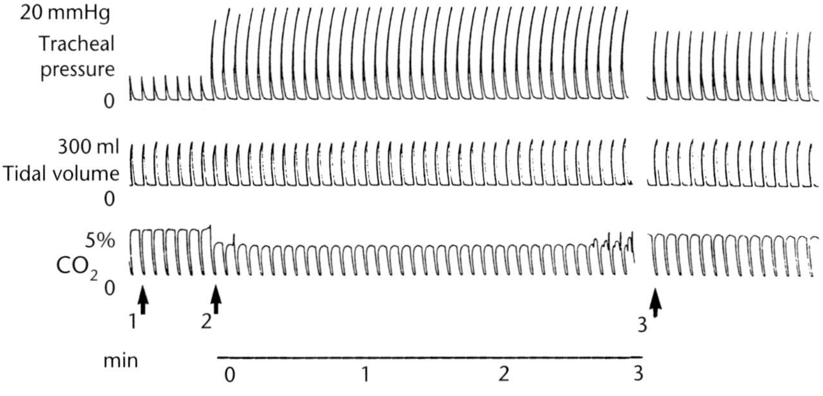

Figure 5.1 Tracheal pressure, tidal volume (vol), and $P_{et}CO_2$ tension in an experimental study in dogs. (1) Endotracheal tube in trachea. (2) Tip of endotracheal tube pushed down into bronchus. (3) Tip of endotracheal tube pulled back into trachea. (Reproduced with permission from Gandhi, S.K., Munshi, C.A., Coon, R. & Bardeen-Henschel, A. (1991). Capnography for detection of endobronchial migration of an endotracheal tube. *J. Clin. Monit.*, **7**: 35–38.)

additional six cases capnography contributed to the diagnosis. However, 32 of the 154 patients (20.8%) were not monitored with capnography.

Biphasic capnographic waveforms

The time capnogram is an expression of the $\dot{V}/\dot{Q}$ ratio. Initially with exhalation the anatomical dead-space gas is assessed (infinite $\dot{V}/\dot{Q}$, zero CO_2 concentration). This is followed by gas from well-ventilated, low-resistance regions of the lung (relatively high $\dot{V}/\dot{Q}$, low CO_2 concentration). Later the poorly ventilated, high-resistance regions of the lung (relatively low $\dot{V}/\dot{Q}$, high CO_2 concentrations) are delivered. Often a positive slope (upward to the right) of the alveolar "plateau" portion of the waveform is evident. If a biphasic waveform occurs, the usual continuum of rising CO_2 concentrations has been disrupted, because a biphasic separation of the pulmonary ventilation into a low-resistance, high $\dot{V}/\dot{Q}$ region and a high-resistance, low $\dot{V}/\dot{Q}$ region has occurred.

Unilateral pathophysiologic conditions that cause unilateral hypoventilation or high-airway resistances would result in a biphasic waveform. For example, obstruction of a main-stem bronchus by an external or internal tumor, congenital stenosis, secretions, or by a malfunctioning or malpositioned endotracheal tube could result in a biphasic waveform. Similarly, unilateral compression of a lung by air, blood, or fluid could cause a biphasic capnogram. Clinical scenarios include ventilation in the lateral decubitus position with the non-dependent lung having a relatively high $\dot{V}/\dot{Q}$ ratio and a low airway resistance relative to the dependent lung, or unilateral lung compression by severe kyphoscoliosis. Gilbert and Benumof (1989) reported a case where the transient endobronchial advancement of the tube tip during part of each ventilatory cycle produced a biphasic capnogram that was easily remedied by pulling back the endotracheal tube. Of course, intervening spontaneous breaths during controlled ventilation, a much more common circumstance, must be ruled out.

Positioning of double-lumen tubes

The measurement and comparison of $P_{et}CO_2$ individually for each lung during double-lumen tube ventilation may identify or confirm pathophysiologic defects within the individual lung. For example, Bhavani-Shankar *et al.* (1999) identified an unexpected pulmonary artery thrombus in the putatively normal lung prior to planned contralateral pneumonectomy by measuring an unexpectedly large P_aCO_2–$P_{et}CO_2$ gradient when attempted unilateral ventilation resulted in hypoxemia. After embolectomy $P_{et}CO_2$ sampling using the working lumen of a fiberscope with its tip placed distal to the carina allowed confirmation of the correction of the prior large P_aCO_2–$P_{et}CO_2$ gradient. However, others have noted no significant alteration in $P_{et}CO_2$ or the capnogram when a double-lumen tube was malpositioned (de Vries & Haanschoten, 1992; Cohen *et al.*, 1995).

Blind endotracheal tube placement with capnography

Many techniques to facilitate blind nasal tracheal intubation use the detection of significant exhaled gas flow from the spontaneously breathing patient to indicate the proximity of the tube tip to the glottic opening. Audible breath sounds at the tube tip, magnified by electronic amplification or by the attachment of whistle devices, have been used. However, successful placement may often be associated with an explosive cough and the spraying of secretions from the tube. Connecting the breathing circuit to the tube permits oxygen delivery to the pharynx during placement and facilitates side-stream capnometry. While King and Wooten (1989) recommended closure of the mouth and occlusion of the contralateral nares, dilution of the exhaled CO_2 concentration unless the tube tip is immediately at the vocal folds is actually desirable. The capnogram (Figure 5.2) initially is triangular in shape with a low maximum concentration, attenuated phase II, and severely down-sloping phase III (Bhavani-Shankar & Philip, 2000). As the tube approaches the glottic opening the maximum CO_2

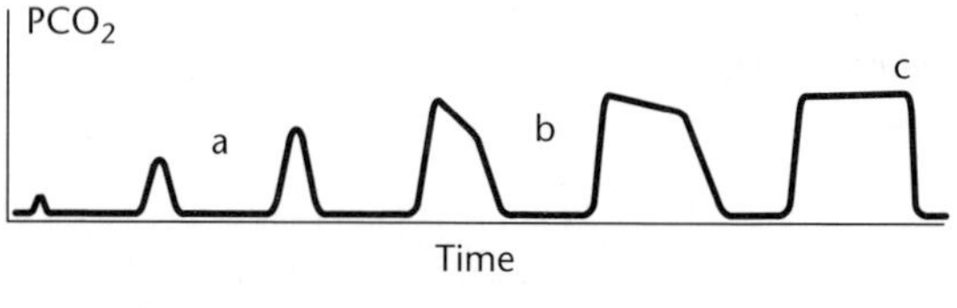

Figure 5.2 A hypothetical capnogram during blind nasal intubation of the trachea in a spontaneously breathing patient. (a) Initially, the waveform is triangular in shape with a low maximum CO_2 concentration, an attenuated phase II, and a severely down-sloping phase III. (b) As the tube approaches the glottic opening the maximum CO_2 concentration increases and but the waveform still shows phase III decay. (c) Finally, when a tracheal position is reached and the airway sealed by cuff inflation, the idealized phase III plateau or an ascending phase III is seen.

concentration increases and the waveform is one commonly seen with leakage around the endotracheal tube from cuff deflation where phase III rapidly decays. Finally, when a tracheal position is achieved and the airway is sealed by cuff inflation, the idealized phase III plateau or an ascending phase III is seen. Omoigui *et al.* (1991) found that viewing the capnogram during the procedure was inconvenient and attached a voltage-controlled oscillator that generates an audio tone increasing in pitch with greater $P_{et}CO_2$ concentration. An antisialagogue is helpful in minimizing the aspiration of secretions into the capnometer sampling line.

When accidental partial extubation occurs in a spontaneously breathing patient, the reverse of the above procedure may be evident on the capnogram. If the endotracheal tube tip slowly migrates out of the glottic opening and progressively further from the glottis, the gas sampled by the capnograph is progressively diluted. The progression of waveforms illustrated in Figure 5.2 may be seen, but in right-to-left order.

The laryngeal mask airway and capnography

The difference between $P_{et}CO_2$ and P_aCO_2 during spontaneous ventilation in adults when the airway is managed with a laryngeal mask airway (LMA) is similar to when an endotracheal tube is used (Hicks *et al.*, 1993). However, $P_{et}CO_2$ does not accurately reflect P_aCO_2 in spontaneously breathing children (Spahr-Schopfer *et al.*, 1993). Subsequently, Chhibber *et al.* (1996) demonstrated that in infants and children weighing more than 10 kg, when the airway is managed with an LMA during controlled ventilation, $P_{et}CO_2$ is as accurate an indicator of P_aCO_2 as when an endotracheal tube is used. For smaller pediatric patients in whom the dead-space to tidal volume ratio is greater, vigilance in monitoring and adjusting ventilation is required.

References

Bhavani-Shankar, K. & Philip, J.H. (2000). Defining segments and phases of a time capnogram. *Anesth. Analg.*, **91**: 973–977.

Bhavani-Shankar, K., Russell, R., Aklog, L. & Mushlin, P.S. (1999). Dual capnography facilitates detection of a critical perfusion defect in an individual lung. *Anesthesiology*, **90**: 302–304.

Birmingham, P.K., Cheney, F.W. & Ward, R.J. (1986). Esophageal intubation: a review of detection techniques. *Anesth. Analg.*, **65**: 886–891.

Bosman, Y.K. & Foster, P.A. (1977). Endotracheal intubation and head position in infants. *S. Afr. Med. J.*, **52**: 71–73.

Caplan, R.A., Posner, K.L., Ward, R.J. & Cheney, F.W. (1990). Adverse respiratory events in anesthesia: a closed claims analysis. *Anesthesiology*, **72**: 828–833.

Chhibber, A.K., Kolano, J.W. & Roberts, W.A. (1996). Relationship between end-tidal and arterial carbon dioxide with laryngeal mask airways and endotracheal tubes in children. *Anesth. Analg.*, **82**: 247–250.

Cohen, E., Neustein, S.M., Goldofsky, S. & Camunas, J.L. (1995). Incidence of malposition of polyvinylchloride and red rubber left-sided double-lumen tubes and clinical sequelae. *J. Cardiothorac. Vasc. Anesth.*, **9**: 122–127.

Conrady, P.A., Goodman, L.R., Lainge, F. & Singer, M.M. (1976). Alteration of endotracheal tube position. Flexion and extension of the neck. *Crit. Care. Med.*, **4**: 7–12.

DeBoer, S., Seaver, M. & Arndt, K. (2003). Verification of endotracheal tube placement: a comparison of confirmation techniques and devices. *J. Emerg. Nurs.*, **29**: 444–450.

Deluty, S. & Turndorf, H. (1993). The failure of capnography to properly assess endotracheal tube location. *Anesthesiology*, **78**: 783–784.

de Vries, J.W. & Haanschoten, M.C. (1992). Capnography does not reliably detect double-lumen endotracheal tube malplacement. *J. Clin. Monit.*, **8**: 236–237.

Ezri, T., Hazin, V., Warters, D., Szmuk, P. & Weinbroum, A.A. (2003). The endotracheal tube moves more often in obese patients undergoing laparoscopy compared with open abdominal surgery. *Anesth. Analg.*, **96**: 278–282.

Gandhi, S.K., Munshi, C.A. & Kampine, J.P. (1986). Early warning sign of accidental endobronchial intubation: a sudden drop or sudden rise in P_ACO_2? *Anesthesiology*, **65**: 114–115.

Gandhi, S.K., Munshi, C.A., Coon, R. & Bardeen-Henschel, A. (1991). Capnography for detection of endobronchial migration of an endotracheal tube. *J. Clin. Monit.*, **7**: 35–38.

Gilbert, D. & Benumof, J.L. (1989). Biphasic carbon dioxide elimination waveform with right mainstem bronchial intubation. *Anesth. Analg.*, **69**: 829–832.

Hicks, I., Soni, N. & Shephard, J. (1993). Comparison of end-tidal and arterial carbon dioxide measurements during anaesthesia with the laryngeal mask airway. *Br. J. Anaesth.*, **71**: 734–735.

Keenan, R.L. & Boyan, C.P. (1985). Cardiac arrest due to anesthesia: a study of incidence and causes. *J. Am. Med. Assoc.*, **253**: 2373–2377.

King, H.K. & Wooten, D.J. (1989). Blind nasal intubation by monitoring end-tidal CO_2. *Anesth. Analg.*, **69**: 412–413.

Knapp, S., Kofler, J., Stoiser, B., *et al.* (1999). The assessment of four different methods to verify tracheal tube placement in the critical care setting. *Anesth. Analg.*, **88**: 766–770.

McCoy, E.P., Russell,W.J. & Webb, R.K. (1997). Accidental bronchial intubation: an analysis of AIMS incident reports from 1988 to 1994 inclusive. *Anaesthesia*, **52**: 24–31.

Morray, J.P., Geiduschek, J.M., Caplan, R.A., Posner, K.L., Gild, W.M. & Cheney, F.W. (1993). A comparison of pediatric and adult anesthesia closed malpractice claims. *Anesthesiology*, **78**: 461–467.

Murray, I.P. & Modell, J.H. (1983). Early detection of endotracheal tube accidents by monitoring carbon dioxide concentration in respiratory gas. *Anesthesiology*, **59**: 344–346.

Omoigui, S., Glass, P., Martel, D.L.J., Watkins, K., Williams, K.L., Whitefield, S.M. & Wooten, L.L. (1991). Blind nasal intubation with audio-capnometry. *Anesth. Analg.*, **72**: 392–393.

Riley, R.H. & Marcy, J.H. (1985). Unsuspected endobronchial intubation – detection by continuous mass spectrometry. *Anesthesiology*, **63**: 203–204.

Riley, R.H., Finucane, K.E. & Marcy, J.H. (1986). Early warning sign of accidental endobronchial intubation: a sudden drop or sudden rise in P_ACO_2? In reply. *Anesthesiology*, **65**: 115.

Salem, M.R. (2001). Verification of endotracheal tube position. *Anesthesiol. Clin. North Am.*, **19**: 813–839.

Salem, M.R. & Wafai, Y. (1997). Practical confirmation of endotracheal intubation in the trauma patient. *Anesthesiol. New*, **23(1)**: 4, 9–11, 12, 30–33.

Solazzi, R.W. & Ward, R.J. (1984). The spectrum of medical liability cases. In: Pierce, E.C. & Cooper, J.B. (eds) *International Anesthesiology Clinics*, Vol. 22. Little, Brown and Company, Boston; pp. 43–59.

Spahr-Schopfer, I.A., Bissonnette, B. & Hartley, E.J. (1993). Capnometry and the pediatric laryngeal mask airway. *Can. J. Anaesth.*, **40**: 1038–1043.

Sum-Ping, S.T. (1987). Esophageal intubation. *Anesth. Analg.*, **66**: 483.

Sum-Ping, S.T., Mehta, M.P. & Anderton, J.M. (1989). A comparative study of methods of detection of esophageal intubation. *Anesth. Analg.*, **69**: 627–632.

Sum-Ping, S.T., Mehta, M.P. & Symreng, T. (1991). Reliability of capnography in identifying esophageal intubation with carbonated beverage or antacid in the stomach. *Anesth. Analg.*, **73**: 333–337.

Tobias, J.D. & Higgins, M. (1995). Capnography during transtracheal needle cricothyrotomy. *Anesth. Analg.*, **81**: 1077–1078.

VENTILATION: MONITORING

SECTION
1c

CAPNOGRAPHY DURING ANESTHESIA 6

J.M. Goldman, J.S. Gravenstein, D.A. Paulus & A. Hamburger

Introduction

Anesthetic practice involves the administration of drugs that can interfere with the central control of ventilation (inhalation and local anesthetics, narcotics, sedatives, anxiolytic drugs), with the transmission of impulses from and to the muscles of breathing (subarachnoid and epidural blocks), and with the integrity of the neuromuscular junction (neuromuscular blocking drugs). The surgeon's work can hinder breathing by interfering with the airway or the lungs. The position of the patient during an operation or examination can hamper gas exchange. Finally, the vicissitudes of breathing equipment and anesthesia machines can impose troubles or result in malfunction. It is, therefore, no wonder that many disasters in anesthesia can be traced to problems with respiration. Consequently, anesthesiologists have monitored their patients' breathing by listening to the lungs or over the trachea, by counting respiratory rate, by watching chest movement and tidal volume and by employing pulse oximetry and capnography. While pulse oximetry generates invaluable data related to oxygen (O_2) content in arterial blood it fails to offer breath-by-breath information of basic respiratory gas exchanges. How capnometry develops such data is discussed in great detail in several subsequent chapters. Here we wish to focus on issues relating to capnography specific to anesthesia and the operating room.

The importance of capnography in anesthesia is illustrated by the fact that the American Society of Anesthesiologists (ASA) in its "Standards for Basic Anesthetic Monitoring" writes:[1] "During all anesthetics, the patient's oxygenation, ventilation, circulation and temperature shall be continually evaluated." It goes on to discuss oxygenation and then writes the following about ventilation:

[1]http://www.asahq.org/publicationsAndServices/standards/02.pdf (Accessed July 20, 2004).

To ensure adequate ventilation of the patient during all anesthetics

Methods

1 Every patient receiving general anesthesia shall have the adequacy of ventilation continually evaluated. Qualitative clinical signs, such as chest excursion, observation of the reservoir breathing bag and auscultation of breath sounds are useful. Continual monitoring for the presence of expired carbon dioxide (CO_2) shall be performed unless invalidated by the nature of the patient, procedure or equipment. Quantitative monitoring of the volume of expired gas is strongly encouraged.

2 When an endotracheal tube or laryngeal mask is inserted, its correct positioning must be verified by clinical assessment and by identification of CO_2 in the expired gas. Continual end-tidal CO_2 analysis, in use from the time of endotracheal tube/laryngeal mask placement, until extubation/removal or initiating transfer to a postoperative care location, shall be performed using a quantitative method such as capnography, capnometry or mass spectroscopy.

3 When ventilation is controlled by a mechanical ventilator, there shall be in continuous use a device that is capable of detecting disconnection of components of the breathing system. The device must give an audible signal when its alarm threshold is exceeded.

4 During regional anesthesia and monitored anesthesia care, the adequacy of ventilation shall be evaluated, at least, by continual observation of qualitative clinical signs.

Equipment

Evidence of official recognition of capnography in anesthesia practice also comes from the Food and Drug Administration (FDA), which published checkout procedures to be followed by anesthesiologists before commencing with putting an anesthesia to use (reprinted as an Appendix to this chapter). We offer the following comments to this important document.

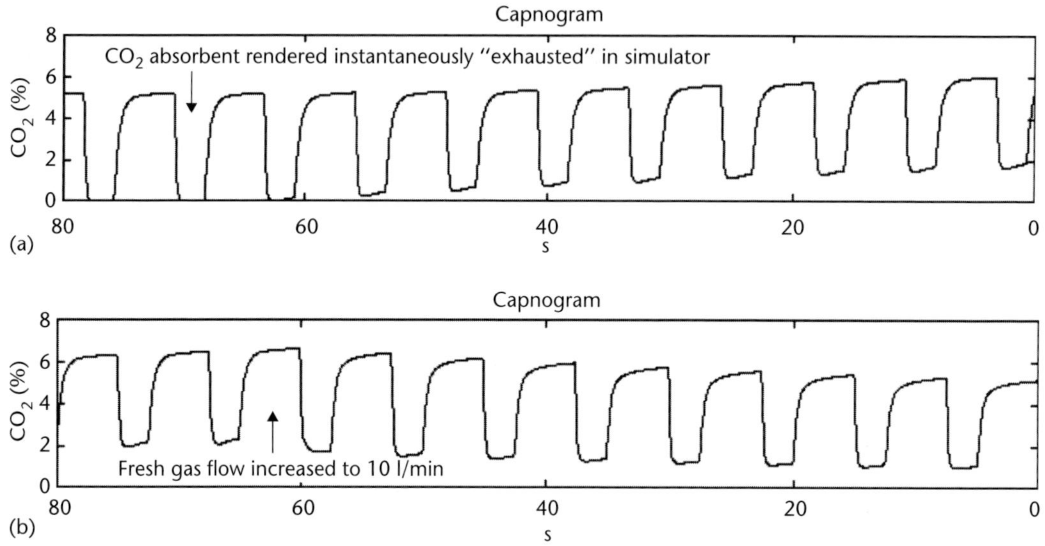

Figure 6.1 (a) Capnogram illustrating exhausted absorbent and (b) resulting capnogram from increased gas flow. Normally, previously exhaled gas is rebreathed after being scrubbed of CO_2 by the CO_2 absorbent. When the CO_2 absorbent is "exhausted", CO_2 will appear in the inspiratory gas and be detected as an elevation of the capnogram above baseline. Rebreathing of CO_2 will produce an increase of $P_{et}CO_2$ as well. (Generated with BreathSim software; Goldman *et al.*, 1996.)

The FDA lists capnography under "relevant standards". The FDA also mentions alarms incorporated in the equipment. It is a good technique to set the alarm levels close to the gas concentration you are going to use. Assume that you are going to use 50% O_2 and that the O_2 alarm default value is 25%. You do not want to wait for the O_2 concentration to drop from 50% to 25% before the alarm sounds. Set the alarm level to, for example, 40% to get an early warning. Similarly, upper and lower limits of CO_2 alarms should be set to bracket values expected during an anesthetic or in the intensive care unit with a patient requiring mechanical or assisted ventilation.

The document refers to the CO_2 absorber. It is often impossible to verify by inspection that the CO_2 absorbent is adequate because the color indicator can fail to show the state of exhaustion of the absorbent. However, if you detect CO_2 in the inspired gas, you need to go through the differential diagnosis of exhausted absorber versus valve incompetence, gas channeling through a non-exhausted absorber or monitor failure. When circle systems are used, the exhaled CO_2 must either be vented to the outside or be absorbed. Consequently, when (a high) fresh gas flow matches the inspired volume, all exhaled gas will be delivered to the scavenging system and the CO_2 absorber will sit idle. When the fresh gas flow supplies only enough gas to match the patient's uptake of gas (e.g. 300 ml/min O_2 for the average adult at rest), the patient would rebreathe all exhaled gas unless an absorbent removes the CO_2. Assuming a respiratory quotient (RQ) of 1, our patient would generate 300 ml/min CO_2. Every 100 g absorbent (typically either soda lime or Baralyme) removes approximately 20 liters CO_2. Absorbers come in different sizes, but most will scrub the respired gas for several hours before inspired CO_2 values begin to appear on the capnogram (Figure 6.1). We do not attempt to estimate the life expectancy of the CO_2 absorbent, because too many unknown variables complicate the calculation (the age of the absorbent and its ability to regenerate during idle time, the RQ and CO_2 production of the patient, the variable fresh gas flow in relation to the patient's minute ventilation). Instead, we monitor the inspired CO_2 concentration. If it inches up it is time to exchange the CO_2 absorber, or increase the fresh gas flow, or fix an incompetent valve.

Let us now examine a simple diagram to identify some of the potential trouble spots of anesthesia equipment (Figure 6.2).

Breathing circuit

The breathing circuit is comprised of hoses that can be disconnected from the machine or from the patient. The ventilator can be disconnected from the breathing circuit; the fresh gas supply can also be disconnected from the breathing circuit. Figure 6.2 shows arrows indicating the different sites of potential disconnection. The consequences of a disconnection will depend on whether the patient can breathe spontaneously – in which case an anesthetized

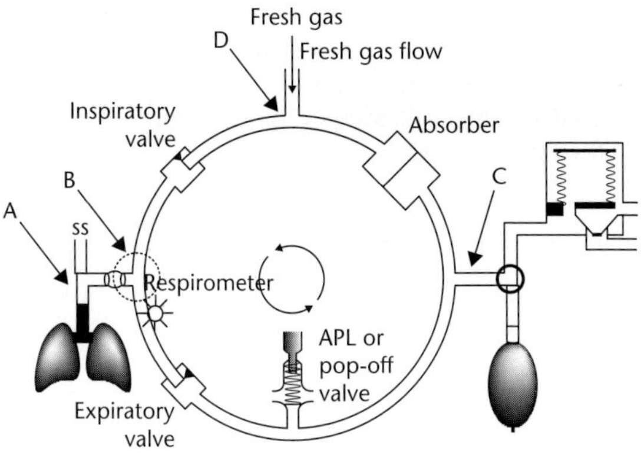

Figure 6.2 *Basic concept of an anesthesia circle system.* The patient's lungs are shown on the left. As the patient's exhaled gas passes under tube (ss), a sample (often as much as 200 ml/min) is aspirated and carried to the side-stream gas analyzer where a time-based capnogram will be generated. An alternative is to let the gas pass through a main-stream cuvette that contains a CO_2 sensor and a flow meter, thus collecting the information necessary for a volume-based capnogram. The gas then enters the breathing circuit. The exhaled gas will now pass the respirometer where the expired volume can be measured (if it had not been measured already). On its way to the breathing bag or ventilator bellows the exhaled gas passes the APL or pop-off valve. When the system is connected to the ventilator (as shown here), the APL valve will be closed. Otherwise it will be adjusted to enable excess gas to escape late in expiration – as long as the patient is breathing spontaneously, or with manual ventilation, during inspiration. The ventilator bellows shows an escape valve that opens late in expiration should enough pressure develop to overcome the small resistance offered by the valve. When the ventilator compresses the bellows with the beginning of inspiration, the expiratory valve will close and the inspiratory valve open. The gas now passes through the CO_2 absorber, receives fresh gas (which may contain anesthetic gases) on its way to the patient, thus concluding the circle. However, it must pass once again past sensors, which can now analyze the inspired gas. The arrows show common sites for leaks in the system. A: between endotracheal tube and breathing circuit. The CO_2 sensors have also been disconnected. B: between Y-piece (identified by the stippled circle) and breathing circuit. The CO_2 sensors are still connected to the patient but disconnected from the breathing circuit. C: between ventilator and breathing circuit. D: between fresh gas inlet and breathing circuit.

patient, now breathing room air – might wake up. If the patient is depending on mechanical ventilation a disconnection will interrupt ventilation of the patient's lungs. Such disconnections have led to many deaths in operating rooms and intensive care units. Multiple alarms (sensing tidal volume and pressures and CO_2), therefore, are now incorporated in modern anesthesia machines to help identify disconnections.

Disconnection with mechanical ventilation

Capnography is the best monitor to identify complete breathing circuit disconnects. Depending on the make and model of the anesthesia machine, some ventilators (piston driven or bellows descending on expiration) continue to work after a disconnection. During the expiratory cycle they will aspirate room air and then deliver the inspiratory tidal volumes through the disconnection instead of to the patient. With a complete disconnection adjacent to the CO_2 sampling (which is usually located at the endotracheal tube) not only will there be no capnographic tracing, but the capnogram will show a zero baseline. Time- and volume-based instruments will be equally effective in detecting the existence of such a disconnection. The capnometer may not easily identify partial disconnections that reduce tidal volume. Typically, the primary capnographic evidence in this case will be increasing end-tidal PCO_2 ($P_{et}CO_2$). In contrast, measurement of exhaled tidal volume is a sensitive indicator of leaks and partial disconnects during mechanical ventilation.

It is rare indeed if the capnogram misleads in case of disconnection. However, one such example was presented by Ginosar and Baranov (1997) who observed prolonged "phantom" square wave capnographic tracings after a patient was disconnected from a Siemens Servo 900c (MEDECO, Inc. Boise, ID, USA) ventilator, which had not been turned off. The gas analyzer aspirated CO_2 containing gas from the expiratory tube and the continuous operation of the ventilator interrupted the plateau of the capnogram, thus generating a series of soon diminishing phantom square wave capnographic tracings.

Disconnection with spontaneous ventilation

Capnography will continue to detect expired CO_2 (and thus miss the disconnection) as long as the patient's tidal volume passes side- or main-stream (Figure 6.2) sampling ports. The patient will be breathing room air without anesthetic agents delivered by the anesthesia machine.

Leak with mechanical ventilation

The most common leak occurs at the endotracheal tube around an incompletely filled endotracheal tube cuff (arrow A in Figure 6.2) and thus cannot be blamed on a machine fault. Other leaks, usually small, can arise with defective breathing tubes or leaks in the CO_2 absorber canister. Canister leaks are usually caused by misalignment of the canister housing after absorbent replacement or when CO_2 absorber granules cause the canister not to fit tightly. During the build-up of inspiratory pressure some of the tidal volume will be delivered to the room and the rest to the patient. However, most of the patient's expired volume (low pressure during expiration) will still pass the sampling site (time-based capnography) or the capnographic sensor (on airway or volumetric capnography) regardless of the position of the large leak. The time-based capnogram can look normal or can present low end-tidal ($P_{et}CO_2$) values should the expired volume be too low to deliver adequate alveolar gas. The volumetric capnogram will reveal a reduced expired volume and if both inhaled and exhaled volumes are recorded, the difference and the leak is distal to the bi-directional inline flow sensor, differences between the inhaled and exhaled volume will become more apparent than the tidal volumes alone.

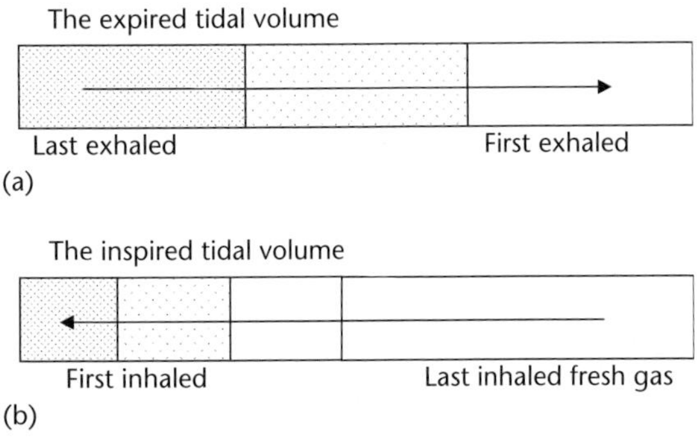

Figure 6.3 Diagrammatic presentation of CO_2 in the expired volume (a). If part of this volume enters the inspiratory hose (b), CO_2 will be present in the inspired volume. Density of shading represents the average concentration of CO_2.

Leak with spontaneous ventilation

These are difficult to detect because the low pressure generated by spontaneous ventilation will not force gas through the leak. (See Appendix at the end of this chapter for the FDA recommended machine check-out test that is designed to detect leaks in the breathing circuit.)

Inspiratory valve incompetence

While the ventilator will deliver the desired inspiratory volume to the patient (the expiratory valve is assumed to work normally), a portion of the expired gas will enter the inspiratory breathing hose. Figure 6.3 depicts this fact and shows how the next inspired volume will first contain decreasing concentrations of CO_2. The resultant time-based capnogram shows a characteristic – and easily overlooked – slurred inspiratory slope (Figure 6.4). Breen and Bradley (1997) demonstrated the phenomenon on the volume-based

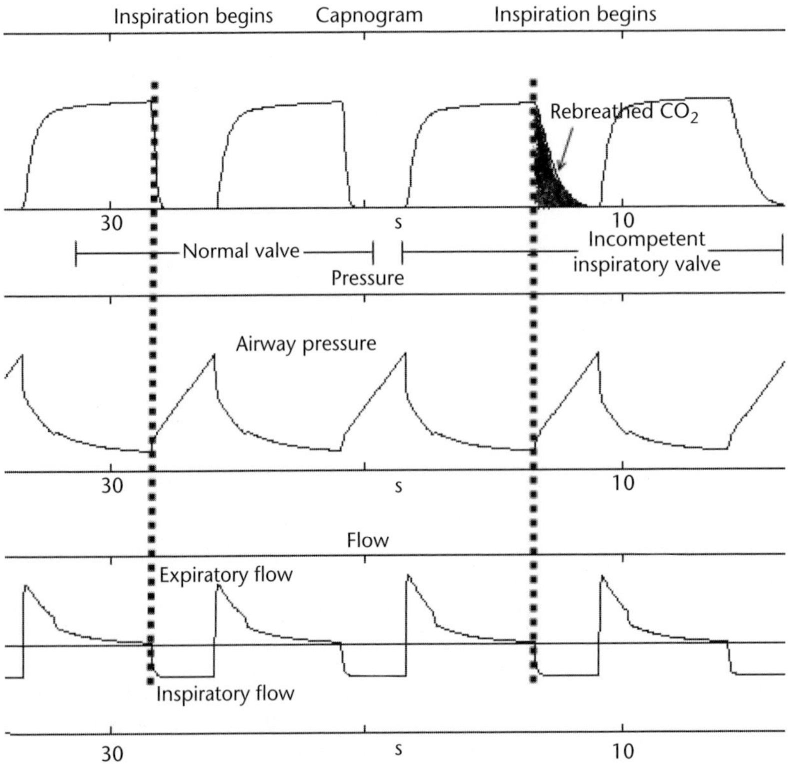

Figure 6.4 Illustration of the difference between normally functioning and incompetent inspiratory valves. Note that the CO_2 tracing in the normal capnogram rapidly drops to baseline at the start of inspiration (marked by increase in airway pressure (center tracing) and inspiratory flow (bottom tracing). When the inspiratory valve is incompetent, exhaled CO_2 from the previous breath enters the inspiratory limb of the circle breathing system, and is rebreathed at the next breath. The presence of CO_2 in the inspiratory limb is evident from the widened capnogram (shaded area). Generated with BreathSim software. (Goldman *et al.*, 1996.)

capnogram (Figure 6.5) in which both inspired and exhaled volumes were recorded.

Expiratory valve incompetence

During expiration, the expiratory hose is normally filled with CO_2 rich gas much of which can be pushed back into the patient with the next inhalation, should the valve be incompetent. Capnograms will show CO_2 in the inspired gas (Figure 6.6). The volume-based capnogram (Figure 6.7) will show normal inspired and expired volumes. Identical appearing capnograms can be obtained with exhausted CO_2 absorber which leads to rebreathing of exhaled CO_2. A clinically useful maneuver can distinguish between exhausted CO_2 absorber and incompetent expiratory valve. Increasing the fresh gas flow high enough to prevent rebreathing will correct the problem should exhausted absorber be the culprit – but it will not correct the abnormal capnogram should an incompetent expiratory valve have led to the appearance of CO_2 in the inspired gas. Incidentally, increasing the fresh gas flow may also affect the capnogram when the inspiratory valve has become incompetent – but not strikingly so.

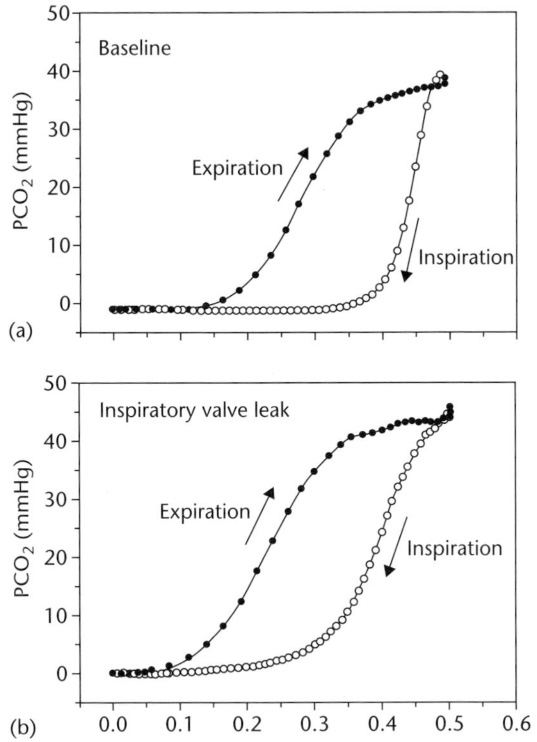

Figure 6.5 Volume-based capnograms with competent (a) and incompetent (b) inspiratory valve. The area defined by the expiratory and inspiratory limbs of the capnogram represents the exhaled CO_2 volume. Observe that the leaky inspiratory valve leads to some rebreathing and thus to a reduced exhaled CO_2 volume. (Reproduced with permission from Breen, P.H. & Bradley, P.J. (1997). Carbon dioxide spirogram (but not capnogram) detects leaking inspiratory valve in a circle circuit. *Anesth. Analg.*, **85**: 1372–1376.)

Side-stream versus main-stream capnography

The most common instrumentation-related capnography problems are caused by blocked and leaking gas

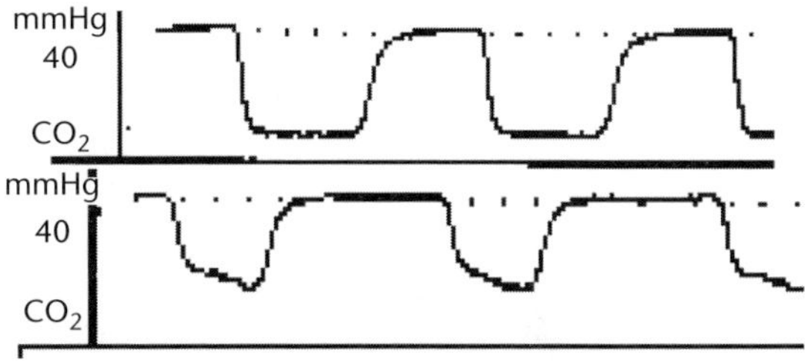

Figure 6.6 Incompetent expiratory valve leads to rebreathing of CO_2 in this time-based capnogram. Observe that the capnogram does not return to baseline, indicating the presence of CO_2 in the inspired gas. In the circle breathing system, all exhaled gas is directed down the expiratory limb. An incompetent expiratory valve allows expiratory-limb gas to flow backward and mix with inspiratory limb gas at the Y-piece and CO_2 sampling site. Note that rebreathing of expired limb gases elevates the baseline of the capnogram throughout inspiratory period. The appearance of the capnogram cannot be distinguished from one generated when the CO_2 absorber is exhausted. However, in modern anesthesia machines a respirometer will notice two-way gas flow in the expiratory tube and will issue an appropriate rebreathing alarm.

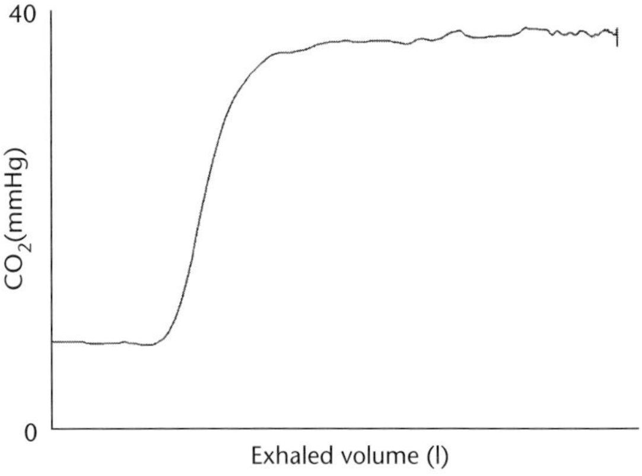

Figure 6.7 Volume based capnogram with an incompetent expiratory valve. Observe the presence of CO_2 in the deadspace, that is, the last inhaled gas. Inhaled and exhaled tidal volumes will not differ.

sample catheters in side-stream systems. Blockages are usually caused by filtration systems that are designed to trap water and other liquids before they can be aspirated internally and produce costly damage to the instrument. Fortunately, blockages usually generate an alarm or warning message and may be easily corrected (i.e. by having spare filters near the instrument). Leaking sample lines produce abnormal capnogram morphologies.

Figure 6.8 shows a "church steeple" appearance of the capnogram, which can sometimes be seen during mechanical ventilation with fairly high-peak inspiratory pressures (Tripathi & Pandey, 2000). A leak in the sampling tube – usually between the sampling tube and the gas analyzer – enables aspiration of room air during low pressure in the breathing circuit (during expiration). This dilutes the exhaled CO_2 and generates the "roof of the church". With onset of mechanical inspiration the positive pressure in the sampling tube now prevents aspiration of air and end-tidal CO_2 reaches the analyzer ("steeple of the church"), which however quickly gives way to fresh inspiratory gas. Abnormal capnogram shown in Figure 6.8(a) was caused by room air entrainment through cracked capnograph sample line connector (Figures 6.8(b) and 6.9). Replacement of water trap/filter assembly corrected the capnogram.

It is important to recognize that a large body of capnography-related literature is devoted to diagnosing problems with an older generation of anesthesia machines. The classic or traditional pneumatic anesthesia machine is slowly being replaced by more complex electromechanical and pneumatic anesthesia "workstations". The newer systems rely on electronic flow sensing and other technologies to improve the reliability and precision of pulmonary ventilation and delivery of anesthetic agents. Unfortunately, we are still learning about the subtleties of gas flow patterns – and hence capnographic patterns – in some of these new systems. The following example is illustrative of this new complexity.

The capnogram shown in Figure 6.10 was recorded from a mechanically ventilated, normal, healthy adult with zero end-expiratory pressure undergoing an intra-abdominal procedure under general anesthesia with muscle relaxant. Note the abnormal alveolar plateau of the capnogram that appeared shortly after the start of the anesthetic. When 2–4 cm of positive end-expiratory pressure (PEEP) was added (with an

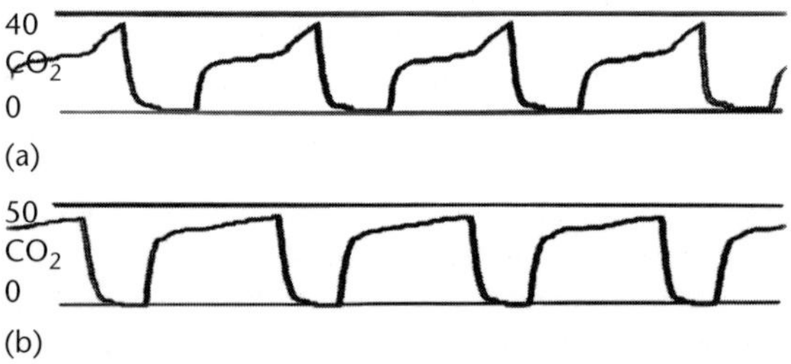

Figure 6.8 (a) A time-based capnogram obtained during mechanical ventilation. The upswing (the "steeple of the church") is generated by a leak – usually between the sampling capillary and the capnograph. The leak enables the gas analyzer to aspirate room air during exhalation (that is when the pressure in the breathing circuit and the sampling capillary is low), thus diluting the sampled CO_2 and generating the "roof of the church". The positive pressure generated early during inspiration stops the aspiration of air and pushes the last CO_2 in the sampling tube towards the analyzer, generating the "steeple". (b) A time-based capnogram after the leak was removed. The volume-based capnogram deprives us of such interesting shapes as it does not remove gas from the breathing circuit and thus cannot be affected by leaks in a sampling tube.

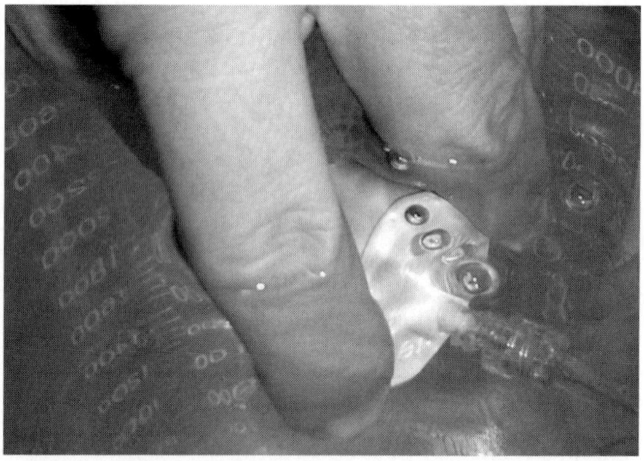

Figure 6.9 Aqua-Knot® II water trap, used in the GE Medical Systems SAM® capnograph, pressurized with air and submerged. Bubble trail reveals crack in Luer connector that permitted the entrainment of air during operation.

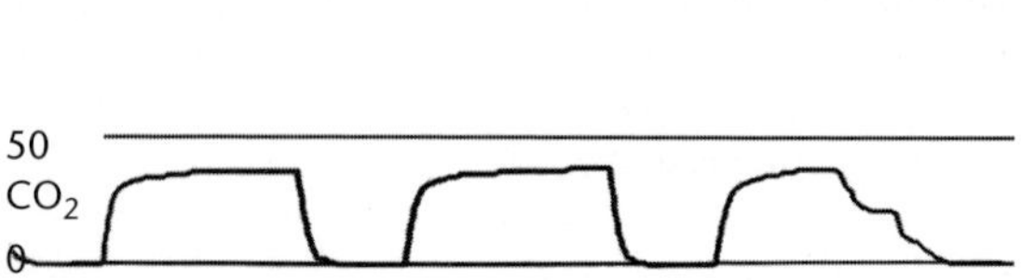

Figure 6.10 Healthy adult patient undergoing intra-abdominal procedure under general with mechanical ventilation using the Draeger Medical Systems Fabius GS anesthesia workstation. Unlike traditional bellows ventilators, the piston-driven ventilator in the Fabius GS produces zero end-expiratory pressure, which given the flow characteristics of its breathing system, may produce a capnogram with an abnormal alveolar plateau. The figure illustrates the change in the alveolar plateau when 2 cm PEEP was removed.

integrated PEEP/adjustable pressure limiting (APL) valve on the Draeger Fabius GS machine) the capnogram normalized. The appearance of the capnographic abnormality was easily reproduced by modulating PEEP. There was no other evidence of ventilatory problems. As we continue to gain experience with these new anesthesia systems, we will have to expand our understanding of the scope of machine-generated capnographic abnormalities.

Position- and anesthesia-related problems

Living in a world of gravity, our ventilation falls under its spell. When we stand, abdominal content and diaphragm are pulled down and the lower levels of the lungs receive the lions share of perfusion, while the upper lung fields excel in ventilation. These ventilation/perfusion ($\dot{V}/\dot{Q}$) inequalities tend to cancel out, resulting in a reasonably close overall ventilation to perfusion of 1. Upon lying supine, as most surgical patients do, the distribution shifts, the diaphragm no longer travels downward as much and the total functional residual capacity (FRC) can be substantially reduced. With spontaneous breathing we manage to compensate for these conditions. However, once we paralyze the diaphragm and impose mechanical ventilation, conditions change markedly. Now the upper segments of the lungs receive a disproportionate share of ventilation resulting in an overall increase of ventilation over perfusion. The addition of anesthetic drugs and with it a decrease in pulmonary blood flow exaggerates the problem leading to a varying degree of deadspace ventilation (areas of the lung ventilated but not adequately perfused). If we add to these conditions mechanical ventilation with large tidal volumes and slow respiratory rates – as is common in general anesthesia – the deadspace ventilation becomes even more pronounced. During spontaneous breathing tidal volume are moved with nary a change in pressures in the lung; with mechanical ventilation sizable inspiratory pressures are needed to expand the lung. These pressures compress some capillaries more than others leading to blood being shunted to the spared capillaries. To make matters worse, anesthetics can interfere with the physiologic hypoxic pulmonary vasoconstriction, which ordinarily causes blood to be diverted to well ventilated areas. Some positions used for surgical procedures aggravate the situation. Face-down, lateral, steep head-down or the infamous kidney role all can further hamper normal pulmonary blood flow and ventilation. It is against this background that blood gases and comparisons of arterial and end-tidal CO_2 values need to be evaluated in anesthesia.

Establishment of an airway

Capnography holds first place, both chronologically and as to importance, with the establishment of an airway. A separate section deals with this (see Ventilation: Airway management). Briefly, as outlined in the ASA minimal monitoring standards (see above), capnography is the best method to demonstrate continued gas exchange taking place, whether the patient is breathing spontaneously, is ventilated by bag and mask, has a supralaryngeal (or supraglottic) airway or an endotracheal tube or a tracheostomy. Remember that the stomach can deliver some CO_2 from a gastric bubble, for example, after drinking a carbonated beverage. However, such a bubble is soon exhausted and CO_2 will disappear from the ventilated stomach, while continued capnograms of normal size point to ongoing ventilation of the lungs.

Pulmonary pathology

In several chapters of this book the reader will find discussions of how capnographic data are affected by pulmonary pathology. In anesthesia we often see patients with chronic obstructive disease or asthma who exhibit the typical capnograms with sloping expired values brought about by the slow emptying of partially obstructed segments of the lungs. The PCO_2 in arterial blood (P_aCO_2) and PCO_2 in expired gas (P_ECO_2) differences increase. It is essential to be aware of the potentially large $P_{et}CO_2$–P_aCO_2 difference in the presence of increased airway resistance. Figure 6.11(a) demonstrates the falsely low $P_{et}CO_2$ produced when mechanical inspiration terminates expiration. Note the marked rise in $P_{et}CO_2$ revealing the presence of hypercarbia when expiration is allowed to continue for several seconds. In contrast, Figure 6.11(b) illustrates the flat stable alveolar plateau present in the healthy patient. Halogenated anesthetic vapors tend to relax the smooth muscles of the respiratory tract and we often see an improvement in the capnographic pattern. Anesthesiologists are on their guard taking care of asthmatic patients with irritable airways lest stimulation under light anesthesia causes acute bronchospasm.

One lung ventilation

When the anesthesiologist inserts a double lumen endotracheal tube for a thoracotomy and the patient is put into a lateral position, $\dot{V}/\dot{Q}$ abnormalities will be introduced as the lower lung will receive more blood flow and the upper one more ventilation. Once the surgeon opens the chest, and ventilation to the upper lung is discontinued and allowed to collapse, ventilation of the upper lung and its perfusion may not be decreased

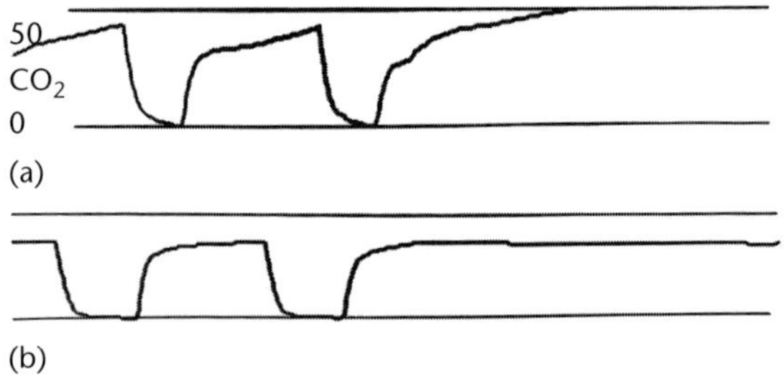

Figure 6.11 Capnogram with steep alveolar plateau. (a) In the presence of a steep alveolar plateau, the displayed $P_{et}CO_2$ of 38 mmHg markedly underestimates the P_aCO_2. Pausing the ventilator for a few seconds provided additional time for slower-emptying alveoli to contribute their CO_2 to the measured gas sample. (b) Normal control with ventilator pause.

in a coordinated fashion. As hypoxic vasoconstriction sets in – provided this mechanism is not depressed by anesthetics – the $\dot{V}/\dot{Q}$ abnormalities will tend to improve. Nevertheless, we usually see the expected increase in the difference between arterial and end-tidal CO_2 and O_2 tensions.

If a properly placed endotracheal tube slips into a main stem bronchus, the story will be different because a tidal volume originally matched for ventilation of two lungs will suddenly be directed into only one lung. Peak inspiratory pressure will increase. Pulmonary blood delivery of CO_2 into this large tidal volume will cause a particularly flat alveolar plateau and end-tidal values to be reduced – at least for a time.

Special anesthesia problems

Laparoscopy

In the setting of laparoscopic surgery, the surgeons use peritoneal insufflation with gas in order to provide a view of the anatomic structures. The gas chosen is CO_2, due to its nonflammable character and because it is absorbed relatively promptly. This constant insufflation (usually at pressures not exceeding 15 mmHg) presents several challenges to the anesthesiologist. On the one hand with the inflation of some 4 l of CO_2 into the abdominal cavity, the diaphragm is pushed up, and compliance and FRC decrease. On the other hand, the addition of CO_2 to the metabolically generated gas imposes an extra burden on gas exchange. Capnography is a reliable indicator for this increased CO_2 load. Studies have shown that on average the anesthesiologist will need to increase minute ventilation by 1.5-fold in order to maintain a relatively constant P_aCO_2. In fact, at the end of CO_2 insufflation it takes on average 8 min for a return to baseline, and over 16 h before the CO_2 exhaled is solely due to metabolic production again (Kazama *et al.*, 1996; Gandara *et al.*, 1997).

When the end-tidal values decrease in the face of increased CO_2 load, the anesthesiologist needs to make a differential diagnosis. Is the decrease a consequence of a drop in pulmonary blood flow, for example, secondary to elevated ventilatory pressures or dissection of CO_2 into the mediastinum with compression of intrathoracic veins and a decrease in preload or is it the result of CO_2 gas embolism? Based on anecdotal evidence and case reports the consequences of CO_2 gas emboli seem to have a lower mortality rate than air emboli, thanks to the rapid absorption of CO_2 emboli. Many studies have shown that transesophageal echocardiography or even transthoracic Doppler are more sensitive tools than capnography for the detection of small emboli of minimal clinical consequence. The capnograph remains the best noninvasive tool in the detection of a major embolus. Gas emboli occur not only during laparoscopic procedures but have also been detected by transesophageal echocardiography during endoscopic vein harvesting for coronary artery bypass grafting (Mann *et al.*, 1997; Bhavani-Shankar, 2000; Lin *et al.*, 2003). Of course, air embolism (see Chapter 21, Embolism) can occur with many different operations in which veins are opened that lie above the level of the right heart. Again, capnography will be helpful in demonstrating the increase in deadspace (see Chapter 21).

Neurosurgical anesthesia

As CO_2 exerts such a profound effect on cerebral circulation, the control of arterial CO_2 tension receives more attention during neurosurgical procedures than during any other anesthetic. Several factors affect cerebral blood flow. Among them are the anesthetics. Halothane has the worst reputation of allowing an increase in cerebral blood flow while thiopental and etomidate enjoy the double advantage of decreasing O_2 consumption and cerebral blood flow. Other factors are shown in the well-known diagram depicting the acute effects of hyper- and hypocarbia on cerebral blood flow (Figure 6.12). Briefly, it shows that cerebral perfusion pressure (i.e. mean arterial pressure minus intracranial or cerebral venous pressure) does not lead to changes in cerebral blood flow (and thus changes in intracranial volume) as long as the perfusion pressure falls somewhere between 70 and 150 mmHg. In chronically hypertensive patients these values are likely to be higher. Very low partial pressure of oxygen (PO_2) leads to a frantic attempt to bring more blood into the brain – causing swelling of the brain. While autoregulation works spectacularly well over a considerable range of perfusion pressures, it fails to compensate for the acute effects of changing CO_2 tensions. Observe the almost linear increase of cerebral blood flow with increasing P_aCO_2. In years gone by many patients were routinely hyperventilated during anesthesia. Today, we

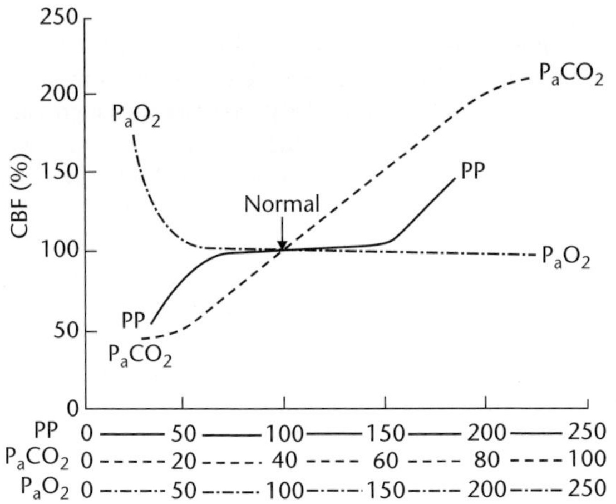

Figure 6.12 The acute effects of hyper- and hypocarbia on cerebral blood flow (CBF). PP: perfusion pressure. All pressures in mmHg.

recognize the benefit of normal CO_2 levels and normal cerebral perfusion (Brian Jr, 1998).

The picture is importantly changed in patients with intracranial pathology, which can cause the affected tissue to lose its autoregulation. In neurosurgical anesthesia, therefore, we strive to maintain a normal P_aCO_2 but attempt to lower it should the brain swell and should the patient be at risk of suffering herniation of the brain with its devastating effects. Capnography plays an important role in neurosurgical anesthesia, however, the clinician must be aware of circumstances that might lead to $\dot{V}/\dot{Q}$ disturbances and thus to enlarged differences between end-tidal and arterial PCO_2 values as discussed extensively in other chapters of this book. Therefore, analysis of arterial blood gases may be necessary to ensure accurate determination of P_aCO_2 in the presence of elevated intracranial pressure.

Cardiovascular operations

When cardiac surgery interferes with pulmonary blood flow, end-tidal CO_2 will be proportionally reduced. Indeed, this phenomenon has been used to assess pulmonary blood flow by monitoring end-tidal CO_2 pressures (Maslow *et al.*, 2001). The authors observed a reasonably good correlations until the $P_{et}CO_2$ values exceeded about 35 mmHg. They assumed that with even better perfusion areas of deadspace ventilation were now opened up and thus the elimination of CO_2 rose with improved pulmonary blood flow (Figure 6.13). Thus, when minute ventilation and CO_2 production remain constant, end-tidal CO_2 can become a clinically useful monitor for cardiac output. Boccara *et al.* (2001) suggest that end-tidal CO_2 can predict unclamping hypotension in patients whose end-tidal CO_2 decreases by more than 15% during clamp.

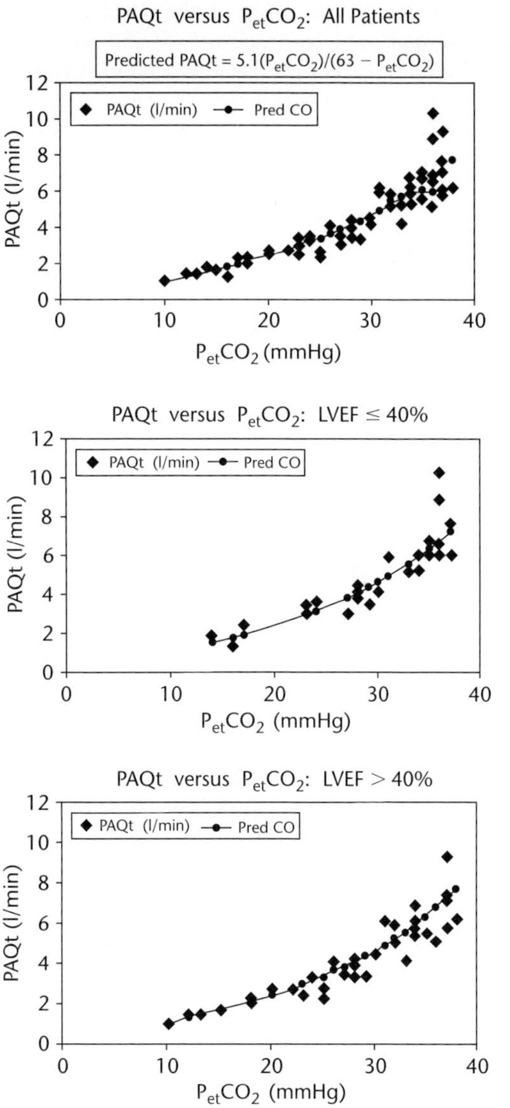

Figure 6.13 End-tidal CO_2 and pulmonary artery blood flow (PAQt). The line shows the calculated pulmonary flow. Observe that the good fit of low $P_{et}CO_2$ values and pulmonary flow. See text for explanation. PAQt = 5.1($P_{et}CO_2$)/(63 − $P_{et}CO_2$). Regression analysis revealed an *r* value of 0.88 ($P < 0.0001$). When data obtained from patients with left ventricular ejection fraction (LEVF) ≤ 40% and < 40% were plotted separately, statistical relationships were similar. (Reproduced with permission from Maslow, A., Stearns, G., Bert, A., Feng, W., *et al.* (2001). End-tidal carbon dioxide during weaning from cardiopulmonary bypass in patients without significant lung disease. *Anesth. Analg.*, **92**: 306–313.)

During aortic surgery the clamping of the aorta leads to complex cardiovascular adjustments and decrease of cardiac output and a concomitant decrease in CO_2 delivery to the lungs. If ventilation remains unchanged, end-tidal CO_2 values will decline, only to rise again with unclamping of the aorta and with reperfusion of ischemic vascular beds and the liberation of acidic metabolites that had accumulated during the cessation of peripheral perfusion (Johnston *et al.*, 2002). Of course, during cardiopulmonary bypass and the cessation of pulmonary blood flow capnography will fall silent as no CO_2 is being delivered.

Capnographic changes after tourniquet release

Release of a lower extremity tourniquet will increase P_aCO_2 as tissue acids circulate and are buffered by the blood. In patients that are breathing spontaneously, minute ventilation increases noticeably until P_aCO_2 normalizes. When ventilation is mechanically controlled, $P_{et}CO_2$ will increase and track the changes in P_aCO_2. Therefore, some clinicians increase minute ventilation to facilitate elimination of the acid load (Deen *et al.*, 1982).

High-frequency jet ventilation

A special circumstance arises during high-frequency jet ventilation (HFJV), which finds use when large pressure fluctuations in the trachea and bronchial tree need to be avoided. In HFJV very small tidal volumes at respiratory rates of 100 breaths/min or more are employed. No CO_2 can be collected under these circumstances. However, it is usually possible to interrupt the high-frequency ventilation and interpose a few slow breaths that enable the demonstration of end-tidal CO_2 pressures.

A clinical perspective

Assuming that artifacts from faulty valves or leaks or equipment malfunction have been ruled out and assuming that the collection of end-tidal gases proceeds without problems, capnographic data can show low, normal, or high end-tidal values. The clinician will need to examine the patient and these data and, whether low, normal, or high, must always first worry about the adequacy of ventilation. Given the patient's weight and temperature, we can estimate a tidal volume and respiratory rate (see also Table 1.1). Volumetric capnography facilitates this assessment by deadspace ventilation and enabling the calculation of effective alveolar ventilation. There are essentially three scenarios to be considered (with lots of gray areas between them).

Low (<34 mmHg) $P_{et}CO_2$

Because we tend to hyperventilate patients, hyperventilation is the most common cause of hypocapnia. If hyperventilation is ruled out, consider several other potential causes of decreased CO_2 delivery to the lungs. These include cardiovascular depression from deep anesthesia, low-preload (hypovolemia or increased venous capacitance and reduced venous return) compression of vessels (e.g. surgeon compressing the vena cava, etc.), pneumothorax, pulmonary embolism, or cardiac disease. Hypocapnia is one of the most important signals of trouble during anesthesia! It deserves a careful and systematic differential diagnosis and rapid correction.

Normal (34–44 mmHg) $P_{et}CO_2$

A normal capnogram with normal respiratory parameters is reassuring indeed. Unfortunately, we can feel reassured *only* if the effective alveolar ventilation is indeed appropriate for the patient. The patient's lungs might actually be hyperventilated and the examination of an arterial blood gas might show a much higher than expected P_aCO_2 as can occur with deadspace ventilation with or without a pulmonary shunt. If a large $P_aCO_2 - P_{et}CO_2$ difference is found, once again the search for an explanation must begin. Ventilation might well have to be increased, because the factors responsible for the difference between $P_aCO_2 - P_{et}CO_2$ will also affect O_2 and anesthetic vapors – if not to the same degree, depending on their individual venous to arterial differences. Conclusion: a normal capnogram is welcome – but it should not lull you to sleep.

High (>44 mmHg) $P_{et}CO_2$

Again, first check if ventilation is okay. This is so important because automatically increasing ventilation to correct hypercarbia can obscure for a time the early and best evidence of malignant hyperthermia or one of the rarer hypermetabolic syndromes. Due to the critical nature of malignant hyperthermia, it is imperative that it be diagnosed at its earliest stages. Tachycardia, often the first symptom, should cause the anesthesiologist to run through a differential diagnosis. By frequency of occurrence it might be due to sympathetic outflow from surgical stimulation; by gravity of consequence we must always include malignant hyperthermia as a potential explanation of a change in heart rate. Many minutes before a change in temperature can be detected, end-tidal CO_2 will increase (often 3–4-fold). It is the pathognomonic sign of increased CO_2 production by hypermetabolic muscle tissue. Therefore, end-tidal CO_2 monitoring is an important noninvasive device that can point to the early stages of malignant hyperthermia (Baudendistel *et al.*, 1984). CO_2 production and malignant hyperthermia and other much rarer conditions are covered extensively in subsequent chapters.

References

Baudendistel, L., Goudsouzian, N., Cote, C. & Strafford, M. (1984). End-tidal CO_2 monitoring: its use in the diagnosis and management of malignant hyperpyrexia. *Anaesthesia*, **39**: 1000–1003.

Bhavani-Shankar, K., Steinbrook, R.A., Brooks, D.C. & Datta, S. (2000). Arterial to end-tidal carbon dioxide pressure difference during laparoscopic surgery in pregnancy. *Anesthesiology*, **93**: 370–373.

Boccara, G., Jaber, S., Eliet, J., Mann, C. & Colson, P. (2001). Monitoring of end-tidal carbon dioxide partial pressure changes during infrarenal aortic cross-clamping: a non-invasive method to predict unclamping hypotension. *Acta Anaesthesiol. Scand.*, **45**: 188–193.

Breen, P.H. & Bradley, P.J. (1997). Carbon dioxide spirogram (but not capnogram) detects leaking inspiratory valve in a circle circuit. *Anesth. Analg.*, **85**: 1372–1376.

Brian Jr, J.E. (1998). Carbon dioxide and the cerebral circulation. *Anesthesiology*, **88**: 1365–1386.

Deen, L., Nyst, C.L. & Zuurmond, W.W. (1982). Metabolic changes after tourniquet release. *Acta. Anaesthesiol. Belg.*, **33**: 107–114.

Gandara, M.V., de Vega, D.S., Escriu, N., Olmedilla, C., Perez-Mencia, M.T., Zueras, R. & Lopez, A. (1997). Respiratory changes during laparoscopic cholecystectomy. A comparative study of three techniques. *Rev. Esp. Anestesiol. Reanim.*, **44**: 177–181.

Ginosar, Y. & Baranov, D. (1997). Prolonged "phantom" square wave capnograph tracing after patient disconnection or extubation. Potential hazard associated with the Siemens Servo 900c ventilator. *Anesthesiology*, **86**, 729–735.

Goldman, J.M., Ward, D.R. & Daniel, L. (1996). BreathSim, a mathematical model-based simulation of the anesthesia breathing circuit, may facilitate testing and evaluation of respiratory gas monitoring equipment. *Biomed. Sci. Instrum.*, **32**: 293–298.

Johnston, W.E., Conroy, B.P., Miller, G.S., Lin, C.Y. & Deyo, D.J. (2002). Hemodynamic benefit of positive end-expiratory pressure during acute descending aortic occlusion. *Anesthesiology*, **97**: 875–881.

Kazama, T., Ikeda, K., Kato, T. & Kikura, M. (1996). Carbon dioxide output in laparoscopic cholecystectomy. *Br. J. Anaesth.*, **76**: 530–535.

Lin, S.M., Chang, W.K., Tsao, C.M., Ou, C.H., Chan, K.H. & Tsai, S.K. (2003). Carbon dioxide embolism diagnosed by transesophageal echocardiography during endoscopic vein harvesting for coronary artery bypass grafting. *Anesth. Analg.*, **96**: 683–685.

Mann, C., Boccara, G., Fabre, J.M., Grevy, V. & Colson, P. (1997). The detection of carbon dioxide embolism during laparoscopy in pigs: a comparison of transesophageal Doppler and end-tidal carbon dioxide monitoring. *Acta, Anaesthesiol. Scand.*, **41**: 281–286.

Maslow, A., Stearns, G., Bert, A., Feng, W., *et al.* (2001). End-tidal carbon dioxide during weaning from cardiopulmonary bypass in patients without significant lung disease. *Anesth. Analg.*, **92**: 306–313.

Tripathi, M. & Pandey, M. (2000). Atypical "tails-up" capnograph due to breach in the sampling tube of side-stream capnometer. *J. Clin. Monit. Comput.*, **16**: 17–20.

Appendix

This checkout, or a reasonably equivalent, should be conducted before administration of anesthesia. These recommendations are only valid for an anesthesia system that conforms to current and relevant standards and includes an ascending bellows ventilator and at least the following monitors: capnograph, pulse oximeter, O_2 analyzer, respiratory volume monitor (spirometer) and breathing system pressure monitor with high- and low-pressure alarms. This is a guideline which users are encouraged to modify to accommodate differences in equipment design and variations in local clinical practice. Such local modifications should have appropriate peer review. Users should refer to the operator's manual for the manufacturer's specific procedures and precautions, especially the manufacturer's low-pressure leak test (step 5).

Emergency ventilation equipment

1 Verify backup ventilation equipment is available and functioning.

High-pressure system

2 Check O_2 cylinder supply:
   (a) Open O_2 cylinder and verify at least half full, about 1000 psi.*
   (b) Close cylinder.

3 Check central pipeline supplies:
   (a) Check that hoses are connected and pipeline gauges read about 50 psi.

Low-pressure systems

4 Check initial status of low-pressure system:
   (a) Close flow control valves and turn vaporizers off.
   (b) Check fill level and tighten vaporizers' filler caps.

*The FDA uses "psi", which stands for pounds per square inch, a delightfully quaint, historically interesting and scientifically cumbersome measure of pressure. Multiply psi by 70.31 to obtain g/cm^2. If you prefer newtons per square millimeter (N/mm^2), multiply psi by 0.006895.

5 Perform leak check of machine low-pressure system:
- (a) Verify that the machine master switch and flow control valves are OFF.
- (b) Attach "suction bulb" to common fresh gas outlet.
- (c) Squeeze bulb repeatedly until fully collapsed.
- (d) Verify bulb stays fully collapsed for at least 10 s.
- (e) Open one vaporizer at a time and repeat (c) and (d) as above.
- (f) Remove suction bulb and reconnect fresh gas hose.

6 Turn on machine master switch and all other necessary electrical equipment.

7 Test flow meters:
- (a) Adjust flow of all gases through their full range, checking for smooth operation of floats and undamaged flow tubes.
- (b) Attempt to create a hypoxic O_2/N_2O mixture and verify correct changes in flow and/or alarm.

Scavenging system

8 Adjust and check scavenging system:
- (a) Ensure proper connections between the scavenging system and both APL (pop-off) valve and ventilator relief valve.
- (b) Adjust waste gas vacuum (if possible).
- (c) Fully open APL valve and occlude Y-piece.
- (d) With minimum O_2 flow, allow scavenger reservoir bag to collapse completely and verify that absorber pressure gauge reads about zero.
- (e) With the O_2 flush activated allow the scavenger reservoir bag to distend fully, and then verify that absorber pressure gauge reads $<10\,cmH_2O$.

Breathing system

9 Calibrate O_2 monitor:
- (a) Ensure monitor reads 21% in room air.
- (b) Verify low O_2 alarm is enabled and functioning.
- (c) Reinstall sensor in circuit and flush breathing system with O_2.
- (d) Verify that monitor now reads greater than 90%.

10 Check initial status of breathing system:
- (a) Set selector switch to "Bag" mode.
- (b) Check that breathing circuit is complete, undamaged and unobstructed.
- (c) Verify that CO_2 absorbent is adequate.
- (d) Install breathing circuit accessory equipment (e.g. humidifier, PEEP valve) to be used during the case.

11 Perform leak check of the breathing system:
- (a) Set all gas flows to zero (or minimum).
- (b) Close APL (pop-off) valve and occlude Y-piece.
- (c) Pressurize breathing system to about $30\,cmH_2O$ with O_2 flush.
- (d) Ensure that pressure remains fixed for at least 10 s.
- (e) Open APL (pop-off) valve and ensure that pressure decreases.

Manual and automatic ventilation systems

12 Test ventilation systems and unidirectional valves:
- (a) Place a second breathing bag on Y-piece.
- (b) Set appropriate ventilator parameters for next patient.
- (c) Switch to automatic ventilation (Ventilator) mode.
- (d) Fill bellows and breathing bag with O_2 flush and then turn ventilator ON.
- (e) Set O_2 flow to minimum, other gas flows to zero.
- (f) Verify that during inspiration bellows delivers appropriate tidal volume and that during expiration bellows fills completely.
- (g) Set fresh gas flow to about 5 l/min.
- (h) Verify that the ventilator bellows and simulated lungs fill and empty appropriately without sustained pressure at end expiration.
- (i) Check for proper action of unidirectional valves.
- (j) Exercise breathing circuit accessories to ensure proper function.
- (k) Turn ventilator OFF and switch to manual ventilation (Bag/APL) mode.
- (l) Ventilate manually and assure inflation and deflation of artificial lungs and appropriate feel of system resistance and compliance.
- (m) Remove second breathing bag from Y-piece.

Monitors

13 Check, calibrate and/or set alarm limits of all monitors:
- (a) capnometer;
- (b) pulse oximeter;
- (c) O_2 analyzer;
- (d) respiratory volume monitor (spirometer);
- (e) pressure monitor with high- and low-airway alarms.

Final position

14 Check final status of machine:
- (a) vaporizers off,
- (b) automatic fill limiter (AFL) valve open,
- (c) selector switch to "bag",
- (d) all flow meters to zero,
- (e) patient suction level adequate,
- (f) breathing system ready to use.

If an anesthesia provider uses the same machine in successive cases, steps 1–9 need not be repeated or may be abbreviated after the initial checkout. http://www.fda.gov/cdrh/humfac/ anesckot.html

MONITORING DURING MECHANICAL VENTILATION 7

J. Thompson & N. Craig

The clinical applications of both time and volumetric capnography during mechanical ventilation are reviewed. A number of applications are discussed at length in other chapters and the reader is advised to consult those chapters for greater detail.

Clinical applications of end-tidal carbon dioxide monitoring

Continuous monitoring of end-tidal carbon dioxide ($ETCO_2$) is a well-established standard of care in the operating room (OR). The exhaled CO_2 in conjunction with its associated capnogram provides early detection of potentially dangerous clinical changes in the patient. Continuous monitoring of $ETCO_2$ has been responsible for the prevention of adverse events including displacement of the endotracheal tube, hypoventilation, and the disruption of the integrity of the ventilator circuit (Cote *et al.*, 1986). Although it is not yet mandated for all patients receiving mechanical ventilatory support outside of the OR, its use in the intensive care unit (ICU) and emergency room setting has become more widespread (Society of Critical Care Medicine, 1988; ACEP, 1995). $ETCO_2$ can be useful to monitor the mechanically ventilated patient when used in conjunction with other monitors of the patients' clinical status. The American Association for Respiratory Care has published guidelines for the use of capnography in the clinical settings during mechanical ventilation (see Table 7.1) (AARC, 2003).

Table 7.1 Indications for capnography during mechanical ventilation

Section	Indication
4.1	Evaluation of the exhaled (CO_2), especially $ETCO_2$, which is the maximum partial pressure of CO_2 exhaled during a tidal breath (just prior to the beginning of inspiration) and is designated $P_{et}CO_2$
4.2	Monitoring severity of pulmonary disease and evaluating response to therapy, especially therapy intended to improve the ratio of dead space to V_d/V_t and the matching of $\dot{V}/\dot{Q}$, and possibly, to increase coronary blood flow
4.3	Use as an adjunct to determine that tracheal rather than esophageal intubation has taken place (low or absent cardiac output may negate its use for this indication); colorimetric CO_2 detectors are adequate devices for this purpose
4.4	Continued monitoring of the integrity of the ventilatory circuit, including the artificial airway
4.5	Evaluation of the efficiency of mechanical ventilatory support by determination of the difference between the arterial partial pressure for CO_2 (P_aCO_2) and the $P_{et}CO_2$
4.6	Monitoring adequacy of pulmonary, systemic, and coronary blood flow
4.6.1	Estimation of effective (non-shunted) pulmonary capillary blood flow by a partial rebreathing method
4.6.2	Use as an adjunctive tool to screen for pulmonary embolism (Evidence for the utility of dead space determinations as a screening tool for pulmonary embolism is at present not conclusive.)
4.6.3	Monitoring the matching of $\dot{V}/\dot{Q}$ during independent lung ventilation for unilateral pulmonary contusion
4.7	Monitoring inspired CO_2 when CO_2 gas is being therapeutically administered
4.8	Graphic evaluation of the ventilator-patient interface: evaluation of the shape of the capnogram may be useful in detecting rebreathing of CO_2, obstructive pulmonary disease, waning neuromuscular blockade (curare cleft), cardiogenic oscillations, esophageal intubation, cardiac arrest, and contamination of the monitor or sampling line with secretions or mucus
4.9	Measurement of the volume of CO_2 elimination to assess metabolic rate and/or alveolar ventilation

Reproduced with permission from AARC Clinical Practice Guideline (2003). Capnography/capnometry during mechanical ventilation – 2003 revision and update. *Respir. Care*, **48**: 534–539.

$ETCO_2$ is a reflection of alveolar CO_2 (partial pressure of carbon dioxide in alveolar gas, P_ACO_2) and thus represents arterial CO_2 (partial pressure of carbon dioxide in arterial blood, P_aCO_2). In contrast to arterial blood gas (ABG) measurement, $ETCO_2$ monitoring is a less invasive, less costly, real-time measurement of exhaled CO_2. However, $ETCO_2$ monitoring is affected by changes in metabolism or CO_2 production, cardiovascular function, respiratory function, and monitor limitations.

Metabolic changes and CO_2 production

Changes in the metabolic rate of the patient result in a change in CO_2 production and thus CO_2 elimination. $ETCO_2$ monitoring can be used as an indicator of CO_2 production provided circulation and ventilation are relatively stable (Hess, 1990). Conditions that increase metabolism include fever, sepsis, pain, and seizures. Under these conditions CO_2 production will increase resulting in an elevation in $ETCO_2$. A decrease in metabolism occurs in patients who are hypothermic or patients who are sedated and paralyzed. These conditions lower CO_2 production and can cause a decrease in the $ETCO_2$. In patients who are mechanically ventilated and unable to alter minute ventilation in response to changes in CO_2 production alterations, changes in $ETCO_2$ can alert the clinician to the need for adjustments in ventilation in response to changes in CO_2 production.

Cardiovascular function

CO_2 transport to the lungs is dependent on adequate cardiovascular function. Any factor that alters cardiovascular function can affect CO_2 transport to the lungs. In the absence of changes in the respiratory status of the patient, $ETCO_2$ may alert the clinician to changes in the cardiovascular function of the patient. Hypovolemia, hypotension, and pulmonary tension can cause a gradual decrease in $ETCO_2$, whereas cardiac arrest will result in a gradual disappearance of monitored $ETCO_2$. Under the condition of complete cardiovascular collapse, the $ETCO_2$ will disappear until circulation is restored. Studies have suggested that monitoring $ETCO_2$ is useful in the evaluation of the effectiveness of cardiopulmonary resuscitation (CPR).[1] With the initiation of CPR and the restoration of pulmonary blood flow there should be a rise in $ETCO_2$. It has also been suggested that the $ETCO_2$ measurement may decrease when chest compressions are less effective (Falk *et al.*, 1988).

Respiratory function

Changes in respiratory function will affect the removal of CO_2 from the lungs to the environment. Obstructive lung diseases, pneumonia, neuromuscular disorders, central nervous system disorders with impaired respiratory function will alter the $ETCO_2$ value. $ETCO_2$ and P_aCO_2 are generally closely matched in lungs with low ventilation and perfusion ($\dot{V}/\dot{Q}$) mismatching. In a number of patients admitted to the ICU for mechanical ventilatory support there may be no access for arterial sampling. Monitoring $ETCO_2$ may be the only available guide for establishing adequate ventilation. The $ETCO_2$ and its associated capnogram can serve as a useful guide for determining the ventilation requirements of the patient. Capnometry without the capnogram in this setting can be of questionable validity. Variations from a normal capnogram may help in the diagnosis of an underlying clinical or technical problem. In a normal appearing capnograph, there is a steep rise in CO_2 followed by a near horizontal plateau which represents alveolar gas. The absence of the plateau can suggest changes in physiologic condition or mechanical problems.

Even with arterial access, blood gas sampling may not provide instantaneous information needed when acute events arise. This is particularly true in patients with cerebral hypertension as a result of trauma. These patients are typically managed with some degree of hyperventilation, as increases in the P_aCO_2 of the patient with head trauma may cause cerebral vasodilation, and also precipitation and increase in intracranial pressure (Kerr *et al.*, 1996). Optimal management of head injured patients at risk for intracranial hypertension requires close monitoring of $ETCO_2$ to detect sudden changes in P_aCO_2. A gradient between P_aCO_2 and $ETCO_2$ will widen with impairment of lung function. The wider the gradient, the more impaired lung function.

Mechanical ventilatory support using P_aCO_2–$ETCO_2$ gradient

In normal individuals, the gradient between arterial and alveolar CO_2 (a–ACO_2) varies between 2 and 5 mmHg (Nunn, 1969). Comparison of the gradient between arterial and end-tidal CO_2 (a–$ETCO_2$) can offer valuable information regarding the patients' clinical status. The gradient is widened by abnormalities

[1] See Chapter 20 on cardiopulmonary resuscitation.

in the $\dot{V}/\dot{Q}$ ratio. Normally the overall $\dot{V}/\dot{Q}$ ratio is 0.8 and is altered by dead-space V_d/V_t ventilation or shunt perfusion.

Dead space-ventilation is characterized by a high $\dot{V}/\dot{Q}$ ratio. In dead space-ventilation alveoli that are ventilated but not well perfused. If there is abnormal perfusion to areas of the lung that are well ventilated, the $ETCO_2$ will decrease. Dead space-ventilation may be caused by physiologic conditions such as pulmonary emboli, hypovolemia, and hemorrhage. Therapies may be initiated to improve systemic perfusion and thus improve pulmonary circulation. As pulmonary circulation improves the a-$ETCO_2$ gradient should narrow and can indicate a positive response to therapy.

Shunt perfusion is characterized by a low $\dot{V}/\dot{Q}$ ratio. Shunt occurs when there exists normal perfusion to alveoli that are not adequately ventilated. Examples of increasing shunt include many pulmonary disease states including pneumonia and atelectasis. Mechanical ventilation strategies aimed at optimizing lung function and decreasing the widened gradient includes positive end-expiratory pressure (PEEP).

The a-$ETCO_2$ gradient can be a useful tool for optimizing PEEP in patients with increasing lung disease. At the appropriate level of PEEP the a-$ETCO_2$ should be at its most narrow point. The phenomena of overdistension can occur when the optimal PEEP is exceeded. In a patient who has had a gradient that has narrowed while PEEP has been gradually increased may have a widened gradient once optimal PEEP has been exceeded (Blanch *et al.*, 1987). One limitation of this technique is the frequency of arterial sampling necessary to assess the gradient.

Diseases such as asthma can produce a widened gradient because of airway obstruction leading to uneven emptying of alveoli, gas trapping, and potentially auto-PEEP. In this disease state the capnograph will provide useful information about responses to therapies (Sabato & Hanson, 2000). The $ETCO_2$ just as a number does not give adequate information regarding the physiologic state of the patient. The abnormal appearing slope of the curve may change with bronchodilator therapy or changes in mechanical ventilation tailored to providing optimal emptying times. Auto PEEP can lead to increasing dead space as overdistension can alter perfusion leading to an increase in dead space-ventilation.

Monitoring integrity of the airway and the breathing circuit

Continuous monitoring of the $ETCO_2$ in the ICU setting just as in the OR can be used to monitor the position and patency of the endotracheal tube. In patients who are mechanically ventilated and moving spontaneously there is a risk for dislodging the endotracheal tube resulting in inadequate ventilation. Changes in head position can dramatically change the position of the endotracheal tube especially in the neonatal or pediatric patient. Likewise in a patient who is chemically paralyzed, moving the patient for procedures such as an X-ray can put the patient at risk for endotracheal tube displacement. In this situation $ETCO_2$ may acutely disappear.

Continuously monitoring $ETCO_2$ can alert the clinician to a partial or total occlusion of the endotracheal tube. Although $ETCO_2$ monitoring should not take the place of the alarms on the mechanical ventilator, changes in the capnograph may alert the clinician to the need for an early intervention such as suctioning. Another condition that may produce an acute fall in $ETCO_2$ in an otherwise stable patient is the partial or complete kinking of the endotracheal tube. In addition to problems with the endotracheal tube, any disruption of the integrity of the ventilator circuit will result in an immediate change in the $ETCO_2$ (Palmon *et al.*, 1996).

Transport of mechanically ventilated patient

The technology of $ETCO_2$ monitoring has been shown to be useful in the inter- or intra-hospital setting (Williamson *et al.*, 1993). When transport is required inadvertent extubation can occur at any point of the process including during the transport itself, during a transfer to and from the bed, and during any procedure. In addition to monitoring the position of the $ETCO_2$ often access to arterial blood gas sampling is not possible and $ETCO_2$ becomes your only tool for monitoring adequacy of ventilation. When patients are transported they are often manually ventilated. During manual ventilation it is difficult to maintain control of ventilation. Although $\dot{V}/\dot{Q}$ abnormalities may be present depending on the patients' condition, in this setting a trend of the $ETCO_2$ may alert the clinician to changes in the ventilatory requirements of the patient. A rise in the expired CO_2 may lead one to question changes in the pulmonary status of the patient. Similarly, a drop may also raise questions about overventilation of the patient as well as questions about the patients' pulmonary and cardiac status. In the patient with pulmonary hypertension or cerebral hypertension where hyperventilation is critical $ETCO_2$ will provide close monitoring of the adequacy of ventilation and rapid detection of hypoventilation.

Weaning from mechanical ventilation

$ETCO_2$ monitoring alone may not be a reliable tool in the patient weaning from mechanical ventilation. Without knowing the a-$ETCO_2$ gradient a patient weaning from mechanical ventilatory support with a consistent $ETCO_2$ may have an under appreciated increase in dead space (Morley *et al.*, 1993). In the patient with a stable or improving respiratory status it may be a useful tool provided there is a comparison of the a-$ETCO_2$ gradient at the start of weaning. $ETCO_2$ monitoring has been shown to correlate well with P_aCO_2 in post-operative patients without parenchymal lung disease (Healey *et al.*, 1987). Other measures of patient status including vital signs, respiratory rate, and SpO_2 must be closely followed.

Special procedures: monitoring the therapeutic administration of CO_2

In the newborn setting, therapeutic administration of CO_2 in the ventilator circuit has been used in the pre-operative management of patients with hypoplastic left heart syndrome. In this patient population maintaining a balance between pulmonary and systemic blood flow is critical. Excessive pulmonary blood flow can lead to a compromise of systemic perfusion resulting in hypoperfusion and metabolic acidosis. One treatment strategy is aimed at increasing pulmonary vascular resistance with the addition of inspired CO_2. CO_2 is added to the inspiratory limb of a continuous flow ventilator to produce a respiratory acidosis to increase pulmonary vascular resistance while minute ventilation and Vt are maintained at constant levels (Bradley *et al.*, 2001; Tabbutt *et al.*, 2001). $ETCO_2$ is monitored and alarmed to maintain a specific range of P_aCO_2 and to avoid significant respiratory acidosis. Sudden changes in $ETCO_2$ can alert the clinician to changes in the clinical status of the patient. Additionally, inspired CO_2 concentrations should be monitored and alarmed to avoid inadvertent alteration of the inspired CO_2.

Use of $ETCO_2$ in patients without an artificial airway

Continuous $ETCO_2$ monitoring may have a role in the spontaneously breathing patient without an artificial airway. The use of side-stream technology and sampling via a nasal cannula makes it possible to monitor patients who are not mechanically ventilated (Flanagan *et al.*, 1995). The use of $ETCO_2$ has expanded to the pediatric setting as advances in the technology have allowed for lower sampling flow rates in patients with small tidal volumes (V_d/V_t) and faster respiratory rates. It may provide a tool to monitor respiratory function in a variety of disease conditions and may limit the need for invasive measure of P_aCO_2 by arterial puncture in the awake patient. The disease states may include a variety of conditions including asthma, bronchiolitis, and neuromuscular diseases. The relationship of the $ETCO_2$ to the P_aCO_2 value may be difficult to determine depending on the degree of pulmonary disease or the cardiovascular status of the patient. Therefore, the clinician must be aware of the effect on the measured $ETCO_2$ caused by conditions of hypoventilation, mouth breathing, or low V_d/V_t that may give a lower $ETCO_2$ reading. As a trend without arterial access to compare the a-$ETCO_2$ gradient, it can alert the clinician to impending respiratory failure when used as a tool in conjunction with other tools of physical assessment such as other vital sign measures including SpO_2.

In the patient with asthma or other diseases with changes in airway resistance $ETCO_2$ and the evaluation of the capnogram can be a useful tool when evaluating responses to bronchodilator therapy. Changes in the slope of the curve can suggest a positive response to bronchodilator therapy (You *et al.*, 1994).

Pediatric patient with diseases such as bronchiolitis may be monitored for response to therapy and adequacy of ventilation. In addition to airway obstruction and atelectasis patients with bronchiolitis are often at risk for developing apnea. $ETCO_2$ monitoring can rapidly detect the cessation of breathing with a decrease in exhaled CO_2 (Toubas *et al.*, 1990).

Patients with neuromuscular disease who may develop muscle fatigue may benefit from $ETCO_2$ monitoring. Complaints of fatigue and sleepiness in patients with neuromuscular disease may be a result of nocturnal hypercapnia. Capnography is used as a tool to detect respiratory insufficiency. Pulse oximetry alone does not provide adequate monitoring of the patient with respiratory insufficiency who may be receiving supplemental oxygen. Rising of $ETCO_2$ may indicate the onset of muscle fatigue and suggest the need for increased respiratory support such as non-invasive ventilation. Patients who are already receiving non-invasive ventilatory support may be monitored for adequacy of assisted ventilation (Kotterba *et al.*, 2001).

Another application of $ETCO_2$ monitoring may be as a diagnostic tool for patients with obstructive sleep apnea. Apnea will cause an immediate reduction in $ETCO_2$. When spontaneous respirations return, $ETCO_2$ will reappear (Magnan *et al.*, 1993).

An area under current investigation is $ETCO_2$ monitoring for diabetic ketoacidosis (DKA). Patients with DKA hyperventilate to lower P_aCO_2 and lessen the severity of acidosis. If $ETCO_2$ can be monitored and sufficiently approximate P_aCO_2 this could be an important diagnostic and/or therapeutic tool (Garcia *et al.*, 2003).

Clinical applications of volumetric CO_2

Volumetric capnography or volumetric CO_2 ($\dot{V}CO_2$) is the measurement of CO_2 as a function of volume as opposed to time. Three important parameters provided by volumetric CO_2 measurement are CO_2 production $\dot{V}CO_2$ or more accurately CO_2 elimination, alveolar ventilation (V_{alv}), and physiological dead space ($V_d/V_{t\ phy}$). With the Enghoff modified Bohr equation $V_d/V_{t\ phys}$ can be calculated, assuming that alveolar and arterial levels are equal. In the future, methods to extrapolate alveolar PCO_2 from the volumetric capnogram may obviate the need for arterial sampling. All three parameters can offer important information on the physiologic state of the patient. Its use has become more widespread in evaluating adequacy of ventilation and determining optimal ventilator support as well as a potentially useful tool in weaning from mechanical ventilation.

CO_2 production

Changes in $\dot{V}CO_2$ reflect changes in $\dot{V}/\dot{Q}$ so it can be a sensitive indicator of changes in the patients' condition. When CO_2 production increases with constant minute ventilation, P_aCO_2 will increase. As CO_2 elimination equals CO_2 production during steady state, the observation of $\dot{V}CO_2$ on a breath-to-breath basis provides the clinician instantaneous feedback on ventilator adjustments (Taskar *et al.*, 1995). If increasing minute ventilation (VE) has resulted in the increased elimination of CO_2, then $\dot{V}CO_2$ will increase until a steady state has been reached. In patients with asthma, changes in minute ventilation that result in an increase in CO_2 elimination will be reflected as an increase in $\dot{V}CO_2$. If an increase in $\dot{V}CO_2$ is not observed than the ventilator adjustments made by the clinician have not improved elimination of CO_2 and may suggest an increase in air trapping in this disease state. Observing $\dot{V}CO_2$ may guide determining optimal PEEP. Optimizing PEEP in the patient with significant lung disease should be accomplished without compromising pulmonary perfusion. CO_2 removal is compromised when perfusion is compromised. The $\dot{V}CO_2$ level can be observed while the PEEP level is incrementally increased. When a decrease in $\dot{V}CO_2$ is observed perfusion is compromised and optimal PEEP has been exceeded.

Predicting ventilatory requirements

Alveolar minute ventilation can be used as a guide for predicting the P_aCO_2 that may result from adjusting ventilation parameters. Using the formula:

$$\text{Desired } P_aCO_2 = \frac{V_{alv} \times P_aCO_2}{\text{adjusted } V_{alv}},$$

one can predict the change in alveolar minute ventilation needed to reach a specific goal for P_aCO_2. This is useful in finely controlling the P_aCO_2 in patients with intracranial hypertension in whom a very tight range of P_aCO_2 is necessary for maintaining hyperventilation to limit cerebral vasodilation. Likewise in the patient in whom the ventilation plan is to employ a strategy of permissive hypercapnea, gradually altering ventilation to a precise P_aCO_2 allows for a gradual elevation in PCO_2 to allow time for the body to buffer pH and prevent significant respiratory acidosis.

Weaning from mechanical ventilation

Observing the $\dot{V}CO_2$ during weaning from mechanical ventilation can be a useful tool in determining the patient's ability to take over the work done by the mechanical ventilator. As support is withdrawn if the patient can successfully maintain the alveolar minute ventilation necessary to sufficiently remove CO_2 then the $\dot{V}CO_2$ should remain consistent. A stable $\dot{V}CO_2$ verifies that the $\dot{V}/\dot{Q}$ relationship has not changed.

During the weaning process if the patient is unable to maintain adequate alveolar ventilation the $\dot{V}CO_2$ will decrease and will indicated an inability to remove CO_2. In additon V_d/V_t is an important indicator in this evaluation. An improvement in V_d/V_t is an indicator of improvement in pulmonary disease and a patients' readiness to wean from mechanical ventilation. Although work of breathing is an important evaluation in patients who are being weaned from ventilatory support, it is a subjective indicator. A more objective indicator of work of breathing is the V_d/V_t. As ventilator support is withdrawn, if the patient continues to maintain the same minute ventilation, if the V_d/V_t increases the patients' ability to remove CO_2 is being compromised. This is often associated with a more rapid shallow breathing pattern. The use of V_d/V_t as a predictor for successful extubation has been studied. One study by Hubble *et al.* (2000) in the pediatric setting determined a V_d/V_t of $\leq .5$ is a predictor of extubation success. A V_d/V_t of $>.65$ was associated with the need for additional respiratory support after extubation. V_d/V_t as a predictor of mortality has been studied in patients with congenital diaphragmatic hernia who required extracorporeal membrane oxygenation (ECMO) support. Interestingly, a V_d/V_t of $>.6$ was associated with an increase in mortality rate (Arnold *et al.*, 1995).

Continuous $ETCO_2$ and volumetric CO_2 monitoring have become important clinical tools for the ICU patient. This tool has allowed us to better assess complicated patients with the varying ventilator strategies gives the clinician a better understanding of the relationship between the ventilator and the patient.

References

AARC Clinical Practice Guideline (2003). Capnography/capnometry during mechanical ventilation – 2003 revision and update. *Respir. Care*, **48**: 534–539.

American College of Emergency Physicians (1995). Expired carbon dioxide monitoring. *Ann. Emerg. Med.*, **25**: 441.

Arnold, J.H., Bower, L.K. & Thompson, J.E. (1995). Respiratory deadspace measurements in neonates with congenital diaphragmatic hernia. *Crit. Care Med.*, **23**: 371–375.

Blanch, L., Fernandez, R., Benito, S., Mancebo, J. & Net, A. (1987). Effects of PEEP on the arterial minus end-tidal carbon dioxide gradient. *Chest,* **92**: 451–454.

Bradley, S.M., Simsic, J.M. & Atz, A.M. (2001). Hemodynamic effects of inspired carbon dioxide after the Norwood procedure. *Ann. Thorac. Surg.*, **72**: 2088–2094.

Cote, C.J., Liu, L.M., Szyfelbein, S.K., Firestone, S., Goudsouzian, N.G., Welch, J.P. & Daniels, A.L. (1986). Intraoperative events diagnosed by expired carbon dioxide monitoring in children. *Can. Anaesth. Soc., J.* **33**: 315–320.

Falk, J.L., Rackow, E.C. & Weil, M.H. (1988). End-tidal carbon dioxide concentration during cardiopulmonary resuscitation. *New Engl. J. Med.*, **318**: 607–611.

Flanagan, J.F., Garrett, J.S., McDuffee, A. & Tobias, J.D. (1995). Noninvasive monitoring of end-tidal carbon dioxide tension via nasal cannulas in spontaneously breathing children with profound hypocarbia. *Crit. Care Med.*, **23**: 1140–1142.

Garcia, E., Abramo, T.J., Okada, P., Guzman, D.D., Reisch, J.S. & Wiebe, R.A. (2003). Capnometry for noninvasive continuous monitoring of metabolic status in pediatric diabetic ketoacidosis. *Crit. Care Med.*, **31**: 2539–2543.

Healey, C.J., Fedullo, A.J., Swinburne, A.J. & Wahl, G.W. (1987). Comparison of noninvasive measurements of carbon dioxide tension during withdrawal from mechanical ventilation. *Crit. Care Med.*, **15**: 764–767.

Hess, D. (1990). Capnometry and capnography: technical aspects, physiologic aspects, and clinical applications. *Respir. Care*, **35**: 557–576.

Hubble, C.L., Gentile, M.A., Tripp, D.S., Craig, D., Meliones, J.N. & Cheifetz, I.M. (2000). Deadspace to tidal volume ratio predicts successful extubation in infants and children. *Crit. Care Med.*, **28**: 2034–2040.

Kerr, M.E., Zempsky, J., Sereika, S., Orndoff, P. & Rudy, E. (1996). Relationship between arterial carbon dioxide and end-tidal carbon dioxide in mechanically ventilated adults with severe head trauma. *Crit. Care Med.*, **24**: 785–796.

Kotterba, S., Patzold, T., Malin, J.B., Orth, M. & Rasche, K. (2001). Respiratory monitoring in neuromuscular disease. *Clin. Neurol. Neurosurg*, **103**: 87–91.

Magnan, A., Philip-Joet, F., Rey, M., Reynaud, M., Porri, F. & Arnaud, A. (1993). End-tidal CO_2 analysis in sleep apnea syndrome: conditions for use. *Chest,* **102**: 129–131.

Morley, T.F., Giaimo, J., Maroszan, E., Bermingham, J., Gordon, R., Griesback, R., Zappasodi, S.J. & Giudice, J.C. (1993). Use of capnography for assessment of the adequacy of alveolar ventilation during weaning from mechanical ventilation. *Am. Rev. Respir. Dis.*, **148**: 339–344.

Nunn, J.F. (1969). *Applied Respiratory Physiology*, 3rd edition. Butterworths & Co Ltd, London.

Palmon, S., Maywin, L., Moore, L. & Kirsch, J. (1996). Capnography facilitates tight control of ventilation during transport. *Crit. Care Med.*, **24**: 608–611.

Sabato, K. & Hanson, J.H. (2000). Mechanical ventilation for children with status asthmaticus. *Resp. Care Clin. North Am.*, **6**: 171–188.

Society of Critical Care Medicine: Task Force on Guidelines (1988). Recommendations for services and personnel for delivery of care in a critical care setting. *Crit. Care Med.*, **16**: 809–811.

Tabbutt, S., Ramamoorthy, C. & Montenegro, L.M. *et al.* (2001). Impact of inspired gas mixtures on preoperative infants with hypoplastic left heart syndrome during controlled ventilation. *Circulation,* **104**: I-159–I-164.

Taskar, V., John, J., Larsson, A., Wetterberg, T. & Jonson, B. (1995). Dynamics of carbon dioxide elimination following ventilator resetting. *Chest,* **108**: 196–202.

Toubas, P.L., Duke, J.C., Sekar, K.C. & McCaffree, M.A. (1990). Microphonic versus end-tidal carbon dioxide nasal airflow detection in neonates with apnoea. *Pediatrics,* **6**: 950–954.

Williamson, J.A., Webb, R.K., Cockings, J. & Morgan, C. (1993). The capnograph: applications and limitations-an analysis of 2000 incident reports. *Anaesth. Intens. Care,* **21**: 551–557.

You, B., Peslin, R., Duvivier, C., Vu, V.D. & Grilliat, J.P. (1994). Expiratory capnograpy in asthma: evaluation of various shape indices. *Eur. Respir. J.*, **7**: 318–323.

CAPNOGRAPHY IN TRANSPORT 8

M.A. Frakes

Introduction

Both interhospital and intrahospital transport add a variable, and often a difficulty, to the care of critically ill patients. In addition to continuing to treat the patient's disease, attention must be paid to the logistics of moving the patient and monitoring equipment, to the added stressors of that move on the patient and providers, and to the barriers presented by the transport environment.

The potential for unplanned events and patient deterioration during transport is well documented. About two-third of patients experience adverse physiologic changes during intrahospital transport, and equipment failures complicate up to 13.4% of transports (Indek *et al.*, 1988; Hurst *et al.*, 1992; Evans & Winslow, 1995; Waydhas *et al.*, 1995). Some of the physiologic changes are likely related to the patient's illness, as changes occur with similar frequency in acuity-matched patients not undergoing transport. Mortality is higher for intensive care unit (ICU) patients experiencing intrahospital transport compared with APACHE score-matched patients who do not travel. That increase, however, does not exceed predicted mortality rates for those patients (Hurst *et al.*, 1992; Szem *et al.*, 1995). Similar comparisons for interhospital transport are difficult because that transport generally brings the patient to therapeutic services that would otherwise be unavailable. The use of specially trained transport teams with proper equipment may reduce the incidence of unplanned events, particularly those related to equipment issues (Edge *et al.*, 1994; Stearley, 1998; Frakes, 2002).

Respiratory changes are particularly common during the transport of intubated patients. A number of studies have demonstrated that changes in partial pressure of carbon dioxide in arterial blood (P_aCO_2) tension and pH occur in between 70% and 100% of such patients. Manual ventilation without minute ventilation monitoring seems to provide the least ventilatory stability, but changes are even observed in patients ventilated with transport ventilators. Although both hyperventilation and hypoventilation occur, unintentional respiratory alkalosis is induced at least 2.5 times as often as respiratory acidosis (Braman *et al.*, 1987; Gervais *et al.*, 1987; Hurst *et al.*, 1989; Martin *et al.*, 1997; Beker *et al.*, 1998). There is physiologic evidence that hemodynamic changes may correlate with the blood gas changes. Hyperventilation can result in air trapping and increased intrathoracic pressures with a resultant hypotension from decreased preload. Both myocardial alkalosis and acidosis are arrhythmogenic and can adversely affect cardiac function (Braman *et al.*, 1987).

The transport environment itself, particularly the interhospital transport environment further contributes to the opportunity for mishap. Transport necessarily involves an increased number of patient movements, each increasing the risk for unplanned removal of medical devices, particularly, endotracheal (ET) tubes. Transport vehicle noise complicates patient assessment as ambient noise compromises pulmonary examination and monitoring. Lung sound intensity is generally between 22 and 30 dB, while transport vehicle noise levels can be as high as 100 dB in helicopters and 84 dB in ground ambulances (Hunt *et al.*, 1991; Patel *et al.*, 1998; Price & Goldsmith, 1998). The accuracy of breath sound assessments in ground transport vehicles has been shown to be barely half as accurate as in a traditional environment and only 0.09% sensitive as an exam tool (Brown *et al.*, 1997). Helicopter medical teams are probably unable to evaluate even the simple presence or absence of lung sounds in flight (Hunt *et al.*, 1991).

Capnography and capnometry provide useful information that can help to optimize patient monitoring in this challenging environment and may help to stave off complications during transport. This chapter will review specific clinical applications of that technology: assuring proper ET tube placement, monitoring airway circuit integrity, monitoring the consistency of mechanical ventilation, aiding in evaluating cardiac output, and evaluating patients in cardiac arrest.

ET tube placement

Transport personnel are often called upon to intubate patients. Esophageal intubation, including detected misplacements, may occur with up to 40% of all intubation attempts, but it is undetected esophageal intubation that is a clinical catastrophe with the potential for anoxic injury and death (Stewart *et al.*, 1985; MacLeod *et al.*, 1991; Katz *et al.*, 1998; Frakes, 2001). Even experienced intubators can overlook an esophageal ET tube placement, with such cases accounting for about 15% of all catastrophic anesthesia incidents (Hussain & Raphael, 1997; Bhende, 1999). The incidence of undetected esophageal intubation in transport has been reported between 0% and 61.7% (Stewart *et al.*, 1985; MacLeod *et al.*, 1991; Katz *et al.*,1998; Frakes, 2001).

Capnometry and capnography aid in the confirmation of correct ET tube placement. End-tidal carbon dioxide ($ETCO_2$) measurement accurately detects esophageal intubation because carbon dioxide (CO_2) is exhaled through the trachea and not the esophagus (Bhende, 1999). Overall, capnometry is 93% sensitive and 97% specific in detecting tracheal intubation. Due to the relationship between cardiac output and $ETCO_2$ tension, measurement is better in patients with a pulse, where sensitivity is near 100%. For patients in cardiac arrest, specificity is between 86% and 100% and sensitivity between 70% and 100% (MacLeod *et al.*, 1991; Bhende *et al.*, 1992a, b; Bozeman *et al*, 1996). Chest compression adequacy seems to relate to measurement reliability in arrest (Ward & Yearly, 1998a). When the ET tube is not, in fact, endotracheal, end-tidal partial pressure of carbon dioxide ($P_{et}CO_2$) will be near zero and the waveform will be disorganized, lacking the characteristic square shape (Frakes, 2001).

Colorimetric and quantitative capnometry are similarly reliable for evaluating ET tube placement (MacLeod *et al.*, 1991; Bhende, 1992a; Kelly *et al.*, 1992; Knapp *et al.*, 1999; Li, 2001). Capnography adds an important additional measure of certainty (Bozeman *et al.*, 1996; Ward & Yearly, 1998a; Puntervoll *et al.*, 2002). Without a waveform for analysis, colorimetric or quantitative capnometry can give false positive readings with the esophageal intubation of a patient whose stomach contains CO_2 from carbonated beverages or artificial respiration (Bhende, 1999; Puntervoll *et al.*, 2002). Evaluating the $ETCO_2$ reading after six ventilations have been given through the ET tube to wash out the CO_2, increases accuracy (Bozeman *et al.*, 1996; Ward & Yearly, 1998a; Puntervoll *et al.*, 2002). The caution is that six ventilations will put at least 3 l of gas into the stomach. Waveform capnography will show a distorted waveform if the ET tube is in the esophagus, and provides better assurance of correct placement than does capnometry alone.

Although less commonly performed than oral intubation, blind nasotracheal intubation is an available option for airway capture. Continuous capnometry is a useful method for facilitating proper placement of a nasotracheal tube in spontaneously breathing patients because the $P_{et}CO_2$ value increases as the tube approaches the larynx and decreases with direction toward the esophagus (Bozeman *et al.*, 1996; Chan *et al.*, 1998).

Capnography is fast becoming a standard of care for intubators. The American Heart Association recommends a non-physical examination technique such as $ETCO_2$ detection for confirming ET tube placement (Cummings & Hazinski, 2000). Similarly, the American Society of Anesthesiologists (1998–2000) describes capnometry as essential for evaluating ET tube or laryngeal mask placement, and for monitoring any patient receiving inhaled anesthetic. The Transport Nurses Association, American College of Emergency Physicians, and National Association of Emergency Medical Services Physicians all specifically recommend capnography as part of post-intubation monitoring for all patients (Rogovin & Hamm, 2003; American College of Emergency Physicians, 2003; National Association of Emergency Medical Services Physicians, 2003).

Monitoring ventilation

Once an ET tube is in place, the mechanical ventilation circuit must be monitored and continued correct placement of the ET tube must be assured. ET tube migration or circuit integrity interruption affects patient oxygenation and ventilation and can be as catastrophic as an undetected esophageal intubation, especially for patients with inadequate spontaneous breathing.

Unplanned extubation occurs in as many as 14.5% of out-of-hospital transports of intubated patients (National Flight Nurses Association (NFNA), 1995; Holleran, 1996; Benumof, 1998; Bhende, 1999; Frakes, 2001). Even when lung sounds cannot be evaluated, capnography will rapidly demonstrate an unplanned extubation by a sudden $P_{et}CO_2$ decrease and loss of the characteristic waveform shape (Frakes, 2001). However, only frank changes in ET tube position are detected by capnographic monitoring. As long as there is a closed inspiratory/expiratory system, the capnogram will maintain a normal shape. Capnography does not detect supraglottic ET tube placement when the cuff seals off the hypopharynx, and it shows bronchial intubation in only about 4% of patients with that misplacement (Deluty & Turndorf, 1993; Werman & Falcone, 1998; Ahrens *et al.*, 1999). A normal waveform with a slowly rising $P_{et}CO_2$ from the associated hypoventilation is more likely to suggest bronchial placement than the waveform shape.

The use of volume-based capnography to detect bronchial intubaton is not widely reported, but should be a fairly sensitive indicator. Evaluation of other ventilatory information, such as lung sounds, inspiratory pressures, and measured volumes, is clinically useful until a radiological confirmation of ET tube position can be made.

Disconnection of the ventilator circuit may demonstrate a change in the capnogram frequency, depending on the patient's spontaneous breathing pattern, and will likely show a $P_{et}CO_2$ change (Frakes, 2001). End-tidal changes in hypoventilating patients precede pulse oximetry changes, and can provide sufficient advance warning to prevent patient deterioration (Miner *et al.*, 2002; Vargo *et al.*, 2002).

The capnogram and $P_{et}CO_2$ values will respond to other abnormalities in the mechanical ventilation circuit as well. They are as follows:

- Partial obstruction of the ET tube can be detected early by waveform changes. The waveform changes from the characteristic square shape to one with a prolonged expiratory upslope or an increasingly sloped alveolar plateau as expiratory resistance increases. These changes will precede changes in the $P_{et}CO_2$ value itself, which requires that the tube be occluded by at least half (Bozeman *et al.*, 1996; Bhende, 1999).
- An expiratory leak in the circuit or the ET tube cuff will result in a premature return of the exhaled waveform to the baseline as well as a loss of the expected square shape (Ward & Yearly, 1998a; Bhende, 1999; Frakes, 2001).
- Lost minute ventilation from an air leak will increase $P_{et}CO_2$ with a normal waveform, while machine failures causing CO_2 rebreathing will both increase $P_{et}CO_2$ and show a rising capnogram baseline (Bozeman *et al.*, 1996; Bhende, 1999; Frakes, 2001).

In addition to monitoring airway technology, capnometry also provides useful physiologic information about ventilation and perfusion that augments patient care during transport. P_aCO_2 levels are affected by both metabolic and ventilatory changes. Ventilation is a primary method of managing acid base balance, and minute ventilation has an inverse relationship with P_aCO_2 (Benumof, 1998; Ward & Yearly, 1998a, b). As both are ventilatory parameters with similar normal values, the use of $ETCO_2$ measurements as a substitute for P_aCO_2 tension is often considered. If this were possible, the advantages of breath-to-breath measurement, avoidance of an arterial puncture, and cost savings would be dramatic. However universal use of capnometry in that fashion is ill advised.

Although the alveolar to end-tidal carbon dioxide gradient [$P_{(alv-et)}CO_2$] is generally 3–5 mmHg, changes in pulmonary dead space and other factors affect the difference. Physiologic dead space is anatomical space other than the pharynx, trachea, and bronchi that is ventilated but not perfused. The $P_{(alv-et)}CO_2$ gradient is an almost perfect measure of that space, widening as dead space increases. The relationship is so effective that it can be used to modify the Bohr equation for the dead space fraction to $V_d/V_t = [P_{(alv-et)}CO_2/P_aCO_2]$ (NFNA, 1995; Kline *et al.*, 1997; Ward & Yearly, 1998a; Frakes, 2001).

When pulmonary blood flow decreases for any reason, dead space increases. Cardiac output is directly related to pulmonary blood flow, so decreased cardiac output increases pulmonary dead space. Causes include cardiac dysfunction, the application of positive end-expiratory pressure (PEEP), and hypovolemia. Pulmonary blood flow can also be decreased by non-cardiac sources, such as pulmonary emboli and patient positioning (Bozeman *et al.*, 1996; Ward & Yearly, 1998a; Bhende, 1999; Frakes, 2001).

Other factors, some of which are likely related at least in part to pulmonary blood flow alterations and some with a less clear physiology, also change the gradient. Age, smoking, general anesthesia, and major systemic disease increase the alveolar to end-tidal difference, and it may be as high as 20 mmHg in patients with severe pulmonary disease. The gradient can also be negative in some cases. That change is common in pregnant women lying supine, in exercising individuals, and it has been found in 8.1% of post-cardiac surgery patients and 4% of multiple trauma patients (Shankar *et al.*, 1986; 1987; Russell *et al.*, 1993; Drew *et al.*, 1998).

Accordingly, overall correlation between P_aCO_2 and $P_{et}CO_2$ is reported between $r = 0.59$ and 0.96, and the literature supporting the use of capnometry to estimate P_aCO_2 tension has similar variability. Correlations between P_aCO_2 and $P_{et}CO_2$ tensions generally are better in patients without lung or systemic disease, and in patients with more stable vital signs. Worsening acuity seems to worsen correlation, as does the use of vasopressors, and patients being monitored during transport generally trend toward higher acuity (Cheng *et al.*, 1986; Morley *et al.*, 1993; Kline *et al.*, 1997; Prause *et al.*, 1997; Sharma *et al.*, 1997). When studied specifically in patients experiencing interhospital transport, correlation was poor ($r = 0.59$), the mean gradient was 12.9, and relationships worsened in patients with underlying disease (Prause *et al.*, 1997). Another chapter in this book (Chapter 23) discusses the relationship of $P_{et}CO_2$ and P_aCO_2 in greater detail.

Single patient correlations have also been found inadequate. After establishing the $P_{(alv-et)}CO_2$ gradient for a patient, 18–27% of subsequent $P_{et}CO_2$ changes failed to match arterial changes (Cheng *et al.*, 1986; Healey *et al.*, 1987; Niehoff *et al.*, 1988; Domsky & Perov, 1993). However, using capnometry to main-tain consistent ventilation has been shown to be useful in some cases, particularly in patients undergoing neurosurgery and in those being transported with closed head injuries (Engoren, 1993; Martin *et al.*, 1997).

It appears that for the relatively short duration of a transport, whether in or out of the hospital, capnometry is a useful part of a complete constellation of patient monitors that can be used to guide maintenance of pre-transport care. Over the course of a transport, a number of variables potentially affecting $P_{(alv-et)}CO_2$ are minimized. Patients are generally maintained in the same position through transport and transport is generally not of a sufficient duration for a substantial metabolic change or the progression of major systemic disease. Accordingly, $ETCO_2$ changes during transport are most likely related to changes in pulmonary blood flow or minute ventilation. If the patient is transported with careful monitoring of blood pressure and cardiogram as a measure of pulmonary blood flow, continuous capnometry should be a good reflection of minute ventilation. When blood pressure and cardiogram are stable, a change in $P_{et}CO_2$ probably reflects a minute ventilation change. Thus, capnometry can be useful in maintaining consistent ventilation. The use of capnometry to establish ventilation parameters without a baseline blood gas or other hemodynamic information and monitors, however, is probably not appropriate.

Evaluating cardiac output and arrest

Another, similar, useful role for capnometry as a supplemental tool, where patient assessment is difficult, is the ability to reflect cardiac output. In the transport environment, if ventilation is consistent, capnometry provides a gross breath-to-breath indicator of cardiac output. If a patient does not have continuous blood pressure monitoring, but has minute ventilation monitoring and pulse oximetry, capnometry can provide a suggestion of changing cardiac output between the cycles of the non-invasive cuff. At the extremes of this are patients in arrest. A number of patients with the so-called pulseless electrical activity (PEA), actually have cardiac activity. More than eight of ten patients believed to be in PEA have synchronous cardiac wall motion, and over 40% have a measurable aortic pulse pressure (Bocka *et al.*, 1988; Paridis *et al.*, 1992; Cantineau *et al.*, 1994). Capnometry can help to distinguish between PEA and very low cardiac output arrest states (Sanders *et al.*, 1985; Isserles & Breen, 1991; Cummings, & Hazinski, 2000). During the course of the arrest, worsening end-tidal values may help to detect rescuer fatigue, and to optimize chest compression (White & Asplin, 1994; Ward & Yealy, 1998a).

Survival from out-of-hospital cardiac arrest is under 3%, and the annual cost of futile resuscitation efforts has been estimated at over $1 billion (Levine *et al.*, 1997). $ETCO_2$ measurements have been found to be useful in evaluating resuscitation efforts. Relying on the correlation between cardiac output and $P_{et}CO_2$, several studies have demonstrated relationships between $ETCO_2$ measurements and outcomes in arrest. Sanders *et al.* (1985) showed that arrest survivors had an average $P_{et}CO_2$ of 18 mmHg 20 min into the arrest, while non-survivors averaged 6 mmHg at the same time. There were no survivors with a value under 10 mmHg. Similarly, another study found that survivors averaged a $P_{et}CO_2$ of 19 mmHg, while non-survivors averaged 5 mmHg. A value of 15 mmHg had the best sensitivity and specificity with a 91% positive and negative predictive value. However, four of the patients resuscitated had values under 10 mmHg (Callaham & Barton, 1990). Rare survivors with low $P_{et}CO_2$ values are not uncommon in the literature and complicate the predictive value of this tool. Others have found no survivors with a $P_{et}CO_2$ under 14 or 10 mmHg (Varon *et al.*, 1991; Cantineau *et al.*, 1994). A large evaluation of 150 arrests showed that a $P_{et}CO_2$ of 10 mmHg or less at 20 min into the resuscitation was 100% sensitive and specific for survival (Levine *et al.*, 1997). In making decisions using capnometry, recall that resuscitation chemistry can change $P_{et}CO_2$ measures. Sodium bicarbonate both contains and produces CO_2, causing a transient $P_{et}CO_2$ rise usually lasting under 2 min (Niemann, 1984; Ward & Yealy, 1998a). High-dose epinephrine administration decreases $P_{et}CO_2$ (Ward & Yealy, 1998a). Another chapter in this book (Chapter 20) discusses the use of capnography in cardiopulmonary resuscitation (CPR) in greater detail.

Potential measurement errors

When using capnography for any clinical decision, the user must be aware of any possible sources of error. Of the potential errors with capnography, two are particularly important in the transport environment: oxygen concentration and altitude.

Patients are more likely to receive high oxygen concentrations during transport. High oxygen concentrations falsely lower $P_{et}CO_2$ reading by up to 10% as interactions between CO_2 and the greater number of oxygen molecules change the infrared absorption of the gas sample. This problem can be minimized by recalibrating the detector with an appropriate reference gas, activating a compensatory selector available on some machines, or by using narrow band infrared sources. (Bozeman *et al.*, 1996; Ward & Yealy, 1998a; Bhende, 1999; Frakes, 2001).

Changes in atmospheric pressure can also be important. Pressure changes vary the intermolecular forces between CO_2 molecules, increasing infrared absorption by about 0.5% for every 1% change in pressure. The error is usually insignificant, as weather-related atmospheric pressure changes are generally under 20 mmHg, or about 2% at sea level (Bozeman *et al.*, 1996; Frakes, 2001). However, pressure-induced variation is a greater possibility outside the hospital, particularly in air transport. A fixed wing aircraft cabin pressurized to 5000 ft represents a pressure change of about 17% from sea level, and would result in a measurement change of around 9%. A transport over mountainous terrain in a non-pressurized cabin could also cause a notable change (Holleran, 1996; Benumof, 1998; Frakes, 2001). This error can be avoided by recalibrating the capnometer at the appropriate altitude or by using a unit that automatically measures and adjusts for the pressure (Bozeman *et al.*, 1996).

Conclusion

Capnography offers monitoring and decision-making advantages during patient transport. As with use in other clinical settings, caution must be exercised in acquiring and interpreting the information, but capnography is helpful in monitoring ventilation circuits, ensuring ET tube placement, and in evaluating cardiac output and arrest states.

References

Ahrens, T., Wijeweera, H. & Ray, S. (1999). Capnography: A key underutilized technology. *Crit. Care Nurse Clin. North Am.*, **11**: 49–62.

American College of Emergency Physicians. Policy statement: Verification of endotracheal tube placement. Available online at http://www.acep.org/index.cfm?id=4293. Accessed 12/18/03.

American Society of Anesthesiologists. (1998–2000). Standards for basic anesthetic monitoring. Available online at: http://asahq.org/standards/02.html and http://www.asahq.org/newsletters/1999/03_99/evolution_0399.html

Beker, A., Ipekoglu, Z. & Tureyen, K., *et al.* (1998). Secondary insults during intrahospital transport of neurosurgical intensive care patients. *Neurosurg. Rev.*, **21**: 98–101.

Benumof, J.L. (1998). Interpretation of capnography. *Am. Assoc. Nurse. Anesth. J.*, **66**: 169–176.

Bhende, M. (1999). Capnography in the pediatric emergency department. *Pediatr. Emerg. Care*, **15**: 64–69.

Bhende, M.S., Thompson, A.E. & Cook, D.R., *et al.* (1992a). Validity of a disposable end-tidal CO_2 detector in verifying endotracheal tube placement in infants and children. *Ann. Emerg. Med.*, **21**: 142–145.

Bhende, M.S., Thompson A.E. & Orr, R.A. (1992b). Utility of an end-tidal CO_2 detector during stabilization and transport of critically ill children. *Pediatrics*, **89**: 1043–1044.

Bocka, J.J., Overton, D.J. & Hauser, A. (1988). Electromechanical dissociation in human beings: an ecohocardiographic evaluation. *Ann. Emerg. Med.*, **17**: 450–452.

Bozeman, W.P., Hexter, D. & Liang, H.K., *et al.* (1996) Esophageal detector device versus detection of end-tidal carbon dioxide level in emergency intubation. *Ann. Emerg. Med.*, **27**: 595–599.

Braman, S.S., Dunn, S.M., Amico, C.A. & Millman, R.P. (1987). Complications of intrahospital transport in critically ill patients. *Ann. Intern. Med.*, **107**: 469–473.

Brown, L.H., Gough, J.E., Bryan-Bert, D.M. & Hunt, R.C. (1997). Assessment of breath sounds during ambulance transport. *Ann. Emerg. Med.*, **29**: 228–231.

Callaham, M. & Barton, C. (1990). Prediction of outcome of cardiopulmonary resuscitation from end-tidal carbon dioxide concentration. *Crit. Care Med.*, **18**: 358–362.

Cantineau, J.P., Merck, P. & Lambert, Y., *et al.* (1994). Effect of epinephrine on end-tidal carbon dioxide pressure during prehospital cardiopulmonary resuscitation. *Am. J. Emerg. Med.*, **12**: 267–270.

Chan, Y.K., Zuraidah, S., Tan, P.S.K. (1998). Use of capnography delaying the diagnosis of tracheal intubation. *Anesthesia*, **53**: 1207–1208.

Cheng, E.Y., Renschler, M.F. & Mihm, F.G., *et al.* (1986). Noninvasive respiratory monitoring of patients weaning from mechanical respiratory support. *Anesth. Analg.*, **65**: S29.

Cummings, R.O., Hazinski, M.F. (eds) (2000). Emergency cardiac care guidelines. *Circulation*, **102(suppl. I)**: I1–I384.

Deluty, S. & Turndorf, H. (1993). Failure of capnography to properly assess ET tube location. *Anesthesiology*, **78**: 783–784.

Domsky, M.F. & Perov, S. (1993). End-tidal carbon dioxide does not reflect arterial carbon dioxide in hemorrhagic shock. *Anesth. Analg.*, **76**: S85.

Drew, K., Brayton, M., Ambrose, A. & Bernard, G. (1998). End-tidal carbon dioxide monitoring for weaning patients: a pilot study. *Dim. Crit. Care Nurs.*, **17**: 127–134.

Edge, W.E., Kanter, R.K., Weigle, C.G. & Walsh, R.F. (1994). Reduction in morbidity in interhospital transport by specialized pediatric staff. *Crit. Care Med.*, **22**: 1186–1191.

Engoren, M. (1993). Efficacy of capnometry in ventilatory management of cardiac patients. *J. Cardiothorac. Vasc. Anesth.*, **7**: 538–540.

Evans, A. & Winslow, E.H. (1995). Oxygen saturation and hemodynamic response in critically ill, mechanically ventilated adults during intrahospital transport. *Am. J. Crit. Care*, **4**: 106–111.

Frakes, M.A. (2001). Measuring end-tidal carbon dioxide: clinical applications and usefulness. *Crit. Care Nurs.*, **21**: 23–37.

Frakes, M.A. (2002). Flight team management of in-place endotracheal tubes. *Air Med. J.*, **21**: 29–31.

Gervais, H.W., Eberle, B. & Konietzke, D., *et al.* (1987). Comparison of blood gases of ventilated patients during transport. *Crit. Care Med.*, **15**: 761–763.

Healey, C.J., Fedullo, A.J. & Swinburne, A.J. (1987). Comparison of noninvasive measurements of carbon dioxide tension during withdrawal from mechanical ventilation. *Crit. Care Med.*, **15**: 764–768.

Holleran, R.S. (1996). *Flight Nursing: Principles and Practice*, 2nd edtion. St. Louis, Mosby.

Hunt, R.C., Bryan, D.M. & Brinkley, S., *et al.* (1991). Inability to assess breath sounds during air medical transport by helicopter. *J. Am. Med. Assoc.*, **265**: 1982–1984.

Hurst, J.M., Davis, K., Branson, R.D. & Johannigman, J.A. (1989). Comparison of blood gases during transport using two methods of ventilatory support. *J. Trauma*, **29**: 1637–1640.

Hurst, J.M., Davis, K. & Johnson, D.J., *et al.*(1992). Cost and complications during in-hospital transport of critically ill patients: a prospective cohort study. *J. Trauma*, **33**: 582–585.

Hussain, S. & Raphael, D.T. (1997). Analysis of a straight-line capnographic waveform. *Anesth. Analg.*, **85**: 463–466.

Indek, M., Peterson, S., Smith, J. & Brotman, S. (1988). Risk, cost, and benefit of transporting ICU patients for special studies. *J. Trauma*, **28**: 1020–1025.

Isserles, S.A. & Breen, P.H. (1991). Can changes in end-tidal pCO_2 measure changes in cardiac output? *Anesth. Analg.*, **73**: 808–814.

Jones, N.L., Robertson, D.G. & Kane, J.W. (1979). Difference between end-tidal and arterial CO_2 in exercise. *J. Appl. Physiol.*, **47**: 954–960.

Katz, S.H., Falk, S.H. & Wash, M. (1998). Misplaced endotracheal tubes by paramedics in an urban emergency medical services system. *Acad. Emerg. Med.*, **5**: 429 [abstract].

Kelly, J.S., Wilhoit, R.D. & Brown, R.E., *et al.* (1992). Efficacy of the FEF colorimetric end-tidal carbon dioxide detector in children. *Anesth. Analg.*, **75**: 45–50.

Kline, J., Meek, S. & Boudrow, D., *et al.* (1997). Use of the alveolar dead space fraction and plasma d-dimers to exclude acute pulmonary embolism in ambulatory patients. *Acad. Emerg. Med.*, **4**: 856–863.

Knapp, S., Kofler, J. & Stoiser, B., *et al.* (1999). The assessment of four different methods to verify tracheal tube placement in the critical care setting. *Anesth. Analg.*, **88**: 766–770.

Levine, R.L., Wayne, M.A. & Miller, C.C. (1997). End-tidal carbon dioxide and outcome of out of hospital cardiac arrest. *New. Engl. J. Med.*, **337**: 301–306.

Li, J. (2001). Capnography alone is imperfect for endotracheal tube placement confirmation during emergency intubation. *J. Emerg. Med.*, **20**: 223–229.

MacLeod, B.A., Heller, M.B. & Gerard, J., *et al.* (1991). Verification of endotracheal tube placement with colorimetric end-tidal CO_2 detection. *Ann. Emerg. Med.*, **20**: 267–270.

Martin, S.E., Agudelo, W.E. & Oschner, M.G. (1997). Monitoring hyperventilation in patients with closed head injury during air transport. *Air. Med. J.*, **16**: 15–18.

Miner, J.R., Heegarard, W. & Plummer, D. (2002). End-tidal carbon dioxide monitoring during procedural sedation. *Acad. Emerg. Med.*, **9**: 275–280.

Morley, T.F., Giaimo, J. & Maroszan, E., *et al.* (1993). Use of capnography for assessment of the adequacy of alveolar ventilation during weaning from mechanical ventilation. *Am. Rev. Respir. Dis.*, **148**: 339–344.

National Association of Emergency Medical Services Physicians. Position paper: Verification of endotracheal tube placement following intubation. Available online at http://www.naemsp.org. Accessed 12/18/03.

National Flight Nurses Association (1995). *Flight Nurse Advanced Trauma Course.* NFNA, Des Plaines, IL.

Niehoff, J., DelGuercio, C. & LaMorte, W., *et al.* (1988). Efficacy of pulse oximetry and capnometry in postoperative ventilatory weaning. *Crit. Care. Med.*, **16**: 701–705.

Niemann, J.T. (1984). Effects of acidemia and sodium bicarbonate therapy in advanced cardiac life support. *Ann. Emerg. Med.*, **13**: 781–782.

Paridis, N.A., Martin, G.B. & Goetting, M.G., *et al.* (1992). Aortic pressure during human cardiac arrest: identification of pseudo-electromechanical dissociation. *Chest*, **101**: 123–128.

Patel, S.B., Callahan, T.F. & Callahan, M.G., *et al.* (1998). An adaptive noise reduction stethoscope for auscultation in high noise environments. *J. Acoust. Soc. Am.*, **103**: 2483–2491.

Prause, G., Hetz, H. & Lauda P., *et al.* (1997). A comparison of the end-tidal CO_2 documented by capnometry and the arterial pCO_2 in emergency patients. *Resuscitation*, **35**: 145–148.

Price, T.G. & Goldsmith, L.J. (1998). Changes in hearing acuity in ambulance personnel. *Prehosp. Emerg. Care*, **2**: 308–311.

Puntervoll, S.A., Soreide, E., Jacewicz, W. & Bjelland, E. (2002). Rapid detection of oesophageal intubation: take care when using colorimetric capnometry. *Acta Anaesthesiol. Scand.*, **46**: 455–457.

Rogovin, C., Hamm, M.L. Airway management and rapid sequence intubation. In: Arndt, K. (ed.) Air and surface transport nurses association standards for critical care and specialty rotor-wing transport. Lexington, KY: Myers; 2003. p. 15.

Russell, G.B., Graybeal, J.M. & Strout, J.C. (1993). Stability of arterial to end-tidal carbon dioxide gradients during postoperative cardiorespiratory support. *Can. J. Anaesth.*, **40**: 206–210.

Sanders, A.B., Ewy, G.A. & Bragg, S., *et al.* (1985). Expired pCO_2 as a prognostic indicator of successful resuscitation from cardiac arrest. *Ann. Emerg. Med.*, **14**: 948–955.

Shankar, K.B., Moseley, H., Kumar, Y., *et al.* (1986). Arterial to end tidal carbon dioxide tension difference during cesarean section anesthesia. *Anaesthesia*, **41**: 698–702.

Shankar, K.B., Moseley, H., Kumar, Y., *et al.* (1987). Arterial to end tidal carbon dioxide tension difference during anesthesia for tubal ligation. *Anaesthesia*, **42**: 482–486.

Sharma, S.K., McGuire, G.P. & Cruise, C.J.E. (1995). Stability of the arterial to end-tidal carbon dioxide difference during anesthesia for prolonged neuro-surgical procedures. *Can. J. Anaesth.*, **42**: 498–503.

Stearley, H.E. (1998). Patient outcomes: intrahospital transportation and monitoring of critically ill patients by a specially trained ICU nursing staff. *Am. J. Crit. Care*, **7**: 282–287.

Stewart, R.D., Paris, P.M. & Winter, P.M., *et al.* (1985). Field endotracheal intubation by paramedical personnel: success rates and complications. *Chest*, **253**: 2373–2377.

Szem, J., Hydo, L. & Fischer, E., *et al.* (1995). High-risk intrahospital transport of critically ill patients. *Crit. Care Med.*, **23**: 1660–1666.

Vargo, J.J., Zuccaro, G. & Dumont, J.A., *et al.* (2002). Automated graphic assessment of respiratory activity is superior to pulse oximetry and visual assessment for the detection of early respiratory depression during therapeutic upper endoscopy. *Gastrointest. Endosc.*, **55**: 826–831.

Varon, A.J., Morrina, J. & Civetta, J.M. (1991). Clinical utility of a colorimetric end-tidal CO_2 detector in cardiopulmonary resuscitation and emergency intubation. *J. Clin. Monit.*, **7**: 289–293.

Ward, K.R. & Yealy, D.M. (1998a). End-tidal carbon dioxide monitoring in emergency medicine. Part 2: Clinical applications. *Acad. Emerg. Med.*, **5**: 637–646.

Ward, K.R. & Yealy, D.M. (1998b). End-tidal carbon dioxide monitoring in emergency medicine. Part 1: Basic principles. *Acad. Emerg. Med.*, **5**: 628–636.

Waydhas, C., Schneck, G. & Duswald, K.H. (1995). Deterioration of respiratory function after intrahospital transport of critically ill surgical patients. *Intens. Care Med.*, **21**: 784–789.

Werman, H.A. & Falcone, R.E. (1998). Glottic positioning of the ET tube tip: a diagnostic dilemma. *Ann. Emerg. Med.*, **31**: 643–646.

White, R.D. & Asplin, B.R. (1994). Out of hospital quantitative monitoring of end-tidal carbon dioxide pressure during CPR. *Ann. Emerg. Med.*, **23**: 25–30.

CAPNOGRAPHY AS A GUIDE TO VENTILATION IN THE FIELD

9

D.P. Davis

Introduction

It has become increasingly apparent that partial pressure of end-tidal carbon dioxide ($P_{et}CO_2$) monitoring is a necessary tool for guiding ventilation of patients in the prehospital setting. In fact, recent data suggest that hyperventilation may be at least as detrimental as hypoxia in patients with severe traumatic brain injury (TBI) (Davis *et al.*, 2004a; b). The unique challenges of the prehospital environment dictate the requirements for an ideal $P_{et}CO_2$ monitor. Clearly, the device must be rugged and lightweight, with a long battery life. Displays must be visible in both bright sun and at night, and the ideal device should be portable enough to remove from the ambulance or aircraft and carry to the patient. The limited training and experience of many prehospital personnel necessitate simplicity. Lastly, the cost of such a device becomes an important issue. In an intensive care unit (ICU) or operating room, $P_{et}CO_2$ monitoring is performed on a daily basis, justifying the cost of a sophisticated monitor. In a prehospital system, each ambulance or aircraft must be supplied with a device for use in the relatively infrequent event of an intubation, resulting in a lower "bang for the buck".

Throughout this chapter, it is important to keep in mind the differences between $P_{et}CO_2$, alveolar CO_2 (P_ACO_2) and arterial partial pressure of carbon dioxide (P_aCO_2), as extremes of temperature and altitude and the potential for sensor interference by condensation or various body fluids may significantly affect the performance of these devices (Bhende & LaCovey, 2001). Here we present the evidence for use of $P_{et}CO_2$ monitoring to guide prehospital ventilation and review each type of device available, discussing the advantages and disadvantages of each.

Evidence for prehospital $P_{et}CO_2$ monitoring

Avoiding hyperventilation

Perhaps the best justification for $P_{et}CO_2$ monitoring in the out-of-hospital environment is to avoid the detrimental effects of hyperventilation, especially in the setting of TBI. The ability of hyperventilation to decrease intracranial pressure (ICP) was recognized several decades ago, leading to its routine use in treating intracranial hypertension (Whitwam *et al.*, 1966; Rossanda, 1968; Johnston *et al.*, 1970; Cruz, 1993). Unfortunately, the lowering of ICP from a decrease in cerebral blood volume comes at the expense of an even greater decrease in cerebral blood flow, potentially leading to ischemia (Stringer *et al.*, 1993; Skippen *et al.*, 1997; Forbes *et al.*, 1998; Bao *et al.*, 2000). While global measures of cerebral perfusion may or may not fall below the ischemic threshold, regional and local ischemia has been documented with even a moderate degree of hyperventilation (McLaughlin & Marion, 1996; Ausina *et al.*, 1998; Schneider *et al.*, 1998; Coles *et al.*, 2002; Imberti *et al.*, 2002; Marion *et al.*, 2002). More importantly, a randomized trial documented an increase in mortality with routine use of hyperventilation (PCO_2 target of 25 mmHg) in patients with severe TBI (Muizelaar *et al.*, 1991). This has led to recommendations against the routine use of hyperventilation in severe TBI except for refractory ICP elevation or impending herniation (The Brain Trauma Foundation, 2000).

It is important to note that in this randomized trial, hyperventilation was performed over the first 5 days of admission, and the significance of a relatively brief period of prehospital hyperventilation is unclear (Muizelaar, 1991). Recent evidence suggests that hyperventilation leads to ischemia almost immediately, with a decrease in cerebral perfusion below ischemic levels and a rise in extracellular glutamate and lactate within the first half-hour (Bao, 2000; Marion, 2002; Sarrafzadeh *et al.*, 2002). In addition, current models of both ischemic and TBI suggest an immediate period during which the brain is especially vulnerable to secondary insults (Forbes *et al.*, Marion *et al.*, Van Santbrink *et al.*, 2003). This underscores the importance of avoiding hyperventilation in the prehospital environment.

A recently completed prospective trial evaluated the impact of paramedic rapid sequence intubation (RSI) on outcome in patients with severe TBI (Davis *et al.*,

2003; Davis *et al.*, submitted). Each trial patient was matched to two non-intubated, historical controls from the County trauma registry on the following parameters: age, gender, mechanism of injury, trauma center, and abbreviated injury scores (AIS) for head/neck, face, chest, abdomen, extremities, and skin. There were no statistically significant differences between trial patients and controls with regard to the matching parameters, arrival vital signs, base deficit, incidence of invasive procedures (craniotomy, thoracotomy, or laparotomy), or the actual head-injury diagnoses on computed tomography (contusion, subdural hematoma, epidural hematoma, subarachnoid hemorrhage, cerebral edema, or skull fracture). Over 98% of trial patients were successfully intubated with either an endotracheal (ET) tube or a combitube, and less than 1% of patients were hypoxic upon arrival. Nevertheless, the mortality in trial patients was 32% versus only 24% for matched controls (Davis *et al.*, 2003; Davis *et al.*, submitted).

Two of the most important clues as to the potential cause of this mortality increase with paramedic RSI were revealed through analysis of data downloaded from handheld capnometer/oximeter devices. Most paramedics were given standardized ventilation parameters (800 cc tidal volume at 12 breaths per minute) and were allowed to practice with a spirometer and stopwatch during the training session. One agency instituted the use of capnometry/oximetry during the trial period, with paramedics instructed to target an $P_{et}CO_2$ value of 30–35 mmHg and to avoid values below 25 mmHg. Data from these devices revealed a high incidence of desaturations during the RSI procedure and routine hypocapnia despite the target parameters (Dunford *et al.*, 2003; Davis *et al.*, 2004a, b, c). Logistic regression analysis revealed a strong association between $P_{et}CO_2$ and mortality, and matched controls analysis revealed an adverse effect of both low $P_{et}CO_2$ values and severe desaturations defined as pulse oxygen saturation (SpO_2) values below 70%. Subsequent analysis documented an association between arrival $P_{et}CO_2$ and outcome, confirming the importance of prehospital ventilation parameters on the injured brain (Davis *et al.*, submitted).

Does $P_{et}CO_2$ monitoring avoid hyperventilation?

In theory, the presence of $P_{et}CO_2$ data should lead to a low incidence of hyperventilation, regardless of whether manual or mechanical ventilation is used. Thus, the high incidence of hypocapnia we observed despite the presence of capnometry to guide ventilation has led to concerns that these devices do not prevent hyperventilation (Davis *et al.*, 2004c). Indeed, multiple investigators have observed a high incidence of hypocapnia in the prehospital environment, especially with manual ventilation (Braman *et al.*, 1987; Gervais *et al.*, 1987; Hurst *et al.*, 1989; Tobias *et al.*, 1996; Helm *et al.*, 2002; Thomas *et al.*, 2002). In a separate analysis, however, a lower incidence of arrival hypocapnia was documented ($PCO_2 < 25$ mmHg) in patients undergoing capnometry (Davis *et al.*, 2004b). Furthermore, the lowest rates of arrival hypocapnia were documented in patients transported by aeromedical crews, who have been using capnometry for many years. Interestingly, the cohort of patients intubated by ground paramedics but transported by aeromedical crews was the only group with improved outcomes versus matched controls (Poste *et al.*, 2004). This suggests that $P_{et}CO_2$-guided ventilation requires some degree of experience but that hyperventilation can be avoided with use of capnometry.

It is useful to inspect the ventilation patterns we observed with paramedics using capnometry (Davis *et al.*, 2004c). A linear relationship was observed between respiratory rate and $P_{et}CO_2$ value. The mean value for maximum ventilation rate was quite elevated at 36 breaths per minute, with a mean minimum $P_{et}CO_2$ value of 23.6 mmHg. Nevertheless, combined values for $P_{et}CO_2$ over time reveal an upswing toward the end of the prehospital course, suggesting that paramedics were eventually able to utilize the capnometry data to slow respiratory rate and achieve a less detrimental $P_{et}CO_2$ value (Figure 9.1). A sample graph demonstrating very mild hyperventilation is displayed in Figure 9.2. Of note, a deep desaturation with bradycardia is also documented for this particular patient.

The potential reasons for prehospital hyperventilation merit some discussion. In one study, hypocapneic patients were more significantly injured, with lower $P_{et}CO_2$ values associated with higher head/neck AIS, lower arrival systolic blood pressure (SBP), and lower post-intubation SpO_2 values (Davis *et al.*, 2004b). Thus, the excitement and anxiety of caring for critical patients may result in a natural tendency toward excessively high respiratory rates. This did not appear to be an attempt to raise SpO_2 values, as there was not an association between SpO_2 and respiratory rate (Davis *et al.*, 2004c). It is also possible that the tendency toward hyperventilation despite $P_{et}CO_2$ monitoring reflects the residual belief in its therapeutic benefits on the injured brain. The occurrence of prehospital hyperventilation also reflects a failure of the scientific community to recognize the importance of optimal ventilation in the immediate post-injury

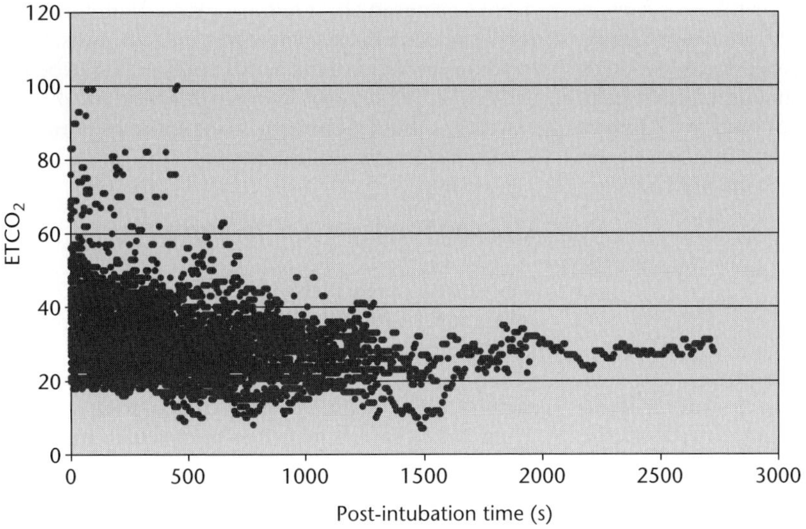

Figure 9.1 Combined data for all patients undergoing capnometry as part of the San Diego Paramedic RSI Trial. Hypocapnia was extremely common, with end-tidal CO_2 ($ETCO_2$) values below 25 mmHg in over half of all patients. Note the upswing in $ETCO_2$ values at the end of the prehospital course. (Adapted from Davis *et al.*, 2004c.)

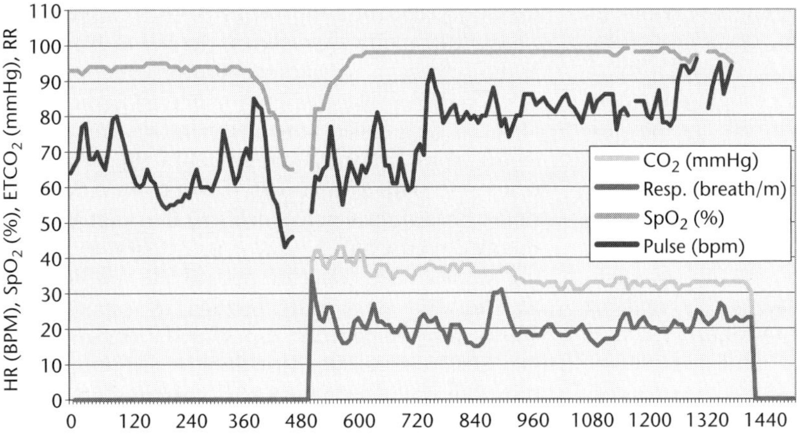

Figure 9.2 Sample capnometry-oximetry graph from patient with severe head trauma undergoing RSI by paramedics. Note the deep desaturation with corresponding bradycardia prior to intubation.

period. Additional research and education should focus on these issues.

Avoiding injurious ventilation

While $P_{et}CO_2$-guided ventilation may appear to have the most direct impact on avoiding the reflex cerebral vasoconstriction in response to hypocapnia, it is possible that lower $P_{et}CO_2$ values are a surrogate marker for injurious ventilation patterns that may ultimately play a greater role in patient outcomes. Positive-pressure ventilation leads to a rise in intrathoracic pressure, which may decrease cerebral perfusion by obstructing venous return and lowering cardiac output (Pepe *et al.*, 2002). In addition, an elevated mean intrathoracic pressure can be transmitted in a retrograde fashion via the jugular venous system, leading to a paradoxical rise in ICP. Hyperventilation, especially when produced by high respiratory rates, can quickly raise intrathoracic pressure and exacerbate hypocapnia-driven ischemia.

In addition to its effects on cerebral and systemic hemodynamics, overaggressive ventilation can be detrimental to the critically ill patient through pro-inflammatory cytokine release, bacterial endotoxin translocation, and endothelial cell apoptosis (Tremblay *et al.*, 1997; Chiumello *et al.*, 1999; ARDS Network, 2000; Slutsky & Ranieri, 2000; Uhlig, 2002; Zhang *et al.*, 2002; Imai *et al.*, 2003; Wilson *et al.*, 2003). Data from the ICU document an increase in multi-organ dysfunction syndrome and death with high tidal volumes and absence of positive end-expiratory pressure (PEEP).

The most profound rise in injurious cytokines occurs in the first hour of ventilation, an observation with significance to prehospital personnel. While $P_{et}CO_2$ is not a substitute for airway pressure monitoring, it is likely that the high ventilation rates and low $P_{et}CO_2$ values observed in previous studies represent injurious ventilation patterns, especially without the use of PEEP.

Devices available

Colorimetric capnometry

Qualitative capnometry is the simplest form of $P_{et}CO_2$ monitoring available, with a limited ability to guide ventilation. Qualitative capnometers rely on the tendency of CO_2 to form acid in solution. A paper filter impregnated with dyes that change color with lower pH values is the basis for this technology. When exhaled gasses pass through this filter, the resultant filter color change indicates the presence of CO_2, confirming tracheal positioning of the ET tube. Although the intensity of color change provides a crude estimate as to the CO_2 concentration, the inability to determine an accurate value for $P_{et}CO_2$ and the poor sensitivity in detecting breath-to-breath changes prohibit the use of these devices to guide ventilation. If concerns arise that the ET tube has become misplaced, however, the qualitative capnometer can be used again to reconfirm tracheal placement, although the absence of color change might indicate that the qualitative capnometer is no longer usable. Details regarding the use of qualitative capnometry to confirm ET tube placement are provided elsewhere in this book.

Semi-quantitative capnometry

In recent years, several semi-quantitative capnometers that provide a rough estimate of $P_{et}CO_2$ have been developed for prehospital use. Rather than provide an actual $P_{et}CO_2$ value, however, a series of stacked bars are used, with each bar representing an approximate range of $P_{et}CO_2$ values. The manufacturers recommend a target number of bars as reflective of an optimal $P_{et}CO_2$ range; additional bars represents hypercapnia, while a lower number of bars represents hypocapnia. These devices are simple to use, rugged, lightweight, and relatively inexpensive.

Semi-quantitative capnometry can be used to initially confirm tracheal positioning of an ET tube. It remains to be seen, however, as to whether use of these devices leads to optimized ventilation and better outcomes. The technology by which CO_2 concentration is measured is not as accurate, with hypo and hypercapnia a possibility even if the target number of bars is achieved. In addition, prehospital personnel might not find the system of stacked bars as useful in guiding ventilation as an actual number. Nevertheless, their affordability could lead to widespread use. Future research should determine their ultimate utility in avoiding extremes of ventilation.

Quantitative capnometry

The most accurate method of measuring $P_{et}CO_2$ concentration involves continuous infrared spectrophotometric analysis of expired gasses, either with a diverting (side-stream) or non-diverting (main-stream) method. Quantitative capnometry has great potential in guiding ventilation in the prehospital arena. An end-tidal value is provided for each breath, with multiple studies demonstrating reasonable clinical accuracy. It is important to understand, however, the physiological limitations to this method, especially with use of a side-stream sampling port. The most physiologically pertinent estimate of $P_{et}CO_2$ is derived from a sample of expired gas taken at the end of expiration, as this represents the closest approximation to alveolar gas. This becomes increasingly important in the setting of auto-PEEP, either from intrinsic airway constriction or resistance to expiration created by the airway circuit itself. With greater obstruction to flow, the expiratory phase is prolonged, delaying the point at which the measured expired value comes closest to reflecting alveolar CO_2 concentration. While this does not significantly affect interpretation of capnography, where this phenomenon can easily be recognized, it may underestimate the true alveolar CO_2 concentration with use of a capnometer, depending on clinical circumstances. Particularly in patients with obstructive lung disease – as discussed extensively elsewhere in this book – the reported $P_{et}CO_2$ might not reflect alveolar concentrations of CO_2, resulting in a large, undetected arterial to $P_{et}CO_2$ difference.

More sophisticated capnometry permits for the capture of volumetric data, allowing for measurements of $P_{et}CO_2$ and respiratory rate to be combined with those for tidal volume and minute ventilation. Clearly, this would allow optimal control of ventilation, potentially minimizing the adverse effects of both hypocapnia and barotrauma. These devices are currently more expensive and less portable, limiting their prehospital application. As a result, there are few data on their out-of-hospital use. It is likely that they will evolve and become an important part of field ventilation, however, and educational strategies designed to introduce capnometry to prehospital personnel should consider incorporating their principles to facilitate their future integration.

Using the waveform

Capnography, the graphical representation of the CO_2 concentration throughout the breath, provides the most information currently available with regard to adequacy of ventilation. In addition, specific patterns can be easily recognized, allowing for early diagnosis of certain conditions and potential problems with ventilation. Perhaps the most important application of capnography in this regard is the early recognition of auto-PEEP from a variety of etiologies. "Stacking" of breaths due to a combination of a prolonged expiratory phase and excessively high respiratory rates is easily identified.

Several capnography patterns can provide valuable clues as to the underlying pathophysiology. A tension pneumothorax or rigid chest wall from significant burns can produce a characteristic pattern of a shortened expiratory phase in combination with a decrease in compliance or increase in peak airway pressures. A cuff leak will result in a gradual downslope replacing the expiratory plateau. A right mainstem intubation can lead to a relatively high, narrow expiratory complex. Most concerning is a sudden absence or truncated expiratory complex, indicating proximal migration of the ET tube into the hypopharynx. Examples of these waveforms are displayed elsewhere in this text.

Recommended prehospital use of end-tidal carbon dioxide monitoring

Guiding ventilation

The primary role for $P_{et}CO_2$ monitoring in EMS is to guide ventilation during transport; applications such as the use of $P_{et}CO_2$ monitoring for ET tube confirmation and CPR are discussed in other chapters. Although the optimal target $P_{et}CO_2$ value has not yet been defined, the most important consideration is to avoid hypocapnia. The measured value for $P_{et}CO_2$ appears to underestimate P_aCO_2 by approximately 5 mmHg, depending upon the metabolic state, dilution of $P_{et}CO_2$ by dead space gasses with higher respiratory rates, and degree of underlying lung disease in a given patient. Thus, a target $P_{et}CO_2$ value of 35 mmHg is recommended, which is above the physiologic threshold for the initiation of brain ischemia (Coles *et al.*, 2002). It is interesting to note that improved outcomes versus matched controls were observed with higher $P_{et}CO_2$ and arrival PCO_2 values, a pattern that continued into the range of hypercapnia (Davis *et al.*, 2004a, b; Davis *et al.*, submitted). This is consistent with recent evidence suggesting that permissive hypercapnia may lead to increased cerebral perfusion and improved outcomes (Manley *et al.*, 2000). Again, these data may reflect higher $P_{et}CO_2$ and P_aCO_2 values as surrogate markers for non-injurious ventilation strategies.

Strategies must be developed to modify ventilation parameters in response to capnometry data. The propensity of prehospital personnel to use excessively high respiratory rates suggests that the number of breaths per minute should be decreased first in response to hypocapnia (Davis *et al.*, 2004c). On the other hand, the mounting evidence against tidal volumes in excessive of 10 cc/kg, especially in the absence of PEEP, would suggest that hypocapnia be addressed by lower volume ventilation (Tremblay *et al.*, 1997; Chiumello *et al.*, 1999; ARDS Network, 2000; Slutsky & Ranieri, 2000; Uhlig, 2002; Zhang *et al.*, 2002; Imai *et al.*, 2003; Wilson *et al.*, 2003). This provides some justification for volumetric capnometry, which allows optimal tidal volume and respiratory rate parameters to be achieved in association with eucapnia.

The application of $P_{et}CO_2$-guided ventilation by prehospital personnel represents a fundamental departure from traditional ventilation strategies, which were either undefined or incorporated the use of estimated tidal volumes and respiratory rates. Thus, significant education must accompany the introduction of field $P_{et}CO_2$ monitoring. As discussed above, there appears to be a learning curve associated with this ventilation strategy (Davis *et al.*, 2004b). In addition, the increased vigilance required for optimal capnometry-guided ventilation may exceed the capabilities of a small team of prehospital personnel. Thus, it remains to be seen whether further experience with these devices will result in normocapnia and improved patient outcomes or if ventilators will ultimately be required to achieve target ventilation parameters.

A lower target $P_{et}CO_2$ may be justified in a patient with suspected transtentorial herniation. Clinical evidence that could justify a target $P_{et}CO_2$ value as low as 25 mmHg includes a non-reactive pupil or hypertension with bradycardia, suggesting markedly elevated ICP. It is doubtful, however, that a patient with signs of herniation in the immediate post-injury period will be salvageable with or without hyperventilation. In addition, other strategies for ICP control, such as the use of hypertonic saline or mannitol, may have more benefit without the associated risk of ischemia.

Troubleshooting

Sudden changes in either the $P_{et}CO_2$ value or the expiratory complex on capnography can indicate an immediate problem, such as tension pneumothorax or misplacement of the ET tube. Unusual expiratory complex morphology may suggest underlying lung disease or a problem with the airway circuit, such as a ruptured ET tube cuff or excessive airway resistance.

End-tidal CO_2 monitoring with ventilators

Ventilators offer several advantages to the prehospital provider and will likely play a larger role in the future of out-of-hospital medicine (Austin *et al.*, 2002). Ventilators are far more precise with regard to the delivered tidal volume and desired respiratory rate. Thus, capnometers can be most useful when determining optimal parameters upon initiation of mechanical ventilation. Any subsequent change in $P_{et}CO_2$ should then initiate a search for problems with the patient or the airway circuit. In addition, ventilators permit hands-free airway management, allowing more attention to be given to patient care and monitoring. Finally, mechanical ventilators allow more sophisticated modes of ventilation, including spontaneous respirations that can restore the negative intrathoracic pressure that accompanies inspiration, augmenting venous return and preventing the rise in ICP associated with positive-pressure ventilation (Austin *et al.*, 2002). In this situation, $P_{et}CO_2$ monitoring can be used to determine whether an under-sedated patient is "over-breathing" the ventilator. In addition to the specific capnographic patterns noted above, an erratic pattern of normal expiratory complexes intercalated with small, narrow complexes indicate an under-sedated patient who is coughing or "bucking" against the ventilator. A change in ventilator mode, the administration of a sedative, or neuromuscular blockade can reverse this pattern.

Summary

A growing body of literature suggests that prehospital ventilation patterns are of utmost importance in the management of the critically ill patient. The detrimental effects of hyperventilation on the injured brain, the hemodynamic compromise that accompanies positive-pressure ventilation, and injurious ventilation strategies are all potential contributors to outcome in intubated patients. Furthermore, the initial resuscitation period appears to be extremely important in this regard. Advances in the technology for $P_{et}CO_2$ monitoring, including both capnometry and capnography, has allowed these devices to be small and durable enough to be carried into the field, where they can help avoid hyperventilation and injurious ventilation strategies.

References

ARDS Network (2000). Ventilation with lower tidal volumes as compared with traditional tidal volumes for acute lung injury and the acute respiratory distress syndrome. *New Engl. J. Med.*, **342**: 1301–1308.

Ausina, A., Baguena, M. Nadal, M., Manrique, S., Ferrer, A., Sahuquillo, J. & Garnacho, A. (1998). Cerebral hemodynamic changes during sustained hypocapnia in severe head injury: can hyperventilation cause cerebral ischemia? *Acta Neurochir.* **Suppl.** (Wien). **71**: 1–4.

Austin, P.N., Campbell, R.S., Johannigman, J.A. & Branson, R.D. (2002). Transport ventilators. *Respir. Care Clin.*, **8**: 119–150.

Bao, Y., Jiang, J., Zhu, C., Lu, Y., Cai, R. & Ma, C. (2000). Effect of hyperventilation on brain tissue oxygen pressure, carbon dioxide pressure, pH value and intracranial pressure during intracranial hypertension in pigs. *Chin. J. Traumatol.*, **3**: 210–213.

Bhende, M.S. & LaCovey, D.C. (2001). End-tidal carbon dioxide monitoring in the prehospital setting. *Prehosp. Emerg. Care*, **5**: 208–213.

Braman, S.S., Dunn, S.M. & Amieo, C.A. (1987). Complications of intrahospital transport in critically ill patients. *Ann. Int. Med.*, **107**: 469–473.

Chiumello, D., Pristine, G. & Slutsky, A.S. (1999). Mechanical ventilation affects local and systemic cytokines in an animal model of acute respiratory distress syndrome. *Am. J. Respir. Care Med.*, **160**: 109–116.

Coles, J.P., Minhas, P.S., Fryer, T.D., Smielewski, P., Aigbirihio, F., Donovan, T., Downey, S.P., Williams, G., Chatfield, D., Matthews, J.C., Gupta, A.K., Carpenter, T.A., Clark, J.C., Pickard, J.D. & Menon, D.K. (2002). Effect of hyperventilation on cerebral blood flow in traumatic head injury: clinical relevance and monitoring correlates. *Crit. Care Med.*, **30**: 1950–1959.

Cruz, J. (1993). Combined continuous monitoring of systemic and cerebral oxygenation in acute brain injury: preliminary observations. *Crit. Care Med.*, **21**: 1225–1232.

Davis, D.P., Dunford, J.V., Hoyt, D.B., Ochs, M., Holbrook, T. & Fortlage, D. (2004). The impact of hypoxia and hyperventilation on outcome following paramedic rapid sequence intubation of patients with severe traumatic brain injury. *J. Trauma* [in press].

Davis, D.P., Dunford, J.V., Ochs, M., Park, K. & Hoyt, D.B. (2004). The use of quantitative end-tidal capnometry to avoid inadvertent severe hyperventilation in head-injured patients following paramedic rapid sequence intubation. *J. Trauma*, **56**: 808–814.

Davis, D.P., Dunford, J.V., Ochs, M., Heister, R. & Hoyt, D.B. (2004). Ventilation patterns in patients with severe traumatic brain injury following paramedic rapid sequence intubation. *Neuro. Crit. Care* [in press].

Davis, D.P., Hoyt, D.B., Ochs, M., Fortlage, D., Holbrook, T., Marshall, L.K. & Rosen, P. (2003). The effect of paramedic rapid sequence intubation on outcome in patients with severe traumatic brain injury. *J. Trauma*, **54**: 444–453.

Davis, D.P., Ochs, M. & Poste, J.C., *et al.* (2004). Paramedic rapid sequence intubation of patients with severe traumatic brain injury is associated with an increase in mortality [submitted].

Dunford, J.V., Davis, D.P., Ochs, M., Doney, M. & Hoyt, D.B. (2003). The incidence of transient hypoxia and heart rate reactivity during paramedic rapid sequence intubation. *Ann. Emerg. Med.*, **42**: 721–728.

Forbes, M.L., Clark, R.S., Dixon, C.E., Graham, S.H., Marion, D.W., DeKosky, S.T., Schiding, J.K. & Kochanek, P.M. (1988). Augmented neuronal death in CA3 hippocampus following hyperventilation early after controlled cortical impact. *J. Neurosurg.*, **88**: 549–556.

Gervais, H.W., Eberle, B., Konietzke, D., Hennes, H.J. & Dick, W. (1987). Comparison of blood gases of ventilated patients during transport. *Crit. Care Med.*, **15**: 761–763.

Helm, M., Hauke, J. & Lampl, L. (2002). A prospective study of the quality of pre-hospital emergency ventilation in patients with severe head injury. *Br. J. Anaesth.*, **88**: 345–349.

Hurst, J.M., Davis, K., Branson, R. & Johannigman, J.A. (1989). Comparison of blood gases during transport using two methods of ventilatory support. *J. Trauma*, **29**: 1637–1640.

Imai, Y., Parodo, J., Kajikawa, O., de Perrot, M., Fischer, S., Edwards, V., Cutz, E., Liu, M., Keshavjee, S., Martin, T.R., Marshall, J.C., Ranieri, V.M. & Slutsky, A.S. (2003). Injurious mechanical ventilation and end-organ epithelial cell apoptosis and organ dysfunction in an experimental model of acute respiratory distress syndrome. *J. Am. Med. Assoc.*, **289**: 2104–2112.

Imberti, R., Bellinzona, G. & Langer, M. (2002). Cerebral tissue PO_2 and $SjvO_2$ changes during moderate hyperventilation in patients with severe traumatic brain injury. *J. Neurosurg.*, **96**: 97–102.

Johnston, I.H., Johnston, J.A. & Jennett, B. (1970). Intracranial-pressure changes following head injury. *Lancet*, **2**: 433–436.

Manley, G.T., Hemphill, J.C., Morabito, D., Derugin, N., Erickson, V., Pitts, L.H. & Knudson, M.M. (2000). Cerebral oxygenation during hemorrhagic shock: perils of hyperventilation and the therapeutic potential of hypoventilation. *J. Trauma*, **48**: 1025–1033.

Marion, D.W., Puccio, A., Wisniewski, S.R., Kochanek, P., Dixon, C.E., Bullian, L. & Carlier, P. (2002). Effect of hyperventilation on extracellular concentrations of glutamate, lactate, pyruvate, and local cerebral blood flow in patients with severe traumatic brain injury. *Crit. Care Med.*, **30**: 2619–2625.

McLaughlin, M.R. & Marion, D.W. (1996). Cerebral blood flow and vasoresponsivity within and around cerebral contusions. *J. Neurosurg.*, **85**: 871–876.

Muizelaar, J.P., Marmarou, A., Ward, J.D., Kontos, H.A., Choi, S.C., Becker, D.P., Gruemer, H. & Young, H.F. (1991). Adverse effects of prolonged hyperventilation in patients with severe head injury: a randomized clinical trial. *J. Neurosurg.*, **75**: 731–739.

Pepe, P.E., Raedler, C., Lurie, K.G. & Wigginton, J.G. (2002). In: Brasel K, (ed.) *Emergency Ventilatory Management in Severe Hemorrhagic States: Elemental or Detrimental?* American Association for the Surgery of Trauma. Orlando, FL; University of Vermont; p. 80.

Poste, J.C., Davis, D.P., Hoyt, D.B. & Ochs, M. (2004). Air medical transport of severely head-injured patients undergoing paramedic rapid sequence intubation. *Air Med. J.*, **23**: 36–40.

Rossanda, M. (1968). Prolonged hyperventilation in treatment of unconscious patients with severe brain injuries. *Scand. J. Clin. Lab. Invest.*, **Suppl. 102**: XIII, E.

Sarrafzadeh, A.S., Sakowitz, O.W., Callsen, T.A., Lanksch, W.R. & Unterberg, A.W. (2002). Detection of secondary insults by brain tissue PO_2 and bedside microdialysis in severe head injury. *Acta Neurochir.*, **Suppl. 81**: 319–321.

Schneider, G.H., Sarrafzadeh, A.S., Kiening, K.L., Bardt, T.F., Unterberg, A.W. & Lanksch, W.R. (1998). Influence of hyperventilation on brain tissue-PO_2, PCO_2, and pH in patients with intracranial hypertension. *Acta Neurochir.*, **Suppl. 71**: 62–65.

Skippen, P., Seear, M., Poskitt, K., Kestle, J., Cochrane, D., Annich, G. & Handel, J. (1997). Effect of hyperventilation on regional cerebral blood flow in head-injured children. *Crit. Care Med.*, **25**: 1402–1409.

Slutsky, A.S. & Ranieri, V.M. (2000). Mechanical ventilation: lessons from the ARDSNet trial. *Respir. Res.*, **1**: 73–77.

Stringer, W.A., Hasso, A.N., Thompson, J.R., Hinshaw, D.B. & Jordan, K.G. (1993). Hyperventilation-induced cerebral ischemia in patients with acute brain lesions: demonstration by xenon-enhanced CT. *Am. J. Neuroradiol.*, **14**: 475–484.

The Brain Trauma Foundation (2000). The American Association of Neurological Surgeons. The Joint Section on Neurotrauma and Critical Care. Initial management. *J. Neurotrauma*, **17**: 463–469.

Thomas, S.H., Orf, J., Wedel, S.K. & Conn, A.K. (2002). Hyperventilation in traumatic brain injury patients: inconsistency between consensus guidelines and clinical practice. *J. Trauma*, **52**: 47–52; discussion 52–53.

Tobias, J.D., Lynch, A. & Garrett, J. (1996). Alterations of end-tidal carbon-dioxide during the intrahospital transport of children. *Ped. Emerg. Care.*, **12**: 249–251.

Tremblay, L., Valenza, F., Ribeiro, S.P., Li, J. & Slutsky, A.S. (1997). Injurious ventilatory strategies increase cytokines and c-fos m-RNA expression in an isolated rat lung model. *J. Clin. Invest.*, **99**: 944–952.

Tremblay, L.N., Miatto, D., Hamid, Q., Govindarajan, A. & Slutsky, A.S. (2003). Injurious ventilation induces widespread pulmonary epithelial expression of tumor necrosis factor-alpha and interleukin-6 messenger RNA. *Crit. Care Med.*, **30**: 1693–1700.

Uhlig, S. (2002). Ventilation-induced lung injury and mechanotransduction: stretching it too far? *Am. J. Physiol. Lung. Cell. Mol. Physiol.*, **282**: L892–L896.

van Santbrink, H., vd Brink, W.A., Steyerberg, E.W., Carmona Suazo, J.A., Avezaat, C.J. & Maas, A.I. (2003). Brain tissue oxygen response in severe traumatic brain injury. *Acta. Neurochir. (Wien)*. **145**: 429–438.

Whitwam, J.G., Boettner, R.B., Gilger, A.P. & Littell, A.S. (1966). Hyperventilation, brain damage and flicker. *Br. J. Anaesth.*, **38**: 846–852.

Wilson, M.R., Choudhury, S., Goddard, M.E., O'Dea, K.P., Nicholson, A.G. & Takata, M. (2003). High tidal volume upregulates intrapulmonary cytokines in an *in vivo* mouse model of ventilator-induced lung injury. *J. Appl. Physiol.*, **95**: 1385–1393.

Zhang, H., Downey, G.P., Suter, P.M., Slutsky, A.S. & Ranieri, V.M. (2002). Conventional mechanical ventilation is associated with bronchoalveolar lavage-induced activation of polymorphonuclear leukocytes. *Anesthesiology*, **97**: 1426–1433.

TIME AND VOLUMETRIC CAPNOGRAPHY IN THE NEONATES 10

G. Schmalisch

Introduction

Systematic investigations of pulmonary function in neonates were first performed in the 1950s after suitable electronic devices had become available. These enabled the measurements and recording of fast and small respiratory signals (Gerhardt & Bancalari, 1991). The pioneering work of Karlberg *et al.* (1954), Nelson *et al.* (1962), and Cook *et al.* (1955) helped to set the stage for new insight in neonatal pulmonary pathophysiology. The interest of pulmonary researchers in capnography was not unanticipated because of the crucial role of alveolar gas exchange in the newborn. Noninvasive capnography provides information about the amount of the exhaled carbon dioxide (CO_2) and airway dead-space.

The first measurements of CO_2 in the expired air were performed using breathing bags for gas collection (Nelson *et al.*, 1962). However, in the 1960s different types of commercial capnographs developed for adults were adapted for measurements in neonates. These first capnographs were bulky and cumbersome to use. Furthermore, the main-stream airway adaptors were heavy and in ventilated infants could easily displace a neonatal endotracheal tube (ET). However, the main problem was the dead-space of the airway adaptors, which could exceed the tidal volume of a preterm infant. This made long-term measurements possible only by using a side-stream device. Furthermore, this problem was magnified if a pneumotachograph was used in series to measure airflow and volume to perform a volumetric capnography.

Meanwhile, a new generation of capnographs has become available, and many of the past problems have been resolved. Lightweight infrared (IR) main-stream sensor with a dead-space <1 ml enable reliable measurements even in preterm infants (Meredith & Monaco, 1990; Arsowa *et al.*, 1997). Some manufacturers already offer a combined sensor to measure CO_2 and airflow simultaneously so that the transition from the time-based capnography to the volume-based capnography is not burdened by an increased apparatus dead-space. For dead-space-free measurements in neonates, special low-flow side-stream capnographs were developed making long-term monitoring possible (Hagerty *et al.*, 2002). Despite this rapid technological progress, neonatology capnography has not been embraced by clinicians for the assessment of alveolar gas exchange and airway dead-space because of remaining technical (Kirpalani *et al.*, 1991; Proquitté *et al.*, 2003) and methodological problems (Ream *et al.*, 1995; Wenzel *et al.*, 1999b; Tirosh *et al.*, 2001). The aim of this survey is to highlight the current possibilities and limitations of capnography in these very young patients.

Techniques of capnography in neonates

Devices

The measuring ranges of the CO_2 fraction (FCO_2) or the corresponding partial pressure (PCO_2) in the breathing gas are identical in neonates and adults. However, the CO_2 production in neonates (about 15 ml/min) is much lower than in adults (about 200 ml/min). The much lower amount of exhaled CO_2 makes capnography in neonates more difficult, because there are objective limits in the size of the analyzer chamber or the magnitude of suction flow by side-stream measurements.

In general, we have to distinguish between discontinuous and continuous CO_2 measurements. The first technique is historically the oldest method and commonly based on the collection of the exhaled gas in breathing bags (so-called Douglas bag). In spontaneously breathing infants special dead-space-reduced exhalation valves are necessary. Nelson *et al.* (1962) developed a special valve (Rhan sampler) for neonates with a dead-space of 1. 3 ml. Beside the mechanical dead-space, the most important problems of such valves are the necessary opening pressure and the increased expiratory resistance that hampers the breathing. Lum *et al.* (1998) have recently shown that in ventilated infants the Douglas bag method for dead-space measurement is relatively simple but cumbersome. Furthermore,

Table 10.1 Measuring techniques for capnography in neonates and infants

Measuring Principle	Mode of operation	References
Chemical volumetric method from *Haldane and Scholander* (Scholander, 1947)	• Chemical binding of CO_2 on 10% potash lye and subsequent measurement of absorbed gas volume. • Precise, only discontinuous measurements of the mean expiratory CO_2 concentration and the CO_2 production. • Very time consuming and cumbersome technique; was widely used in neonates in the past but has been completely replaced by fast CO_2 analyzers that enables on-line measurements.	Karlberg *et al.* (1954); Cook *et al.* (1957); Stahlman & Meece (1957); Nelson *et al.* (1962)
Mass spectrometer	• Gas sample is aspirated into a high-vacuum chamber and ionized by an electronic beam. The ions are than accelerated by an electric field into a final chamber, which has a magnetic field to separate the ionized gas stream on the basis of mass-to-charge ratios and directed toward metal plates that produce a current proportional to the gas concentrations. • Mass spectrometers are bulky and expensive to use. And they are used mainly in specialized lung function laboratories. However, only side-stream measurements are possible. • The main advantage of this technique is the ability to analyze several breathing gases simultaneously.	Strang (1961); Hunt *et al.* (1974); Gerhardt *et al.* (1978); Badgwell & Heavner (1991); Bouferrache *et al.* (1998); Bouferrache *et al.* (2000); Behrends *et al.* (2001); Gustafsson *et al.* (2003)
IR spectrography	• The amount of IR rays absorbed in an analyzer chamber is proportional to the CO_2 concentration in the sample, provided that there is no interference by other polyatomic gases (e.g. anesthetic gases) or water vapor. To reduce this cross-sensitivity to other gases and vapors, special precautions in the construction of the CO_2 analyzer were introduced. • This technique provided the first low cost and compact main-stream sensors – now in combination with a pneumotachograph for volumetric capnography. • IR spectrography is currently the most important and most frequently used technique for capnography in neonates.	Proenca & Wenner (1962); Thibeault *et al.* (1968); Krauss & Auld (1969); Rigatto & Brady (1972); Evans *et al.* (1977a); Dumpit & Brady (1978); Schulze *et al.* (1981); McEvedy *et al.* (1988); Meredith & Monaco (1990); Hopper *et al.* (1994); Arnold *et al.* (1995); Tobias & Meyer (1997); Wenzel *et al.* (1999c); Rozycki *et al.* (1998); Wu *et al.* (2003)
Raman spectroscopy	• The gas sample is aspirated into an analyzing chamber and illuminated by a high-intensity monochromatic argon laser beam that causes a light scattering of low intensity (Raman scattering). The spectrum of Raman scattering lines can be used to identify all types of molecules in the gas phase so that continuous CO_2 measurements are possible. • This side-stream technique is rarely used for capnography	Rich & Sconzo (1991)

this method failed if there was an unknown bias flow through the ventilator. In neonates this collection technique has several technical difficulties and can only measure mean CO_2 values over the sampling period. Nevertheless, it provides accurate CO_2 measurements and it is used as reference method to validate new techniques (Lum *et al.*, 1998). Fast continuous CO_2 measurements that enable us to analyze the exhaled CO_2 during the breathing cycle are much better for diagnostic purposes. Therefore, in neonates they are now used exclusively for clinical and research purposes.

As shown in Table 10.1, nearly all measuring principles used in adults have been applied for measurements in neonates. Currently, IR spectrography is the most frequently used technique because only this measuring principle makes possible miniaturized low cost main- and side-stream sensors optimized for measurements in neonates.

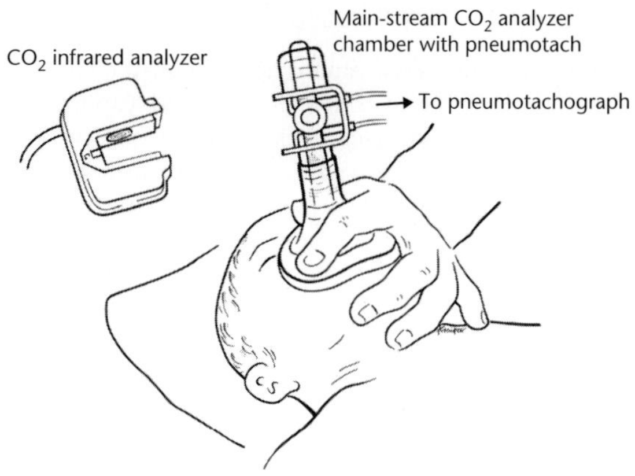

Figure 10.1 Volumetric capnography in a newborn using a face mask connected to a main-stream sensor.

Main- and side-stream measurements

Depending on the capnograph used, the CO_2 can be measured in the main-stream and side-stream. Several studies, in particular in infants, have shown that main-stream measurements are superior to side-stream measurements from the technical point of view (Pascucci *et al.*, 1989). Main-stream sensors have a faster response time so that reliable single breath CO_2 measurements even at high respiratory rates are possible. However, main-stream measurements are difficult in infants who are not intubated. Figure 10.1 shows the main-stream measurement in a spontaneously breathing newborn using a face mask connected to a CO_2 sensor with integrated pneumotach for volumetric capnography. The main problem with this technique is the additional equipment dead-space (i.e. face mask and CO_2 analyzer chamber). The apparatus dead-space leads to a rebreathing of the exhaled CO_2, which must be considered, mainly in very small infants. Due to its influence on ventilatory pattern and gas exchange this technique can be used in neonates only for short-term measurements (Schmalisch *et al.*, 2001a).

Side-stream measurements without a face mask (e.g. by nasal tubes (Weese-Mayer *et al.*, 2000)) are dead-space free and therefore enable long-term measurements, but their accuracy is commonly lower than that of main-stream measurements particularly at high respiratory rates. As discussed above in neonates with a minute ventilation of about 200 ml/min/kg body weight the suction flow must be much lower to prevent a dilution by surrounding air that will occur when the expiratory gas flow falls below the suction flow. However a low suction flow means a long delay time and a distortion of the CO_2 signal by gas mixing in the tube. Therefore, the sampling tube should be as short as possible. Meanwhile a micro-stream capnometer using a suction flow of 30 ml/min and a miniaturized small sample chamber has been developed, which improves the measurement accuracy in intubated and spontaneously breathing patients (Casati *et al.*, 2000; Singh *et al.*, 2001; Hagerty *et al.*, 2002). Nevertheless, for precise time-synchronized measurements with other respiratory signals this technique is less suitable, because the delay time of the suction tube is affected by pressure changes in the system and changes in the resistance of the tube so that numerical compensations provide only approximations.

Which technique should be used in neonates? This depends on the clinical situation. Provided that the additional apparatus dead-space is tolerable, main-stream measurements have uncontested advantages. However, not only technical properties decide the successful clinical use of capnography – it is necessary to consider the clinical settings. Therefore, side-stream measurements will be used,

- if the apparatus dead-space is not tolerable (e.g. measurements in ventilated preterm infants or small animals with a tidal volume <5 ml) or long-term investigations (e.g. sleep studies);
- if there is a need for a direct access to the airways (e.g. for endoscopy);
- if simultaneously other sensors with high dead-space are used inline with the ET (e.g. main-stream gas analyzers of tracer gases); or
- if side-stream gas sampling is already in use (e.g. the frequently used nasal spectacle or multiplex gas sampling from different ventilated patients).

Thus, despite technical disadvantages, side-stream measurements will continue to serve in many clinical settings.

Time- and volume-based capnograms

While the time-based capnogram is a strip chart and theoretically infinite, the volume-based capnogram describes a loop of each cycle that can be averaged over a high number of recorded cycles using a suitable averaging technique (Schmalisch *et al.*, 2001c). The informative potential of both presentations differs considerably.

In the past, only time-based capnograms were recorded. Several investigators have described the changes in the waveform of the time-based capnogram that are characteristic of specific clinical situations (Cote *et al.*, 1986; Arsowa *et al.*, 1993; Santos *et al.*, 1994). Some typical patterns measured in neonates are shown in Figure 10.2.

An important question is the presence of a more or less steep alveolar plateau at the end of expiration. Only if the capnogram shows a plateau that differs significantly from phase II, can we assume that PCO_2 in arterial blood ($P_{et}CO_2$) reflects the alveolar CO_2 pressure. However, the time-based capnogram does not give any information about the volume of exhaled alveolar gas. Furthermore, in ventilated patients the ventilator-imposed expiratory pause can exceed the actual expiratory flow. CO_2 diffusion from the lungs or dilution of gas in the ventilator makes any interpretation of "end-tidal" values doubtful.

These pitfalls in capnography can be avoided by volumetric capnography. Furthermore, this technique allows the calculation of the CO_2 production and the different dead-spaces as shown in the following. The disadvantage of volumetric capnography is the higher technical expense of simultaneous ventilatory measurements and the necessity of exact compensation of any time delay between airflow and CO_2 signal. In the past the volumetric capnography in the main-stream was only possible by use of a CO_2 analyzer and a pneumotachograph in series, which considerably increases the apparatus dead-space (Wenzel *et al.*, 1999a). Meanwhile, combined low dead-space sensors have become available (dead-space <1 ml) making use of this technique possible in ventilated and spontaneously breathing neonates.

Nevertheless, the advantage of volumetric capnography comes with a price: the two respiratory signals (CO_2 and respiratory gas flow) have to be measured in-phase and without any artifacts. Experience has shown that the acquisition of artifact-free data requires extra efforts and the correlative evaluation of two respiratory signals is more difficult than one signal. If either the volume channel or the airflow cannot be correctly measured, we have to revert back to time-based capnography.

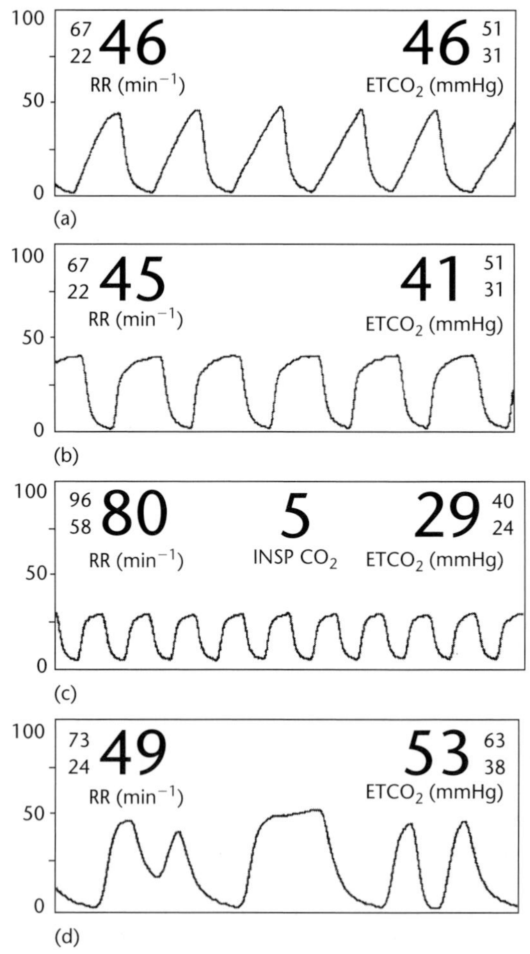

Figure 10.2 Typical pattern of time-based capnograms in ventilated newborns. Capnogram of a premature baby with respiratory distress syndrome before (a) and after (b) administration of surfactant. (c) Rebreathing due to high respiratory rate (RR) and too large-apparatus dead-space. (d) Superimposition of the respiratory cycles of the ventilator by spontaneous breathing. $ETCO_2$: end-tidal PCO_2. (Reproduced with permission from Arsowa, S., Schmalisch, G. & Wauer, R.R. (1993). Techniques and clinical application of capnography in newborn infants and infants. *Padiatr. Grenzgeb.*, **31**: 295–311.)

$P_{et}CO_2$

In infants with normal pulmonary function and matching ventilation-to-perfusion ratio ($\dot{V}/\dot{Q}$), $P_{et}CO_2$ can be a good estimation of the PCO_2 in arterial blood (P_aCO_2) (McDonald *et al.*, 2002; Wu *et al.*, 2003). However, several physiologic factors (e.g. high respiratory rate, incomplete expiration, pulmonary inhomogeneities, disturbed $\dot{V}/\dot{Q}$ ratio), technical factors (e.g. too slow response time, gas dilution by surrounding air) and diseases can affect the $P_{et}CO_2$

and make it unreliable for blood gas interpretation. It appears that in neonatology, $P_{et}CO_2$ measurement may not substitute for arterial or transcutaneous blood gases but can be helpful in monitoring the trend of the PCO_2 or to detect technical artifacts (e.g. unintended extubation) (Rozycki *et al.*, 1998).

Nevertheless, the continuous measurement of $P_{et}CO_2$ in spontaneously breathing infants can help to recognize hypoventilation, hyperventilation, and apnea. In mechanically ventilated infants a sudden decrease in $P_{et}CO_2$ can indicate disconnection, endotracheal leaks, obstructions of the ET, or ventilator malfunction.

The difference ($P_{a-et}CO_2$) between P_aCO_2 and $P_{et}CO_2$ in infants is normally <6 mmHg if ventilation and perfusion are almost evenly matched. However, when the alveoli are not properly ventilated (shunt perfusion) or the perfusion of the lungs is decreased or regionally interrupted (dead-space ventilation), the $P_{a-et}CO_2$ difference will grow. An increase of the $P_{a-et}CO_2$ is one the most sensitive indicators of acute pulmonary embolism (Napolitano, 1999).

Alveolar ventilation and dead-spaces

Only one part of the total ventilated gas – the alveolar ventilation – takes part in gas exchange with pulmonary capillary blood. The difference between the minute ventilation and the alveolar ventilation is the dead-space ventilation in which gas exchange is negligible. Dead-space consists of conducting airways (anatomic dead-space), nonperfused or underperfused alveoli (alveolar dead-space) and the apparatus dead-space.

The first calculations of alveolar ventilation and dead-space in neonates were performed by Karlberg *et al.* (1954), Cook *et al.* (1957), and Nelson *et al.* (1962) using the Scholander method (Scholander, 1947). These investigators assumed that alveolar CO_2 can be approximated by the arterial CO_2. Chu *et al.* (1967) were the first to use a rapid capnograph to measure the $P_{et}CO_2$ in neonates and to calculate the anatomic and physiologic dead-space using the Bohr equation:

$$V_{D\,ana} = V_{ex} \times \frac{P_{et}CO_2 - \text{mean } PCO_2}{P_{et}CO_2}$$

or the Bohr–Enghoff equation by substituting arterial CO_2 for $P_{et}CO_2$:

$$V_{D\,phys} = V_{ex} \times \frac{P_aCO_2 - \text{mean } PCO_2}{P_aCO_2},$$

where mean PCO_2 is the CO_2 tension of the mixed expired air. The difference of both dead-spaces represents the alveolar dead-space:

$$V_{D\,alv} = V_{D\,phys} - V_{D\,ana}.$$

Fletcher *et al.* (1981) were the first to develop the calculation of the different dead-spaces from the CO_2-volume plot from a single breath. This single breath CO_2 test ($SBCO_2$-test) is now commercially available (Arnold *et al.*, 1996) and is used for capnography in neonates (Wenzel *et al.*, 1999c) and older infants (Ream *et al.*, 1995).

The basic concept is shown in Figure 10.3. The three dead-spaces can be derived from ratios of the areas X, Y, and Z. With this technique it is important to recognize the problem surrounding the definition of $V_{D\,ana}$, which is not well-defined. Fletcher (1984) recognizes $V_{D\,ana}$ shown in Figure 10.3 when the areas *p* and *q* are equal. Using this definition it is easy to understand that this dead-space will differ from a dead-space defined by a CO_2 threshold at the beginning of phase II or by dead-space calculated using Bohr's equations (Figure 10.4). Thus, the estimations of dead-spaces are strongly method depended (Kars *et al.*, 1997).

Furthermore, the determination of dead-spaces by the $SBCO_2$-test can be foiled if there is no alveolar plateau or if the transition from phase II to III cannot be clearly identified. In contrast, the dead-space calculations by the Bohr or the Bohr–Enghoff equations are independent of the shape of the capnogram. This means that the failure rate of capnography to determine airway dead-spaces depends on the method used (Wenzel *et al.*, 1999b).

Clinical applications

Operating room

Capnography has become the standard monitoring modality in the pediatric operating room (Bhavani-Shankar *et al.*, 1992; Mather, 1994; Bhende & Thompson, 1995; Roberts *et al.*, 1995; Nosovitch *et al.*, 2002). We see continuous technologic improvements in the measuring techniques (Casati *et al.*, 2000; Hagerty *et al.*, 2002). For intraoperative monitoring commonly time-based capnography is used and the shape of the capnogram provides robust qualitative data (Benumof, 1998) and the $P_{et}CO_2$ (Domsky *et al.*, 1995; Wilson *et al.*, 1996).

Several anesthesiologists strongly recommend the use of capnography in every newborn requiring tracheal intubation because capnography can instantly identify life-threatening conditions before irreversible damage is done. Widely discussed in the literature are failed intubation (Bhende *et al.*, 1992a; Ong, 1998), failed ventilation (McQuillen & Steele, 2000; Hsieh *et al.*, 2001) and failure of the respirator or respiratory circuit (French & Kennedy, 1998).

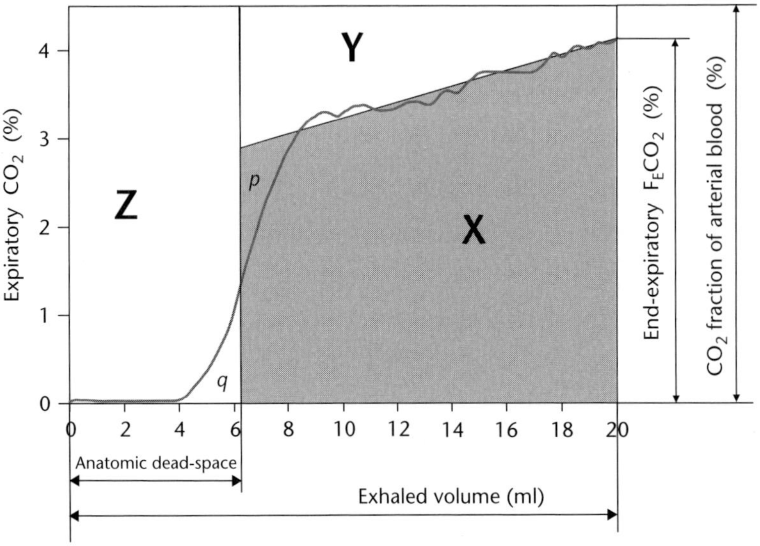

Figure 10.3 Evaluation of the volumetric capnogram by Fletcher's method. The area X corresponds to the exhaled amount of CO_2 and the areas Z + Y to the nonexhaled CO_2 as a consequence of the anatomic (X) and alveolar (Y) dead-spaces. Thus, for the physiological dead space it holds that $V_{D\,phys} = V_T \times (Y + Z)/(X + Y + Z)$. F_ECO_2: fractional concentration of CO_2 in expired gas.

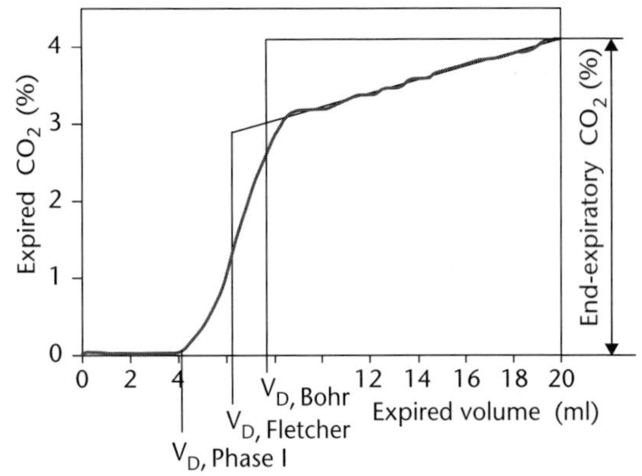

Figure 10.4 Dependence of the determined anatomic dead space from the method used.

Table 10.2 Differential diagnostic causes of absent end-expiratory CO_2

Immediately after intubation CO_2 only minimal or absent

- Inadvertent esophageal intubation

Exhaled CO_2 present, then suddenly absent

- Accidental tracheal extubation
- Disconnection of breathing circuit
- Cardiac arrest
- Apneic spells
- Complete obstruction of ET
- Disconnection of the CO_2 sample tube
- Water condensation or secretions in the sampling tube
- Failure of the capnograph

What information can the capnogram offer the anesthetist? At first we look for the presence of exhaled CO_2. If end-expiratory CO_2 is not present, failure to ventilate the patient's lungs must be assumed. Table 10.2 presents typical causes of absent CO_2.

Second, independent of whether time- or volume-based capnography is used, the shape of the capnogram must be compared with a typical pattern by looking at the inspiratory CO_2 baseline, the steepness of phase II and the alveolar plateau of phase III, and the decline of the capnogram at the beginning of the next inspiration. Third, depending on the capnograph used, we look for characteristic parameters derived from the capnogram, for example, $P_{et}CO_2$, CO_2 production, $P_{a-et}CO_2$, and the dead-spaces.

Inspiratory baseline

During inspiration fresh CO_2-free gas flows through the main-stream sensor or is aspirated by the sample port. The CO_2 level should be zero otherwise there is a rebreathing of CO_2 from the patient (high apparatus dead-space, valve malfunction or exhausted CO_2 absorber). CO_2 rebreathing can occur if the tidal volume is relatively low compared to the apparatus dead-space (Figure 10.2(c)). This is mainly a problem in very small infants or in non-intubated infants during mask ventilation.

The expiratory CO_2 increase (phase II)

During expiration the first gas comes from the CO_2-free anatomic dead-space. After that in healthy lungs, the CO_2 curve rises with a steep upward slope. The phase II can be prolonged when the delivery of CO_2 from the lung is delayed, for example, due to pulmonary inhomogeneities, high resistances of the small airways, and mechanical obstructions, such as a blocked or kinked ET. In neonates a prolonged phase II can also be caused by technical problems related to the capnograph. In infants with a high respiratory rate the response time of the CO_2 analyzer can be too slow or in side-stream devices the sampling flow rate too low.

The alveolar plateau (phase III)

Theoretically, the shape of the alveolar plateau is one of the most interesting parts of the capnogram, because the steepness of the slope is a function of morphometric structure and respiratory mechanics. This was shown in the past by several computer simulations and experimental studies (Schwardt *et al.*, 1991; Jeng *et al.*, 2000; Whiteley *et al.*, 2002). The phase III contains gas from the well-ventilated, low resistance regions of the lung. Later, gas from poorly ventilated, high-resistance regions is exhaled, which causes the alveolar plateau to slope. Thus, the steepness of the alveolar plateau is commonly used as an indicator for inhomogeneities in the alveolar time constants and the $\dot{V}/\dot{Q}$ ratio. However, in neonates this interpretation should be used with caution, because the plateau (if it exits at all) is often small and the steepness is also a function of lung growth (Ream *et al.*, 1995). Therefore, the diagnostic value of a phase III analysis is often limited. Nevertheless, the appearance of a phase III in the capnogram indicates that alveolar gas was sampled.

The decrease of the CO_2 at the beginning of inspiration

After expiration the fresh gas from the breathing circuit rinses out the CO_2 from the previous exhalation and there should be a quick decrease of the end-expiratory CO_2 at the beginning of inspiration. In the past several techniques (e.g. tracheal gas insufflation (Dassieu *et al.*, 2000; Davies & Woodgate, 2002)) were developed to reduce rebreathing and dead-space ventilation so that the tidal volume is more efficiently used for gas exchange. A delayed decrease of the CO_2 may be caused by a leaking inspiratory valve or a respiratory circuit with a low flow, so that CO_2 can be accumulated in the inspiratory circuit. Technical failures can represent a slow response time of the CO_2 analyzer.

Emergency medicine and transport

In emergency medicine, critically ill infants often require tracheal intubation before transportation to the hospital. The intubation must be done quickly and the ET must be positioned correctly. Failure to recognize an unintentional esophageal intubation may be catastrophic and can lead to severe hypoxia and to permanent neurologic injury (Bhende *et al.*, 1992b; Roberts *et al.*, 1995). Such intubation failure can occur even in the hands of the most experienced personnel (Nakayama *et al.*, 1990).

As stated above, CO_2 monitoring and the measurement of $P_{et}CO_2$ is probably the best way to detect esophageal intubation or displacement of the ET at a later stage. Furthermore, Roberts *et al.* (1995) investigated the time for correct placement of the ET. A clinical assessment of the position of the endotracheal took 97 s but only 1.6 s using capnography.

Due to the vicissitudes of transport, inadvertent extubation can occur at any time. The vibrations and noisy environments of the ambulance or helicopter make assessment of tube positions difficult. In these situations when the patient is in critical condition, and time is of the essence, the use of capnography offers essential help. The use of portable CO_2 monitors during transport provide an effective visual check of ET position and indirectly gives information about the ventilatory status and the circulation. In neonatology pulse oximetry is widely used for monitoring during transport whereas the CO_2 measurements of the exhaled air can sound an alarm before hypoxemia can be recognized.

Intensive care

Capnography also plays a significant role in the monitoring of neonates and children in intensive care units (ICU). In contrast to the operating room or during transport, the duration of mechanical ventilation in the ICU is usually prolonged. Variables monitored subserve not only ventilator adjustments but also diagnosis and prognosis (e.g. optimal time of weaning (Hubble *et al.*, 2000). Ventilatory support in newborn infants must carefully balance the amount of support (oxygen and pressure/volume) and its toxicities (Rozycki *et al.*, 1998). Therefore, continuous monitoring of blood gases is an essential part in the optimization of respiratory support or mechanical ventilation. In neonates a low P_aCO_2 can contribute to the development of chronic lung diseases and periventricular leukomalacia, whereas high levels can cause enhanced cerebral blood flow and increase the risk of periventricular hemorrhage. Although arterial blood gas analysis provides the most accurate data, the number of arterial samplings must be limited to prevent excess blood loss. Alternative noninvasive methods are the transcutaneous PCO_2 ($P_{tc}CO_2$) measurement or the end-tidal CO_2 measurement.

Patient safety

As already stated, capnography can identify disconnections in the ventilatory circuit instantaneously before O_2 and CO_2 levels change in the blood and corrective measures can be taken before irreversible damage is caused by prolonged hypoxia. An alarm is commonly activated if $P_{et}CO_2$ falls to zero. However, during mechanical ventilation there is often a spontaneous breathing with a measurable $P_{et}CO_2$ (see Figure 10.2(d)). Circuit disconnections distal to the CO_2 sampling site can be identified instantaneously as CO_2 concentration falls to zero, whereas, circuit disconnection proximal to the sampling site may not be detected due to spontaneous breathing. If spontaneous breathing is adequate, the $P_{et}CO_2$ can reach normal values, but low $P_{et}CO_2$ values will alert the clinician to potentially inadequate spontaneous ventilation.

In addition to end-tidal CO_2 monitoring, the shape of the capnogram is also examined in the ICU to detect partially kinked or obstructed ETs, which are characterized by prolonged phase II and steeper phase III, and irregular height of the CO_2 tracings (Cote *et al.*, 1986). Because accidental kinking or displacement of the ET can occur in the ICU during positioning, bathing, or while changing the bed (Bhende *et al.*, 1995) the capnograph should never be turned off during these activities.

CO_2 monitoring

Measurement of $P_{et}CO_2$ provides a noninvasive method for immediate estimation of P_aCO_2 without the time delay associated with performing an arterial blood gas analysis. $P_{et}CO_2$ monitoring has several advantages for patients requiring intensive care (Rozycki *et al.*, 1998; McDonald *et al.*, 2002):

- Decreased blood loss by arterial sampling.
- Lower risk of infection.
- Decreased costs.

In intubated neonates with normal respiratory and cardiovascular physiology, $P_{et}CO_2$ values approximate P_aCO_2 values. However in critically ill patients the ventilation and pulmonary perfusion ratio is often abnormal so that the $P_{a-et}CO_2$ difference is increased. Nevertheless, McDonald *et al.* (2002) and Wu *et al.* (2003) have recently shown in large clinical studies in critically ill mechanically ventilated infants that $P_{et}CO_2$ correlates with P_aCO_2 and provides a clinically relevant, reliable estimation of ventilation for most of the infants. Similar results were found by Rozychi *et al.* (1998) investigating 45 newborn infants receiving mechanical ventilation. They suggest that capnography in these patients may be useful for trending or screening patients for abnormal arterial CO_2 values. In contrast, Tobias and Meyer (1997) found in intubated infants that $P_{et}CO_2$ does not accurately predict P_aCO_2 and that $P_{tc}CO_2$ measurements are more accurate. However, $P_{tc}CO_2$ measurements are not well-tolerated in tiny infants with fragile skin and are affected by acidosis and hypoxia (Bhat *et al.*, 1981). Low cardiac output, hypothermia, size of tidal volume and lung disease can adversely affect the $P_{a-et}CO_2$ difference. However, McDonald *et al.* (2002) showed that in most of the patients $P_{a-et}CO_2$ is small enough so that $P_{et}CO_2$ monitoring enables the clinician to monitor ventilation. This means that changes in P_aCO_2 can be assumed to occur in parallel with those of $P_{et}CO_2$, thus, avoiding repeated blood gas measurements.

If the goal of mechanical ventilation is to avoid hypocapnia or hypercapnia, rather than achieving a specific level or range of P_aCO_2, then continuous $P_{et}CO_2$ measurements may be pertinent to clinical treatment (Rozycki *et al.*, 1998). A new concept of mechanical ventilation in neonates is permissive hypercapnia, with lower tidal volumes and thus decreased potential for lung injury (Thome & Carlo, 2002). However, this technique requires careful P_aCO_2 monitoring to prevent unintentional side effects. Based on this approach Rozycki *et al.* (1998) have demonstrated that mainstream CO_2 monitoring can point to a P_aCO_2 within prescribed parameters (P_aCO_2 between 34 and 55 mmHg) 91% of the time.

Furthermore, the arterial–alveolar CO_2 difference can be used as a minimally invasive monitor of pulmonary blood flow. A reduction in the cardiac output causes a reduction in the pulmonary blood flow, which produces a high $\dot{V}/\dot{Q}$ ratio and an increased alveolar deadspace resulting in lower $P_{et}CO_2$ and an increased $P_{a-et}CO_2$ difference. As pulmonary blood flow increases, thereby improving $\dot{V}/\dot{Q}$ ratio, the $P_{et}CO_2$ increases and $P_{a-et}CO_2$ becomes small. Sanders *et al.* (1989) have shown that $P_{a-et}CO_2$ monitoring can advantageously be used to predict successful resuscitation after cardiac arrest. During cardiac arrest circulation and $P_{et}CO_2$ gradually disappears and an increase in the $P_{et}CO_2$ indicates an effective cardiopulmonary resuscitation. Recently, Berg *et al.* (1996) confirmed these observations in an animal model.

Weaning

In long-term mechanically ventilated infants weaning from the respirator presents a critical situation. Weaning of mechanical ventilation often requires multiple blood gas analyses. The practice is not only invasive but also means a blood loss that can lead to anemia in premature infants (Obladen & Maier, 1995). For these infants noninvasive capnography can be very helpful. In addition to the $P_{et}CO_2$ and the $P_{a-et}CO_2$ the capnography gives also information about the breathing pattern, and importantly the consistency of breathing before extubation (Hubble *et al.*, 2000). Monitoring the capnogram enables us gradually to reduce ventilatory support to the lowest point that is compatible with comfortable breathing and adequate alveolar ventilation. The stability of the $P_{et}CO_2$ and the proper shape of the capnogram indicate the patient's readiness to be weaned from mechanical ventilation. However, if the patient becomes distressed or the alveolar gas exchange is insufficient, ventilatory support can be returned immediately to the previous settings.

Recently Hubble *et al.* (2000) showed the high diagnostic value of capnogram-derived parameters able to predict successful extubation in infants and children. In a clinical study of 45 pediatric patients they found that the ratio of physiologic dead-space and tidal volume ($V_{D\,phys}/V_T$) ≤ 0.5 reliably predicts a successful extubation, whereas ($V_{D\,phys}/V_T$) > 0.65 identifies patient at risk for respiratory failure following extubation. They suggest the calculation of the pulmonary dead-spaces in ventilated patients may permit earlier extubation or reduce unexpected extubation failures.

Arnold *et al.* (1995) investigated the predictive value of dead-space in neonates with congenital diaphragmatic hernia. Using capnographic measurements in 30 neonates they found that the respiratory dead-space can be easily quantified in these infants by the Bohr–Enghoff method, and that a physiologic dead-space fraction of >0.60 is associated with a 15-fold increase in mortality rate. Furthermore, they could show that in infants treated with extracorporeal membrane oxygenation (ECMO), the survivors manifested a significant decrease in $V_{D\,phys}/V_T$ before ECMO decannulation.

Lung function testing

Capnography plays an important role not only at the bedside in ventilated patients but also in lung function testing in spontaneously breathing infants. This is not surprising, because capnography is a simple noninvasive technique to obtain information on alveolar ventilation and the dead-spaces of the respiratory system. Furthermore the shape of the capnogram (mainly the steepness of phase III) gives information about airway obstructions and pulmonary inhomogeneities (Yaron *et al.*, 1996). For these reasons capnography has become an integral component of modern equipment for infant respiratory function testing (e.g. Spiroson, ECO MEDICS, Dürnten, CH).

In spontaneously breathing neonates volumetric capnography requires an airtight face mask, which has disadvantages:

- We usually do not know exactly the apparatus dead-space after application of the face mask (approximately 50% of the mask volume (Morris, 1999)).
- The measured anatomic dead-space encompasses the apparatus dead-space, which varies with the type of equipment in use.
- Especially in infants with low tidal volume the apparatus dead-space of the face mask leads to a significant CO_2 rebreathing, which affects the blood gases and the PCO_2 of the breathing air as well as the breathing pattern. This imposes limits on the duration of the measurement (Katz *et al.*, 1991; Schmalisch *et al.*, 2001a).

Morris (1999) described for neonates a technique to determine *in vivo* the effective dead-space of a face mask by water displacement. However, this technique is too cumbersome for clinical use. Therefore, in spontaneously breathing neonates $V_{D\,ana}$ is of limited value for lung function testing. More informative is the alveolar dead-space determined by Fletcher's method and the shape of the capnogram. Severe airway obstruction such as bronchial asthma and laryngo–tracheobronchitis can affect the shape of the capnogram resulting in a prolongation of phase II and increased steepness of phase III.

Similar to other tidal breathing measurements in neonates (Bates *et al.*, 2000) capnography for lung function testing is hampered by missing reference values. Unfortunately, despite repeated efforts over the last 50 years to establish reference values for capnographic parameters in healthy infants (Cook *et al.*, 1955; Nelson *et al.*, 1962; Evans *et al.*, 1977b) these values are highly specific to the equipment used and the behavioral state of the specific population studied and cannot be recommended for general use. Furthermore, knowledge about the biological development (i.e. the influence of growth and maturation) and clinical/diagnostic value of most of the parameters remain sparse. Thus, it is currently difficult to compare capnographic parameters from different laboratories. This problem needs to be addressed urgently in the near future once equipment, evaluation techniques and measurement conditions for capnography in neonates have been standardized.

Sleep laboratory

Isolated measurements of lung function are only brief snap-shots and they may be of limited value if disturbed lung function depends on the behavior of the infant. The extensive sequence of changes in sleep organization during the perinatal period, the length and time spent in sleep by the neonates and the fact that many respiratory disorders are sleep related indicate the need for sleep studies in this age.

In neonates many cardiorespiratory disorders are caused by apnea. Apnea is defined as the cessation of respiration originating from the central nervous system or obstruction of the airway (Morielli *et al.*, 1993). In premature infants apnea is a very common phenomenon. The incidence lies between 59% and 79% with an inverse relationship to the gestational age (Henderson-Smart, 1981). If apnea is associated with hypoxemia and/or bradycardia the cerebral hemodynamics can be affected (Jenni *et al.*, 1996; Payer *et al.*, 2003). Therefore, the quantification of apnea during sleep and the detection of hypoxia or bradycardia are essential goals of sleep studies in this age.

Capnography is used in the sleep laboratory both to detect the breathing movements by CO_2 in the exhaled gas and to measure the $P_{et}CO_2$. Transthoracic impedance measurements or breathing belts are commonly used to monitor the breathing by chest wall movements (Brouillette *et al.*, 1987). However, they can only detect central apnea. Obstructive apnea (i.e. breathing efforts without air flow) can only be recognized by simultaneous airflow measurements with the help of a pneumotachograph (Bates *et al.*, 2000), nasal thermistor (Trang *et al.*, 2002), or CO_2 measurements. As face masks are unsuitable for long-term measurements in neonates, side-stream capnography has been shown to be a reliable method for the detection of central and obstructive apnea during sleep (Smith *et al.*, 1993; Weese-Mayer *et al.*, 2000). Furthermore, capnography can be used as a reliable monitor to detect sleep apnea syndromes characterized by excessive daytime somnolence, tiredness, episodes of asphyxia during the night or non-refreshing sleep (Magnan *et al.*, 1993).

For the use in the sleep laboratory the capnograph has to fulfill special requirements:

- The device must be quiet so that sleep is not disturbed.
- The CO_2 measurement in the nasal prongs should not affect the sleeping infant or respiration by increased airway resistance and should be insensitive to head movements.
- The side-stream gas sampling must have a long-term reliability (no collection of water rainout in the tube for the duration of measurement).
- The capnograph must be compatible with commonly used polysomnographic measurement equipment.

The advantages of capnography in the measurements of CO_2 during sleep are obvious.

Blood gas sampling is not practical during sleep, because it would considerably disturb the sleep. The use of $P_{tc}CO_2$ measurement may be more accurate to predict true P_aCO_2, however, capnography has a better long-term stability and is simpler to perform during sleep (Hand *et al.*, 1989; Sivan *et al.*, 1992; Morielli *et al.*, 1993). Both techniques have methodological limitations. $P_{et}CO_2$ is affected by changes in pulmonary perfusion and dead-space ventilation whereas $P_{tc}CO_2$ is subject to changes in peripheral perfusion (Stock, 1988). Thus, neither technique can reliably predict true P_aCO_2, however both are useful for trend monitoring. Furthermore, capnography is the only technique fast enough to detect breath-to-breath changes in the expired and hence presumably blood gases. Vos *et al.* (1993) have shown that nocturnal $P_{et}CO_2$ recording detects obstructive apneas and hypopneas and is especially helpful to identify hypopneas that are accompanied by only small dips in oxygen saturation.

Current methodological and technical limitations of capnography in neonates

Technical limitations

Relatively higher respiratory rates and smaller tidal volumes encountered in neonates, as compared to older infants and adults, make capnography much more difficult. The technical requirements of the capnograph for use in neonates are higher, e.g.:

- minimal dead-space of main-stream sensors because of the low tidal volume,
- low suction flow of side-stream monitors because of the low breathing flow,
- fast response time of the CO_2 analyzer because of the short exhalation times especially in preterm neonates with stiff lungs,
- high sample rate to get a sufficient graphic resolution of the capnogram especially in infants with high respiratory rate.

Dead-space

In the past the importance of apparatus dead-space on the breathing pattern and on the measuring results themselves was often underestimated in neonates although it had been documented in several studies (Fleming *et al.*, 1982; Dolfin *et al.*, 1983; Katz *et al.*, 1991; Emralino & Steele, 1997). The apparatus dead-space is of particular interest for capnographic measurements because it can lead to rebreathing of exhaled CO_2 with the potential of generating false inspiratory and expiratory CO_2 measurements. Rebreathing, of course, can raise P_aCO_2 (McEvedy *et al.*, 1990). This was a significant problem in the past using volumetric capnography by serial connection of a CO_2 analyzer and a pneumotachograph where the resulting dead-space was often at least 30% of the tidal volume (Wenzel *et al.*, 1999b). Meanwhile, combined sensors for volumetric capnography have become available (e.g. neonatal sensor of the CO_2SMO+, Novametrix, USA) with dead-spaces of about 1 ml, which allows reliable measurements in neonates. Nevertheless, if the tidal volume is not more than 5 ml (e.g. ventilated preterm newborn <1000 g) a dead-space of 1 ml is an undesirable load. Technical limitations in the miniaturization of main-stream sensors compel us to use dead-space-free measuring techniques. To prevent rebreathing in neonates, Evans *et al.* (1977a) used a bias flow of 3 l/min, similar to dead-space-free ventilatory measurements by the flow-through technique (Foitzik *et al.*, 2001; Schmalisch *et al.*, 2001a). However, the bias flow reduces the CO_2 concentration of the analyzed breathing gas and can cause a loss in the precision of CO_2 measurements.

Side-stream sampling

Recently a micro-stream technology (e.g. NBP-75, Nellcor Puritan Bennett, Plesanton, CA, USA) was developed for side-stream measurements in neonates. It utilizes low aspiration sampling flows and rapid response time (Colman & Krauss, 1999; Casati *et al.*, 2001; Singh *et al.*, 2001). Hagerty *et al.* (2002) have shown, in 20 ventilated neonates without pulmonary disease that this micro-stream capnography correlates well with the P_aCO_2, as demonstrated by normal $P_{a-et}CO_2$ differences. Casati *et al.* (2000) demonstrated in 20 spontaneously breathing adults that micro-stream capnometer provides a more accurate $P_{et}CO_2$ measurement than conventional side-stream capnometers.

When a side-stream capnograph is used the sampling tube needs special care to prevent measuring errors. During mechanical ventilation water droplets and secretions can accumulate in the breathing circuit. Depending on the site of the sample port, the contaminant can enter the sampling tubes and increase flow resistance in the tubing, thus, significantly affecting accuracy of the CO_2 measurement. In the extreme, the sample port or the sampling tube can be completely occluded. Some capnographs either increase the sampling flow or, to clear the contaminant from the tube, reverse the flow (purge) when they sense a drop in pressure from a flow restriction. If this fails the sampling port and/or the tube has to be replaced.

Occasionally, liquids enter the CO_2 analyzer chamber despite the presence of a water trap. This can affect the performance of the CO_2 monitor and produce abnormal capnograms. Cleaning the CO_2 analyzer chamber is often difficult. Positioning of the sampling tube upwards away from the patient decreases the risk of liquids in the tubes and the analyzer chamber.

When capnograms are abnormal, the clinician should ensure that there is not a system fault. In clinical practice a common, but less accurate, bedside method to check the capnograph is to record a normal CO_2 tracing (e.g. one's own) to confirm the proper functioning of the capnometer (Bhavani-Shankar *et al.*, 1992).

Response time

It is an essential prerequisite of all physiologic measurements that the response time of the measuring and recording system must be sufficiently high so that magnitude and shape of the signal are not falsified. Thus, especially for measurements in neonates a capnograph should have a rapid time for accurate measurements. The delay time of a capnograph has two components – the transit time and rise time. In side-stream measurements the transit time is the time taken by the gas sample to travel from the sample port to the CO_2 analyzer. This time depends on the suction flow, length and diameter of the tube. The transit time can be numerically corrected provided that it is nearly constant. The rise time is the time of the CO_2 analyzer taken from 10 to 90% of the final value. The possibilities of improving the rise time by signal filtering are marginal and are limited by the rapid increase of the noise in the signal (Wong *et al.*, 1998). Too long rise time results in errors in $P_{et}CO_2$ measurements and distortions in the capnogram, which escalate with increasing respiratory rate, for example, prolonged phase II and a steeper phase III (Brunner & Westenskow, 1988).

Main-stream capnographs are generally faster than side-stream capnographs because they are not affected by the dynamic problems of the sample tube.

Capnographs used in neonates have currently rise times $T_{10-90\%}$ of about 50–80 ms depending on the airflow used for testing. For preterm neonates with low expiratory flow and respiratory rates of 60/min and higher (this means expiratory times $t_E < 500$ ms) it is doubtful that this rise time is sufficient to reflect the capnogram accurately in these small infants. Because low-flow CO_2 sensors with rise times <10 ms are still not available it is difficult to verify the dynamic errors of the current CO_2 sensors for measurements in neonates.

In the past in preterm infants, side-stream devices often did show sinusoidal capnograms without clear alveolar plateau. Sinusoidal shapes may have several causes, such as sampling flow too high for volume of CO_2 produced, signal distortions by turbulence produced by gas sampling and transport, long sampling tubes and CO_2 sampling from an unsuitable site (Schena *et al.*, 1984; Pascucci *et al.*, 1989; Badgwell, 1992; Badgwell *et al.*, 1993). It is very likely that in the past the rise time of the CO_2 analyzers was too long for low breathing flows for an accurate measurement of the capnogram in neonates. Therefore, older measuring results from neonates should be viewed with reservations.

Sampling rate

The use of equipment developed for measurements in adults have been often shown to be inappropriate for measurements in neonates. This is particularly true for capnography. High suction flow, long rise time and high volume of the analyzer chamber exemplify the often underestimated features. The relatively low sampling rate translates into insufficient digital resolution. Special technical features are required to deal with the challenges presented by the signals from neonates. These include optimized digital signal processing thresholds for breath detection and dead bands to stabilize the volume integration to deal with the signal-to-noise ratio in capnography for neonates (Schmidt *et al.*, 1998; Schmalisch *et al.*, 2001b).

A sampling rate of 50/s of CO_2 and gas flow may be sufficient in adults with an expiratory time of some seconds. However that would provide only 25 sample values, in a preterm newborn with an expiratory time of 500 ms and would put into doubt our ability to cleanly distinguish phase I, II, and III, of volumetric capnograms. Furthermore, we have to consider that in contrast to a time-based CO_2 curve the distances between sampling points in the volume-based CO_2 curve are not equidistant. For tidal breathing signals in neonates a sampling rate of at least 200 Hz is required (Bates *et al.*, 2000) as this is necessary for a precise evaluation and for an accurate graphic presentation of the signals or loops presented in suitable scales.

As already shown, the graphic assessment of a capnogram is an essential prerequisite for a valid interpretation of capnogram-derived parameters. The small size of the displays of the current monitors (which often have only a low number of sampling points) may be helpful for monitoring purposes. However, the commonly offered hard copy of small diagrams are mostly insufficient for a quantitative evaluation. For a manually quantitative evaluation a print out in A4 size is necessary, which requires a high-digital resolution in the amplitudes and the time (Frey *et al.*, 2000).

Peculiarities of capnography in small lungs

The developing lung and the breathing pattern of neonates differ in many respects from adults and this may also influence CO_2 measurements significantly. It is essential to understand these age-related deviations to minimize misleading interpretations of the capnogram.

Small airways

In healthy adult lungs there is a rapid rise of CO_2 concentration during phase II and only a negligible contribution of the upper airways to the gas exchange. In neonates the diameter of the airways are much small and the smaller the airway diameter the higher the impact on the exhaled CO_2. This may explain why we have in neonates an exaggerated phase II and a reduced or even missing phase III (Tirosh *et al.*, 2001; Proquitté *et al.*, 2003).

The effect of the airway diameter on the capnogram was investigated in small animals (Gaertner & Barnikol, 1990). Despite the morphological differences between the animal and human lungs, Weiler *et al.*, (1987) showed that in small guinea pigs with airway diameter <2 mm no anatomic dead-space was measured whereas in large guinea pigs with airways >3 mm an anatomic dead-space could be measured. Obviously, with a larger airway diameter the ratio between inner surface and volume suffices to prevent a fast CO_2 exchange between gas and tissue. However in much smaller airways at the end of inspiration a nearly complete equilibration is possible between the inner-bronchial PCO_2 and the PCO_2 of the tissue. Consequently, phase I disappears because the gas exchange is very fast (Gaertner & Barnikol, 1990).

Lung growth during infancy also affects phase III (if there is any) of the capnogram as shown by several computer simulations (Schwardt *et al.*, 1991; Neufeld *et al.*, 1992). Ream *et al.* (1995) confirmed these results by capnographic measurements in 44 infants. They showed a morphometric decrease in the alveolar airway cross-section is associated with an increase of the phase III slope. This may explain the steeper slope of the phase III in small infants compared to adults. However, the steeper phase III the more difficult is it to distinguish between phase II and III and the more difficult is the calculation of the dead-spaces from the volumetric capnogram by Fletcher's method (Figure 10.3).

Fletcher's method developed for adults requires a clear subdivision of the capnogram in the phases I, II, and III. It is, therefore, often difficult to apply Fletcher's method to measurements in small lungs. The Bohr and Bohr–Enghoff equations can be used independently from the shape of the volumetric capnogram; however, the more the capnogram differs from a step function the more unreliable will be the calculated dead-spaces. Currently we have no special techniques for capnograms in which the three phases cannot be clearly distinguished.

Missing alveolar plateau

Fletcher's method fails if there is no distinct phase III in the volumetric capnogram. Furthermore, a missing alveolar plateau may indicate that the measured $P_{et}CO_2$ does not reflect the alveolar CO_2 pressure. A recently published study of spontaneously breathing preterm infants by Tirosh *et al.* (2001) has shown that with decreasing gestational age the number of capnograms without alveolar plateau increased significantly. The influence of the stiffness of the lungs on the incidence of capnograms without alveolar plateau was investigated by Proquitté *et al.* (2003) in 21 ventilated newborn piglets (body weight 560–1435 g). Mainstream capnographic measurements were performed in healthy lungs and in surfactant-depleted lungs after lung lavage by saline. As shown in Figure 10.5 before lavage 10% of all capnograms did not show an alveolar plateau whereas in the surfactant-depleted lungs the incidence was about 50%. In this study it was also shown that the incidence of capnograms without alveolar plateau increased considerably with decreasing exhalation time (Figure 10.5). If the exhalation time was shorter than 200 ms an alveolar plateau was not seen in more than 75% of all recorded files.

This high rate of missing plateaus in Figure 10.5 illustrates the current problems of capnography in small, stiff lungs. The explanations remain speculative. Likely, it is caused by both the technical limitations of the current technique (mainly the too long response time) and the physiological peculiarities of CO_2 exchange in small lungs. For further capnographic investigations in small stiff lungs it is crucial to avoid the current technical limitations and to shorten the response time of the sensor and to improve time resolution of the signals.

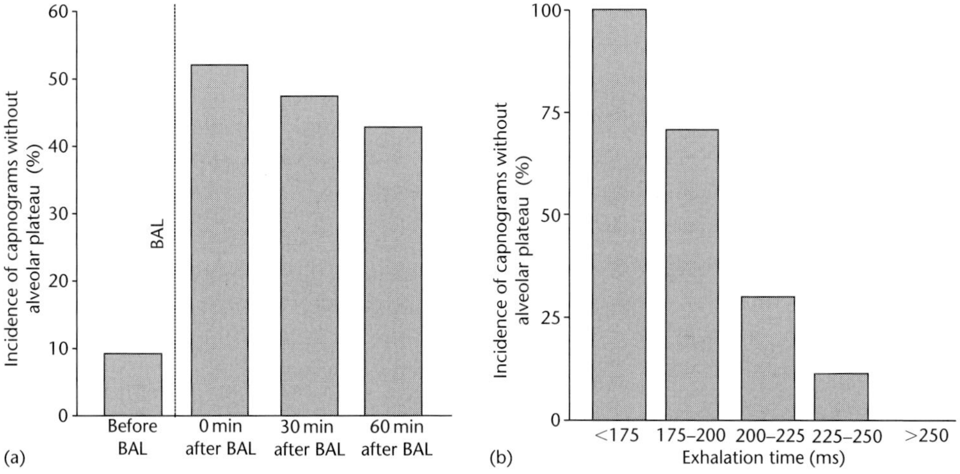

Figure 10.5 Effect of surfactant depletion by bronchoalveolar lavage (BAL) on the incidence of capnograms without an alveolar plateau in newborn piglets (a) and increase of the drop out rate with decreasing exhalation time (b). (Reproduced with permission from Proquitté, H., Krause, S., Rüdiger, M., Wauer, R.R. & Schmalisch, G. (2004). Current limitations of volumetric capnography in surfactant-depleted small lungs. *Pediat. Crit. Care Med.*, **5**: 75–80.)

Incomplete expiration

Beside morphological differences between adult and newborn lungs there are also significant differences in the breathing strategy. Adults and older infants breathe from an end-expiratory lung volume determined by the opposing recoil of the lungs and chest wall. Neonates have a highly compliant chest wall that can cause several problems during breathing, among them a small end-expiratory lung volume, low oxygen stores, and a high risk for airway occlusion and atelectasis (Stark *et al.*, 1987). Therefore, infants compensate for this mechanical disadvantage by actively maintaining lung volume above the resting volume. Kosch and Stark (1984) have shown in the past that flow braking and a preterm onset of inspiration before the complete expiration provide a neonatal breathing strategy dynamically to increase lung volume (Figure 10.6).

Tidal breathing measurements in 99 neonates (Schmalisch *et al.*, 2003) have shown that an incomplete expiration due to a premature onset of inspiration was seen in about 50% of all neonates. There was no statistically significant difference between healthy neonates and neonates with chronic lung diseases.

An incomplete expiration shortens or even suppresses mainly phase III of the capnogram and thus, hampers capnographic measurements in this age. In mechanically ventilated infants the expiratory time can be adapted easily to the exhalation time of the patient so that an incomplete expiration can be avoided. In contrast, during spontaneous breathing the investigator cannot influence the tidal breathing pattern, which must be considered in the interpretation of the capnographic measurements.

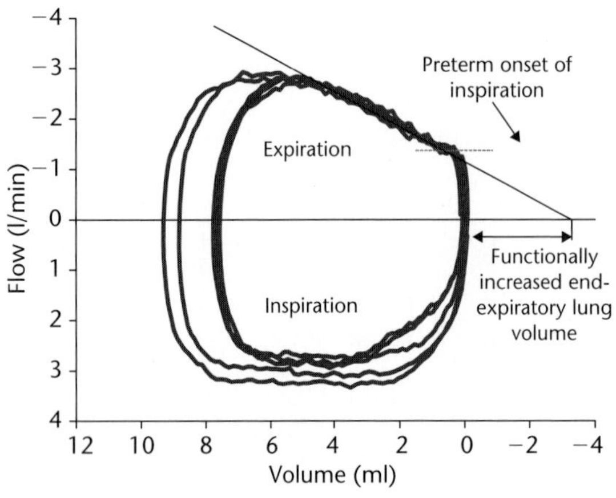

Figure 10.6 Tidal breathing flow–volume loops of a spontaneously breathing newborn with incomplete expiration to increase functionally the end-expiratory lung volume.

Conclusion and outlook

Capnography is a fascinating, noninvasive technique to collect information about breathing and alveolar gas exchange. Its use in spontaneously breathing neonates and in mechanically ventilated infants is attractive. Currently the most important clinical application in neonates is to monitor mechanical ventilation. Several clinical studies have shown that capnography is effective in correctly positioning the ET, the early detection of accidental tracheal extubation and disconnection of breathing circuit and the CO_2 monitoring before irreversible damage is caused by prolonged hypoxia.

Compared with the simpler time-based capnography, the volumetric capnography measurements have a much higher informative potential and enable the calculation of the different dead-spaces, which did show a high predictive value in ventilated neonates. However, this technique requires accurate and artifact-free volume measurements. Volumetric capnography in spontaneously breathing neonates is more expensive and only possible with the help of a face mask. Due to the relatively high-apparatus dead-space of a face mask, only short term measurements can be performed.

Main-stream and flow reduced side-stream capnographs are currently in clinical use. Main-stream capnographs are more accurate than side-stream capnographs, however, in neonates with very small tidal volume the additional apparatus dead-space of the main-stream sensor can result in unacceptable rebreathing. Dead-space-free CO_2 measurements (e.g. for long-term studies in spontaneously breathing infants) are only possible by side-stream measurements.

Despite continuous technological progress we still face technical limitations in correctly measuring the fast CO_2 signals of neonates. For this age we will need faster CO_2 sensors with an integrated pneumotachograph for volumetric capnography. Furthermore, the gas exchange in small lungs differs from that of adult lungs due to the greater impact of the small airways on gas exchange. Particularly in neonates or small animals in which the phase II is widen and phase III reduced or absent we will need imaginative physiological concepts to interpret such capnograms.

Finally, after improvement in the technical and methodological prerequisites for volumetric capnography more clinical research is necessary to demonstrate the value and diagnostic possibilities of this new technique.

References

Arnold, J.H., Bower, L.K. & Thompson, J.E. (1995). Respiratory deadspace measurements in neonates with congenital diaphragmatic hernia. *Crit. Care Med.*, **23**: 371–375.

Arnold, J.H., Thompson, J.E. & Arnold, L.W. (1996). Single breath CO_2 analysis: description and validation of a method. *Crit. Care Med.*, **24**: 96–102.

Arsowa, S., Schmalisch, G. & Wauer, R.R. (1993). Techniques and clinical application of capnography in newborn infants and infants. *Padiatr. Grenzgeb.*, **31**: 295–311.

Arsowa, S., Schmalisch, G. & Wauer, R.R. (1997). Simultaneous measurements of end-expiratory and transcutaneous carbon dioxide partial pressure in ventilated premature and newborn infants. *Klin. Padiatr.*, **209**: 47–53.

Badgwell, J.M. (1992). Respiratory gas monitoring in the pediatric patient. *Int. Anesthesiol. Clin.*, **30**: 131–146.

Badgwell, J.M. & Heavner, J.E. (1991). End-tidal carbon dioxide pressure in neonates and infants measured by aspiration and flow-through capnography. *J. Clin. Monit.*, **7**: 285–288.

Badgwell, J.M., Kleinman, S.E. & Heavner, J.E. (1993). Respiratory frequency and artifact affect the capnographic baseline in infants. *Anesth. Analg.*, **77**: 708–712.

Bates, J.H., Schmalisch, G., Filbrun, D. & Stocks, J. (2000). Tidal breath analysis for infant pulmonary function testing. ERS/ATS task force on standards for infant respiratory function testing. European Respiratory Society/American Thoracic Society. *Eur. Respir. J.*, **16**: 1180–1192.

Behrends, M., Kernbach, M., Brauer, A., Braun, U., Peters, J. & Weyland, W. (2001). In vitro validation of a metabolic monitor for gas exchange measurements in ventilated neonates. *Intensive Care Med.*, **27**: 228–235.

Benumof, J.L. (1998). Interpretation of capnography. *American Association of Nurse Anesthetists J.*, **66**: 169–176.

Berg, R.A., Henry, C., Otto, C.W., Sanders, A.B., Kern, K.B., Hilwig, R.W. & Ewy, G.A. (1996). Initial end-tidal CO_2 is markedly elevated during cardiopulmonary resuscitation after asphyxial cardiac arrest. *Pediatr. Emerg. Care*, **12**: 245–248.

Bhat, R., Kim, W.D., Shukla, A. & Vidyasagar, D. (1981). Simultaneous tissue pH and transcutaneous carbon dioxide monitoring in critically ill neonates. *Crit. Care Med.*, **9**: 744–749.

Bhavani-Shankar, K., Moseley, H., Kumar, A.Y. & Delph, Y. (1992). Capnometry and anaesthesia. *Can. J. Anaesth.*, **39**: 617–632.

Bhende, M.S., Karr, V.A., Wiltsie, D.C. & Orr, R.A. (1995). Evaluation of a portable infrared end-tidal carbon dioxide monitor during pediatric interhospital transport. *Pediatrics*, **95**: 875–878.

Bhende, M.S. & Thompson, A.E. (1995). Evaluation of an end-tidal CO_2 detector during pediatric cardiopulmonary resuscitation. *Pediatrics*, **95**: 395–399.

Bhende, M.S., Thompson, A.E., Cook, D.R. & Saville, A.L. (1992). Validity of a disposable end-tidal CO_2 detector in verifying endotracheal tube placement in infants and children. *Ann. Emerg. Med.*, **21**: 142–145.

Bhende, M.S., Thompson, A.E. & Orr, R.A. (1992). Utility of an end-tidal carbon dioxide detector during stabilization and transport of critically ill children. *Pediatrics*, **89**: 1042–1044.

Bouferrache, B., Filtchev, S., Leke, A., Marbaix-Li, Q., Freville, M. & Gaultier, C. (2000). The hyperoxic test in infants reinvestigated. *Am. J. Respir. Crit. Care Med.*, **161**: 160–165.

Bouferrache, B., Krim, G., Marbaix-Li, Q., Freville, M. & Gaultier, C. (1998). Reproducibility of the alternating breath test of fractional inspired O_2 in infants. *Pediatr. Res.*, **44**: 239–246.

Brouillette, R.T., Morrow, A.S., Weese-Mayer, D.E. & Hunt, C.E. (1987). Comparison of respiratory inductive plethysmography and thoracic impedance for apnea monitoring. *J. Pediatr.*, **111**: 377–383.

Brunner, J.X. & Westenskow, D.R. (1988). How the rise time of carbon dioxide analysers influences the accuracy of carbon dioxide measurements. *Br. J. Anaesth.*, **61**: 628–638.

Casati, A., Gallioli, G., Passaretta, R., Scandroglio, M., Bignami, E. & Torri, G. (2001). End tidal carbon dioxide monitoring in spontaneously breathing, nonintubated patients. A clinical comparison between conventional sidestream and microstream capnometers. *Minerva Anesthesiol.*, **67**: 161–164.

Casati, A., Gallioli, G., Scandroglio, M., Passaretta, R., Borghi, B. & Torri, G. (2000). Accuracy of end-tidal carbon dioxide monitoring using the NBP-75 microstream capnometer. A study in intubated ventilated and spontaneously breathing nonintubated patients. *Eur. J. Anaesthesiol.*, **17**: 622–626.

Chu, J., Clements, J.A., Cotton, E.K., Klaus, M.H., Sweet, A.Y., Tooley, W.H., Bradley, B.L. & Brandorff, L.C. (1967). Neonatal pulmonary ischemia. I. Clinical and physiological studies. *Pediatrics*, **40(suppl.82)**.

Colman, Y. & Krauss, B. (1999). Microstream capnograpy technology: a new approach to an old problem. *J. Clin. Monit. Comput.*, **15**: 403–409.

Cook, C.D., Cherry, R.B., O'Brien, D., Karlberg, P. & Smith, C.A. (1955). Studies of respiratory physiology in the newborn infant. Observations on normal and full-term infants. *J. Clin. Invest.*, **34**: 975–982.

Cook, C.D., Sutherland, J.M., Segal, S., Cherry, R.B., Mead, J., McIlroy, M.B. & Smith, C.A. (1957). Studies of respiratory physiology in the newborn infant. III. measurements of mechanics of respiration. *J.Clin.Invest.*, **36**: 440–448.

Cote, C.J., Liu, L.M., Szyfelbein, S.K., Firestone, S., Goudsouzian, N.G., Welch, J.P. & Daniels, A.L. (1986). Intraoperative events diagnosed by expired carbon dioxide monitoring in children. *Can. Anaesth. Soc. J.*, **33**: 315–320.

Dassieu, G., Brochard, L., Benani, M., Avenel, S. & Danan, C. (2000). Continuous tracheal gas insufflation in preterm infants with hyaline membrane disease. A prospective randomized trial. *Am. J. Respir. Crit. Care Med.*, **162**: 826–831.

Davies, M.W. & Woodgate, P.G. (2002). Tracheal gas insufflation for the prevention of morbidity and mortality in mechanically ventilated newborn infants. *Cochrane Database Syst. Rev.*, CD002973.

Dolfin, T., Duffty, P., Wilkes, D., England, S. & Bryan, H. (1983). Effects of a face mask and pneumotachograph on breathing in sleeping infants. *Am. Rev. Respir. Dis.*, **128**: 977–979.

Domsky, M., Wilson, R.F. & Heins, J. (1995). Intraoperative end-tidal carbon dioxide values and derived calculations correlated with outcome: prognosis and capnography. *Crit. Care Med.*, **23**: 1497–1503.

Dumpit, F.M. & Brady, J.P. (1978). A simple technique for measuring alveolar CO_2 in infants. *J. Appl. Physiol.*, **45**: 648–650.

Emralino, F. & Steele, A.M. (1997). Effects of technique and analytic conditions on tidal breathing flow volume loops in term neonates. *Pediatr. Pulmonol.*, **24**: 86–92.

Evans, J.M., Hogg, M.I. & Rosen, M. (1977a). Correlation of alveolar PCO_2 estimated by infra-red analysis and arterial PCO_2 in the human neonate and the rabbit. *Br. J. Anaesth.*, **49**: 761–764.

Evans, J.M., Hogg, M.I. & Rosen, M. (1977b). Measurement of carbon dioxide output, alveolar carbon dioxide concentration and alveolar ventilation in the neonate. *Br. J. Anaesth.*, **49**: 453–456.

Fleming, P.J., Levine, M.R. & Goncalves, A. (1982). Changes in respiratory pattern resulting from the use of a facemask to record respiration in newborn infants. *Pediatr. Res.*, **16**: 1031–1034.

Fletcher, R. (1984). Airway deadspace, end-tidal CO_2, and Christian Bohr. *Acta Anaesthesiol. Scand.*, **28**: 408-411.

Fletcher, R., Jonson, B., Cumming, G. & Brew, J. (1981). The concept of deadspace with special reference to the single breath test for carbon dioxide. *Br. J. Anaesth.*, **53**: 77–88.

Foitzik, B., Schmidt, M., Proquitte, H. & Schmalisch, G. (2001). Deadspace free ventilatory measurements in newborns during mechanical ventilation. *Crit. Care Med.*, **29**: 413–419.

French, R.A. & Kennedy, R.R. (1998). Disconnect alarm failure in detection of common gas outlet disconnection. *Anaesth. Intens. Care*, **26**: 665–670.

Frey, U., Stocks, J., Sly, P. & Bates, J. (2000). Specification for signal processing and data handling used for infant pulmonary function testing. ERS/ATS task force on standards for infant respiratory function testing. European Respiratory Society/American Thoracic Society. *Eur. Respir. J.*, **16**: 1016–1022.

Gaertner, T. & Barnikol, W.K. (1990). Measurement of phase I volume breath by breath in spontaneously breathing guinea pigs. *J. Appl. Physiol.*, **69**: 747–755.

Gerhardt, T., McCarthy, J. & Bancalari, E. (1978). Aminophylline therapy for idiopathic apnea in premature infants: effects on lung function. *Pediatrics*, **62**: 801–804.

Gerhardt, T.O. & Bancalari, E. (1991). Measurement and monitoring of pulmonary function. *Clin. Perinatol.*, **18**: 581–609.

Gustafsson, P.M., Kallman, S., Ljungberg, H. & Lindblad, A. (2003). Method for assessment of volume of trapped gas in infants during multiple-breath inert gas washout. *Pediatr. Pulmonol.*, **35**: 2–49.

Hagerty, J.J., Kleinman, M.E., Zurakowski, D., Lyons, A.C. & Krauss, B. (2002). Accuracy of a new low-flow sidestream capnography technology in newborns: a pilot study. *J. Perinatol.*, **22**: 219–225.

Hand, I.L., Shepard, E.K., Krauss, A.N. & Auld, P.A. (1989). Discrepancies between transcutaneous and end-tidal carbon dioxide monitoring in the critically ill neonate with respiratory distress syndrome. *Crit Care Med.*, **17**: 556–559.

Henderson-Smart, D.J. (1981). The effect of gestational age on the incidence and duration of recurrent apnoea in newborn babies. *Aust. Paediatr., J.*, **17**: 273–276.

Hopper, A.O., Nystrom, G.A., Deming, D.D., Brown, W.R. & Peabody, J.L. (1994). Infrared end-tidal CO_2 measurement does not accurately predict arterial CO_2 values or end-tidal to arterial PCO_2 gradients in rabbits with lung injury. *Pediatr. Pulmonol.*, **17**: 189–196.

Hsieh, V.K.S., Lee, C.L., Lin, C.C., Wu, S.N., Ko, F.Y., Huang, Y.F. & Huang, T.C. (2001). Quantitative analysis of end-tidal carbon dioxide during mechanical and spontaneous ventilation in infants and young children. *Pediatr. Pulmonol.*, **32**: 453–458.

Hubble, C.L., Gentile, M.A., Tripp, D.S., Craig, D.M., Meliones, J.N. & Cheifetz, I.M. (2000). Deadspace to tidal volume ratio predicts successful extubation in infants and children. *Crit. Care Med.*, **28**: 2034–2040.

Hunt, C.E., Matalon, S., Wangensteen, O.D. & Leonard, A.S. (1974). Mass spectrometer evaluation of ventilation-perfusion abnormalities in respiratory distress syndrome. *Pediatr. Res.*, **8**: 621–627.

Jeng, D.R., Wu, G., Cruz, J.C., Han, D. & Flores, X.F. (2000). Diffusion-convection equation solved in parallel regions of the lung. *Ann. Biomed. Eng.*, **28**: 453–462.

Jenni, O.G., Wolf, M., Hengartner, M., Siebenthal, K., Keel, M. & Bucher, H.U. (1996). Impact of central, obstructive and mixed apnea on cerebral hemodynamics in preterm infants. *Biol. Neonate*, **70**: 91–100.

Karlberg, P., Cook, C.D., O'Brien, D., Cherry, R.B. & Smith, C.A. (1954). Studies of respiratory physiology in newborn infants. II. Observations during and after respiratory distress. *Acta Paediatr.*, **43**: 387–411.

Kars, A.H., Bogaard, J.M., Stijnen, T., de Vries, J., Verbraak, A.F. & Hilvering, C. (1997). Dead space and slope indices from the expiratory carbon dioxide tension-volume curve. *Eur. Respir. J.*, **10**: 829–1836.

Katz, S.M., Hertzberg, T. & Lagercrantz, H. (1991). CO_2-sensitivity in newborn and young infants tested by the rebreathing method. Methodological aspects. *Biol. Neonate*, **59**: 126–132.

Kirpalani, H., Kechagias, S. & Lerman, J. (1991). Technical and clinical aspects of capnography in neonates. *J. Med. Eng. Technol.*, **15**: 154–161.

Kosch, P.C. & Stark, A.R. (1984). Dynamic maintenance of end-expiratory lung volume in full-term infants. *J. Appl. Physiol.*, **57**: 1126–1133.

Krauss, A.N. & Auld, P.A. (1969). Ventilation-perfusion abnormalities in the premature infant: triple gradient. *Pediatr. Res.*, **3**: 255–264.

Lum, L., Saville, A. & Venkataraman, S.T. (1998). Accuracy of physiologic deadspace measurement in intubated pediatric patients using a metabolic monitor: comparison with the Douglas bag method. *Crit. Care Med.*, **26**: 760–764.

Magnan, A., Philip-Joet, F., Rey, M., Reynaud, M., Porri, F. & Arnaud, A. (1993). End-tidal CO_2 analysis in sleep apnea syndrome. Conditions for use. *Chest*, **103**: 129–131.

Mather, S.J. (1994). Capnography in babies and small children. *Anaesthesia*, **49**: 1096–1097.

McDonald, M.J., Montgomery, V.L., Cerrito, P., Parrish, C.J., Boland, K.A. & Sullivan, J.E. (2002). Comparison of end-tidal CO_2 and $PaCO_2$ in children receiving mechanical ventilation. *Pediatr. Crit. Care Med.*, **3**: 244–249.

McEvedy, B.A., McLeod, M.E., Kirpalani, H., Volgyesi, G.A. & Lerman, J. (1990). End-tidal carbon dioxide measurements in critically ill neonates: a comparison of sidestream and mainstream capnometers. *Can. J. Anaesth.*, **37**: 322–326.

McEvedy, B.A., McLeod, M.E., Mulera, M., Kirpalani, H. & Lerman, J. (1988). End-tidal, transcutaneous, and arterial pCO_2 measurements in critically ill neonates: a comparative study. *Anesthesiology*, **69**: 112–116.

McQuillen, K.K. & Steele, D.W. (2000). Capnography during sedation/analgesia in the pediatric emergency department. *Pediatr. Emerg. Care*, **16**: 401–404.

Meredith, K.S. & Monaco, F.J. (1990). Evaluation of a mainstream capnometer and end-tidal carbon dioxide monitoring in mechanically ventilated infants. *Pediatr. Pulmonol.*, **9**: 254–259.

Morielli, A., Desjardins, D. & Brouillette, R.T. (1993). Transcutaneous and end-tidal carbon dioxide pressures should be measured during pediatric polysomnography. *Am. Rev. Respir. Dis.*, **148**: 1599–1604.

Morris, M.G. (1999). A simple new technique to measure the effective dead space of the face mask with a water volumeter in infants. *Eur. Respir. J.*, **14**: 1163–1166.

Nakayama, D.K., Gardner, M.J. & Rowe, M.I. (1990). Emergency endotracheal intubation in pediatric trauma. *Ann. Surg.*, **211**: 218–223.

Napolitano, L.M. (1999). Capnography in critical care: accurate assessment of ARDS therapy? *Crit. Care Med.*, **27**: 862–863.

Nelson, N.M., Prod'hom, L.S., Cherry, R.B., Lipsitz, P.J. & Smith, C.A. (1962). Pulmonary function in the newborn infant: 1. Methods: ventilation and gaseous metabolism. *Pediatrics*, **30**: 963–974.

Neufeld, G.R., Schwardt, J.D., Gobran, S.R., Baumgardner, J.E., Schreiner, M.S., Aukburg, S.J. & Scherer, P.W. (1992). Modelling steady state pulmonary elimination of He, SF6 and CO_2: effect of morphometry. *Respir. Physiol.*, **88**: 257–275.

Nosovitch, M.A., Johnson, J.O. & Tobias, J.D. (2002). Noninvasive intraoperative monitoring of carbon dioxide in children: end-tidal versus transcutaneous techniques. *Paediatr. Anaesth.*, **12**: 48–52.

Obladen, M. & Maier, R.F. (1995). Recombinant erythropoietin for prevention of anemia in preterm infants. *J. Perinat. Med.*, **23**: 119–126.

Ong, B.C. (1998). Oesophageal intubation in an infant for oesophageal dilatation. *Paediatr. Anaesth.*, **8**: 273–274.

Pascucci, R.C., Schena, J.A. & Thompson, J.E. (1989). Comparison of a sidestream and mainstream capnometer in infants. *Crit. Care Med.*, **17**: 560–562.

Payer, C., Urlesberger, B., Pauger, M. & Muller, W. (2003). Apnea associated with hypoxia in preterm infants: impact on cerebral blood volume. *Brain Dev.*, **25**: 25–31.

Proenca, J. & Wenner, J. (1962). Zur Bestimmung der alveolären CO_2-Spannung im Säuglingsalter. *Klin. Wochenschrift*, **40**: 898–903.

Proquitté, H., Krause, S., Rüdiger, M., Wauer, R.R. & Schmalisch, G. (2004). Current limitations of volumetric capnography in surfactant-depleted small lungs. *Pediat. Crit. Care Med.*, **5**: 75–80.

Ream, R.S., Schreiner, M.S., Neff, J.D., McRae, K.M., Jawad, A.F., Scherer, P.W. & Neufeld, G.R. (1995). Volumetric capnography in children. Influence of growth on the alveolar plateau slope. *Anesthesiology*, **82**: 64–73.

Rich, G.F. & Sconzo, J.M. (1991). Continuous end-tidal CO_2 sampling within the proximal endotracheal tube estimates arterial CO_2 tension in infants. *Can. J. Anaesth.*, **38**: 201–203.

Rigatto, H. & Brady, J.P. (1972). Periodic breathing and apnea in preterm infants. I. Evidence for hypoventilation possibly due to central respiratory depression. *Pediatrics*, **50**: 202–218.

Roberts, W.A., Maniscalco, W.M., Cohen, A.R., Litman, R.S. & Chhibber, A. (1995). The use of capnography for recognition of esophageal intubation in the neonatal intensive care unit. *Pediatr. Pulmonol.*, **19**: 262–268.

Rozycki, H.J., Sysyn, G.D., Marshall, M.K., Malloy, R. & Wiswell, T.E. (1998). Mainstream end-tidal carbon dioxide monitoring in the neonatal intensive care unit. *Pediatrics*, **101**: 648–653.

Sanders, A.B., Kern, K.B., Otto, C.W., Milander, M.M. & Ewy, G.A. (1989). End-tidal carbon dioxide monitoring during cardiopulmonary resuscitation. A prognostic indicator for survival. *J. Am. Med. Assoc.*, **262**: 1347–1351.

Santos, L.J., Varon, J., Pic-Aluas, L. & Combs, A.H. (1994). Practical uses of end-tidal carbon dioxide monitoring in the emergency department. *J. Emerg. Med.*, **12**: 633–644.

Schena, J., Thompson, J. & Crone, R.K. (1984). Mechanical influences on the capnogram. *Crit. Care Med.*, **12**: 672–674.

Schmalisch, G., Foitzik, B., Wauer, R.R. & Patzak, A. (2003). Influence of preterm onset of inspiration on tidal breathing parameters in infants with and without CLD. *Respir. Physiol. Neurobiol.*, **135**: 39–46.

Schmalisch, G., Foitzik, B., Wauer, R.R. & Stocks, J. (2001a). Effect of apparatus dead space on breathing parameters in newborns: "flow-through" versus conventional techniques. *Eur. Respir. J.*, **17**: 108–114.

Schmalisch, G., Foitzik, B., Wauer, R.R. & Stocks, J. (2001b). In vitro assessment of equipment and software to assess tidal breathing parameters in infants. *Eur. Respir. J.*, **17**: 100–107.

Schmalisch, G., Schmidt, M. & Foitzik, B. (2001c). Novel technique to average breathing loops for infant respiratory function testing. *Med. Biol. Eng. Comput.*, **39**: 688–693.

Schmidt, M., Foitzik, B., Wauer, R.R., Winkler, F. & Schmalisch, G. (1998). Comparative investigations of algorithms for the detection of breaths in newborns with disturbed respiratory signals. *Comput. Biomed. Res.*, **31**: 413–425.

Scholander, P. (1947). Analyser for accurate estimation of respiratory gases in one-half cubic centimeter samples. *J. Biol. Chem.*, **167**: 235–250.

Schulze, K., Kairam, R., Stefanski, M., Sciacca, R. & James, L.S. (1981). Continuous measurement of minute ventilation and gaseous metabolism of newborn infants. *J. Appl. Physiol.*, **50**: 1098–1103.

Schwardt, J.D., Gobran, S.R., Neufeld, G.R., Aukburg, S.J. & Scherer, P.W. (1991). Sensitivity of CO_2 washout to changes in acinar structure in a single-path model of lung airways. *Ann. Biomed. Eng.*, **19**: 679–697.

Singh, S., Venkataraman, S.T., Saville, A. & Bhende, M.S. (2001). NPB-75: A portable quantitative microstream capnometer. *Am. J. Emerg. Med.*, **19**: 208–210.

Sivan, Y., Eldadah, M.K., Cheah, T.E. & Newth, C.J. (1992). Estimation of arterial carbon dioxide by end-tidal and transcutaneous PCO_2 measurements in ventilated children. *Pediatr. Pulmonol.*, **12**: 153–157.

Smith, T.C., Proops, D.W., Pearman, K. & Hutton, P. (1993). Nasal capnography in children: automated analysis provides a measure of obstruction during sleep. *Clin. Otolaryngol.*, **18**: 69–71.

Stahlman, M.T. & Meece, N.J. (1957). Pulmonary ventilation and diffusion in the human newborn infant. *J. Clin. Invest.*, **36**: 1081–1091.

Stark, A.R., Cohlan, B.A., Waggener, T.B., Frantz, I.D. & Kosch, P.C. (1987). Regulation of end-expiratory lung volume during sleep in premature infants. *J. Appl. Physiol.*, **62**: 1117–1123.

Stock, M.C. (1988). Noninvasive carbon dioxide monitoring. *Crit. Care Clin.*, **4**: 511–526.

Strang, L. (1961). Alveolar gas and anatomical dead-space measurements in normal newborns. *J. Clin. Sci.*, **21**: 107–114.

Thibeault, D.W., Poblete, E. & Auld, P.A. (1968). Alevolar-arterial O_2 and CO_2 differences and their relation to lung volume in the newborn. *Pediatrics*, **41**: 574–587.

Thome, U.H. & Carlo, W.A. (2002). Permissive hypercapnia. *Semin. Neonatol.*, **7**: 409–419.

Tirosh, E., Bilker, A., Bader, D. & Cohen, A. (2001). Capnography in spontaneously breathing preterm and term infants. *Clin. Physiol.*, **21**: 150–154.

Tobias, J.D. & Meyer, D.J. (1997). Noninvasive monitoring of carbon dioxide during respiratory failure in toddlers and infants: end-tidal versus transcutaneous carbon dioxide. *Anesth. Analg.*, **85**: 55–58.

Trang, H., Leske, V. & Gaultier, C. (2002). Use of nasal cannula for detecting sleep apneas and hypopneas in infants and children. *Am. J. Respir. Crit. Care Med.*, **166**: 464–468.

Vos, P.J., Folgering, H.T. & van Herwaarden, C.L. (1993). Nocturnal end-tidal PCO_2 to detect apnoeas and hypopnoeas in sleep-disordered breathing. *Physiol. Meas.*, **14**: 433–439.

Weese-Mayer, D.E., Corwin, M.J. & Peucker, M.R. *et al.* (2000). Comparison of apnea identified by respiratory inductance plethysmography with that detected by end-tidal CO(2) or thermistor. The CHIME Study Group. *Am. J. Respir. Crit. Care Med.*, **162**: 471–480.

Weiler, N., Barnikol, W.K. & Burkhard, O. (1987). Simultane quasi kontinuierliche bestimmung des bronchialvolumens des meerschweinchens mit hilfe des O_2- und CO_2-bronchialplateaus atemzug für astemzug. *Prax. Klin. Pneumol.*, **41**: 537–538.

Wenzel, U., Rudiger, M., Wagner, M.H. & Wauer, R.R. (1999a). Utility of deadspace and capnometry measurements in determination of surfactant efficacy in surfactant-depleted lungs. *Crit. Care Med.*, **27**: 946–952.

Wenzel, U., Wauer, R.R. & Schmalisch, G. (1999b). Comparison of different methods for dead space measurements in ventilated newborns using CO_2-volume plot. *Intens. Care Med.*, **25**: 705–713.

Wenzel, U., Wauer, R.R., Wagner, M.H. & Schmalisch, G. (1999c). In vitro and in vivo assessment of the Ventrak 1550/Capnogard 1265 for single breath carbon dioxide analysis in neonates. *Br. J. Anaesth.*, **83**: 503–510.

Whiteley, J.P., Turner, M.J., Baker, A.B., Gavaghan, D.J. & Hahn, C.E. (2002). The effects of ventilation pattern on carbon dioxide transfer in three computer models of the airways. *Respir. Physiol. Neurobiol.*, **131**: 269–284.

Wilson, R.F., Tyburski, J.G., Kubinec, S.M., Warsow, K.M., Larky, H.C., Wilson, S.R. & Schermerhorn, T. (1996). Intraoperative end-tidal carbon dioxide levels and derived calculations correlated with outcome in trauma patients. *J. Trauma*, **41**: 606–611.

Wong, L., Hamilton, R., Palayiwa, E. & Hahn, C. (1998). A real-time algorithm to improve the response time of a clinical multigas analyser. *J. Clin. Monit. Comput.*, **14**: 441–446.

Wu, C.H., Chou, H.C., Hsieh, W.S., Chen, W.K., Huang, P.Y. & Tsao, P.N. (2003). Good estimation of arterial carbon dioxide by end-tidal carbon dioxide monitoring in the neonatal intensive care unit. *Pediatr. Pulmonol.*, **35**: 292–295.

Yaron, M., Padyk, P., Hutsinpiller, M. & Cairns, C.B. (1996). Utility of the expiratory capnogram in the assessment of bronchospasm. *Ann. Emerg. Med.*, **28**: 403–407.

CAPNOGRAPHY AND SLEEP: TECHNICAL ASPECTS

11

T. Schäfer

Introduction

Multi-cell organisms depend on gas exchange between the organism and its environment ("external respiration") for the oxidation of nutrients ("internal respiration"). The long paths between oxygen-consuming (and carbon dioxide (CO_2) producing) cells and the ambient air are overcome by convection. In the respiratory system this mass transport is affected by gas flow, in the cardiovascular system it is affected by blood flow. Feedback control systems optimize alveolar ventilation to meet the metabolic needs, particularly the CO_2 production and oxygen consumption. This maintains blood gases (partial pressure of carbon dioxide and oxygen, respectively, PCO_2 and PO_2) within tight limits. Hypercapnia results from alveolar ventilation that is too small relative to the CO_2 production (hypoventilation), and hypocapnia results from hyperventilation. There is a multitude of reasons for these deviations from normocapnia, including a failure of the "central" respiratory control by the central nervous system. They may also have "peripheral" causes, for example obstruction of the upper airways, as commonly seen with the obstructive sleep apnea syndrome.

Respiratory measurements are of great significance in sleep medicine. Initially the focus was the recording of respiratory movements and airflow for the detection of apneas. However, respiratory control failures can also lead to disorders that are relevant to sleep medicine. The qualitative or at best semi-quantitative measurement of ventilation is usually not sufficient for the detection of these disorders nor for assessing their treatment. This creates a measurement problem in sleep medicine. Adequate quantitative measurement methods are usable only to a certain extent during sleep.

Pneumotachography is considered the "gold standard" for the measurement of ventilation, that is tidal volumes and respiratory rate. Work of breathing can be determined from esophageal pressure measurements and flow. To differentiate central from obstructive apneas, it has been recommended to use a combination of both methods. To determine the adequacy of ventilation with respect to metabolic activity, that is to determine hypo-, normo-, or hyperventilation the American Academy of Sleep Medicine Task Force in 1999 suggested the measurement of arterial PCO_2. Clinically, however, none of the three measurement methods is very practical. Pneumotachography requires a leak-proof face mask. Esophageal pressure measurements require insertion of an esophageal catheter. Arterial PCO_2 measurement requires repeated arterial blood draws or continual measurement using an arterial catheter, such as the Paratrend 7 (Diametrics). There is a need for noninvasive techniques that allow one to make measurements while minimizing interference with sleep and having minimal side effects. Additionally, these techniques should agree well with the respected gold standard and/or it must be shown that they correlate closely with relevant outcome variables, such as mortality or morbidity.

This chapter will focus on the use of capnography for sleep studies including using end-tidal values for the noninvasive estimation of arterial PCO_2.

Methodological aspects

The term "capnography" describes the continuous recording of CO_2 partial pressure in inspiratory and expiratory gas. A capnometer indicates the inspiratory and expiratory PCO_2 numerically, while a capnograph provided a continuous depiction of PCO_2 as a function of time or volume. The sample gas is acquired using either the mainstream or the sidestream method. For sleep studies the sidestream method is often preferred because the application of the mainstream sensor may not be well tolerated by patients during sleep.

Measurement techniques are ultra red absorption spectrometry (mainstream and sidestream) or mass spectrometry (sidestream only). The former is the preferred technique in the sleep laboratory, due to its lower cost and comparative ease of use. There are deviations in the presence of large PCO_2 values in the gas (Raemer & Calalang, 1991). Usually capnographs need to be calibrated with premixed CO_2 gas mixtures.

The capnogram represents the respiratory PCO_2 waveform (Figure 11.1). The maximum value within each breath, known as the end-expiratory CO_2 arterial pressure, $P_{et}CO_2$ can often be considered an approximation of arterial CO_2 pressure, P_aCO_2 – but only for breaths in which a plateau phase was observed. During slow, prolonged expiration PCO_2 continues to rise slowly and reaches venous PCO_2 after about 13 s (Ulmer *et al.*, 2003).

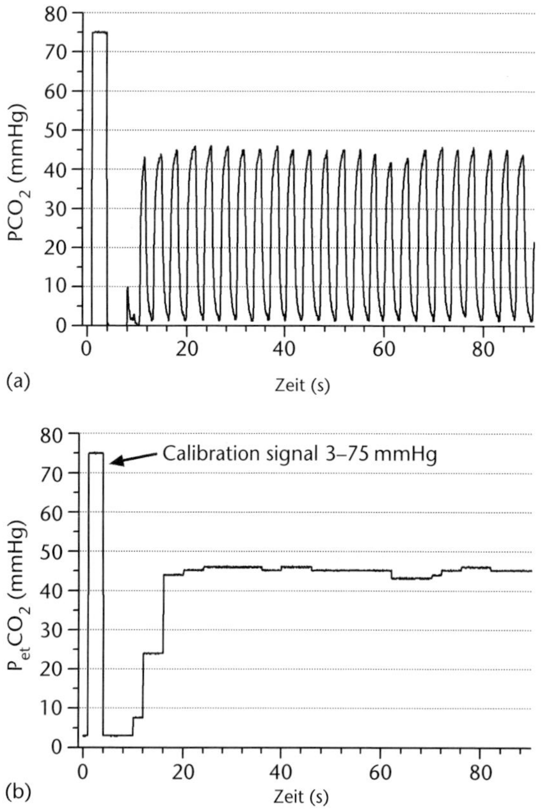

Figure 11.1 (a) Capnogram, starting with a calibration signal. Values vary between the inspiratory PCO_2 and the end-expiratory value (maxima of the waveform). (b) Waveform of $P_{et}CO_2$, as determined from the capnogram.

Recordings are made of either the complete capnogram (Smalhout & Kalenda, 1981) and/or the derived $P_{et}CO_2$ as an estimate of P_aCO_2. The complete waveform is to be preferred because it allows an evaluation of signal quality. A steepening or lack of the plateau phase indicates that the end-expiratory gas may not represent alveolar gas (Figure 11.2).

Advantages of capnography are noninvasiveness and the continuous data acquisition for every breath. Limitations are associated with compromises for the patient interface, with discrepancies between end-expiratory and alveolar PCO_2 (from inhomogeneities and distribution problems in the lung), with significant hypoventilation, and with apneas during which no pure alveolar gas can be acquired and analyzed.

During gas sampling the sampling of room air should be avoided to prevent measurement of erroneously low values. A reliable mainstream measurement is possible in intubated patients. In spontaneously breathing patients this would require using a nasal or face mask with attached mainstream sensor. That is usually not practical in sleep studies for reasons of weight and patient discomfort. The alternative is to use nasal prongs for sidestream measurements. However, they may not provide accurate measurements, particularly with nasal congestion or mouth breathing. The delivery of oxygen through a second pair of nasal prongs or the application of continuous positive airway pressure (CPAP) through a nasal mask (for treatment of sleep apnea) may result in

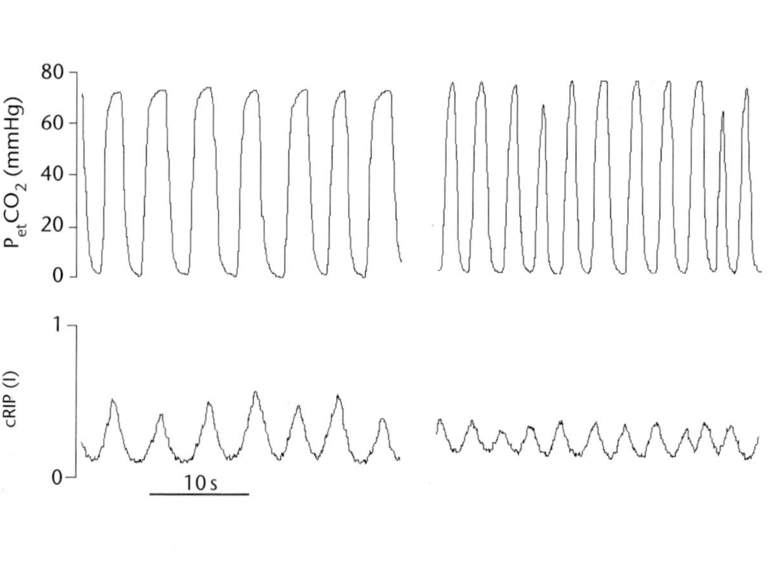

Figure 11.2 Capnogram and tidal volume (as determined by calibrated respiratory inductive plethysmography, cRIP) in a child with severe sleep-related hypoventilation (congenital central hypoventilation syndrome). In the left part of the figure there are still alveolar plateaus, worsening hypoventilation causes the $P_{et}CO_2$ to rise above the range of the capnograph, insufficiently small tidal volumes result in artifacts in the capnogram, as indicated by lacking alveolar plateaus.

erroneously low measurement of PCO_2 (Sanders *et al.*, 1994). This problem can be circumvented by advancing a nasal catheter through the nose into the laryngeal area (Øberg *et al.*, 1995; Waldau *et al.*, 1995).

It is important for long-term sidestream measurements in sleep laboratories to dehumidify the sample gas. This may be achieved through water traps, water permeable tubing, or filters. Depending on sampling tube geometry and sample flow rate there is a delay between volume flow and capnogram. This delay must be considered for the analysis (Figure 11.2). It is also important to make sure the sample pump is not noisy as not to disturb the patient's sleep.

Knowing arterial PCO_2 or a reliable surrogate is important for the diagnosis of hypo- or hyperventilation. It can also aid in finding the cause for central sleep apneas, Cheyne–Stokes respiration and other disorders (Schläfke *et al.*, 1997). Despite its importance, CO_2 monitoring has not become clinical routine yet. The reasons include the lag between new discoveries and their routine application, and the reported technical problems and limitations of indirect PCO_2 monitoring.

Signal quality of capnography during sleep

The capnogram as a qualitative volume flow indicator for apnea detection

The capnogram cannot be used as a quantitative indicator for flow, since it only shares the CO_2 concentration but not the volume or volume per time of the respiration gas. On the other hand, if the expiratory volume exceeds the deadspace, $P_{et}CO_2$ increases. A recent multi-center study of the application of capnography led by the author in the sleep laboratory showed that this qualitative flow signal is as sensitive and specific for determining the apnea index as the currently widely used qualitative flow measurement via thermo-element or thermistor based in measurement and using thresholds of 5, 10, and 20 events per hour, the sensitivity was 97%, 100%, and 92% and the specificity was 94%, 98%, and 98%, respectively (Schäfer *et al.*, 1999). Sidestream measurements were made from a double-lumen nasal prong, increasing the vulnerability to artifacts from oral respiration. Still, alveolar plateaus were detected in 71% of the data collection time (386 min on average of 121 measurements). In another 25% of the data collection time the signal quality was sufficient for determining respiratory rate and for detecting apneas. Unusable signals were present during 4% of the data collection time.

An alternative to capnography is transcutaneous CO_2 monitoring (Hanly, 1997). This method uses pH electrodes, which are placed on the skin. The skin is warmed to 42–44°C increasing its perfusion. CO_2 diffuses through the skin and is measured. There are not sufficient data available to evaluate the utility of this method in sleep studies (American Academy of Sleep Medicine Task Force, 1999). The method is more expensive than capnography, needs to be calibrated before each use, depends on skin condition and perfusion, and needs about 30 min after placement on the skin, before stable measurements are available. It might be that transcutaneous O_2 correlates better than $P_{et}CO_2$ with P_aCO_2 (Sanders *et al.*, 1994; Janssens *et al.*, 2001).

Study of $P_{a\text{-}et}CO_2$ in sleep laboratory patients

We analyzed the difference between $P_{et}CO_2$ and P_aCO_2 in 57 unselected patients (46 men and 11 women) who underwent a polysomnographic study because of suspected sleep-related breathing disorders (Schäfer, 2003). The polysomnography indicated an apnea–hypopnea index (AHI) of less than 5/h in 31 patients, of 5–20/h in 21 patients and of more than 20/h in 5 patients. Thirteen patients had a 1-s forced expiratory volume (FEV_1) of less than 80% of the normal value. $P_{et}CO_2$ was measured via sidestream capnography. P_aCO_2 was determined from capillary blood. Blood was drawn while the patients were awake, either in the evening before the sleep study or in the morning after the sleep study. The mean $P_{a\text{-}et}CO_2$ difference was 0.63 mmHg and the standard deviation was 3.3 mmHg. It can be expected that 95% of the differences are between −6.0 and +7.3 mmHg. A dependence of the $P_{a\text{-}et}O_2$ difference and the absolute PCO_2 value could not be shown. $P_{a\text{-}et}CO_2$ differences recorded in patients with lower FEV_1 (+1.8 ± 3.4 mmHg) were not statistically significantly different than those recorded in patients with a normal FEV_1 (+0.3 ± 3.3 mmHg, *t*-test, $P = 0.65$). On average capnography allowed reasonably accurate estimation of P_aCO_2. The degree of scatter was independent of the absolute PCO_2 value, however, the standard deviation was ±3.3 mmHg. This may mean that small changes in P_aCO_2 cannot be detected with certainty. The sample of patients studied did not show significant hyper- or hypocapnia. Their P_aCO_2 values were between 32 and 48 mmHg. This study did not allow conclusions regarding the sensitivity or specificity for detecting these disorders based on $P_{a\text{-}et}CO_2$ measurements.

Discussion

A recent consensus report did not recommend capnography as a P_aCO_2 surrogate for the detection of hypercapnia due to hypoventilation (American Academy of Sleep Medicine Task Force, 1999). The reason cited for this decision by the Task Force was the contradicting studies comparing arterial with end-expiratory PCO_2. Still, the currently available literature of measurements during sleep remains rather slim. One study of arterial to end-expiratory differences ($P_{a-et}CO_2$) in intensive care patients during mechanical ventilation or under anesthesia (Overview in Hess (1997)) found that typically $P_{et}CO_2$ was several Torr below P_aCO_2. There was a large variability in the differences. Comparisons of $P_{et}CO_2$ during intubation and spontaneous respiration with P_aCO_2 values of blood drawn from radial artery catheters showed $P_{a-et}CO_2$ differences of 7.3 ± 4.0 and 6.5 ± 4.8 mmHg, respectively (Casati *et al.*, 2000). The same group observed an improvement in accuracy when using a new sidestream capnometer with reduced sample flow rate. The $P_{a-et}CO_2$ difference decreased during spontaneous breathing from 7.0 to 4.4 mmHg (Casati *et al.*, 2001). Using a tracheal tube and an oropharyngeal cuff in patients under anesthesia, differences of 4.8 ± 3.0 and 5.4 ± 3.4 mmHg, respectively, were found (Nakata *et al.*, 1998). Particularly patients with lung disorders that result in inhomogenous exhalation and in ventilation/perfusion disorders show elevated and varying $P_{a-et}CO_2$ differences (Raemer *et al.*, 1983; Hoffman *et al.*, 1989; Russell *et al.*, 1990).

So far the only study that looked at the $P_{a-et}CO_2$ difference during sleep and spontaneous breathing and while delivering supplemental oxygen and nasal CPAP (Øberg *et al.*, 1995) found that only 23% (and 15% and 20%, respectively) of the $P_{et}CO_2$ variability could be explained by changes in P_aCO_2. The investigators observed deviations of more than 10 mmHg in 21% of the spontaneously breathing patients, in 46% of the patients receiving oxygen, and in 64% of the patients under CPAP. Our own analysis reported above found better correlations in spontaneously breathing patients.

When performing these comparisons it is important to consider that both capnography and invasive P_aCO_2 measurements are sensitive to errors. Drawing blood can have an effect on respiration. Small changes of tidal volumes result in fast changes of $P_{et}CO_2$, which make comparisons difficult.

Typically, $P_{et}CO_2$ is lower than P_aCO_2. Larger $P_{et}CO_2$ than (average) P_aCO_2 values can only be observed in extreme ventilation/perfusion distributions with late-expiratory emptying of poorly ventilated alveoli or during strenuous physical exercise. Falsely positive detections of hypoventilation and hypercapnia based on capnography are not expected in typical sleep laboratory patients. In these situations elevated $P_{et}CO_2$ usually allow inference of elevation of P_aCO_2. Low $P_{et}CO_2$ measurements do not allow the diagnosis of hyperventilation with low P_aCO_2 values nor do they allow the exclusion of hypoventilation with hypercapnia.

As long as these methodological limitations are considered, capnography can provide important diagnostic information for diseases that are associated with frequent night-time ventilation insufficiencies, for example, congenital central hypoventilation syndrome (Schläfke *et al.*, 1999), in children with suspected upper airway obstruction (Marcus *et al.*, 1992), in patients with Cheyne–Stokes respiration and central sleep apnea (Xie *et al.*, 1995), and in neuromuscular (Kotterba *et al.*, 2001), musculoskeletal and neurological disorders (Schäfer, 2001; Schäfer *et al.*, 2001). A further important area of application is the assessment of therapy in patients with night-time administration of supplemental oxygen and in patients receiving ventilation therapy (Overview in Schläfke *et al.* (1997)). Capnography provides additional diagnostic and therapeutic insight that traditional approaches, such as the analysis of breathing patterns and apneas, do not reveal.

Improved analysis algorithms for capnograms might be able to reject (Figure 11.2) falsely low $P_{et}CO_2$ values, for example, from a lacking alveolar plateau (phase 3), and instead could provide maximum values within certain time intervals (McNulty *et al.*, 1990). The use of pharyngeal catheters might avoid the interference of supplemental oxygen delivery or CPAP with capnography.

Capnography with its $P_{et}CO_2$ values and transcutaneous CO_2 measurements could of course also be treated as if they were independent stand-alone variables. Then the significance would not be measured by their agreement with a reference P_aCO_2, but directly with the degree of morbidity. There are yet no systematic studies of this issue.

References

American Academy of Sleep Medicine Task Force (1999). Sleep-related breathing disorders in adults: recommendations for syndrome definition and measurement techniques in clinical research. The Report of an American Academy of Sleep Medicine Task Force. *Sleep*, **22**: 667–689.

Casati, A., Gallioli, G., Scandroglio, M., Passaretta, R., Borghi, B. & Torri, G. (2000). Accuracy of end-tidal carbon dioxide monitoring using the NBP-75 microstream capnometer. A study in intubated ventilated and spontaneously breathing nonintubated patients. *Eur. J. Anaesthesiol.*, **17**: 622–626.

Casati, A., Gallioli, G., Passaretta, R., Scandroglio, M., Bignami, E. & Torri, G. (2001). End tidal carbon dioxide monitoring in spontaneously breathing, nonintubated patients. A clinical comparison between conventional sidestream and microstream capnometers. *Minerva Anestesiol.*, **67**: 161–164.

Hanly, P.J. (1997). Transcutaneous monitoring of carbon dioxide tension. In: Tobin, M.J. (ed.) *Principles and Practice of Intensive Care Monitoring*. McGraw-Hill, New York; pp. 401–414.

Hess, D.R. (1997). Capnometry. In: Tobin, M.J. (ed.) *Principles and Practice of Intensive Care Monitoring*. McGraw-Hill, New York; pp. 377–400.

Hoffman, R.A., Krieger, B.P., Kramer, M.R., Segel, S., Bizousky, F., Gazeroglu, H., *et al.* (1989). End-tidal carbon dioxide in critically ill patients during changes in mechanical ventilation. *Am. Rev. Respir. Dis.*, **140**: 1265–1268.

Janssens, J.P., Perrin, E., Bennani, I., de Muralt, B., Titelion, V. & Picaud, C. (2001). Is continuous transcutaneous monitoring of PCO_2 ($TcPCO_2$) over 8 h reliable in adults? *Respir. Med.*, **95**: 331–335.

Kotterba, S., Patzold, T., Malin, J.P., Orth, M. & Rasche, K. (2001). Respiratory monitoring in neuromuscular disease – capnography as an additional tool? *Clin. Neurol. Neurosurg.*, **103**: 87–91.

Marcus, C.L., Omlin, K.J., Basinski, D.J., Bailey, S.L., Rachal, A.B., von Pechmann, W.S., *et al.* (1992). Normal polysomnographic values for children and adolescents. *Am. Rev. Respir. Dis.* **146**: 1235–1239.

McNulty, S.E., Roy, J., Torjman, M. & Seltzer, J.L. (1990). Relationship between arterial carbon dioxide and end-tidal carbon dioxide when a nasal sampling port is used. *J. Clin. Monit.* **6**: 93–98.

Nakata, Y., Goto, T., Uezono, S., Sasaki, F. & Morita, S. (1998). Relationship between end-tidal and arterial carbon dioxide partial pressure using a cuffed oropharyngeal airway and a tracheal tube. *Br. J. Anaesth.*, **80**: 253–254.

Øberg, B., Waldau, T. & Larsen, V.H. (1995). The effect of nasal oxygen flow and catheter position on the accuracy of end-tidal carbon dioxide measurements by a pharyngeal catheter in unintubated, spontaneously breathing subjects. *Anaesthesia*, **50**: 695–698.

Raemer, D.B. & Calalang, I. (1991). Accuracy of end-tidal carbon dioxide tension analyzers. *J. Clin. Monit.*, **7**: 195–208.

Raemer, D.B., Francis, D., Philip, J.H. & Gabel, R.A. (1983). Variation in PCO_2 between arterial blood and peak expired gas during anesthesia. *Anesth. Analg.*, **62**: 1065–1069.

Russell, G.B., Graybeal, J.M. & Strout, J.C. (1990). Stability of arterial to end-tidal carbon dioxide gradients during postoperative cardiorespiratory support (see comments). *Can. J. Anaesth.*, **37**: 560–566.

Sanders, M.H., Kern, N.B., Costantino, J.P., Stiller, R.A., Strollo, P.J., Studnicki, K.A., *et al.* (1994). Accuracy of end-tidal and transcutaneous PCO_2 monitoring during sleep. *Chest*, **106**: 472–483.

Schäfer, D. (2001). Schlafbezogene Atmungsstörungen bei Parkinsonsyndromen: Häufigkeit, Art und Behandlungsansätze. *Somnologie*, **5**: 103–114.

Schäfer, T. (2003). Methodik der Atmungsmessung im Schlaf: Kapnographie zur Beurteilung der Ventilation. *Biomed. Tech. (Berl)*, **48**: 170–175.

Schäfer, T., Burmann-Urbanek, M., Glaser, S., Hein, H., Koper, I., Kröger, H., *et al.* (1999). Multicenter-Studie "Kapnographie in der Schlafmedizin". *Somnologie*, **3**: 3–13.

Schäfer, D., Gopon, F., Sidiropoulou, M., Schläfke, M.E. & Greulich, W. (2001). Polygraphic screening after ischemic stroke: a consecutive study on 258 patients. *Somnologie*, **5**: 135–140.

Schläfke, M.E., Hein, H., Kotterba, S., Rasche, K., Rühle, K.H., Sanner, B., *et al.* (1997). Zur Bedeutung des CO_2-Partialdruckes als Meßgröße im Schlaflabor. *Somnologie*, **1**: 184–196.

Schläfke, M.E., Schäfer, C. & Schäfer, T. (1999). Das Undine-Syndrom als kongenitales zentrales Hypoventilationssyndrom (CCHS). *Somnologie*, **3**: 128–133.

Smalhout, B. & Kalenda, Z. (1981). *An Atlas of Capnography*, 2nd edition, vol. 1. Kerckebosch, Zeist, The Netherlands.

Ulmer, W.T., Nolte, D., Lecheler, J. & Schäfer, T. (2003). *Die Lungenfunktion*, 7th edition. Georg Thieme Verlag, Stuttgart; p. 41.

Waldau, T., Øberg, B. & Larsen, V. H. (1995). Reliability of CO_2 measurements from the airway by a pharyngeal catheter in unintubated, spontaneously breathing subjects. *Acta Anaesthesiol. Scand.*, **39**: 637–642.

Xie, A.L., Rutherford, R., Rankin, F., Wong, B. & Bradley, T.D. (1995). Hypocapnia and increased ventilatory responsiveness in patients with idiopathic central sleep apnea. *Am. J. Respir. Crit. Care Med.*, **152**: 1950–1955.

A CASE FOR CARBON DIOXIDE MONITORING IN THE SLEEP LABORATORY 12

R.J. Thomas

Direct monitoring of blood gas is not a standard practice in clinical sleep laboratories due to the invasive nature of the measurement (such as the requirement for an arterial catheter) and the general perception of lack of need for this type of clinical information. Oxymetry has been used as the surrogate for adequate ventilation and oxygenation, which has worked for the most part as the typical patient in the sleep laboratory is medically stable, without multiple reasons for hypoxemia. Thus, disproportionate desaturation after normalizing airflow is taken as a practical marker for hypoventilation, although ideally this requires carbon dioxide (CO_2) measurement in some form.

Oxymetry, airflow monitoring with nasal pressure and CO_2 monitoring provide complementary information. Hypoxemia in the sleep laboratory context is secondary to airway obstruction or hypoventilation, as problems of ventilation–perfusion mismatch are not seen in the typical subject. Nasal flow patterns provide information regarding upper airway characteristics, such as flow limitation (Ayappa *et al.*, 2000). The end-tidal CO_2 signal gives no information about inspiratory flow; breath-to-breath variations can occur secondary to varying upper airway obstruction, but the nasal flow signal is superior for this purpose. Transcutaneous monitoring provides overall trends over time and could be particularly useful during positive airway pressure titrations, especially in those with mixed physiology (Wiedemann & McCarthy, 1989). One such example would be a patient with periodic breathing in non-rapid eye movement (NREM) sleep and hypoventilation in rapid eye movement (REM) sleep. Avoiding hypocapnia is critical to minimize periodic breathing. Adequate ventilation is the target in REM sleep, which may require increases in the inspiratory–expiratory pressure differential with bilevel ventilation. If oxygen (O_2) is added, "disproportionate desaturation" may be lost as a marker of hypoventilation but a transcutaneous partial pressure of CO_2 (PCO_2) trend will give information on the adequacy of ventilation.

End-tidal and transcutaneous CO_2 are complementary options in a sleep laboratory. End-tidal measurements using a main-stream sensor requires using a non-vented mask that is sealed tightly (a practical challenge to maintain throughout the night). Side-stream sampling could be done with a nasal cannula both during diagnostic testing using a divided cannula, or even during titration, although the set-up becomes more cumbersome. Transcutaneous CO_2 measurements have numerous sources of errors but do provide a reasonable trend over several minutes. Clearly, a good end-tidal PCO_2 signal provides a more direct measure of respiration (Levine, 2000). This is possible only when the subject is breathing evenly, such as when positive airway pressure is close to or at an optimum.

Is it important to measure CO_2 in the sleep laboratory? The answer depends on the perspective taken to the pathophysiological approach to sleep-disordered breathing. Those believing in the dominance of the anatomical theory will rely on positive airway pressure to open up the airway, ignoring the contribution of abnormal control that is now well characterized in obstructive disease (Younes, 2003). Those who consider polysomnographically obstructive disease as an interaction of control and anatomy will prefer to have a measure of stabilizing and destabilizing influences. Hypocapnia is destabilizing to the respiratory controller and a primary cause of periodic breathing. Its correction can contribute to stabilization of respiration in patients with mixed or non-obstructive disease (Bradley, 2002). The latter is characterized by distinctive polysomnographic patterns, such as periodic breathing including Cheyne–Stokes respiration, smooth and symmetric desaturations, reduced severity during REM versus NREM sleep, and short (25–30 s) symmetrical cycles of respiratory abnormality (Thomas *et al.*, 2004). Certain conditions impose special risk for complex disease, such as congestive heart failure, chronic renal failure, advanced diabetes, Parkinson's disease, and post-stroke (Bradley & Floras, 2003).

The use of CO_2 for therapy has been limited because of the belief that positive airway pressure works exceedingly well for all types of sleep-disordered breathing.

Complex diseases deserve complex airway pressure modalities, such as bilevel ventilation, proportional pressure, and adaptive servo-controlled pressure ventilation. If the underlying disease can be treated successfully, abnormal control stabilized the problem becomes purely obstructive, allowing standard positive airway pressure to work as well as it can in simple obstructive disease.

Diseases and conditions that can destabilize breathing during sleep include:

1 *Mechanical*: Upper airway, cardiorespiratory mechanics. This includes upper airway obstruction, abnormal neuromuscular apparatus (kyphoscoliosis, neuromuscular disorders such as myopathies).
2 *Gas*: Hypocapnia and hypoxia are destabilizing. The best and relatively pure example of this is high- altitude-related sleep-disordered breathing, where periodic breathing patterns are universal and relatively severe before acclimatization (Rodway *et al.*, 2003).
3 *Chemosensitivity*: Ventilatory response to O_2 and CO_2 has strong genetic influences and may be modified by disease (sleep apnea, heart failure). For example, periodic breathing at altitude is more common in those who have enhanced hypoxic responsiveness (Lahiri *et al.*, 1983). Patients with heart failure who have Cheyne–Stokes respiration have enhanced sensitivity to inhaled CO_2 (Quaranta *et al.*, 1997).
4 *Sleep*: Obstructive disease is vulnerable in REM sleep, while non-obstructive disease is minimal in REM sleep and augmented by cyclic alternating pattern (CAP) type of NREM sleep (Thomas *et al.*, 2004). As the contribution of arousals to respiratory instability is reduced, the more consolidated and stable sleep is (non-CAP electroencephalogram (EEG) morphology). In mathematical models of periodic breathing, repetitive arousals, and the resulting fluctuations in sleep–wake state can maintain periodic cycling of ventilation (Khoo *et al.*, 1991).

Direct inhalation of CO_2 or the addition of dead space and rebreathing CO_2 can reduce periodic breathing, central sleep apnea and Cheyne–Stokes respiration (Andreas *et al.*, 1998; Khayat *et al.*, 2003). More recently, use of CO_2 has been shown to be synergistic with positive airway pressure in the treatment of otherwise uncontrollable mixed disease (Thomas & Daly, 2004). For this purpose, positive airway pressure has been used with approximately 150 ml of dead space or with a prototype device that can add precise percentages of CO_2 into a positive airway pressure circuit. To successfully use CO_2 as a respiratory stabilizer in clinical practice, both end-tidal and transcutaneous monitoring could be required in the sleep laboratory, as one or the other measure has a significant chance for an imprecise signal (e.g. mask leaks, subcutaneous edema in heart failure). Great accuracy is not required, as trends and avoidance of excess are the clinical targets. What is done is not induction of hypercapnia, but prevention of subtle degrees of hypocapnia during sleep.

In conclusion, increasing the concentration of CO_2 in the inhaled gas is a potent stabilizer of sleep–respiration, and to do so will require monitoring of CO_2. This will be especially relevant in patient populations with a high risk of complex sleep-disordered breathing, such as congestive heart failure and chronic renal failure.

References

Andreas, S., Weidel, K., Hagenah, G. & Heindl, S. (1998). Treatment of Cheyne–Stokes respiration with nasal oxygen and carbon dioxide. *Eur. Respir. J.*, **12**: 414–419.

Ayappa, I., Norman, R.G., Krieger, A.C., Rosen, A., O'Malley, R.L. & Rapoport, DM. (2000). Non-invasive detection of respiratory effort-related arousals (RERAs) by a nasal cannula/pressure transducer system. *Sleep*, **23**: 763–771.

Bradley, T.D. (2002). Crossing the threshold: implications for central sleep apnea. *Am. J. Respir. Crit. Care Med.*, **165**: 1203–1204.

Bradley, T.D. & Floras, J.S. (2003). Sleep apnea and heart failure. Part II: Central sleep apnea. *Circulation*, **107**: 1822–1826.

Khoo, M.C., Gottschalk, A. & Pack, A.I. (1991). Sleep-induced periodic breathing and apnea: a theoretical study. *J. Appl. Physiol.*, **70**: 2014–2024.

Khayat, R.N., Xie, A., Patel, A.K., Kaminski, A. & Skatrud J.B. (2003). Cardiorespiratory effects of added dead space in patients with heart failure and central sleep apnea. *Chest*, **123**: 1551–1560.

Lahiri, S., Maret, K. & Sherpa, M.G. (1983). Dependence of high altitude sleep apnea on ventilatory sensitivity to hypoxia. *Respir. Physiol.*, **52**: 281–301.

Levine, R.L. (2000). End-tidal CO_2: physiology in pursuit of clinical applications. *Intens. Care Med.*, **26**: 1595–1597.

Quaranta, A.J., D'Alonzo, G.E. & Krachman, S.L. (1997). Cheyne–Stokes respiration during sleep in congestive heart failure. *Chest*, **111**: 467–473.

Rodway, G.W., Hoffman, L.A. & Sanders, M.H. (2003). High-altitude-related disorders. Part I: Pathophysiology, differential diagnosis, and treatment. *Heart Lung*, **32**: 353–359.

Thomas, R.J., Terzano, M.G., Parrino, L. & Weiss, J.W. (2004). Obstructive sleep-disordered breathing with a dominant cyclic alternating pattern – a recognizable polysomnographic variant with practical clinical implications. *Sleep*, **27**: 229–234.

Thomas, R.J. & Daly, R.W. (2004). Positive airway pressure gas modulation in the treatment of complex sleep-disordered breathing. *Sleep*, **27**: A219.

Wiedemann, H.P. & McCarthy, K. (1989). Noninvasive monitoring of oxygen and carbon dioxide. *Clin. Chest Med.*, **10**: 239–254.

Younes, M. (2003). Contributions of upper airway mechanics and control mechanisms to severity of obstructive apnea. *Am. J. Respir. Crit. Care Med.*, **168**: 645–658.

CAPNOGRAPHY DURING SEDATION 13

E.A. Bowe & E.F. Klein Jr

Introduction

Although ubiquitous during general endotracheal anesthesia, capnometry has not achieved a similar degree of acceptance for patients during sedation. Requirements imposed by institutions, regulatory agencies and professional societies are combining with documented efficacy, improved sampling techniques and decreased implementation costs to increase the use of capnometry in patients undergoing sedation (Cote, 1997).

Conscious sedation

Apparently based on reports of increased morbidity and mortality in children receiving sedation outside the classic operating room setting (Cote *et al.*, 1995; Cote, 1997), *Guidelines for the Elective Use of Conscious Sedation, Deep Sedation, and General Anesthesia in Pediatric Patients*, drafted by the Committee on Drugs of the American Academy of Pediatrics (AAP), were adopted by the AAP and the American Academy of Pediatric Dentistry in 1985 (American Academy of Pediatrics, 1985).

As the guidelines of various professional organizations are written using specific terminology, compliance requires understanding the words and phrases used to describe various stages of sedation. The term "conscious sedation" has been a source of confusion almost since its introduction by the American Dental Association (Sa Rego *et al.*, 1997). The first widely accepted definitions were those proposed by the AAP's Committee on Drugs (Table 13.1).

The initial intent of the AAP's Committee on Drugs was to have the term "conscious sedation" indicate a state of minimal sedation in which the patient responded appropriately to verbal commands and would cry "ouch" in response to a painful stimulus (American Academy of Pediatrics, 2002). Because the AAP definitions have been misinterpreted to imply "conscious sedation" is present when the patient manifests only a reflex withdrawal to pain, the AAP recently recommended adoption of the terminology proposed by the American Society of Anesthesiologists (ASA) (2004) (Table 13.2, Box 13.1). The ASA definitions are those also currently endorsed by the Joint Commission on Accreditation of Healthcare Organizations (JCAHO).[1]

Table 13.1 AAP definitions (American Academy of Pediatrics, 1992)

1. **Conscious sedation,** a medically controlled state of depressed consciousness that: (1) allows protective airway reflexes to be maintained; (2) retains the patient's ability to maintain a patent airway independently and continuously; (3) permits appropriate response by the patient to physical stimulation or verbal command (e.g. open your eyes).
2. **Deep sedation,** a medically controlled state of depressed consciousness or unconsciousness from which the patient is not easily aroused. It may be accompanied by partial or complete loss of protective reflexes, including the ability to maintain a patent airway independently and respond purposefully to physical stimulation or verbal command.

Reproduced with permission from American Academy of Pediatrics (1992). Committee on Drugs. Guidelines for monitoring and management of pediatric patients during and after sedation for diagnostic and therapeutic procedures. *Pediatrics*, **89**: 1110–1115.

Historical statistics

Although there is a paucity of data, the impression of most anesthesia providers is that sedation for diagnostic or therapeutic procedures is increasing in frequency. Clearly most patients would rather have neither pain nor memory of an invasive procedure. In many settings sedation for procedures outside the operating room is provided by individuals with minimal training in sedation techniques; in most circumstances, the individual providing the sedation is working under the direction of a physician who is

[1] http://www.jcaho.com/

Table 13.2 Continuum of depth of sedation*

	Minimal sedation (anxiolysis)	Moderate sedation/ analgesia (conscious sedation)	Deep sedation/ analgesia	General anesthesia
Responsiveness	Normal response to verbal stimulation	Purposeful** response to verbal or tactile stimulation	Purposeful** response following repeated or painful stimulation	Unarousable even with painful stimulus
Airway	Unaffected	No intervention required	Intervention may be required	Intervention often required
Spontaneous ventilation	Unaffected	Adequate	May be inadequate	Frequently inadequate
Cardiovascular function	Unaffected	Usually maintained	Usually maintained	May be impaired

* Monitored anesthesia care does not describe the continuum of depth of sedation, rather it describes "a specific anesthesia service in which an anesthesiologist has been requested to participate in the care of a patient undergoing a diagnostic or therapeutic procedure."

** Reflex withdrawal from a painful stimulus is *not* considered a purposeful response.

Box 13.1 Definition of general anesthesia and levels of sedation/analgesia

Minimal sedation (anxiolysis) is a drug-induced state during which patients respond normally to verbal commands. Although cognitive function and coordination may be impaired, ventilatory and cardiovascular functions are unaffected.

Moderate sedation/analgesia (conscious sedation) is a drug-induced depression of consciousness during which patients respond purposefully** to verbal commands, either alone or accompanied by light tactile stimulation. No interventions are required to maintain a patent airway, and spontaneous ventilation is adequate. Cardiovascular function is usually maintained.

Deep sedation/analgesia is a drug-induced depression of consciousness during which patients cannot be easily aroused but respond purposefully** following repeated or painful stimulation. The ability to independently maintain ventilatory function may be impaired. Patients may require assistance in maintaining a patent airway, and spontaneous ventilation may be inadequate. Cardiovascular function is usually maintained.

** Reflex withdrawal from a painful stimulus is *not* considered a purposeful response.

engrossed in performing the procedure. Government agencies generally require reporting of significant adverse consequences during anesthesia; similarly, most institutions carefully track the number of anesthetics provided in an operating room environment. Comparable reporting of either complications or frequency of sedation is generally lacking.

Differing terminology, voluntary (incomplete) reporting of complications, inability to determine the number of procedures performed, and failure to determine preexisting status of the patient combine to preclude an accurate determination of morbidity and mortality statistics relating to sedation. A 1992 attempt to review morbidity and mortality data for dental patients undergoing sedation or general anesthesia determined that only nine states maintained data regarding these occurrences (Krippaehne & Montgomery, 1992). Excluding cases of local anesthetic toxicity, death occurred in 81% of 43 incidents. State boards ruled that misconduct by a practitioner occurred in over 66% of these cases. Underuse of monitoring and inexperienced resuscitators efforts were deemed to have contributed to the adverse outcomes. Anesthetic-related morbidity during dental office procedures was reviewed in a closed-claim analysis (Jastek & Peskin, 1991). Again, in the absence of data regarding the total number of anesthetics administered, the incidence rate cannot be determined. Ventilatory depression or airway obstruction leading to hypoxia was primarily responsible for the majority of catastrophic (death, hypoxic brain injury) complications. In over 75% of cases the outcome was described as "avoidable," with "timely monitoring and effective response to adverse occurrences."

Under-reporting of complications was recognized by the authors of two retrospective studies involving patients receiving sedation for endoscopy. A nonrandom retrospective analysis of data on 19,363 procedures performed in conjunction with administration of midazolam or diazepam noted "serious cardiac or respiratory complications" occurring in 5.4 per thousand procedures (Arrowsmith *et al.*, 1991). The fact that the reported incidence of complications varied by a factor of 15 between institutions is strong evidence for a reporting bias and suggests that the true incidence is probably substantially higher than what was reported. A retrospective study from England reviewing 11,998 gastroscopies reported that approximately 4% of patients required administration of an antagonist to reverse ventilatory depression and that "cardiorespiratory distress" occurred in approximately 2.5 per thousand patients (Quine *et al.*, 1995). Twice as many deaths were attributed to complications of sedation than to the procedures, but the authors note that because these figures rely on voluntary reporting, they are probably an underestimate. In a prospective study involving endoscopic procedures on patients with comorbid diseases, even when the endoscopists had access to measurements of transcutaneous CO_2 ($P_{tc}CO_2$), four of 101 patients developed hypercarbia ($P_{tc}CO_2 > 70$ mmHg) (Freeman *et al.*, 1993). The authors state that access to values for $P_{tc}CO_2$ likely resulted in greater than usual restraint in the administration of sedatives. Another prospective study involving capnographic monitoring reported that 80 patients undergoing sedation for endoscopy experienced 96 episodes of apnea (Vargo, 2000). Interestingly, over half of all patients who experienced an apneic episode were given additional sedative medication following the apnea. This increased to 80% in patients receiving supplemental oxygen, apparently indicating that the lack of change in oxygen saturation lead the sedation team to interpret the restlessness associated with apnea as being due to discomfort. A prospective study of 74 patients undergoing sedation for procedures in the emergency department (ED) documented ventilatory depression ($ETCO_2 > 50$ mmHg, absent capnograph waveform, or $ETCO_2$ increased by more than 10 mmHg over baseline) in 45% of patients and a need for assisted ventilation in 15% (Minor *et al.*, 2002).

Children constitute a large percentage of patients receiving sedation for procedures. A quality assurance form with voluntary reporting of complications was used to retrospectively review 1140 sedation outcomes in hospitalized children (Malviya *et al.*, 1997). Sixty-three (5.5%) children developed hypoxemia, and most of these episodes were attributed to ventilatory depression; seven (0.6%) occurred as a consequence of upper airway obstruction, two as a result of apnea. A prospective study of 20 children receiving ketamine for sedation in the ED noted maximum $ETCO_2$ values of 47 mmHg during sedation (no attempt was made to correlate $ETCO_2$ with P_aCO_2) and described one patient (5%) who developed upper airway obstruction requiring intervention (Kim *et al.*, 2003). Also in the ED setting, another study of 106 children receiving sedation for painful procedures demonstrated increases in $ETCO_2$ by as much as 22 mmHg (McQuillen & Steele, 2000). Perhaps most importantly, this study noted that the highest $ETCO_2$ values "invariably occurred after the completion of the procedure," – a time during which most patients in other studies did not have $ETCO_2$ monitoring. A study of 21 pediatric oncology patients undergoing sedation for procedures reported that five patients (23.8%) experienced sedation failure (unable to perform the procedure) and three patients (14.3%) experienced significant cardiorespiratory problems (one became apneic, one required two doses of naloxone for ventilatory depression, and one (4.7%) became hypoxic and bradycardic with a subsequent requirement for supplemental oxygen and physical stimulation for over 3 h following the procedure (Marx *et al.*, 1997)). A similar study of 50 children receiving sedation for painful procedures documented increases in $ETCO_2$ to 53 mmHg and one episode (2%) of airway obstruction (Tobias, 1999).

From these results it is apparent that ventilatory depression is a common problem during sedation and in many instances constitutes a greater risk to the patient than the actual procedure that is being performed (Galandiuk & Ahmad, 1998). Accordingly, it seems imperative that these complications be minimized and that any effort to reduce sedation-associated complications will ultimately produce a marked increase in patient safety. Capnography is a relatively inexpensive, non-invasive monitor that has documented efficacy (most studies involving capnography during sedation report that airway obstruction was detected first or solely as a result of monitoring this modality) in detecting hypercarbia, airway obstruction, and apnea sedation.

Hypoventilation and airway obstruction

Essentially all drugs used for sedation depress ventilation; drug combinations may have a synergistic, rather than simply additive, effect on ventilation. Experienced practitioners recognize that the response of a given individual to a particular dosing regimen is unpredictable – doses with minimal effect on one patient can cause profound ventilatory depression in another (Litman *et al.*, 1996). Attempting to categorize sedation into specific levels tends to obscure the fact that even "minimal sedation" is the first step along a path of

Table 13.3 Frequency of respiratory compromise

Author	Patient age	O_2 admin	$S_PO_2 < 90\%$	Apnea/obstruct	Comments
Baily *et al.* (1990)	Adults	No	92%	50%	Apnea > 15 s
Wright (1992)	Adults	No	33%	4%	Apnea > 30 s
Iwasaki *et al.* (1989)	2–5 y/o	No	50%	10%	Obstruction
Croswell *et al.* (1995)	2–4 y/o	Yes	20%	23%	Apnea > 15 s
Litman *et al.* (1996)	1–3 y/o	Yes	0%	0%	

O_2 admin = whether supplemental O_2 was routinely administered. $S_PO_2 < 90\%$ = incidence of $S_PO_2 < 90\%$ during procedure. Apnea/Obsruct = incidence of apnea or airway obstruction detected during the procedure. (Reproduced with permission from Vascello, L.A., & Bowe, E.A. (1999). A case for capnographic monitoring as a standard of care. *J. Oral Maxillofac. Surg.*, **57**: 1342–1347.)

pharmacologic sedation that progresses to general anesthesia. In many instances it is desirable that a patient's level of sedation change during the course of a procedure – "deep sedation/analgesia" during episodes of increased painful stimulation, "moderate sedation" during less stimulating intervals. Numerous studies have documented the frequency of desaturation and airway obstruction/apnea during sedation with various drug regimens (Table 13.3).

Role of pulse oximetry

Acknowledgement of the risks inherent in sedation requires consideration of practice modifications that can reduce this risk. Pulse oximetry is seen by many clinicians as providing an adequate monitor of ventilation during sedation. Hypoxemia secondary to central ventilatory depression and/or airway obstruction occurs when increases in alveolar CO_2 (P_ACO_2) produce decreases in alveolar O_2 (P_AO_2). Because pulse oximeters measure oxygen saturation (S_PO_2) instead of the partial pressure of oxygen in arterial blood (P_aO_2), the shape of the oxyhemoglobin dissociation curve dictates that P_aO_2 will be significantly below 100 mmHg before desaturation will be detected. In patients breathing room air, this occurs with only modest increases in P_ACO_2; in the presence of supplemental O_2, however, S_PO_2 can be maintained at >90% despite truly spectacular increases in arterial carbon dioxide tension (P_aCO_2). Several studies have documented the clinical applicability of this physiological fact (Iwasaki *et al.*, 1989; Croswell *et al.*, 1995; Hart *et al.*, 1997). Recognition of this relationship has lead some to recommend that supplemental oxygen not be administered during sedation to enhance the ability of pulse oximetry to detect hypoventilation. Although this may be effective, it occurs at the expense of increasing the incidence of hypoxic episodes and decreasing the total body oxygen content present at the time of a problem. Because monitoring exhaled carbon dioxide is feasible, relatively inexpensive and non-invasive, it is more logical to attempt directly to monitor something that reflects ventilatory depression.

Sedation guidelines

In October 2002, the American Dental Association adopted *Guidelines for the Use of Conscious Sedation, Deep Sedation and General Anesthesia for Dentists.* These guidelines recommend capnometry or auscultation of breath sounds for all patients undergoing any form of parenteral conscious sedation (American Dental Association, 2003). The American Academy of Pediatric Dentistry's document, *Clinical Guideline on the Elective Use of Conscious Sedation, Deep Sedation and General Anesthesia in Pediatric Dental Patients* (reviewed/revised in May, 1998) includes the statement that, "There shall be continual monitoring of ... expired carbon dioxide concentration via capnography ..." and describes a capnograph as "required" for children undergoing "deep sedation." ("Deep sedation" is defined as a "deeply depressed level of consciousness" and the patient is described as responding only to intense stimulus.)

The AAP *Guidelines for Monitoring and Management of Pediatric Patients During and After Sedation for Diagnostic and Therapeutic Procedures* encourage monitoring ventilation with either capnometry or a precordial stethoscope for all children undergoing more than conscious sedation (American Academy of Pediatrics, 1992).

The American College of Emergency Physicians' *Clinical Policy for Procedural Sedation and Analgesia in the Emergency Department* does not recognize any evidence-based standards regarding capnometry during sedation and makes no specific recommendations regarding capnometry for any level of sedation, but does note that "There is an excellent correlation between P_aCO_2 and $P_{et}CO_2$ even when $P_{et}CO_2$ is measured through a nasal cannula while the patient is receiving oxygen" and notes that "capnometry may be helpful when managing cases where the patient's ventilatory efforts cannot be visualized," but states that there is no evidence to substantiate an advantage for its use (American College of Emergency Physicians, 1998). The guidelines proposed by the Canadian Association of Emergency Physicians, *Procedural Sedation and Analgesia in the Emergency Department*, make no mention of capnography recommending only that "the adequacy of spontaneous ventilations" should be assessed during the procedure and noting that supplemental oxygen administration "may increase oxygen saturation in the face of hypoventilation, and that undetected CO_2 retention may occur (Innes *et al.*, 1999)."

The ASA *Standards for Basic Anesthetic Monitoring* do not make any mention of capnography for patients receiving sedation but do state that "the adequacy of ventilation shall be evaluated, at least, by continual observation of qualitative clinical signs."

Theoretic considerations

Sampling exhaled gases from spontaneously breathing unintubated patients presents problems not encountered when samples are taken from a closed system (e.g. tight-fitting mask or cuffed endotracheal tube). Factors that have been postulated to influence the accuracy of the sample are presented in Table 13.4.

Table 13.4 Factors postulated to decrease precision of $ETCO_2$ monitoring using modified nasal cannulae

- Patient secretions
- Partial airway obstruction
- Small tidal volumes
- Tachypnea
- Large volume of sampling line
- Large diameter of nasal prong tips
- High sampling flow rate
- Dilution of sample by supplemental oxygen administration
- Mouth breathing

Although small tidal volumes, high respiratory rates, and high sampling flow rates are theoretic constraints, numerous studies have documented the efficacy of this sampling technique on infants and children (in whom small tidal volumes, high respiratory rates and high sampling flow rates relative to expiratory flow are the rule rather than the exception). Divided nasal cannulae have been successfully used on children to assess syncope related to hyperventilation (Martion-Torres *et al.*, 2001), the presence of hypoventilation during the post-ictal period (Abramo *et al.*, 1995), severity of metabolic acidosis associated with diabetic ketoacidosis (Fearon & Steele, 2002), the presence of hypercarbia during sedation in the emergency room (McQuillen & Steel, 2002) and dental office (Anderson & Vann, 1988; Iwasaki *et al.*, 1989; Primosch *et al.*, 2000), ventilatory response during ketamine sedation (Kim *et al.*, 2003), comparing the ventilatory depression associated with different sedation protocols (Tobias, 1999), and the presence of hypoventilation in the post-operative period (Tobias *et al.*, 1994). Perhaps most impressive, a study evaluating the significance of position on $ETCO_2$ in neonates (age as low as 30 weeks post-conceptual age, weight as low as 1464 gm) generated adequate data using appropriately sized divided nasal cannulae with a sampling flow rate of 150 ml/min (Kugelman *et al.*, 2002). One study using divided nasal cannulae reported $P_{a-et}CO_2$ increased when oxygen flow rates were 3 l/min or greater. Inspection of the data indicates that $P_{a-et}CO_2$ was unchanged in four of six patients and that the statistical increase in the difference can be attributed to significant (approximately 15 mmHg) reductions in $ETCO_2$, which occurred in the two remaining patients (Kaneko, 1995). Sampling by nasal cannula is not fool-proof; most authors report a low but finite incidence of spuriously low $ETCO_2$ values that is attributed to mouth breathing.

Sampling devices

Almost as soon as capnography became widely utilized on patients undergoing general anesthesia in an operating room setting, clinicians began seeking a way to monitor exhaled CO_2 in spontaneously breathing, non-intubated patients. Although possible with a tight-fitting face mask or laryngeal mask airway, the objective was to have a non-invasive system that could be used on patients receiving supplemental oxygen during sedation. Suggestions included placing an intravenous catheter "close to but not irritating" the nose of a patient receiving supplemental oxygen by standard face mask (Huntington & King, 1986), inserting a CO_2 sampling line with Luer-lock connector into "vent hole" of a Hudson-style oxygen mask (Kempen, 1999b) or inserting a capnometer sampling tube (Ibarra & Lees, 1985; Langer, 1996), intravenous catheter (Goldman, 1987; Shah, 1994), or blunt metal needle (Kempen, 1999a) into standard nasal cannula partially obstructing one of the prongs. Although these devices may provide the ability to determine the presence of CO_2 in the sampled gas, the resulting values

Table 13.5 Efficacy of $ETCO_2$ sampling during spontaneous ventilation in patients who are not intubated

Author	Patient age (mean)	Number of patients (samples)	Supplemental O_2 admin	Device	$P_{et}CO_2$ (mmHg) Mean ± SD (range)	$P_{a-et}CO_2$ (mmHg) Mean ± SD (range)	Comments
Abramo *et al.* (1995)	6.5 years	58 (58)	Not described	DNC[a]	34.0 ± 4.26 (22–42)	2.0 ± 2.6 (range not given)	Reliability not effected by age or respiratory rate
Abramo *et al.* (1997)	6.8 years	166 (166)	Not described	DNC	42.0 ± 11.8 (range not given)	0.3 ± 2.1 (range not given)	Reliable
Bongard *et al.* (1993)	Adults	41 (82)	Face mask, "when necessary"	NTA[b]	39.7 ± 5.1 (range not given)	2.8 ± 2.6 (range not given)	Accurate estimate of P_aCO_2
Casati *et al.* (2001)	69 years	30 (120)	Not described	DNC	31 (SD not given) (18–44) 33 (SD not given) (22–45)	4.4 (SD not given) (0–28)[c] 7(SD not given) (0–22)[d]	
Casati *et al.* (2000)	70 years	20 (60)	No	DNC	No values given	6.5 ± 4.8 (range not given)	
Liu *et al.* (1992)	Adults	25 (25)	Not described	NTA	34.5 ± 8 (20–52)	3.6 ± 6.8 (−4.7–25.1)	
Tobias *et al.* (1994)	7.8 years	30 (55)	Not described	DNC	39.7 ± 3.8 (range not given)	2.2 ± 0.9 (range not given)	Accurate and reliable
Bowe *et al.* (1989)	67 years	21 (21)	3 l/min	DNC	36.5 ± 4.7 (28–44)	2.1 ± 2.2 (range not given)	

[a] DNC, divided nasal cannula.
[b] NTA, nasotracheal airway.
[c] Values when analysis performed with microstream capnometer.
[d] Values when analysis performed with standard capnometer.

are "less reliable" than those obtained in intubated patients (Dunphy, 1988; Urmey, 1988). Initial reports using a capnometer sampling tube sutured 1 cm from the pharyngeal end of a nasal airway (Norman *et al.*, 1986) indicated the presence of a "satisfactory" capnogram, but no data was presented to document its efficacy. A relatively unique suggestion has been to apply two sets of nasal cannula simultaneously (Desmarattes *et al.*, 1990) – one for oxygen administration, the other for sampling exhaled gases. Subsequent work has demonstrated the efficacy of $ETCO_2$ sampling during spontaneous ventilation in patients who are not intubated (Table 13.5).

Divided nasal cannula

The first system with documented ability to obtain samples permitting quantitative determination of $ETCO_2$ in spontaneously breathing, unintubated patients receiving supplemental oxygen relied on modifying a standard set of nasal prongs to permit insufflation of oxygen into one nostril while sampling exhaled gas from the other nostril (Bowe *et al.*, 1989). The $P_{a-et}CO_2$ gradient was comparable during spontaneous ventilation with supplemental oxygen in the pre-operative period (2.1 ± 2.1 mmHg) to that achieved during general endotracheal anesthesia with positive pressure ventilation (3.1 ± 2.8 mmHg). The efficacy of this basic design has been repeatedly documented in studies demonstrating a $P_{a-et}CO_2$ difference generally comparable to that obtained in intubated patients. Sampling via a divided nasal cannula demonstrated good correlation between P_aCO_2 and $P_{et}CO_2$ ($P_{a-et}CO_2 = 2.2 \pm 0.9$ mmHg) in children during the post-operative period (Tobias *et al.*, 1994). In a study of 58 children, the difference between the partial pressure of CO_2 in capillary blood ($P_{cap}CO_2$) and $ETCO_2$ determined using a divided nasal cannula was found to be 1.96 ± 2.6 mmHg (Abramo *et al.*, 1995). In a different study on 166 children who were in a post-ictal state in the ED, the $P_{cap-et}CO_2$ gradient was 0.3 ± 2.1 mmHg (Abramo *et al.*, 1997). Using nasal cannula, 120 samples were obtained on 30 patients undergoing regional anesthesia; resulting $P_{a-et}CO_2$ were compared when the samples were analyzed in a conventional capnometer and a microstream capnometer with a very low aspiration flow rate (Casati *et al.*, 2001). Although the $P_{a-et}CO_2$ was lower using the microstream capnometer (4.4 mmHg versus 7.0 mmHg), both devices appeared to be sufficiently accurate for clinical purposes. With the same microstream technology, $P_{a-et}CO_2$ was compared in awake, non-intubated patients following surgery and compared with the $P_{a-et}CO_2$ obtained during general endotracheal anesthesia with positive pressure mechanical ventilation (Casati *et al.*, 2000). The authors reported comparable values for $P_{a-et}CO_2$ (7.3 ± 4 mmHg when intubated and ventilated, 6.5 ± 5 mmHg when breathing spontaneously). One study on 76 adults receiving supplemental oxygen in the ED began with using divided nasal cannulae to sample exhaled gas, but after 11 patients the authors converted to having the patients exhale through an endotracheal tube adapter (Barton & Wang, 1994). Data regarding the $P_{a-et}CO_2$ for samples obtained using the divided nasal cannula are not presented.

Nasotracheal airway

Subsequent work has also documented the efficacy of sampling via a nasal airway. Most authors have advocated a coaxial system (Liu *et al.*, 1992) that involves insertion of a sampling tube [5 French pediatric feeding tube (Bongard *et al.*, 1994), 10 French (Cheng *et al.*, 1999) or a 12 French (Hou *et al.*, 1993) suction catheter, or special nafion tubing (Oberg *et al.*, 1995)]; one has recommended inserting a 15 mm endotracheal tube adapter connected to an anesthesia circuit directly into the nasal airway (Dominguez, 1999). One study on 41 post-operative patients sampled $P_{et}CO_2$ via a nasotracheal airway containing a 5 French pediatric feeding tube 30 and 60 min after admission to the post-anesthesia care unit. Supplemental oxygen was administered by face mask "when deemed clinically necessary" but no data are available regarding the frequency of oxygen administration. The authors report that the mean $P_{a-et}CO_2$ was 2.8 ± 2.6 mmHg (Bongard *et al.*, 1994). Although $P_{a-et}CO_2$ remained constant during laparoscopy performed under general endotracheal anesthesia, patients undergoing the same procedure while breathing spontaneously experienced a gradual increase in P_aCO_2 without an accompanying increase in $ETCO_2$ (Cheng *et al.*, 1999). Accordingly, when using a nasotracheal airway equipped with a 10 French suction catheter for sampling purposes, the $P_{a-et}CO_2$ increased over time and the correlation between P_aCO_2 and $P_{et}CO_2$ under these conditions was relatively poor ($r = 0.55$ during spontaneous ventilation, $r = 0.85$ during mechanical ventilation). Sampling via a 12 French suction catheter inserted into a nasotracheal airway resulted in lower values for $P_{a-et}CO_2$ during regional anesthesia than general endotracheal anesthesia when positive pressure ventilation was used for comparable procedures (Hou *et al.*, 1993). In a study of 25 intensive care unit patients, sampling was performed using a coaxial nasotracheal sampling catheter (Liu *et al.*, 1992), and the $P_{a-et}CO_2$ was found to be 3.6 ± 6.8 mmHg. Awake or lightly sedated patients might not accept a nasal airway.

Acceptance

As evidenced by the disparity in guidelines (AAP recommends capnometry for all children receiving parenteral sedation; associations of emergency physicians in both Canada and the US do not recommend capnometry for any patients receiving sedation), acceptance of capnometry varies widely based on venue and specialty of sedating physician. Interestingly, the guidelines of anesthesiology specialty societies (The Association of Anaesthetists for Great Britain and Ireland, 2003; The American Society of Anesthesiologists, 2003) do not comment on capnography during regional anesthesia or sedation inside or outside the operating room environment. Many opinion papers advocate capnography for patients undergoing sedation, terming it "the gold standard in the near future (Golnick & Mandeville, 2002)," advocating that capnometry be recommended by the ASA as a standard for all patients undergoing procedural sedation (Sandlin, 2002), and describing capnometry as "quite probably, the most useful assessment tool *not* being used on a daily basis in ambulances throughout the world" (Whitehead, 2003).

Even authors who argue against adopting capnography as a monitoring standard during sedation usually base their objections on the absence of documented improvements in outcomes (American College of Emergency Physicians, 1998; Bennett, 1999). Some evidence suggests that the mortality rate of children undergoing sedation is greater than that for children receiving a general anesthetic. Even if the mortality rate is 100 fold greater, a statistically meaningful comparison of outcomes between those sedated with and without capnographic monitoring would require tens of thousands of patients in each group. Such studies are unlikely to be performed given the fact that we don't even know the number of sedations actually performed.

Conclusion

Available data indicate that divided nasal cannulae are non-invasive, well tolerated by most patients (including children), and capable of providing samples that produce $P_{a-et}CO_2$ differences comparable to those obtained during general endotracheal anesthesia with positive pressure ventilation. Most studies also document that capnometry was more effective in detecting episodes of apnea or airway obstruction than clinical observation or pulse oximetry. Under these circumstances and because sedation can be associated with more severe complications than the procedure itself, the risk-to-benefit ratio clearly favors the use of capnometry during regional anesthesia and sedation either inside or outside of the operating room.

References

Abramo, T.J., Cowan, M.R., Scott, S.M., *et al.* (1995). Comparison of pediatric end-tidal CO_2 measured with nasal/oral cannula circuit and capillary PCO_2. *Am. J. Emerg. Med.*, **13**: 30–33.

Abramo, T.J., Wibee, R.A., Scott, S., *et al.* (1997). Noninvasive capnometry monitoring for respiratory status during pediatric seizures. *Crit. Care Med.*, **25**: 1242–1246.

American Academy of Pediatrics (1985). Committee on Drugs, Section on Anesthesiology. Guidelines for the elective use of conscious sedation, deep sedation, and general anesthesia in pediatric patients. *Pediatrics*, **76**: 317–321.

American Academy of Pediatrics (1992). Committee on Drugs. Guidelines for monitoring and management of pediatric patients during and after sedation for diagnostic and therapeutic procedures. *Pediatrics*, **89**: 1110–1115.

American Academy of Pediatrics (2002). Committee on Drugs. Guidelines for monitoring and management of pediatric patients during and after sedation for diagnostic and therapeutic procedures: addendum. *Pediatrics*, **110**: 836–838.

American College of Emergency Physicians (1998). Clinical policy for procedural sedation and analgesia in the emergency department. *Ann. Emerg. Med.*, **31**: 663–677.

American Dental Association (2003). Guidelines for the use of conscious sedation, deep sedation and general anesthesia for dentists. Available at: http://www.ada.org/prof/ed/guidelines/guidedent.doc. Accessed June 30, 2003.

American Society of Anesthesiologists (2004). Continuum of depth of sedation: definition of general anesthesia and levels of sedation/analgesia. Available at: http://www.asahq.org/publicationsAndServices/standards/20.htm. Accessed July 13, 2004.

Anderson, J.A. & Vann, W.F. (1988). Repiratory monitoring during pediatric sedation: pulse oximetry and capnography. *Pediatr. Dent.*, **10**: 94–101.

Arrowsmith, J.B., Gerstman, B.B., Fleischer, D.E. & Benjamin, S.B. (1991). Results from the American Society for gastrointestinal endoscopy/US Food and Drug Administration collaborative study on complication rates and drug use during gastrointestinal endoscopy. *Gastrointest. Endosc.*, **37**: 421–427.

Bailey, P.L., Pace, N.L., Ashburn, M.A., *et al.* (1990). Frequent hypoxemia and apnea after sedation with midazolam and fentanyl. *Anesthesiology*, **73**: 826–830.

Barton, C.W. & Wang, E.S.J. (1994). Correlation of end-tidal CO_2 measurements to arterial P_aCO_2 in nonintubated patients. *Ann. Emerg. Med.*, **23**: 560–563.

Bennett, J. (1999). A cases against capnographic monitoring as a standard of care. *J. Oral. Maxillofac. Surg.*, **57**: 1348–1352.

Bongard, F., Wu, Y., Lee, T.S., *et al.* (1994). Capnographic monitoring of extubated postoperative patients. *J. Invest. Surg.*, **7**: 259–264.

Bowe, E.A., Boysen, P.G., Broome, J.A. & Klein, E.F. (1989). Accurate determination of end-tidal carbon dioxide during administration of oxygen by nasal cannulae. *J. Clin. Monit.*, **5**: 105–110.

Casati, A., Gallioli, G., Scandroglio, M., *et al.* (2000). Accuracy of end-tidal carbon dioxide monitoring using the NBP-75 microstream capnometer: a study in intubated ventilated and spontaneously breathing patients. *Eur. J. Anaesthesiol.*, **17**: 622–626.

Casati, A., Gallioli, G., Passaretta, R., *et al.* (2001). End tidal carbon dioxide monitoring in spontaneously breathing, non-intubated patients. *Minerva Anestesiol.*, **67**: 161–164.

Cheng, K.I., Tang, C.S., Tsai, E.M., *et al.* (1999). Correlation of arterial and end-tidal carbon dioxide in spontaneously breathing patients during ambulatory gynecologic laparoscopy. *J. Formos. Med. Assoc.*, **98**: 814–819.

Cote, C.J. (1997). Pediatric premedication: from disasters to guidelines. *Am. J. Anesthesiol.*, **24**: 6–9.

Cote, C.J., Alderfer, R.J., Notterman, D.A. & Fanta, K.B. (1995). Sedation disasters: adverse drug reports in pediatrics – FDA, USP, and others. *Anesthesiology*, **83**: A1183.

Croswell, R.J.R., Dilley, D.C., Lucas, W.J. & Vann, W.F. (1995). A comparison of conventional versus electronic monitoring of sedated pediatric dental patients. *Pediatr. Dent.*, **17**: 332–339.

Desmarattes, R., Kennedy, R. & Davis, D.R. (1990). Inexpensive capnography during monitored anesthesia care. *Anesth. Analg.*, **71**: 100–101.

Dominguez, E. (1999). Carbon dioxide monitoring during deep conscious sedation using nasopharyngeal airways. *Anesthesiology*, **91**: 1177–1178.

Dunphy, J.A. (1988). Accuracy of expired carbon dioxide partial pressure sampled from a nasal cannula. II. *Anesthesiology*, **68**: 960.

Fearon, D.M. & Steele, D.W. (2002). End-tidal carbon dioxide predicts the presence and severity of acidosis in children with diabetes. *Acad. Emerg. Med.*, **9**: 1373 – 1378.

Freeman, M.L., Hennessy, J.T., Cass, O.W. & Pheley, A.M. (1993). Carbon dioxide retention and oxygen desaturation during gastrointestinal endoscopy. *Gastroenterology*, **105**: 331–339.

Galandiuk, S. & Ahmad, P. (1998). Impact of sedation and resident teaching on complications of colonoscopy. *Dig. Surg.*, **15**: 60–63.

Goldman, J.M. (1987). A simple, easy, and inexpensive method for monitoring $ETCO_2$ through nasal cannulae. *Anesthesiology*, **67**: 606.

Golnick, J.M. & Mandeville, M. (2002). Considerations for monitoring pediatric sedation. *J. Michigan Dent. Assoc.*, **84**: 34–36.

Hart, L.S., Berns, S.D., Houck, C.S. & Boenning, D.A. (1997). The value of end-tidal CO_2 monitoring when comparing three methods of conscious sedation for children undergoing painful procedures in the emergency department. *Pediatr. Emerg. Care*, **13**: 189–193.

Hou, W.Y., Sun, W.Z., Suscelo, L., *et al.* (1993). Validity and feasibility of nasopharyngeal end-tidal carbon dioxide tension monitorings: a novel approach in spontaneously breathing patients. *J. Formos. Med. Assoc.*, **92**: 553–557.

Huntington, C.T. & King, H. (1986). A simpler design for mass spectrometer monitoring in the awake patient. *Anesthesiology*, **65**: 565–566.

Ibarra, E. & Lees, D.E. (1985). Mass spectrometer monitoring of patients with regional anesthesia. *Anesthesiology*, **63**: 572–573.

Innes, G., Murphy, M., Nijssen-Jordan, C., *et al.* (1999). Procedural sedation and analgesia in the emergency department: Canadian consensus guidelines. *J. Emerg. Med.*, **17**: 145–156.

Iwasaki, J., Vann, W.F., Dilley, D.C., *et al.* (1989). An investigation of capnography and pulse oximetry as monitors of pediatric patients sedated for dental treatment. *Pediatr. Dent.*, **11**: 111–117.

Jastek, J.T. & Peskin, R.M. (1991). Major morbidity or mortality from office anesthetic procedures: a closed-claim analysis of 13 cases. *Anesth. Prog.*, **38**: 39–44.

Joint Commission on Accreditation of Healthcare Organizations. Standards and intents for anesthesia and anesthesia care. In: *Revisions to Anesthesia Care Standards, Comprehensive Accreditation Manual for Hospitals.* Oakbrook Terrace, IL.

Kaneko, Y. (1995). Clinical perspectives on capnography during sedation and general anesthesia in dentistry. *Anesth. Prog.*, **42**: 126–130.

Kempen, P. (1999a). Cost-efficient carbon dioxide monitoring via nasal cannula. *Anesthesiology*, **90**: 633–634.

Kempen, P. (1999b). Cost-efficient end-tidal carbon dioxide monitoring via Hudson-style mask. *Anesthesiology*, **91**: 1176–1177.

Kim, G., Green, S.M., Benmark, T.K. & Krauss, B. (2003). Ventilatory response during dissociative sedation in children: a pilot study. *Acad. Emerg. Med.*, **10**: 140–145.

Krippaehne, J.A. & Montgomery, M.T. (1992). Morbidity and mortality from pharmacosedation and general anesthesia in the dental office. *J. Oral Maxillofac. Surg.*, **50**: 691–698.

Kugelman, A., Bilker, A., Bader, D., *et al.* (2002). Sidestream end-tidal capnometry as related to infant's position and maturation. *Acta Pediatr.*, **91**: 869–873.

Langer, R.A. (1996). Simple modification of a medium concentration (Hudson type) oxygen mask improves patient comfort and respiratory monitoring with capnography. *Anesth. Analg.*, **83**: 202.

Litman, R.S., Berkowitz, R.J. & Ward, D.S. (1996). Levels of consciousness and ventilatory parameters in young children during sedation with oral midazolam and nitrous oxide. *Arch. Pediatr. Adolesc. Med.*, **150**: 671–675.

Liu, S.Y., Lee, T.S. & Bongard, F. (1992). Accuracy of capnography in noninutbated surgical patients. *Chest*, **102**: 1512–1515.

Malviya, S., Voepel-Lewis, T. & Tait, A.R. (1997). Adverse events and risk factors associated with the sedation of children by nonanesthesiologists. *Anesth. Analg.*, **85**: 1207–1213.

Martinon-Torres, F., Rodriguez-Nunez, A., Fernandez-Cebrian, S., *et al.* (2001). The relation between hyperventilation and pediatric syncope. *J. Pediatr.*, **138**: 894–897.

Marx, C.M., Stein, J., Tyler, M.K., *et al.* (1997). Ketamine–midazolam versus meperidine–midazolam for painful procedures in pediatric oncology patients. *J. Clin. Oncol.*, **15**: 94–102.

McQuillen, K.K. & Steele, D.W. (2000). Capnography during sedation/analgesia in the pediatric emergency department. *Pediatr. Emerg. Care*, **16**: 401–404.

Minor, J.R., Heegaard, W. & Plummer, D. (2002). End-tidal carbon dioxide monitoring during procedural sedation. *Acad. Emerg. Med.*, **9**: 275–280.

Norman, E.A., Zeig, N.G. & Ahmad, I. (1986). Better designs for mass spectrometer monitoring of the awake patient. *Anesthesiology*, **64**: 664.

Oberg, B., Waldau, T. & Larsen, V.H. (1995). The effect of nasal oxygen flow and catheter position on the accuracy of end-tidal carbon dioxide measurements by a pharyngeal catheter in unintubated, spontaneously breathing subjects. *Anaesthesia*, **50**: 695–698.

Primosch, R.E., Buzzi, I.M. & Jerrell, G. (2000). Monitoring pediatric dental patients with nasal mask capnography. *Pediatr. Dent.*, **22**: 120–124.

Quine, M.A., Bell, G.D., McCloy, R.F., Charlton, J.E., Devlin, H.B. & Hopkins, A. (1995). Prospective audit of upper gastrointestinal endoscopy in two regions of England: safety, staffing, and sedation methods. *Gut*, **36**: 462–467.

Sa Rego, M.M., Watcha, M.F. & White, P.F. (1997). The changing role of monitored anesthesia care in the ambulatory setting. *Anesth. Analg.*, **85**: 1020–1036.

Sandlin, D. (2002). Capnography for nonintubated patients: the wave of the future for routine monitoring of procedural sedation patients. *J. Perianesth. Nurs.*, **17**: 277–281.

Shah, M.G. (1994). Measurement of carbon dioxide at both nares and mouth using standard nasal cannula. *Anesthesiology*, **81**: 779–780.

The Association of Anaesthetists for Great Britain and Ireland (2003). Recommendations for standards of monitoring during anesthesia and recovery. Available at: http://www.aagbi.org/pdf/Absolute.pdf. Accessed June 30, 2003.

Tobias, J.D. (1999). End-tidal carbon dioxide monitoring during sedation with a combination of midazolam and ketamine for children undergoing painful, invasive procedures. *Pediatr. Emerg. Care*, **15**: 173–175.

Tobias, J.D., Flanagan, J.F.K., Wheeler, T.J., *et al.* (1994). Noninvasive monitoring of end-tidal CO_2 via nasal cannulas in spontaneously breathing children during the perioperative period. *Crit. Care Med.*, **22**: 1805–1808.

Urmey, W.F. (1988). Accuracy of expired carbon dioxide partial pressure sampled from a nasal cannula. I. *Anesthesiology*, **68**: 959.

Vargo, J.J. (2000). Monitoring during procedural sedation. Paper published in the *Proceedings presented at the 54th Post Graduate Assembly in Anesthesiology*, New York City, 2000.

Vascello, L.A. & Bowe, E.A. (1999). A case for capnographic monitoring as a standard of care. *J. Oral Maxillofac. Surg.*, **57**: 1342–1347.

Whitehead, S. (2003). The capnography revolution begins. *J. Emer. Med. Serv.*, **28**: 130.

Wright, S.W. (1992). Conscious sedation in the emergency department: the value of capnography and pulse oximetry. *Ann. Emerg. Med.*, **21**: 551–555.

RESPIRATION AT HIGH- AND LOW-PRESSURE ENVIRONMENTS 14

M.S. Ozcan & T.J. Gallagher

Introduction

The human system displays a wide range of adaptability to varying changes in atmospheric pressure. Man lives, works and plays throughout an extensive range of these high- and low-pressure environments. These supra- and sub-atmospheric pressures encompass temporary situations, such as recreational and commercial diving, mountaineering, skiing and aviation activities. Occupational exposures also include mining and tunnel construction including caissons. Hyperbaric oxygen (O_2) therapy highlights a therapeutic supra-atmospheric environment. Furthermore, we know many choose to inhabit high-altitude regions of the planet.

Table 14.1 Available O_2 at altitude

Altitude (msl) ft	m	Pressure (atm)	PO_2 in air (mmHg)	Predicted P_AO_2 (mmHg)
5000	1524	0.83	122	82
10,000	3048	0.68	99	59
15,000	4572	0.56	79	39
20,000	6096	0.45	72	32
30,000	9144	0.35	55	15

The non-linear changes in available O_2 with increased altitude. The atmospheric pressures are ideal, but will vary slightly with atmospheric and local weather conditions.

Altitude

Altitude and human physiology

As many as 140 million people may inhabit regions of the earth where ambient pressures vary from 0.75 to 0.5 atm, which corresponds to 6000–17,000 ft (≈1800–5000 m) above sea level (msl) (World Health Organization, 1996). Each year over 30 million will travel to high altitude for recreational or commercial purposes. Also, consider that air travel is the single most common setting of altitude exposure for millions every year. The typical commercial airliner pressurizes its cabin to 7000–10,000 ft (≈2000–3000 m) msl. Whatever the reason, the non-acclimated human experiences significant physiologic changes when venturing to high ground.

Excursions to high altitudes mean that the available O_2 decreases in a non-linear manner along with atmospheric pressure (Table 14.1). At sea level the partial pressure of O_2 (PO_2) of air is about 150 mmHg. Compare this to 5000 ft (≈1500 m) msl and 12,000 ft (≈3500 m) msl, which have atmospheric pressures of 632 and 483 mmHg, respectively. The expected PO_2 of air at these altitudes will be 132 and 101 mmHg compared to 150 mmHg at sea level. Once we consider alveolar partial pressure of CO_2 (P_ACO_2 = 40 mmHg), we can anticipate an alveolar partial pressure of O_2 (P_AO_2) of 92 and 61 mmHg, respectively. Climb to 18,000 ft (≈5500 m) msl, where the pressure decreases to 0.5 atm (380 mmHg), and the P_AO_2 drops to 40 mmHg. Although the relative change in atmospheric pressure seems small compared to the changes encountered while diving, the effect on available O_2 remains great.

Acute exposure of the non-acclimated visitor to high altitude will cause early symptoms relatively proportional to the decrease in available O_2. The most sensitive, night vision, first becomes apparent at ambient pressures of 0.8 atm (6000 ft or ≈1800 m) msl, a response not readily appreciated by many private pilots (Pretorius, 1970). At 0.6 atm, perioral numbness, tingling of the fingers or dizziness might be encountered. These symptoms might reflect the hyperventilation, which will be discussed later. The more sensitive individuals may lose consciousness at 15,000 ft (≈4500 m) msl and almost all quickly become unconscious upon sudden exposure to the atmosphere at altitudes above 20,000 ft (≈6000 m) msl. The time to loss of consciousness becomes exponentially shorter with the drop in ambient pressure. While individual variations are common, 2 min or less of sudden exposure to 0.3 atm (the ambient pressure at the summit of Mt. Everest) results in unconsciousness.

Hypoxic respiratory stimulation

The initial excursions to high altitude result in a significant increase in the ventilatory rate and minute ventilation. The principle driving force evolves from the hypoxemia sensed at the carotid and aortic bodies; the carotid being the more important of the two (Lambertsen, 1968; Mcdonald, 1981). This increased ventilation rate also initiates somewhat of a negative feedback loop. The hyperventilation decreases PCO_2, the displacement of which, in turn, permits an increased P_AO_2. Without the hyperventilation to reduce P_ACO_2 and allow more room for O_2, survival would not be possible. The net result can be an increase in blood O_2 values and at least a partial blunting of the hypoxic ventilatory drive. The hypoxic drive becomes active at an ambient PO_2 of about 100 mmHg, which corresponds to an altitude close to 10,000 ft ($\approx$3000 m) msl. At this altitude the arterial PO_2 (P_aO_2) will be about 50 mmHg. Any future changes in ventilation will be directly related to subsequent decreases in P_aO_2 because the PO_2 sits on the steep portion of the oxyhemoglobin dissociation curve.

The hypoxic drive appears to be bi-phasic. After acclimatization it may be blunted, but will once again respond with a further decrease in PO_2 such as excursion to a higher altitude (Weil, 1986). Longtime residents or those born at high altitudes appear to have a blunted, or in some cases even absent response to hypoxemia. However, unlike non-responsive lowlanders or experimental animals with a denervated carotid body, this blunted response does not seem harmful and certainly does not interfere with performance.

In acclimatized individuals, the more brisk the response to hypoxia, the better the physical performance – at least at the mid-altitude range (Schoene *et al.*, 1984). Few data have been collected at the higher altitudes, but some authorities believe that these same brisk responders may actually do worse at the more extreme altitudes. Brisk responders also fare poorly at most cognitive studies carried out at altitude. It has been postulated that hyperventilation with its attendant decreased cerebral blood flow and possible cellular ischemia plays a role.

True acclimatization occurs as a gradual process and may never actually be complete. Studies have clearly demonstrated that continued exposure to altitude and the resulting hypoxemia causes a significant decline in higher cognitive functions (Kennedy *et al.*, 1989). Skill tests at high altitudes are poorly performed, and memory may be altered for as long as 6 months after return to sea level. Many of the most powerful telescopes are located at high altitudes (greater than 12,000 ft or $\approx$4000 m) msl to improve clarity. Various attempts at acclimatization have been undertaken with minimal success. To combat these known decrements in performance, some facilities have taken to enriching the environment with O_2 up to 26% (Gerard *et al.*, 2000). They reported a significant improvement in cognitive function and fewer problems with headaches and other effects of high altitude.

CO_2 respiratory stimulation

Receptors in the medulla are sensitive to changes in PCO_2 while the peripheral receptors play a secondary role (Hultgren, 1997). The brain responds essentially to changes in hydrogen ion concentration. If arterial PCO_2 (P_aCO_2) increases, cerebral spinal fluid (CSF) PCO_2 increases and ultimately the hydrogen ion $[H^+]$ levels in the brain rise. The increased $[H^+]$, in turn, triggers hyperventilation. Studies at altitude have demonstrated reduced CSF bicarbonate levels in both non- and acclimatized subjects. Since lowered CSF bicarbonate values mean higher brain $[H^+]$ levels, hyperventilation will ensue. Three mechanisms have been proposed. One focuses on development of CSF acidosis secondary to hypoxia. A second theory proposes equilibration by the kidney with reduced CSF bicarbonate leading to elevated brain $[H^+]$. Severinghaus *et al.* (1963) and West (1962) both point to an active transport mechanism to reduce the CSF bicarbonate values.

The initial response to PCO_2 changes occurs within the first 24 h and accounts for about 50% of the response. The remainder takes place over about 2 weeks provided one remains at altitude. These changes to CO_2 become important because the increased time at altitude minimizes the hypoxic response. Without this CO_2 effect hyperventilation would be inadequate.

With acclimatization, the ventilatory response increases by a factor of 5 (Wren & Robbins, 1999). Table 14.2 compares the ventilatory response in the non-acclimatized to the acclimatized individual.

It is apparent that the increased hyperventilation in the acclimatized individual results ultimately in a higher P_aO_2. The ability to hyperventilate appears to be unrelated to factors such as age, sex or physical conditioning (Ward *et al.*, 2000). In fact, it is probably genetically driven.

Other respiratory changes

At altitude, diffusion capacity increases by perhaps 20–30% (West, 1962). Proposed mechanisms involve the known increase in pulmonary blood flow. The elevated blood flow to the pulmonary circulation recruits capillaries and small vessels, which were not previously

Table 14.2 P_ACO_2 and P_AO_2 at altitude in acclimatized and non-acclimatized individuals

Altitude (msl) ft	m	PCO_2 (mmHg)	PO_2 (mmHg)
10,000	3048	36 (23)	67 (92)
20,000	6096	24 (10)	40 (53)
30,000	9144	24 (7)	18 (30)

The values in parenthesis represent acclimatized individuals. This helps explain their impaired tolerance to higher altitudes.

Table 14.3 Thoracic volume in native high-altitude dwellers

Altitude (m)	Thoracic volume (ml)
150	10,500
3260	11,000
4000	12,200

The increased lung volumes contribute to improve diffusion in high-altitude natives who also generally have smaller body masses, which contributes to efficient O_2 utilization.

opened. This expanded capillary surface area aids in O_2 transfer. In contrast to increased ambient pressures that decrease lung volumes, altitude has the opposite effect (Table 14.3). Therefore, we can anticipate an increased alveolar surface area for diffusion. The pulmonary hypertension that results with altitude and hypoxemia further increases blood flow.

Cardiovascular system

Significant changes take place within the cardiovascular system after ascent to high altitude. Predictably, and most likely because of hypoxemia, the pulmonary vascular bed undergoes significant vasoconstriction. The concurrent hyperventilation probably, to some degree, blocks this response. Thus, almost all individuals – those acclimatized or not – experience pulmonary hypertension. Usually, O_2 can decrease, if not restore, the pressures toward normal. As the muscularis layer of the pulmonary artery is minimal, the vasoconstriction must be a fairly sensitive and intense response. However, prolonged exposure without supplemental O_2 leads to chronic pulmonary hypertension, which cannot be reversed with supplemental O_2 therapy (Etozzi *et al.*, 1989). Obviously, this means that beyond vasoconstriction, anatomic changes must involve various layers including the intima. Ultimately, these increased pressures lead to right ventricular hypertrophy.

Increased heart rate leads to increased cardiac output. For the same imposed work level, the increases in cardiac output are identical, whether at sea level or altitude. Stroke volume does ultimately decrease perhaps linked to decreased intravascular volume due to dehydration and diuresis. Hypoxemia-induced polycythemia will aid O_2 delivery.

Many athletes move to high altitude to improve their conditioning levels. The primary benefit seems to be the increase in hemoglobin concentrations. However, this can be offset by the fact that the actual degree of physical activity attainable at altitude seems to be less than at sea level. Therefore, ultimate athletic performance depends on the benefits of polycythemia coupled with training at reduced altitudes where increased work levels can be achieved and result in a higher fitness levels (Gore *et al.*, 1996).

Different arrhythmias, including premature atrial contractions (PACs) and premature ventricular contractions, have been noted in high-altitude dwellers. Although not well documented, some of these represent the alkalemia secondary to the hyperventilation. The periodic breathing often experienced by mountaineers and other high-altitude dwellers is often seen in conjunction with atrial arrhythmias.

Hematology

Hematologic changes at altitude primarily involve an increase in red blood cells. Various studies have demonstrated that with the initial exposure to the hypoxemic environment, erythropoietin begins to rise (Reynafarje *et al.*, 1964) within 2 to 3 days; however, red cell numbers take up to 6 months to reach peak levels.

Within 3 weeks, if there is no further change in the altitude, the erythropoietin levels return to normal. However, any further excursions to higher altitudes, which result in further hypoxemia, will once again stimulate erythropoietin production. Return from altitude causes a reduction to sea level values within 24 h. The red blood cell increase usually lasts about 6 weeks after return from altitude.

Concomitant with the blood changes, plasma volume ordinarily decreases due to a significant diuresis, and salt loss takes place so that intravascular volume actually decreases. Increased levels of exercise can stimulate aldosterone, which would help to restore intravascular volume. Also, blood shifts into the central circulation, which is usually well tolerated.

Neurologic

As previously mentioned, alterations also take place in the central nervous system (Hornbein *et al.*, 1989).

Initially, various cognitive functions may deteriorate because of acute hypoxemia. However, hyperventilation will result in a decrease in cerebral blood flow due to vasoconstriction. In some instances, if significant hyperventilation takes place, then PCO_2 values in the range of 20 mmHg or below can result in pathologic vasoconstriction and (at least, temporary) brain cell ischemia. Therefore, long-term central nervous problems, such as memory loss and concentration, may be attributed to both hypoxemia and the intense vasoconstriction.

Complications of altitude

Probably the most common complication developing in high-altitude dwellers is acute mountain sickness (AMS) (Hackett *et al.*, 1986). Typical symptoms include headache, nausea, anorexia, insomnia and occasionally vomiting. These symptoms generally develop within 6–12 h of arrival at altitude. The more abrupt the change in altitude, the more likely the symptoms. AMS can be unpredictable and develop in individuals who have made multiple excursions without difficulty and then suddenly fall victim. The higher the altitude, the more likely the onset of AMS. Although hypoxia has often been ascribed as the cause it does not appear to be part of the actual etiology. A review of the literature indicates that AMS may be more likely to occur in those who are unable to hyperventilate to the same degree as contemporaries at that particular altitude. It may also, in some way, be related to abrupt increases in pulmonary artery pressures.

Prevention for AMS includes a gradual ascent to altitude. As an example, limitations of 5000–6000 ft (≈1500–1800 m) msl from sea level for the first 24 h seems to provide some protection. Acetazolamide has been shown to play a protective role. Acetazolamide induces a metabolic alkalosis, and stimulates hyperventilation. It is also a diuretic and this may have some benefit because with AMS the expected high-altitude diuresis does not take place. Steroids, such as dexamethasone, have been effective in treating the cerebral edema and the accompanying headache often seen. When all else fails, it may be necessary to remove the patient to a lower altitude.

AMS may progress to high-altitude pulmonary edema (HAPE). In general, these patients have had increased pulmonary artery pressures. A breakdown in the pulmonary vascular endothelium leads to leakage of proteins into the pulmonary edema fluid (Hackett *et al.*, 1986). Whereas AMS may occur at 7000–8000 ft (≈2000–2500 m), HAPE usually requires altitudes over 12,000 ft (≈3600 m).

Treatment of HAPE requires descent to lower altitudes. O_2 is beneficial, but not curative. Continuous positive airway pressure (CPAP) can be helpful. Mountaineering expeditions have used portable hyperbaric chambers in an attempt to relieve the symptomology.

Hyperbaric environment

Exposure to increased barometric pressures is part of commercial and sport diving. Tunnel construction work with the use of caissons involves increased environmental pressures. Hyperbaric chamber facilities use the therapeutic benefits of elevated pressures. Compared to altitude, the pressure changes experienced can be tremendous. Each 33 ft (10.1 m) of seawater (fsw) represents one more atmosphere of pressure or 14.2 lb/in.^{2} (34 ft ≈ 10.4 m for fresh water). Divers commonly exceed 100 fsw (30.5 m of seawater (msw)) (or more than 3 atm over sea level). As would be expected, significant physiologic adjustment takes place.

Gas laws

This discussion of hyperbaric environment requires at least a working knowledge of some of the gas laws (Bove, 1997). For instance, Boyle's law states that at a constant temperature gas volume is inversely related to pressure. This phenomenon is used in the treatment of air embolism and also plays a role in its etiology. *Table 14.4 illustrates the point.*

Charles' law states that if pressure remains constant, volume will relate directly to temperature. Charles' law and Boyle's law can be combined into the general gas law, which states that $K = PV/T$, where K is a constant, P equals pressure, V equals volume and T equals temperature.

Table 14.4 Effect of pressure on gas volumes

Depth		Pressure (atm)	Volume (%)
fsw	msw		
Sea level		1	100
33	10	2	50
66	20	3	33
99	30	4	25
132	40	5	20

This shows the relative effect of increased pressure on lung volume and discrete air bubbles.

Particularly, when considering mixed gas mixtures while diving, Dalton's law states that the total pressure of the gas mixture is the sum of all the pressures of the individual gases. $P = P_1 + P_2 + P_3$, etc.

Pulmonary effects

Elevated ambient pressures compress lung volumes. The relationships remain essentially unchanged but volumes significantly decrease. This does not imply, however, that any lung collapse actually occurs.

As the pressures increase, all the inspired and expired gas densities increase. Work of breathing increases. Divers use demand valves with high flow rates to help overcome this resistance. At the deeper depths even this is not sufficient. Below 100 fsw helium can be used. It has 1/7 the density of nitrogen. The partial pressure of any gas increases directly along with the pressure. For example, 100% O_2 at sea level would imply a P_AO_2 of about 673 mmHg ($760 - 47 - 40 = 673$): where 47 mmHg equals water vapor at 37°C and 40 mmHg equals P_ACO_2. The addition of 3 more atm (99 fsw) means the P_aO_2 increases to 2019 mmHg (673×3). PCO_2 does not actually change because CO_2 production does not change. At these pressures O_2 becomes toxic (Butler & Thalmann, 1986). Seizures can develop and can be preceded by nausea, chewing motion, light disturbances and altered mental status. Treatment is symptomatic and the person should be removed from the high O_2 environment. With immediate care these symptoms are self-limited and have no long-term effects. Short-term CO_2 production increases and a lactic acid develops.

Decompression sickness

Any increase in atmospheric pressure will increase the solubility in tissue and blood of all inhaled gases. We will use air with nitrogen and O_2 as our primary example. Although nitrogen is considered inert – more will be dissolved in blood and tissues at the higher pressures experienced by the diver. The amount taken up during the dive depends on the depth, duration and activity level. Upon return to the surface the nitrogen must first move from tissue into blood before it can be exhaled. Failure to follow prescribed ascent rates and decompression stops can result in the nitrogen coming out of solution too rapidly and forming micro-bubbles (Vann & Thalmann, 1993). These micro-bubbles occlude flow to various structures and lead to specific symptoms dependent on the anatomical structures involved. Blood flow to the lung is usually not affected and any change in P_ACO_2 will result from specific breathing patterns.

Air embolism

Air embolism, on the other hand, can affect expired CO_2 (Schaeffer *et al.*, 1958). This is an over pres-sure accident. At depth the diver's lung volume and tidal volume have been decreased by the high environmental pressures. During rapid ascent to the surface, failure to exhale at a proper rate permits the gas in the lungs to expand, according to Boyle's law. Since the gas is under pressure it can rup-ture bronchioles and alveoli, and gain access to the circulation.

Treatment for air embolism consists of placement in a hyperbaric chamber. Recompression to a treatment depth as great as 165 fsw (50.3 msw) or 5 atm is usually considered sufficient to reduce any discrete bubbles to a size that will pass through all the capillaries. Ultimately these very compressed bubbles should then be exhaled.

While in the chamber the patient breathes 100% O_2, which provides a secondary benefit (Moon, 1990). The high O_2 levels achieved in the blood stimulate vasoconstriction, which in turn reduces blood flow to tissue, particularly neural. This can help reduce edema in important structures such as the spinal cord. Less edema or swelling usually contributes to a better outcome.

CO_2 elimination

A major problem in a hyperbaric environment can be elimination of CO_2. Humans can tolerate an acute increase in PCO_2 up to 80 mmHg. Chronic elevations of up to 140 mmHg are also tolerated (Hicking *et al.*, 1994). Minute ventilation will increase by a factor of 8–10. The signs and symptoms of toxic CO_2 levels relate first to the respiratory acidosis. Profound vasodilation ensues; ultimately, narcosis and an anesthesia-like state supervenes.

Sport divers mostly use an open circuit and simply exhale CO_2 into the water. A closed circuit, used by certain military groups, will eliminate any bubbles, which could pinpoint their position. However, they must have an efficient CO_2 removal device, which requires periodic replacement.

Larger structures such as hyperbaric chambers rely on continued ventilation to maintain a safe CO_2 level. When using masks for O_2, many have an overboard dump for the exhaled gases. This minimizes the need for venting. Submarines and submersibles rely on CO_2 scrubbers with a large capacity to remove CO_2.

CO_2 monitoring and ambient pressure

Dependent on the type of technology selected, CO_2 monitoring may be affected by ambient pressure. Infrared analysis and mass spectroscopy are the most common technologies used to monitor end-tidal CO_2. Differences in methods of measurement and units displayed by different commercial monitors (percentage of volume versus partial pressure) complicate the interpretation of data at varying ambient pressures. To meet the standards published by the American Society for Testing and Materials (1992), a capnometer should either provide an automatic compensation for barometric pressure or the accompanying documents should explain that the readings in "concentration units" are correct only under the pressure at which the devise is calibrated.

Capnometers measure either the partial pressures (infrared analyzers) or percent volumes (mass spectroscopes) of gases. Clinicians are accustomed to CO_2 levels expressed as partial pressures. Therefore, monitors that measure percent volumes of gases usually display the partial pressure calculated by the following formula:

$$PCO_2 = \left\{\begin{matrix}\%\text{ volume}\\ CO_2\end{matrix}\right\} \times \left\{\begin{matrix}\text{barometric}\\ \text{pressure}\end{matrix} - 47\,\text{mmHg}\right\}$$

where 47 mmHg = water vapor pressure at 37°C.

Monitors that measure partial pressures are calibrated using a sample gas with known concentration of CO_2. For example, a monitor calibrated at sea level against a sample gas containing 5% of CO_2 by volume might be set to read 38 mmHg by using the following formula:

$$PCO_2 = 0.05 \times 760\,\text{mmHg}$$

To clarify the effect of ambient pressure on partial pressure and concentration of CO_2, let us examine a hypothetical subject who breathes 100% O_2 at steady minute ventilation. Assume that the end-tidal breath has 5% CO_2. Assume a unit volume of end-tidal gas to have 100 molecules of which 5 molecules of CO_2 and 95 molecules of O_2 and water vapor. If the ambient pressure is reduced to 0.50 atm, there will only be a total of 50 molecules in the same unit volume of end-tidal gas. As previously mentioned, CO_2 production does not change with changes in ambient pressure. Therefore, 5 molecules of CO_2 will still be present in the end-tidal gas sample. However, the ratio moves to 5 of 50 (or 10%) rather than the original. If the same subject is now compressed to an ambient pressure of 2 atm, a total of 200 molecules will be present in the same original unit volume. There will be 195 molecules of O_2 and water vapor combined while the same 5 molecules of CO_2 will be produced. The ratio of CO_2 in the end-tidal gas changes to 5 of 200 (or 2.5%).

Altitude

Capnometers with infrared analyzers report the PCO_2 (Dorsch & Dorsch, 1994). If the end-tidal gas sample with a CO_2 concentration of 5% reaches an instrument that is calibrated at sea level, it would display a PCO_2 of 38 mmHg. In this regard, it would display the correct PCO_2 regardless of ambient pressure. If, however, the device was set to display the *fraction* of CO_2 instead of *partial pressure*, the actual ambient pressure must be known and would directly affect the accuracy of the result (James & White, 1984). For example, at 0.5 atm in the previous example, the concentration of CO_2 would now read 10%. It is important to note that this *is* an accurate value, which is physiologically equivalent to an end-tidal CO_2 concentration of 5% at sea level. However, clinicians do not ordinarily think of physiologic values in relation to the barometric pressure.

To avoid errors in clinical management, one of the following steps can be taken. In order of preference, these are:

1. Set adjustment of the device to read partial pressure instead of concentration. After calibration, this will be accurate at any altitude.
2. Calibration at altitude with a known gas CO_2 concentration. This will then display the percentage of CO_2 as it would be measured at sea level.
3. Interpretation of the displayed CO_2 concentration in accordance with the actual barometric pressure. This should prompt the clinician to regard 10% of CO_2 at 0.5 atm equal to 5% at sea level (1 atm). We do not actually encourage this last option because it might lead to confusion among different members of a healthcare team.

Mass spectrometers measure the volume percent of dry gases. Therefore, partial pressure of end-tidal CO_2 ($P_{et}CO_2$) is computed and displayed by the machine using the following formula:

$$PCO_2 = \text{volume ratio of } CO_2 \times \text{barometric pressure}$$

It is obvious that a capnometer using mass spectroscopy has to have the capability of allowing altitude compensation to display accurate values in ambient pressures other than 1 atm.

Hyperbaric chamber

As long as the monitoring device is in the same ambient pressure (i.e. in the chamber) with the patient, the logic discussed above for altitude remains valid in hyperbaric chambers with increased ambient pressures (Arieli *et al.*, 2001; Mummery *et al.*, 2003). However, many chambers place the analyzer outside the chamber, which brings up additional points of interest.

To better understand this concept, let us return to the example of the hypothetical 5 molecules of CO_2 and 195 molecules of O_2 and water combined in the same unit volume of gas. Now as this volume exits the chamber accompanied by an ambient pressure changes to atmosphere, the unit volume *expands* to twice its original volume. This means a final CO_2 concentration of 2.5% at the measurement site. Therefore, although the subject still has an $P_{et}CO_2$ of 38 mmHg *inside* the chamber, it is measured as 17.5 mmHg by the capnometer *outside* the chamber. The actual PCO_2 inside the chamber can be calculated using the following formula:

$$\text{actual } PCO_2 = PCO_2 \times \left(\frac{\text{chamber pressure}}{\text{ambient pressure}} \right)$$

In summary, end-tidal CO_2 can be reliably and accurately monitored at altitude or in the hyperbaric setting by any of the available techniques, provided that the basic physical properties of the gas mixtures and the basic principles of the chosen technique are recognized.

References

American Society for Testing and Materials (1992). Specifications for capnometers (F-1456-92). ASTM, Philadelphia, PA.

Arieli, R., Daskalovic, Y., Eynan, M., Arieli, Y., Ertracht, O. & Shupak, A. (2001). Use of a mass spectrometer for direct respiratory gas sampling from the hyperbaric chamber. *Aviat. Space Environ. Med.*, **72**: 799–804.

Bove, A.A. (1997). *Bove and Davis' Diving Medicine*, 3rd edition, W.B. Saunders Co., Philadelphia, PA; pp. 17–22.

Butler, F.K. & Thalmann, E.D. (1986). Central nervous system oxygen toxicity in closed-circuit scuba divers II. *Undersea Bio. Med. Res.*, **13**: 193–223.

Dorsch, J.A. & Dorsch, S.E. (1994). In: Dorsch, J.A., Dorsch, S.E. & Baltimore, M.D. (eds) *Gas Monitoring, Understanding Anesthesia Equipment*, 3rd edition. Williams & Wilkins, pp. 547–607.

Etozzi, C.A., Poianig, J., Harangozo, A.M., *et al.* (1989). Pressure-induced connective tissues synthesis in pulmonary artery distal segments is dependant on intact endothelium. *J. Clin. Invest.*, **84**: 1005–1012.

Gerard, A.B., Mcelroy, M.D., Taylor, M.J., *et al.* (2000). 6% oxygen enrichment of room air at simulated 5000 m altitude improves neuropsychological function. *High Alt. Med. Biol.*, **1**: 51–61.

Gore, C.J., Hahn, A.G., Watson, D.B., *et al.* (1996). VO_2 max and arterial oxygen saturation at sea level and at 610 m. *Med. Sci. Sport. Exerc.*, **27** [abstract 42].

Hackett, P.H., Bertman, J. & Rodriguez, G. (1986). Pulmonary edema fluid protein in high altitude pulmonary edema. *J. Am. Med. Assoc.*, **256**: 36.

Hicking, K.G., Walsh, J., Henderson, S. & Jackson, R. (1994). Low mortality rate in adult respiratory distress syndrome using low-volume, pressure-limited ventilation with permissive hypercapnia: a prospective study. *Crit. Care Med.*, **22**: 1568–1578.

Hornbein, T.F., Townes, B.D., Schoene, R.B., *et al.* (1989). The cost to the central nervous system of climbing to extremely high altitude. *New Engl. J. Med.*, **321**: 1714–1719.

Hultgren, H. (1997). *High Altitude Medicine*. Hultgren Publications, San Francisco, CA; pp. 15–32, 212–255.

James, M.F.M. & White, J.F. (1984). Anesthetic considerations at moderate altitude. *Anesth. Analg.*, **63**: 1097–1105.

Kennedy, R., Dunlap, W., Banderet, L., *et al.* (1989). Cognitive performance and deficits in a simulated climate of Mount Everest: operation Everest II. *Aviat. Space Environ. Med.*, **60**: 99–104.

Lambertsen, C. (1968). Chemical control of respiration at rest. In: Mountcastle, V. (ed.) *Medical Physiology*. C.V. Mosby, St. Louis; pp. 713–763.

Mcdonald, D. (1981). Peripheral chemoreceptors. In: Hornbein, T. (ed.) *Regulation of Breathing*. Marcel Dekker, New York; pp. 305–319.

Moon, R.E. (1990). Treatment of decompression sickness and arterial gas embolism. In: Bove, A.A. & Davis, J.C. (eds) *Diving Medicine*, W.B. Saunders Co., New York, NY; pp. 184–204.

Mummery, H., Stolp, B.W., Dear, G.L., *et al.* (2003). Effects of age and exercise on physiological dead space during simulated dives at 2.8 ATA. *J. Appl. Physiol.*, **94**: 507–517.

Pretorius, H.A. (1970). Effect of oxygen on night vision. *Aerosp. Med.*, **41**: 560–562.

Reynafarje, C., Ramos, J., Faura, J., *et al.* (1964). Humoral control of the erythropoietic activity in man during and after altitude exposure. *Proc. Soc. Exp. Biol. Med.*, **116**: 649.

Schaeffer, K.E., Nulty, W.P., Carey, *et al.* (1958). Mechanisms in development of intrastitial emphysema and air embolism on decompression from depth. *J. Appl. Physiol.*,**13**: 15–29.

Schoene, R.P., Lahire, S., Hackett, P.H., *et al.* (1984). Relationships of hypoxic ventilatory response and exercise performance on Mt. Everest. *J. Appl. Physiol.*, **56**: 1478–1483.

Severinghaus, J., Mitchell, R., Richardson, D., *et al.* (1963). Respiratory control at high altitude suggesting accurate transport regulation of cerebral spinal fluid pH. *J. Appl. Physiol.*, **18**: 1155–1166.

Vann, R.D. & Thalmann, E.D. (1993). Decompression physiology and practice. In: Bennett, P.B. & Elliott, D.H. (eds) *Physiology of Diving in Compressed Airwork*, 4th edition. W.B. Saunders, London; pp. 376–432.

Ward, M.P., Milledge, J.S. & West, J.B. (2000). *High Altitude Medicine and Physiology*. 3rd edition. Oxford University Press, Arnold, pp. 50–64.

Weil, J.V. (1986). Ventilatory control at high altitude. In: Cherniack, N.S. & Widdicome, J.G. *Handbook of Physiology*, Section 3, Vol. Ii. American Physiologic Society, Bethesda, MD; pp. 703–727.

West, J.B. (1962). Diffusing capacities of lung for carbon monoxide high altitude. *J. Appl. Physiol.*, **17**: 421–426.

World Health Organization. World Health Statistics Annual (1996).

Wren, X. & Robbins, P.A. (1999). Ventilatory responses to hypercapnia and hypoxia after six hours past the hyperventilation in humans. *J. Appl. Physiol.*, **514**: 885–894.

THERAPEUTIC USE OF AMBULATORY CAPNOGRAPHY 15

A.E. Meuret, T. Ritz, B. Dahme & W.T. Roth

Capnometry in the therapy setting: treatment of hypocapnia

Hypocapnia has been linked experimentally to organ injury and a number of organic illnesses and mental disorders. It has been hypothesized that therapeutic hypercapnia would be beneficial for these conditions (Laffey & Kavanagh, 2002). The development of light, user-friendly ambulatory capnometry equipment has opened up new possibilities for the development of behavioral treatments targeting hypocapnia. Patients can use these devices at home as part of a treatment protocol that attempts to modify breathing behavior systematically. Electronic data storage allows control over use of the equipment even in the absence of trained clinical personnel.

Hyperventilation refers to increases in the rate or depth of breathing that produce a higher degree of ventilation than necessary to meet metabolic demand. The end result is that alveolar and arterial carbon dioxide (CO_2) pressures decrease and blood pH increases. Sustained hyperventilation produces a variety of adverse changes including a diminished ability for oxygen to pass from the blood to the organism's cells.

We describe several disorders that have been associated with hypocapnia and to which breathing therapies have been applied that make use of capnography. Although it seems obvious that a therapy to reverse hypocapnia should make use of CO_2 measurements for both validating the effect of instructions about breathing and to evaluate the results, breathing training has often been conducted without any objective measurement of the crucial parameter.

Hyperventilation syndrome

The clinical literature abounds with observations of patients presenting with a miscellany of complaints for which no organic origin is apparent. One group typically feels dyspneic, breathless, dizzy, and lightheaded, and reports chest pain, heart racing, or sweating. It has been proposed that hypocapnia and disturbance of the acid–base balance are the underlying origin of these symptoms (Lum, 1987). Hyperventilation syndrome (HVS) has become a common designation for the constellation of complaints of these patients. HVS has been reported to be present in at least 5%–10% of general medical outpatients (Magarian, 1982). The breathing pattern of these patients is typically described as disorganized, with rapid respiratory rates (RRs), frequent sighing, low partial pressure of CO_2 in arterial blood (P_aCO_2) levels, and emphasis on thoracic rather than abdominal breathing. Patients often feel anxious and depressed. In rare cases, fear of loss of consciousness or dying are reported (Howell, 1997).

Earlier therapeutic approaches considered the utility of measuring partial pressure of CO_2 at end-tidal ($P_{et}CO_2$) levels during therapy sessions. Folgering *et al.* (1980) and van Doorn *et al.* (1982) were among the first to use feedback of $P_{et}CO_2$ levels as a therapeutic tool in HVS. Over the course of 7 weeks, patients were taught to increase $P_{et}CO_2$ levels in the sessions. Feedback was delivered through a two-channel chart recorder while they were breathing into a face mask. Compared to patients receiving breathing training without feedback, the feedback training group improved symptomatically and showed significant, sustained increases in $P_{et}CO_2$ (from approximately 32–39 mmHg).

Similarly, a study by Grossman *et al.* (1985) used within sessions a stationary CO_2 infrared gas analyzer and between sessions during home exercises a portable device that measured RR. The authors demonstrated improvement in both psychologic and physiologic measures, suggesting that changes in respiratory control are the basis of treatment success.

Agreement about criteria for HVS as a distinct diagnostic entity has never been reached (Bass, 1997). Furthermore, recent research (Hornsveld *et al.*, 1996) has questioned the validity of HVS by demonstrating a lack of psychologic and physiologic specificity of the purported signs and symptoms. For these reasons, no attempts have been made to replicate or extend early innovative interventions in treating chronic hypocapnic breathing.

Panic disorder

Abnormalities in respiration have been postulated as a central component in anxiety disorders for several decades based on patient reports of severe respiratory distress during anxiety episodes and on a variety of other clinical and experimental observations. Shortness of breath, together with palpitations and faintness, has been found to be one of the most commonly reported symptoms of panic (McNally *et al.*, 1995). Dyspnea, accompanied by hyperventilation, may contribute to the development and maintenance of panic disorder (PD) (Ley, 1985) and a biological vulnerability due to an abnormal brainstem respiratory control mechanism may trigger a false suffocation alarm resulting in compensatory hyperventilation and panic attacks (Klein, 1993). In addition, hyperventilation may not be limited to the attack itself, but may precede and follow it, giving rise to moderate sustained hypocapnia (Lum, 1987). According to this hypothesis, the cause of seemingly spontaneous panic attacks is often chronic or episodic hyperventilation of which the patient is generally not aware.

Hypocapnia has been repeatedly identified as distinguishing PD patients from other groups during baseline assessment (Munjack *et al.*, 1993; Hegel & Ferguson, 1997). Standardized voluntary hyperventilation generally increases anxiety and produces symptoms similar or identical to panic attacks (Maddock & Carter, 1991), but it remains uncertain whether hyperventilation causes panic attacks or is merely an accompanying phenomenon in some panic patients (Garssen *et al.*, 1996). Other provocation tests such as lactate infusions (Gorman *et al.*, 1989), inhalation of CO_2 (Papp *et al.*, 1997), or administration of other respiratory stimulants such as doxapram (Dopram®) (Abelson & Nesse, 1994) produce panic attacks, which are often accompanied by hypocapnia.

Interestingly, even though breathing training is aimed at changing hypocapnic breathing, $P_{et}CO_2$ levels are seldom measured in therapy studies. Exceptions are studies such as the one by Salkovskis *et al.* (1986). The authors used repeated $P_{et}CO_2$ measurements to test whether patients suffering from panic attacks had lower resting $P_{et}CO_2$ levels before treatment, and whether these levels increased during treatment. Psychologic outcome variables (panic attack frequency and self-report of anxiety and avoidance) showed a marked improvement compared to baseline. $P_{et}CO_2$ levels increased from 35 mmHg at baseline to approximately 41.5 mmHg in the course of the therapy. The authors concluded that respiratory training can restore a patient's $P_{et}CO_2$, and may thus reduce their previously heightened vulnerability to psychologic stressors.

Asthma

Ventilatory changes have often been found to exacerbate asthmatic symptoms. Breathing patterns with deep inspirations, increased minute ventilation, increased respiratory drive, or decreased $P_{et}CO_2$ have all been linked to airway obstruction in asthma (Gayrard *et al.*, 1975; van den Elshout *et al.*, 1991). Hypocapnic breathing can also play a key role in exacerbations of asthma during episodes of stress, anxiety, or panic (Knapp, 1989). The increase in respiratory drive through excessive deep breathing also leads to subjective experience of dyspnea (Mahler *et al.*, 1991). Asthmatics have been shown to respond with excessive increases in respiratory drive to challenges such as physical exercise (Varray & Prefaut, 1992; Ritz *et al.*, 1998) or added resistive loads on air flow (Kelsen *et al.*, 1979). Increased respiratory drive or minute ventilation puts patients at risk of becoming hypocapnic. Using ambulatory monitoring of respiration, we found increased RR and decreased $P_{et}CO_2$ in asthma patients compared to healthy controls (Ritz *et al.*, 2003). Similarly, others have observed statistically significant reductions in $P_{et}CO_2$ in mild chronic asthmatics with no accompanying symptoms of hyperventilation (Osborne *et al.*, 2000). The level of $P_{et}CO_2$ was negatively correlated with airway hyperreactivity to methacholine provocation. Thus, a deep breathing pattern with high minute volume and/or lowered $P_{et}CO_2$ can lead to subjective and physiologic changes contributing to exacerbations of asthma.

Breathing training and biofeedback have long been advocated as adjunctive treatment in asthma (Ritz & Roth, 2003; Ritz, Dahme & Roth, 2004). The Buteyko breathing technique has recently been proposed as a powerful tool to improve asthma patients' quality of life. Patients are taught to breathe slower and shallower to increase their $P_{et}CO_2$ levels. The basic assumption is that decreased $P_{et}CO_2$ leads to a number of autonomic, endocrine and metabolic disturbances, which contribute to the pathophysiology of asthma (Stalmatski, 1999). Three controlled trials of asthmatics demonstrated increases in quality of life as measured by standardized questionnaires and/or a reduction in bronchodilator use (Bowler *et al.*, 1998; Opat *et al.*, 2000; Cooper *et al.*, 2003). Bowler *et al.* reported significant decreases in minute ventilation in the Buteyko breathing training group, but parameters of mechanical lung function and $P_{et}CO_2$ levels remained constant. The two other studies did not incorporate measures of $P_{et}CO_2$, and thus were not able to test the main treatment rationale.

Epilepsy

Cerebral hypoxia accompanying hypocapnic breathing has been hypothesized as a possible cause of seizures in epilepsy (Riley, 1982). A successful strategy of seizure control would therefore be the normalization of P_aCO_2 level, thereby restoring the acid–base balance to control seizure thresholds, particularly in patients intolerant to the physiologic effects of respiratory alkalosis. Fried *et al.* (1984) developed a method to train idiopathic seizure sufferers to self-regulate P_aCO_2 levels through diaphragmatic breathing techniques. They used stationary equipment to measure RR and $P_{et}CO_2$. Visual feedback of both parameters was provided on a video monitor, and the goal for adequate breathing was set at 5% $P_{et}CO_2$ and 12–14 breaths/min.

Following at least 7 months of diaphragmatic breathing training combined with feedback of $P_{et}CO_2$ a group of 18 patients showed significant decreases in RR and seizure frequency, but no significant long-term change in $P_{et}CO_2$. Thus, the hypothesized mechanism of seizure control by CO_2 levels was not tested in this study, and the potential benefits of stable long-term increases in $P_{et}CO_2$ levels were not investigated. In addition, due to incomplete description of the treatment protocol (e.g. no information on duration, number and frequency of training sessions) and data analysis and due to the lack of a treatment-control group, the results have to be interpreted with caution.

New behavioral treatment applications for ambulatory capnometry

Capnometry-assisted breathing training in PD

Given the assumed central role of hypocapnia in panic development, a biofeedback-assisted breathing training has been recently developed aimed at increasing $P_{et}CO_2$ levels during treatment (Meuret *et al.*, 2001; Meuret *et al.*, 2004). Previous breathing training studies have rarely included measurements of $P_{et}CO_2$ levels, and thus were unable to address the validity of their main underlying rationale for change in therapy. We assumed that lasting modifications in breathing behavior and $P_{et}CO_2$ levels would require intensive breathing retraining combined with close monitoring of relevant breathing parameters. Because sufficiently frequent practice sessions were not practical in a clinic environment, training and monitoring methods had to be adapted to a home environment. Training at home would also facilitate the transfer of learned breathing behavior to everyday life situations. The advent of small handheld capnometers with electronic memory is a major step towards implementation of $P_{et}CO_2$ home-training protocols.

This capnometry-assisted breathing therapy is aimed at regulating respiration and thus reducing symptoms in PD. Patients used a light, handheld, battery-operated capnometry device (Capnocount mini, Weinmann Inc.®, Germany) to monitor and modify their $P_{et}CO_2$. When activated, the instrument records $P_{et}CO_2$ and RR every 2 s along with the time and date of the entire measurement in its internal memory. Visual feedback of $P_{et}CO_2$ and RR appears continuously on a small digital display. Stored data can be downloaded through an interface module in the clinic to a computer.

To increase their $P_{et}CO_2$, patients learned to breathe abdominally and regularly at a decreased rate. Prerecorded audiotapes with pacing tones were used to guide the breathing exercises. Increasing tones indicated inspiration, decreasing tones, expiration, and silence, a pause between expiration and inspiration. RR was successively decreased across the 4 weeks of training. The tone pattern was modulated to correspond to a RR of 13 breaths/min in the first treatment week, and rates of 11, 9, and 6 breaths/min in successive following weeks. Patients were instructed to practice this highly standardized breathing twice a day for 17 min. Each exercise consisted of three parts: (A) a baseline period during which patients sat quietly and relaxed with their eyes closed for 2 min, (B) a 10-min paced breathing period during which patients monitored their $P_{et}CO_2$ and RR, and (C) a 5-min transfer phase without pacing tones during which patients maintained this breathing pattern in absence of timing information, but with continued $P_{et}CO_2$ and RR feedback. Timing of these phases and instructions were announced on the tape guiding the exercises. During the second and third exercise period patients were instructed to aim for increased $P_{et}CO_2$ levels by changing their breathing rhythm, pace, and depth of inspiration.

In addition to the twice-daily home exercises, patients attended five individual training and review sessions over 4 weeks. The initial session was mainly educational, while the other sessions served to review progress in the daily exercises. Using a docking station for the portable capnometry device, the therapist downloaded the physiologic data of the exercises recorded during the previous week and presented the data in graphic printouts to the patient (see Figure 15.1) (Meuret *et al.*, 2004). These were discussed in conjunction with the patient's psychologic reports, and the next week's breathing training was modified according to individual needs. The application of new

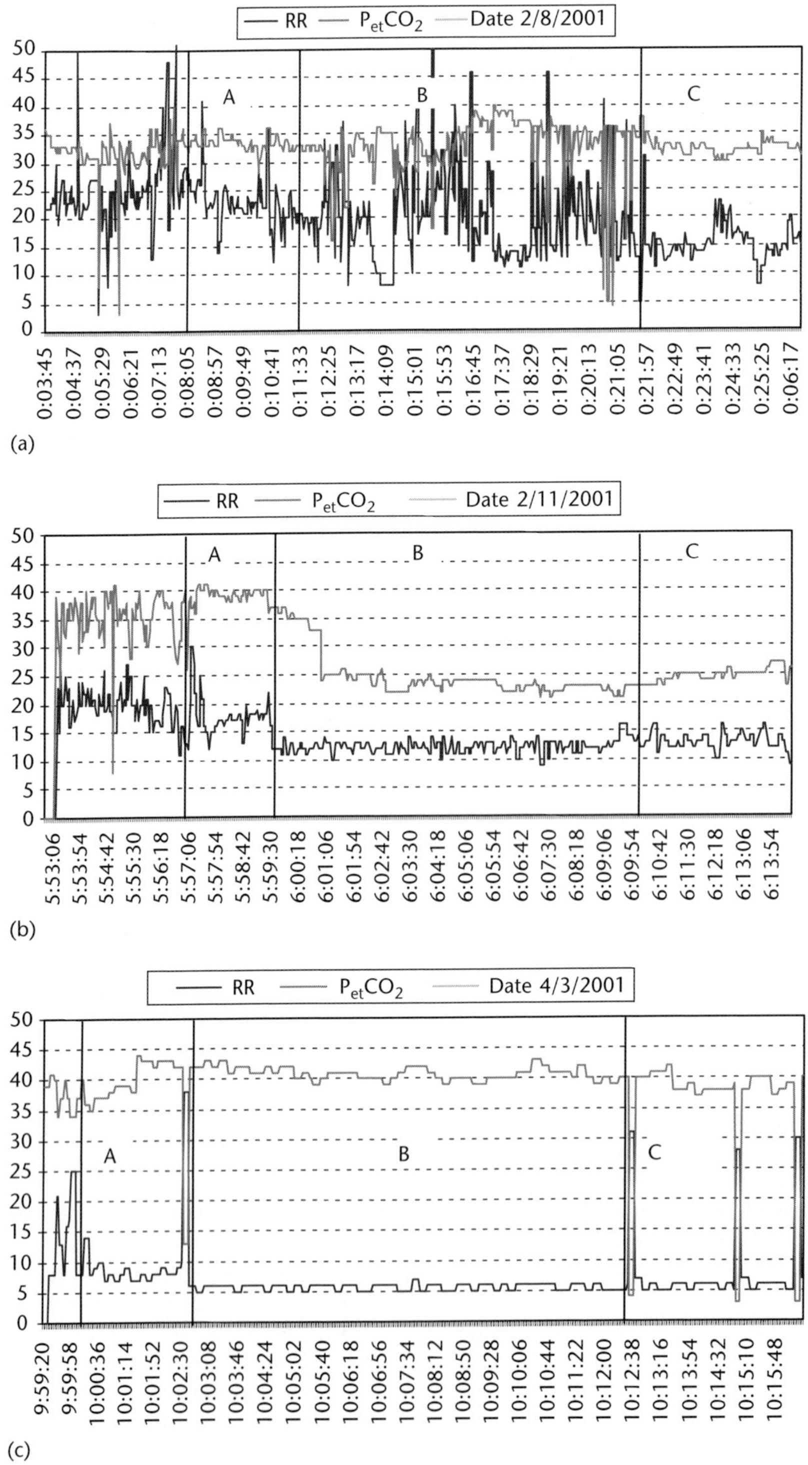

Figure 15.1 Breath-by-breath $P_{et}CO_2$ and RR printouts of exercises performed in the first (a and b) and last treatment week (c) over the course of the biofeedback breathing exercise. Upper line represents $P_{et}CO_2$ and lower line represents RR (A: baseline; B: paced breathing tones with $P_{et}CO_2$ feedback; and C: only $P_{et}CO_2$ feedback).

breathing skills during difficult situations was also planned and reviewed.

Figure 15.1 shows illustrations of $P_{et}CO_2$ and RR at three different times in therapy. The upper panel (a) displays the first home-breathing exercise. As can be seen, $P_{et}CO_2$ levels fluctuate around hypocapnic ranges and RR is increased and irregular. Overall breathing patterns are irregular in pace and rhythm, being interrupted by frequent sighs as indicated by the spikes in momentary RR. The center panel (b) displays $P_{et}CO_2$ and RR after a few days of training. The patient is more able to follow the instructions to breathe at a rate of 13 breaths/min. Nevertheless, $P_{et}CO_2$ decreases markedly to hypocapnic levels (<25 mmHg) with the onset of the paced breathing phase. At this early stage in therapy such seemingly paradoxical effects represent compensatory breathing efforts of the patient: the slowing of RR and efforts to keep it regular lead to compensatory increases in tidal volume, thus decreasing $P_{et}CO_2$ levels. As diary ratings show, the patient often experiences shortness of breath. While this shortness of breath typically increases throughout a 17-min exercise, it gradually abates over the 4 weeks of training. The lower panel (c) of Figure 15.1 shows the progress documented towards the end of the 4-week training. In addition to decreased RRs and increased $P_{et}CO_2$ at baseline, the patient is able to reach and maintain baseline levels of $P_{et}CO_2$ and RR throughout paced breathing. Overall the patient breathes regular in terms of speed and depth.

The results of a recent randomized controlled trial (Meuret *et al.*, submitted) of a 4-week training with follow-up assessments at 2 and 12 months suggest substantial and long-lasting corrections and a positive correlation of respiratory dysregulation and improvement of panic symptomatology. Panic patients had increased their $P_{et}CO_2$ levels by approximately 5 mmHg at 12-month follow-up, they recovered faster from voluntary hyperventilation, and 68% were free of panic attacks for the past 12 months according to criteria of the Diagnostic and Statistical Manual of Mental Disorders (DSM-IV, American Psychiatric Association, 1994). Compliance with the 4-week training protocol was very high, and patients rated the rationale and effectiveness of the treatment as very convincing.

Capnometry-assisted breathing training as an adjunctive treatment for asthma

To overcome some of the deficiencies of earlier hypoventilation training studies in asthma, capnometry-assisted $P_{et}CO_2$-biofeedback training has been adapted to asthma patients (Meuret *et al.*, 2002). Patients with predominantly mild persistent to moderate asthma volunteered for a breathing training intervention, which was presented as an adjunctive behavioral training supplementing their existing medical treatment. They were encouraged to reduce their bronchodilator use, but to keep their other asthma medication constant.

The techniques and protocol followed largely those outlined for panic patients above. The therapy consisted of five individual sessions of respiratory control training over the course of 4 weeks, with additional homework assignments of two 17-min breathing exercises each day. The therapy rationale outlined general as well as asthma-specific adverse effects of overbreathing or hypocapnia. In addition to using the capnometer, patients monitored their lung function and symptoms using a handheld electronic spirometer with diary functions for ratings of symptoms and mood. Measurements of lung function and symptoms were scheduled before and after each exercise, and during the five therapist-guided sessions.

Initial results of a pilot trial (Meuret *et al.*, 2003), including eight patients in the treatment group and four patients in a waiting-list control, demonstrated the usefulness of the capnometry training in initiating long-term increases in $P_{et}CO_2$ levels, although peak flow and spirometric lung function (forced expiratory volume in the first second, FEV1) remained constant. Detailed analysis of within-individual changes in $P_{et}CO_2$ levels and lung function across individual home-training exercises demonstrated no systematic relationship between them (Meuret *et al.*, 2002). Although basal lung function did not change, patients reported improved symptoms and better control of asthma at the end of the 4-week training and the 2-month follow-up. Credibility and acceptance of the training was generally high. Patients reported that the training gave them greater voluntary control over their asthma symptoms, particularly over coughing.

Thus, while capnometry-assisted breathing training has the potential to improve symptoms and perceived asthma control, improvements in basal lung function have yet to be documented. Changes in $P_{et}CO_2$ levels as initiated during our typical breathing exercises are apparently too small to impact basal lung function, at least when measured by spirometric techniques. How hypoventilation training improves asthma control is apparently more complex than initially believed (Walters & Johns, 2001). It remains to be shown whether capnometry-assisted hypoventilation training can improve asthma control by leading to long-term reductions in non-specific hyper-reactivity of the airways, a parameter not included in our pilot study.

Principles and perspectives in the use of capnometry for behavioral therapy

Panic and asthma patients in the above-described studies experienced specific benefits from the repeated use of a portable capnometer. They were able to measure their RR and $P_{et}CO_2$ levels at different times of the day, in situational, and in emotional states. They not only were able to better understand the mechanism of different breathing maneuvers on symptoms and emotions, but also were gradually able to influence and modify these parameters willingly. Patients were able to test these assumptions directly and were able to revalue bodily misconceptions such as fear of suffocation. This can be particularly important in chronic diseases such as asthma where introspective awareness may be altered and patients are no longer able to detect deteriorations in their physiologic state.

Portable capnometry devices facilitate patient's home-training efficiency, self-modification efforts, and treatment compliance by immediate, objective feedback of respiratory parameters. Until recently patients' homework compliance and progress outside the therapists' office have rarely been measured systematically because affordable and portable devices were lacking. Ambulatory capnometry devices with electronic data storage, however, allow therapists to track patients' progress without having to rely exclusively on retrospective self-reports. Self-modification of physiologic parameters require more than in-session "snap-shots". Monitoring throughout therapy can help health professionals tailor the treatment to the patient's individual needs. It also allows easy handling of data, which can be downloaded directly, analyzed, and presented to the patient in therapy sessions. Thus, ambulatory capnometry has the potential significantly to change behavioral treatment of mental disorders and organic diseases that are linked to respiratory disturbances and hypocapnic breathing. More research is needed into the application of hypercapnic breathing in clinical therapy. The general therapeutic goal in treating patients can be expressed as "keep the P_aCO_2 high; if necessary, make it high; and above all, prevent it from being low" (Laffey & Kavanagh, 1999, p. 1286).

References

Abelson, J. & Nesse, R. (1994). Pentagastrin infusions in patients with panic disorder. I. Symptoms and cardiovascular responses. *Biol. Psychiatr.*, **36**: 73–83.

American Psychiatric Association (1994). *Diagnostic and Statistical Manual of Mental Disorders – DSM-IV*, 4th edition. American Psychiatric Association, Washington, D.C.

Bass, C. (1997). Hyperventilation syndrome: a chimera? *J. Psychosom. Res.*, **42**: 421–426.

Bowler, S.D., Green, A.G. & Mitchell, C.A. (1998). Buteyko breathing techniques in asthma: a blinded randomised controlled trial. *Med. J. Aust.*, **169**: 575–578.

Cooper, S., Oborne, J. & Newton, S., *et al.* (2003). Effects of two breathing exercises (Buteyko and Pranayama) in asthma: a randomized controlled trial. *Thorax*, **58**: 674–679.

Folgering, H., Lenders, J. & Rosier, I. (1980). In: Herzog, H. *et al.* (eds) *Biofeedback Control of P_aCO_2, a Prospective Therapy in Hyperventilation. Progress in Respiratory Research, Vol. 14. Asthma*. Karger, Basel; pp. 26–30.

Fried, R., Rubin, S.R., Carlton, R.M. & Fox, M.C. (1984). Behavioral control of intractable idiopathic seizures: self-regulation of end-tidal carbon dioxide. *Psychosom. Med.*, **46**: 315–331.

Garssen, B., Buikhuisen, M. & van Dyck, R. (1996). Hyperventilation and panic attacks. *Am. J. Psychiatr.*, **153**: 513–518.

Gayrard, P., Orehek, J., Grimaud, C. & Charpin, J. (1975). Bronchoconstrictor effects of a deep inspiration in patients with asthma. *Am. Rev. Respir. Dis.*, **111**: 433–439.

Gorman, J., Battista, D. & Goetz, R., *et al.* (1989). A comparison of sodium bicarbonate and sodium lactate infusion in the induction of panic attacks. *Arch. Gen. Psychiatr.*, **46**: 145–150.

Grossman, P., de Swart, J.C. & Defares, P.B. (1985). A controlled study of a breathing therapy for treatment of hyperventilation syndrome. *J. Psychosom. Res.*, **29**: 49–58.

Hegel, M.T. & Ferguson, R.J. (1997). Psychophysiological assessment of respiratory function in panic disorder: evidence for a hyperventilation subtype. *Psychosom. Med.*, **59**: 224–230.

Hornsveld, H.K., Garssen, B., Dop, M.J., van Spiegel, P.I. & de Haes, J.C. (1996). Double-blind placebo-controlled study of the hyperventilation provocation test and the validity of the hyperventilation syndrome. *Lancet*, **348**: 154–158.

Howell, J.B.L. (1997). The hyperventilation syndrome: a syndrome under threat? *Thorax*, **52(suppl. 3)**: S30–S34.

Kelsen, S.G., Fleegler, B. & Altose, M.D. (1979). The respiratory neuromuscular response to hypoxia, hypercapnia, and obstruction to airflow in asthma. *Am. Rev. Respir. Dis.*, **120**: 517–527.

Klein, D.F. (1993). False suffocation alarms, spontaneous panics, and related conditions. An integrative hypothesis. *Arch. Gen. Psychiatr.*, **50**: 306–317.

Knapp, P.H. (1989). Psychosomatic aspects of bronchial asthma: a review. In: Cheren, S. (ed.) *Psychosomatic Medicine: Theory, Physiology, and Practice*, Vol. 2. Innocence: International University Press, Madison, CT, pp. 503–564.

Laffey, J.G. & Kavanagh, B.P. (1999). Carbon dioxide and the critically ill – too little of a good thing. *Lancet*, **354**: 1283–1286.

Laffey, J.G. & Kavanagh, B.P. (2002). Hypocapnia. *New Engl. J. Med.*, **347**: 43–53.

Ley, R. (1985). Agoraphobia, the panic attack and the hyperventilation syndrome. *Behav. Res. Ther.*, **23**: 79–81.

Lum, L.C. (1987). Hyperventilation syndromes in medicine and psychiatry: a review. *J. Roy. Soc. Med.*, **80**: 229–231.

Maddock, R.J. & Carter, C.S. (1991). Hyperventilation-induced panic attacks in panic disorder with agoraphobia. *Biol. Psychiatr.*, **29**: 843–854.

Magarian, G.J. (1982). Hyperventilation syndrome: infrequently recognized common expression of anxiety and stress. *Medicine (Baltimore)*, **61**: 219–236.

Mahler, D.A., Faryniarz, K., Lentine, T., Ward, J., Olmstead, E.M. & O'Connor, G.T. (1991). Measurement of breathlessness during exercise in asthmatics. Predictor variables, reliability, and responsiveness. *Am. Rev. Respir. Dis.*, **144**: 39–44.

McNally, R.J., Hornig, C.D. & Donnell, C.D. (1995). Clinical versus nonclinical panic: a test of suffocation false alarm theory. *Behav. Res. Ther.*, **33**: 127–131.

Meuret, A.E., Wilhelm, F.H. & Roth, W.T. (2001). Respiratory biofeedback-assisted therapy in panic disorder. *Beh. Mod.*, **25**: 584–605.

Meuret, A.E., Ritz, T., Wilhelm, F.H. & Roth, W.T. (2002). Targeting overbreathing in asthma by self-modifications of PCO_2-levels. *Psychophysiology*, **39**: S59.

Meuret, A.E., Wilhelm, F.H., Ritz, T. & Roth, W.T. (2003). Modification of dysfunctional breathing in panic disorder and asthma. *Biol. Psychol.*, **62**: 231.

Meuret, A.E., Wilhelm, F.H. & Roth, W.T. Effects of capnometry-assisted breathing therapy on symptoms and respiration in panic disorder (submitted).

Meuret, A.E., Wilhelm, F.H., & Roth, W.T. (2004). Respiratory feedback for treating panic disorder: concept and illustration. *J. Clin. Psychol.* **60**: 197–207.

Munjack, D.J., Brown, R.A., Cabe, D.D., McDowell, D.E. & Baltazar, P.L. (1993). A naturalistic follow-up of panic patients after short-term pharmacologic treatment. *J. Clin. Psychopharmacol.*, **13**: 156–158.

Opat, A.J., Cohen, M.M., Bailey, M.J. & Abramson, M.J. (2000). A clinical trial of the Buteyko breathing technique in asthma as taught by video. *J. Asthma*, **37**: 557–564.

Osborne, C.A., O'Connor, B.J., Lewis, A., Kanabar, V. & Gardner, W.N. (2000). Hyperventilation and asymptomatic chronic asthma. *Thorax*, **55**: 1016–1022.

Papp, L.A., Martinez, J.M. & Klein, D.F., *et al.* (1997). Respiratory psychophysiology of panic disorder: three respiratory challenges in 98 subjects. *Am. J. Psychiatr.*, **154**: 1557–1565.

Riley, T.I. (1982). Epilepsy – or merely hyperventilation? *Emerg. Med.*, **14**: 162–167.

Ritz, T. & Roth, W.T. (2003). Behavioral interventions in asthma: breathing training. *Beh. Mod.*, **27**: 710–730.

Ritz, T., Dahme, B. & Wagner, C. (1998). Effects of static forehead and forearm muscle tension on total respiratory resistance in healthy and asthmatic participants. *Psychophysiology*, **35**: 549–562.

Ritz, T., Meuret, A., Wilhelm, F. & Roth, W.T. (2003). End-tidal pCO_2 levels in asthma patients in the laboratory and at home. *Biol. Psychol.*, **62**: 233–234 [abstract].

Ritz, T., Dahme, B. & Roth, W.T. (2004). Behavioral interventions in asthma. Biofeedback techniques. *J. Psychosom. Res.*, **56**: 711–720.

Salkovskis, P.M., Jones, D.R. & Clark, D.M. (1986). Respiratory control in the treatment of panic attacks: replication and extension with concurrent measurement of behaviour and PCO_2. *Br. J. Psychiatr.*, **148**: 526–532.

Stalmatski, A. (1999). Freedom from asthma. *Buteyko's Revolutionary Treatment*. Kyle Cathie, London.

van Doorn, P., Folgering, H. & Colla, P. (1982). Control of the end-tidal PCO_2 in the hyperventilation syndrome: effects of biofeedback and breathing instructions compared. *Bul. Eur. Physiopathol. Respir.*, **18(6)**: 829–836.

van den Elshout, F.J.J., van Herwaarden, C.L.A. & Folgering, H.T.M. (1991). Effects of hypercapnia and hypocapnia on respiratory resistance in normal and asthmatic subjects. *Thorax*, **46**: 28–32.

Varray, A. & Prefaut, C. (1992). Importance of physical exercise training in asthmatics. *J. Asthma*, **29**: 229–234.

Walters, E.H. & Johns, D.P. (2001). Unraveling the Buteyko effect. *Med. J. Aust.*, **171**: 64–65.

NON-INVASIVE END-TIDAL CARBON DIOXIDE MONITORING IN CONJUNCTION WITH NON-INVASIVE POSITIVE PRESSURE VENTILATION 16

L. Greenway

Introduction

Non-invasive positive pressure ventilation (NPPV, mechanical ventilation without the use of an endotracheal tube, and intubation) has been available for the treatment of patients in ventilatory failure for over 100 years (Hill, 2001). In the past 20 years, with the advent of microprocessor technology, graphic displays and sophisticated patient interfaces, NPPV has experienced a popularity (Brochard *et al.*, 1990; Meduri *et al.*, 1991; Kramer *et al.*, 1995) that ensures its continued use in the management of respiratory failure far into the future. At the same time continued refinement in non-invasive end-tidal and volumetric carbon dioxide (CO_2) measuring devices has occurred. The application of both main- and side-stream partial pressure of CO_2 at end-tidal expiratory gas ($P_{et}CO_2$) monitoring in combination with NPPV is the focus of the chapter.

The history of both NPPV and $P_{et}CO_2$ will be briefly discussed as well as the current status and recommendation that $P_{et}CO_2$ monitoring be employed for the management of patients with either acute or chronic respiratory failure. Additionally, the limitations of this approach will be discussed as well as future research needed to improve the utilization of these two technologies.

The sophistication of NPPV and the currently available $P_{et}CO_2$ technologies make the combination of these two modalities attractive and potentially beneficial in the management of patients suffering from respiratory failure. The benefit to patient management may be enhanced if both technologies are used early in the management of respiratory failure. The criteria for the use of NPPV are beyond the scope of this chapter, but can be found in a number of other sources (International Consensus Conference, 2001; Mehta & Hill, 2001; AARC, 2003).

History

NPPV as currently applied to acutely ill patients was derived from technologies used for many years as the non-invasive choice of treatment in obstructive sleep apnea (OSA) and obesity hypoventilation syndrome (OHS) in the hospital and home settings. The evolution of bi-level positive airway pressure (inspiratory pressure support and positive end-expiratory pressure) for OSA has lead to the application of this technology in the management of acute and chronic respiratory failure. Continued equipment refinement and improved mask design and practitioner education has made the use of NPPV easier and more patient friendly.

At the same time, the use of $P_{et}CO_2$ monitoring in critically ill patients has improved over the years. Solid-state equipment design and the availability of advanced catheter, dehumidification, and filtering techniques have led to the increased application of side-stream end-tidal monitoring. Similarly, main-stream monitoring of $P_{et}CO_2$ has resolved the problems resulting from moisture in the circuit and allows an easy to use and cost effective application in a wide range of patients. The improvements in main-stream senor design and the reduction of endotracheal adapter weight and dead-space allow $P_{et}CO_2$ monitoring in very low-tidal volume situations that would have precluded its application only a few years ago. The graphic display of the capnogram and time trend information has improved the utility of patient data supplied to the clinician.

$P_{et}CO_2$ monitoring

The accuracy of $P_{et}CO_2$ monitoring has been well established and in the non-diseased lung is 2–7% when compared to measured partial pressure of CO_2 in arterial blood (P_aCO_2) (a–$ADCO_2$) (AARC, 2003). In the diseased lung the a–$ADCO_2$ widens considerably. The reasons for this difference may be explained in part by examining the gas exchange mechanics of the lung. Pulmonary gas exchange is assessed by both the dead-space fraction and oxygen transfer parameters. Abnormalities causing a high ventilation/perfusion ($\dot{V}/\dot{Q}$) ratio in the lung also cause a high

V_d/V_t ratio, because these areas are ventilated and not well perfused. Increases in $PA–aDO_2$ are due to low $\dot{V}/\dot{Q}$ areas or shunt (AARC, 2003).

It is instructive to think of the $a–ADCO_2$ as an efficiency equation. The closer the $P_{et}CO_2$ is to the P_aCO_2 (smaller difference) the more efficient the lung is as an "exhaust" or elimination system for CO_2 (Hoffman *et al.*, 1989). Patients with acute respiratory failure will have a large difference due to their increased dead-space ventilation. As ventilation improves this difference will decrease.

The union of NPPV and $P_{et}CO_2$ in the management of respiratory failure

At the present time, the development of both NPPV and $P_{et}CO_2$, technologies have progressed to a point that their application in patients with acute and chronic respiratory failure is cost effective and technically easy.

Non-invasive measures of P_aCO_2 such as $P_{et}CO_2$ have been misunderstood and characterized as not sufficiently accurate surrogates of P_aCO_2. Sanders *et al.* (1994) studied 41 patients for $P_{et}CO_2$ accuracy using three groups of patients where 19 were spontaneously breathing room air, 13 received supplemental oxygen and 22 received positive pressure ventilatory assistance via mask. (*Note*: Some were studied under more than one condition.) Patients were eligible to be included in the study if they were undergoing polysomnographic evaluation for suspected OSA or nocturnal hypoventilation in the presence of awake hypercapnia or neuromuscular/chest wall disease. $P_{et}CO_2$ was measured with a side-stream capnogram with the catheter suspended in a loose-fitting aerosol mask for the first two groups and either within the mask or attached to port on mask for the support group. They concluded that $P_{et}CO_2$ does not adequately reflect P_aCO_2. The study design compared differences between average absolute value of $P_{et}CO_2$ and P_aCO_2 at three "conditions" (using mostly different subjects) rather than comparing the change in end-tidal to the change in P_aCO_2 for the same subjects which would be a more sensitive measure of the utility of $P_{et}CO_2$ particularly due to the end-tidal–arterial differences in different subjects. Additionally, the impact of leak and the difference resulting from inadequate ventilation were not reflected in this work. Successful $P_{et}CO_2$ monitoring with NPPV depends on understanding and controlling these factors.

Table 16.1 Mask selection

	Complete face mask	Full face mask	Nasal mask
Immediate seal for ventilation required	✓		
Mouth breather	✓	✓	
Claustrophobia	✓	✓	
Facial abnormalities	✓		✓
Eye irritation	✓		
Lack of teeth	✓		
Anxiety	✓	✓	
Access to mouth			✓
Long-term NPPV		✓	✓

Issues affecting the utility of $P_{et}CO_2$ when used with non-invasive ventilation

Several factors can impact both the utility and the results of $P_{et}CO_2$ when used with non-invasive ventilation technology. These include, for example, the selection of the patient interface, management of leaks, whether the patient is a mouth breather, the location of the passive exhalation port and the use of side- or main-stream technologies.

The interface selection

Factors to consider when selecting a patient interface device for use with NPPV include estimated length of NPPV use, and issues such as claustrophobia, dentation, and glaucoma. In terms of the impact of the mask on $P_{et}CO_2$ the choice of a nasal, full face or a mask-covering nose, mouth, and eyes may alter the method used for $P_{et}CO_2$ measurement (Table 16.1).

Fraticelli *et al.* (2003) from Brochard's group studied several mask designs and found that the lack of P_aCO_2 increase with the larger dead-space mask configurations represented an important finding. They noted:

> "the most important clinical implication of these results is the possibility to choose different interfaces in the acute patient, based on the patients physiognomy and mask tolerance, with the aim to limit air leaks regardless of their dead-space."

Schettino *et al.* (2003) compared face masks of internal areas using a bench model comprised of a one compartment lung model, mannequin head with fixed dead-space and a constant CO_2 infuser. Masks studied included those with a built in exhalation valve and others with either no exhalation value or the valve disabled. They reported a slight increase in the rebreathed CO_2 (e.g. 2.9–3.4 mmHg) in one design, which they indicated was statistically significant. However, Hill questioned the clinical significance of these findings in a commentary in the same journal.

> "Indeed, some of the observations (by Schettino) are of doubtful clinical significance. For example, most of the rebreathing in this model system was attributable to the dead-space in the mannequin's upper airway and not to the masks themselves. Furthermore, it is difficult to conceive of how a difference as small as 2–3 ml in the amount of CO_2 rebreathed per breath between the masks could be clinically significant, even if it is statistically significant"
>
> (Hill, 2003).

Short-term use

Immediate ventilation requires the use of a quick and easy to apply interface device. Therefore, a mask that covers the nose, mouth, and eyes (i.e. Total Face Mask™, Respironics, Inc.) is often used in emergency situations and is seen most frequently because it is quick and easy to apply (Criner *et al.*, 1994; Liesching *et al.*, 2003) Due to the exhalation ports usually built in to masks of this type, it is not possible to measure exhaled CO_2 with a main-stream sensor because exhaled gases are cleared by the continuous flow generated to compensate for the mask leak before the exhaled gas can reach the main-stream sampling location. To correct this issue, a side-stream $P_{et}CO_2$ monitoring device and cannula will need to be used. Once the patient has stabilized, conversion to a smaller mask, such as a full or nasal mask, and mask-stream $P_{et}CO_2$ monitoring may be helpful.

Long-term use

The full face mask (Figure 16.1) or the nasal mask is often selected for patients requiring ventilation longer than a few hours. These masks can be employed with main-stream $P_{et}CO_2$ monitoring as long as there is no exhalation ports in the mask itself and the inspiratory flow and mask leak are well controlled. These masks will offer patients increased movement and flexibility and facilitate frequent removal and reapplication of the interface.

Leak management

The presence of large leaks (generally those over 20 l/min) will increase the elimination of exhaled gases. While many non-invasive ventilators are capable of compensating for substantial leaks and some level of leak is recommended to assure that the interface has not been applied too tightly, too large a leak will cause both the capnogram and the $P_{et}CO_2$ to be dampened. If the leak cannot be minimized, side-stream monitoring through a cannula can be employed to reduce the impact of the leak.

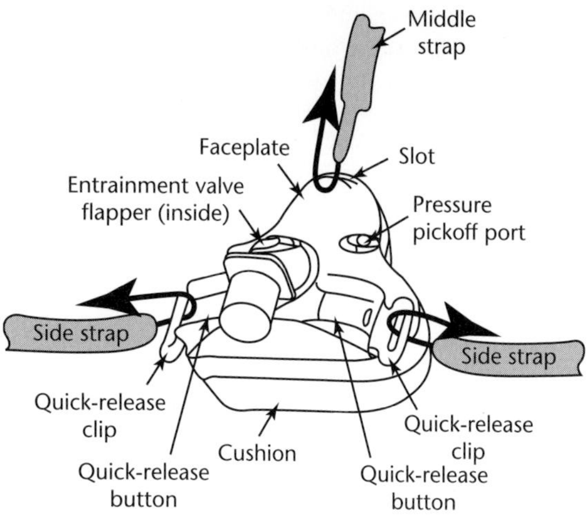

Figure 16.1 Image3™ disposable full face mask. (Image courtesy of Respironics, Inc., Murrysville, PA.)

Rebreathing

Rebreathing may be assessed by observation of the capnogram for evidence of an upward trend observed on the capnogram over time. The potential for CO_2 rebreathing during bi-level ventilation has been noted in the past (Ferguson & Gilmartin, 1995; Lofaso *et al.*, 1995; Renaghan, 2000) but its clinical significance has not been established and "has not been shown to be deleterious in any way" (Schettino *et al.*, 2003; Hill, 2003).

Facial configuration

To help ensure an appropriate seal and maximum patient comfort, it is important to take into account the patient's facial features when selecting an interface. Always assess the skin of the face to determine the appropriate mask fit to prevent tissue damage. Many conditions, such as age or chronic oral steroid use, can cause the facial skin to become fragile. Designs such as the Total Face Mask™ (Respironics, Inc., Murrysville, PA, USA) exert little pressure on the face and may be indicated in situations where the skin is delicate.

It is extremely important to be proactive in the management of the patients requiring NPPV to ensure that the patient interface is properly sized and fitted. Reducing the headgear tension can many times lead to resolution of a leak at the same time greatly improving patient comfort. The mask pressure applied to the tissues of the face maybe enough to cause tissue necrosis (e.g. bridge of nose) (Smurthwaite & Ford, 1993). A comfortable fit and frequent evaluation by all care providers of the skin will help to prevent facial breakdown.

Mouth breather

A mouth breather will require the use of a mask that covers the mouth and nose in order to ensure ventilation. If a patient breathes via the mouth only at night you may alternate masks to accommodate day/night variation. This will allow the patient the freedom to speak and eat during the day. Should a nasal mask be used there may be times when $P_{et}CO_2$ values do not reflect exhaled gases because these gases exiting the mouth will not be seen by the capnograph and not exit via the exhalation port by way of the nose.

Location of the exhalation port

The positioning of the exhalation port relative to the measurement site for $P_{et}CO_2$ can greatly alter the values (Figure 16.2). Ports located in the mask will generally flush out the exhaled CO_2 gas prior to reaching the main-stream sampling port location. In some cases it may alter the ability to obtain a side-stream sample as well. Main-stream monitoring can only be effectively performed in circuits where the exhalation port is located distal to the sampling location. As side-stream methods generally employ a nasal cannula this will reduce the effect of the location of the exhalation port unless the flow is too large.

Side-stream versus main-stream sampling

Side-stream monitoring affords a great deal of flexibility in terms of the selection of sampling locations, however the introduction of moist gases into the measurement area and even into small diameter tubes can result in technical problems as the moisture condenses. Methods have evolved to address this including filters and alternative tubing designs. The most effective way to address moisture problems is the use of main-stream monitoring where the "optical bench" samples the gas as it passes through the breathing circuit. This does limit the choices of the sampling site, particularly in non-invasive ventilation where there is only a single limb. This is an area where technological developments may provide a means to reposition the main-stream sensor and possibly better address leaks.

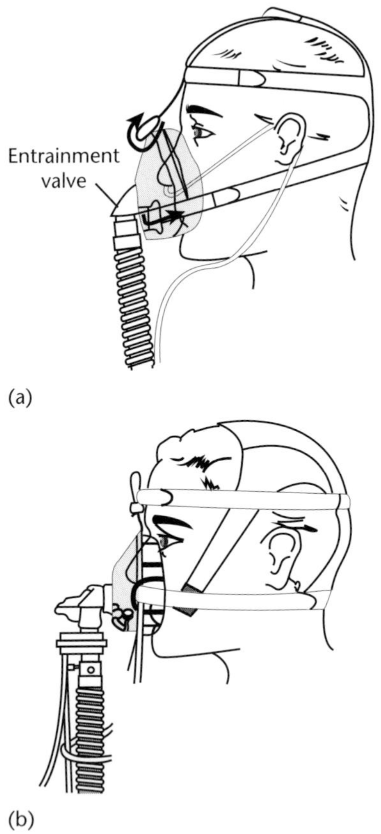

Figure 16.2 Disposable full face mask applied to subject with (a) nasal cannula and (b) main-stream gas sensor and airway adapter. (Images courtesy of Respironics, Inc., Murrysville, PA.)

Future directions

Three areas of research need to further mature before end-tidal CO_2 monitoring will be accepted as a routine practice with NPPV.

1 The clinical utility of using continuous $P_{et}CO_2$ in invasively ventilated patients needs to be more widely established. The $P_{et}CO_2$ to arterial P_aCO_2 difference needs to be studied in different disease states and at varying levels of ventilatory support. Ideally, $P_{et}CO_2$ and a–ADCO_2 should be measured and monitored in individual patients over the course of their ventilatory management before the $P_{et}CO_2$ can be used reliably as an indicator of P_aCO_2 and the effectiveness of ventilatory support. Work conducted on volumetric capnography may be helpful to the extent that this approach is applicable to NPPV.

2 The application of $P_{et}CO_2$ monitoring with NPPV as a qualitative tool will need to be better

understood. This will require monitoring patients during various phases of non-invasive ventilatory management. The $P_{et}CO_2$ to arterial P_aCO_2 difference will need to be understood in the context of changes in $\dot{V}/\dot{Q}$ relationships in the lung as the underlying pulmonary disease changes over time. In the patient with acute or chronic respiratory insufficient the relationship between NPPV and a-$ADCO_2$ has yet to be fully understood and appreciated by clinicians.

3 In a recent editorial, Kacmarek (2003) describes important considerations when using NPPV including the education of all the care team members, the patient interface, the importance of mask fit, leak management and humidity. Each of these issues will need to be more thoroughly addressed in light of the addition of an end-tidal CO_2 monitor before $P_{et}CO_2$ monitoring with NPPV will become common place in the management of patients with acute ventilatory failure. Plant *et al.* (2000) further detail the importance of specific focused training of the health care staff. In answer to the question, "Is NPPV an easy technique to apply in the ward?" they state, "Whenever it (NPPV) is delivered, specific training is necessary for its optimal administration". This is true both on the medical ward, the intensive care unit, and in the emergency department. The addition of $P_{et}CO_2$ monitoring adds a new level of complexity to patient management that will require further specific training in its application and usefulness.

Conclusion

NPPV and $P_{et}CO_2$ monitoring can be used together to manage patients with acute or chronic respiratory failure. Although experience using $P_{et}CO_2$ monitoring with NPPV is lacking, along with a clear understanding of its utility in patient management, it is believed that the use of $P_{et}CO_2$ monitoring early on, in patients requiring NPPV will offer important clinical information and aid the clinician in rapidly achieving therapeutic pressure levels. This will effectively enable the practitioner to set the ventilator to maximize CO_2 elimination and rapidly minimize the patient's work of breathing two of the key objectives of non-invasive ventilation.

References

AARC (2003). Clinical practice guideline, capnography/capnometry during mechanical ventilation 2003, revision and update. *Respiratory Care*, **48**: 534–539.

Brochard, L., Isabey, D. & Piquet, J., *et al.* (1990). Reversal of acute exacerbations of chronic obstructive lung disease by inspiratory assistance with a face mask. *New Engl. J. Med.*, **323**: 1523–1530.

Criner, G.J., Travaline, J.M., Brennan, K.J. & Kreimer, D.T. (1994). Efficacy of a new full face mask for noninvasive positive pressure ventilation. *Chest*, **106**: 1109–1115.

Ferguson, G.T. & Gilmartin, M. (1995). CO_2 rebreathing during BiPAP ventilatory assistance. *Am. J. Respir. Crit. Care Med.*, **151**: 1126–1135.

Fraticelli, A., Lellouche, F., Taille, S., Qader, S. & Brochard, L. (2003). Comparison of different interface during NIV in patients with acute respiratory failure. *Am. J. Respir. Crit. Care Med.*, **167**: A389.

Hill, N. (2003). What mask for noninvasive ventilation: is deadspace an issue? *Crit. Care Med.*, **31**: 2247–2248.

Hill, N.S. (ed.) (2001). *Noninvasive Positive Pressure Ventilation – Principles and Applications.* Futura Publishing Co., Armonk, NY.

Hoffman, R.A., Krieger, B.P., Kramer, M.R., Segel, S., Bizousky, F., Gazeroglu, H. & Sackner, M.A. (1989). End-tidal carbon dioxide in critically ill patients during changes in mechanical ventilation. *Am. Rev. Respir. Dis.*, **140**: 1265–1268.

International Consensus Conferences in Intensive Care Medicine (2001). Noninvasive positive pressure ventilation in acute respiratory failure. *Am. J. Respir. Crit. Care Med.*, **163**: 283–291.

Kacmarek, R. (2003). Noninvasive positive-pressure ventilation: the little things do make the difference! *Respiratory Care*, **48**: 919–921.

Kramer, N., Meyer, T.J., Meharg, J., Cece, R.D. & Hill, N.S. (1995). Randomized, prospective trail of noninvasive positive pressure ventilation in acute respiratory failure. *Am. J. Respir. Crit. Care Med.*, **151**: 1799–1806.

Liesching, T.N., Cromier, K., Nelson, D., Short, K., Sucov, R., Mecharg, A.J. & Hill, N.S. (2003). Total Face Mask™ vs standard full face mask for noninvasive therapy of acute respiratory failure. *Am. J. Respir. Crit. Care Med.*, **167**: A996.

Lofaso, F., Brochard, L., Touchard, D., Hang, T., Harf, A. & Isabey, D. (1995). Evaluation of carbon dioxide rebreathing during pressure support ventilation with airway management system (BiPAP) devices. *Chest*, **108**: 772–778.

Meduri, G.U., Abou-Shala, N., Fox, R.C., Jones, C.B., Leeper, K.V. & Wunderink, R.G. (1991). Noninvasive face mask mechanical ventilation in patients with acute hypercapnic respiratory failure. *Chest*, **100**: 445–454.

Mehta, S. & Hill, N.S. (2001). Noninvasive ventilation. *Am. J. Respir. Crit. Care Med.*, **163**: 540–577.

Plant, P., Owen, J. & Elliott, M. (2000). A multicentre randomized controlled trail of the early use of non-invasive ventilation for acute exacerbations of chronic obstructive pulmonary disease. *Lancet*, **355**: 1931–1935.

Renaghan, D. (2000). Capnometric analysis of carbon dioxide rebreathing during non-invasive positive pressure ventilation with BiPAP. *Crit. Care Med.*, **28**: A177.

Sanders, M.H., Kern, N.B., Costantino, J.P., *et al.* (1994). Accuracy of end-tidal and transcutaneous PCO_2 monitoring during sleep. *Chest*, **106**: 472–483.

Schettino, G.P., Chatmongkolchart, S., Hess, D.R. & Kacmarek, R.M. (2003). Position of exhalation port and mask design affect CO_2 rebreathing during noninvasive positive pressure ventilation. *Crit. Care Med.*, **31**: 2178–2182.

Smurthwaite, G.J. & Ford, P. (1993). Skin necrosis following continuous positive airway pressure with a face mask. *Anaesthesia*, **48**: 147–148.

VENTILATION: WEANING

SECTION

1d

END-TIDAL CARBON DIOXIDE MONITORING IN POST-OPERATIVE VENTILATOR WEANING 17

J. Varon & P.E. Marik

Premature extubation after general anesthesia significantly increases post-operative morbidity. The evaluation of the suitability for weaning and extubation includes a clinical examination assessing the patient's alertness, ability to follow commands and to lift his/her head of the bed. These simple steps are the best method for assessing the level of consciousness and muscle strength. Clinical examination, however, is inadequate to determine the adequacy of arterial oxygenation and ventilation (Semmes *et al.*, 1985). Clinical and experimental studies have repeatedly demonstrated the insensitivity of clinical evaluation for detection of potentially life threatening events such as major changes in oxygen arterial saturation (SaO_2), alveolar ventilation and esophageal intubation (Semmes *et al.*, 1985; Vaghadia *et al.*, 1989; Cote *et al.*, 1991). Pulse oximetry is now regarded as the standard of care in patients undergoing anesthesia and provides a continuous, non-invasive, and accurate method of estimating the arterial oxygenation. A number of methods are available to monitor adequacy of ventilation each with its own utility and its own limitations.

Assessing ventilation adequacy

Several laboratory techniques are commonly used as adjuncts to clinical assessment of the adequacy of ventilation. The most direct is the measurement of the partial pressure of carbon dioxide in arterial blood (P_aCO_2). However, blood gas analysis requires an arterial puncture, which is expensive, and provides only intermittent P_aCO_2 data. Transcutaneous measurement of CO_2 tension can provide continuous data but requires adequate cardiovascular function and peripheral perfusion to be well correlated with P_aCO_2. Other disadvantages include its long warm-up and slow response time, and the risk of skin burns.

Under normal conditions P_aCO_2 is related to mixed venous partial pressure of CO_2 (PCO_2) ($P_aCO_2 = 0.8\ P_vCO_2$). However, mixed venous blood sampling requires invasive hemodynamic monitoring and is therefore not practical. Intravascular CO_2 electrodes are under development but are not yet ready for routine clinical use. This technology may also incorporate an oxygen or pH electrode with the CO_2 electrode.

Another method to assess the adequacy of ventilation makes use of capnometry.

Under normal conditions there is a small difference ($\approx$6 mmHg) between P_aCO_2 and partial pressure of carbon dioxide at end-tidal ($P_{et}CO_2$). At sea level (atmospheric pressure = 760 mmHg) a normal value for $P_{et}CO_2$ is about 38 mmHg. The most important determinants of $P_{et}CO_2$ are alveolar ventilation, pulmonary perfusion (i.e. cardiac output) and CO_2 production (Adrogue *et al.*, 1989).

The assessment of $P_{et}CO_2$ may be misleading if not considered in the context of changing hemodynamics and ventilatory pattern. In the mechanically ventilated patient, alterations in the ventilation and perfusion ($\dot{V}/\dot{Q}$) can occur due to changes in tidal volume (V_d/V_t), positive end-expiratory pressure (PEEP), the development of atelectasis or pulmonary edema or due to patient repositioning. Morley observed that $P_{et}CO_2$ was useful as a predictor of P_aCO_2 only in patients without significant parenchymal lung disease (Morley *et al.*, 1993). Prause and colleagues (1997) found that $P_{et}CO_2$ was useful for the adjustment of ventilatory parameters in pre-hospital emergency care patients only if they had no major cardiopulmonary disease. In a 1985–1991 literature review of the efficacy on non-invasive blood gas monitoring in the adult critical care unit, the Technology Subcommittee of the Working Group of Critical Care (Ontario Ministry of Health) concluded that changes in $P_{et}CO_2$ need to be interpreted with extreme caution (Ontario Ministry of Health, 1992).

Clinical applications of end-tidal CO_2 in operative patients

Verification of endotracheal tube placement

Weaning

The important role played by capnometry in verification of endotracheal tube placement is discussed in

Table 17.1. Standard indices for weaning success

Index	Value suggesting success
Minute ventilation (V_E)	<10 l/min
Tidal volume (V_T)	5 ml/kg
Vital capacity (V_C)	$2 \times V_T$
Maximal voluntary ventilation (MVV)	$2 \times V_E$

detail in another chapter. Here we will focus on the procedures useful in weaning patients from the ventilator. Successful weaning during the post-operative period requires that the clinician ensure that the patient is clinically stable and without clinically significant residual effects of the anesthetic agents utilized during surgery. A number of ventilatory parameters have been evaluated to predict the success of weaning. Some of the standard indices predicting weaning success are depicted in Table 17.1.

The Tobin index is commonly used to predict weaning success and is calculated as follows:

$$\text{Tobin index} = \frac{f}{V_T}$$

where f = frequency and V_T = tidal volume. Successful weaning is usually accomplished if the Tobin index <100 breaths/min/l (Yang & Tobin, 1991).

When $P_{et}CO_2$ values are considered in combination with the standard parameters to assure adequate ventilation prior to extubation, the chance of successful extubation increases. In a prospective study, Morley and associates (1993) studied the reliability of end-tidal CO_2 ($ETCO_2$) monitoring as a reflection of arterial CO_2 tension during weaning from mechanical ventilation. Capnographic monitoring of their patients provided reasonable estimates of arterial CO_2 tension during weaning. Saura and colleagues (1996) in a prospective study to evaluate the relationship between P_aCO_2 and $P_{et}CO_2$ before and during weaning with continuous positive airway pressure ventilation, found that $P_{et}CO_2$ could detect clinically relevant hypercapnic episodes. However, there was a high incidence of false positives that led to arterial blood gas sampling. Withington *et al.* (1991) found that, after a gradient between P_aCO_2 and $P_{et}CO_2$ was established, $P_{et}CO_2$ was a useful parameter in the weaning of post-cardiac surgery patients.

Some clinicians utilize $P_{et}CO_2$ as a marker of the metabolic rate and, therefore, as a way of determining optimal ventilator settings during the weaning process (Taskar *et al.*, 1995). Patients with high metabolic rates (i.e. sepsis) may be difficult to wean under these conditions making it often difficult to predict the success of weaning.

Special considerations of $P_{et}CO_2$ in critically ill patients

Cardiopulmonary bypass weaning

$P_{et}CO_2$ has been used as a surrogate marker for pulmonary blood flow (Maslow *et al.*, 2001). When used in these circumstances, a $P_{et}CO_2$ that exceeds 30 mmHg is usually associated with a cardiac output greater than 4.0 l/min.

Conclusion

$P_{et}CO_2$ monitoring serves as a useful adjunct in weaning post-operative patients from mechanical ventilation.

References

Adrogue, H.J., Rashad, M.N., Gorin, A.B., Yacoub, J. & Madias, N.E. (1989). Assessing acid–base status in circulatory failure. Differences between arterial and central venous blood. *New Engl. J. Med.*, **320**: 1312–1316.

Bhende, M.S., Thompson, A.E. & Howland, D.F. (1991). Validity of a disposable end-tidal carbon dioxide detector in verifying endotracheal tube position in piglets. *Crit. Care Med.* **19**: 566–568.

Carlon, G.C., Ray, Jr, C., Miodownik, S., Kopec, I. & Groeger, J.S. (1988). Capnography in mechanically ventilated patients. *Crit. Care Med.*, **16**: 550–556.

Cote, C.J., Rolf, N., Liu, M.N., *et al.* (1991). A single-blind study of combined pulse oximetry and capnography in children. *Anesthesiology*, **74**: 980–987.

Hoffman, R.A., Krieger, B.P., Kramer, M.R., Segel, S., Bizousky, F., Gazeroglu, H. & Sackner, M.A. (1989). End-tidal carbon dioxide in critically ill patients during changes in mechanical ventilation. *Am. Rev. Respir. Dis.*, **140**: 1265–1268.

Maslow, A., Stearns, G., Bert, A., Feng, W., Price, D., Schwartz, C., MacKinnon, S., Rotenberg, F., Hopkins, R., Cooper, G., Singh, A. & Loring, S. (2001). Monitoring end-tidal carbon dioxide during weaning from cardiopulmonary bypass in patients without significant lung disease. *Anesth. Analg.* **92**: 306–313.

Morley, T.F., Giaimo, J. Maroszan, E., Bermingham, .J., Gordon, R., Griesback, R., Zappasodi, S.J. & Giudice, J.C. (1993). Use of capnography for assessment of the adequacy of alveolar ventilation during weaning from mechanical ventilation. *Am. Rev. Respir. Dis.*, **148**: 339–344.

Ontario Ministry of Health (1992). Technology Subcommittee of the Working Group on Critical Care, Ontario Ministry of Health. *Can. Med. Assoc. J.*, **146**: 703–712.

Prause, G.,H., Hetz, P., Lauda, H., Pojer, F., Smolle-Juettner, F. & Smolle, J. (1997). A comparison of the end-tidal CO_2 documented by capnometry and arterial PCO_2 in emergency patients. *Resuscitation*, **35**: 145–148.

Saura, P., Blanch, L., Lucangelo, U., Fernandez, R., Mestre, J. & Artigas. A. (1996). Use of capnography to detect hypercapnic episodes during weaning from mechanical ventilation. *Intensive. Care Med.*, **22**: 374–381.

Semmes, B.J., Tobin, M. J., Snyder, V. & Grenvik, A. (1985). Subjective and objective measurement of tidal volume in critically ill patients. *Chest*, **87**: 577–579.

Smalhout, B. & Kalenda, A. (1981). *An Atlas of Capnography*. Kerckebosch, Zeist, The Netherlands..

Szaflarski, N.L. & Cohen, N.H. (1991). Use of capnography in critically ill adults. *Heart Lung*, **20**: 363–372.

Taskar, V., John, J., Larsson, A., Wetterberg, T. & Johnson, B. (1995). Dynamics of carbon dioxide elimination following ventilator resetting. *Chest*, **8**: 196-202.

Vaghadia, H., Jenkins, L.C. & Ford, R.W. (1989). Comparison of end-tidal carbon dioxide, oxygen saturation and clinical signs for the detection of oesophageal intubation. *Can. J. Anesth.*, **36**: 560-564.

Withington, D.E., Ramsay, J.G., Saoud, A.T. & Bilodeau, J. (1991). Weaning from ventilation after cardiopulmonary bypass: evaluation of a non-invasive technique. *Can. J. Anaesth.*, **38**: 15–19.

Yang, K.L. & Tobin, M.J. (1991). A prospective study of indexes predicting the outcome of trials of weaning from mechanical ventilation. *New Engl. J. Med.*, **324**: 1445–1450.

CAPNOGRAPHY TO OPTIMIZE AND MINIMIZE MECHANICAL VENTILATION 18

D.S. Hamel & I.M. Cheifetz

Importance of rapid and successful liberation from mechanical ventilation

Minimizing the duration of mechanical ventilation is crucial in the management of critically ill infants, children, and adults. Few clinicians would disagree that mechanical ventilation, while life saving, is not without real risk (Meade *et al.*, 1970; DeRobertis *et al.*, 2001).

Overall, the application of mechanical ventilation has many adverse pulmonary, cardiac, and neuromuscular effects. Prolonged mechanical ventilation is associated with increased ventilator induced lung injury (VILI), airway injury, nosocomial pneumonia, excessive use of pharmacologic sedation, prolonged length of intensive care unit (ICU) and hospital admission, increased costs, increased physiologic stress, and possibly increased mortality (Orlowski *et al.*, 1980; Benjamin *et al.*, 1990; Pierson, 1990; Tobias *et al.*, 1994; Manthous *et al.*, 1998; Suematsu *et al.*, 2000). High peak airway pressure, inadequate positive end-expiratory pressure (PEEP), repeated alveolar collapse and expansion, and repetitive derecruitment can create a stress activated signaling cascade (Figure 18.1). The ultimate result of this cascade is VILI and possibly multiorgan system dysfunction/failure. The effects of mechanical ventilation on the body's immune system and organ function are extremely complex (Margolin & Groeger, 2002; Zhang *et al.*, 2002). The consequences of barotrauma, volutrauma, atelectotrauma, and biotrauma can be significant and are variable among individual patients. Multiple lung protective strategies have been proposed in the medical literature; however, the most optimal method to minimize VILI and its consequences is to minimize the length of mechanical ventilation.

Stress activated signaling cascade

Stress failure of plasma membranes

↓

Necrosis

↓

Liberation of preformed inflammatory mediators

↓

Loss of compartmentalization

↓

Spread of mediators

↓

Spread of bacteria throughout body

↓

Pulmonary edema

↓

Impairment of type II surfactant producing pnuemocytes

↓

Local production of inflammatory cytokines

↓

Systemic release of bacteria, endotoxins and cytokines

↓

May lead to multiple organ system dysfunction/failure

Figure 18.1 *VILI.* The stress activated signaling cascade in response to mechanical ventilation can be extremely complex. This cascade results in VILI and possibly multiorgan system dysfunction/failure.

Clinical debate continues as to whether a patient should be "weaned" or "liberated" from mechanical ventilation. Weaning implies a gradual reduction in the amount of ventilatory support provided to the patient. Liberation from mechanical ventilation implies the use of an extubation readiness test to withdraw mechanical ventilation as soon as the patient meets extubation criteria regardless of the level of ventilatory support. Regardless of the terminology employed, the goal must be to minimize the length of mechanical ventilation for each patient to the shortest possible time frame. The clinical difficulty becomes the balance of minimizing the length of ventilation while maintaining an acceptable extubation failure rate. While a relative consensus concerning the timing of intubation and the initiation of mechanical ventilation has existed for some time, the management, weaning and extubation of mechanically ventilated patients has been primarily subjective and determined by institutional and/or individual practices and preferences (Esteban *et al.*, 1995; Sinha & Donn, 2000; Soo Hoo & Park, 2002). A myriad of adversities makes weaning and liberation from mechanical ventilation an extremely important clinical issue.

Weaning from mechanical ventilation is a process requiring ongoing clinical assessment and planning by multidisciplinary members of the patient care team (Henneman *et al.*, 2001). The contributions made by physicians, nurses, and respiratory care practitioners provide a comprehensive evaluation of the strategy as well as patient response. Complications result from mechanical ventilation even under the best of circumstances; therefore, ventilator management strategies should be implemented with weaning towards prompt and successful extubation as a primary goal. Careful consideration must be given to provide optimal weaning and extubation strategies which begin on the first day that success is considered likely (Manthous, 2002). With recent advances in technology, clinicians are provided with measurable and consistent data, thus, allowing for a more objective approach to total ventilator management.

Potentially even more complex than weaning is the accurate identification of patients who can be successfully extubated. This is an everyday challenge in most neonatal, pediatric, and adult ICUs. Patients are at risk for continued ventilator associated lung injury if their ability to breathe unassisted is not recognized. However, the ideal extubation timing for a patient with acute lung injury has been elusive, and the techniques utilized have traditionally been more art than science. Although prolonged mechanical ventilation has significant risks, failed extubation also potentially increases morbidity and mortality. Reintubation results in prolonged intubation, increased risk for VILI and nosocomial pneumonia, prolonged ICU and hospital admission, increased costs, and increased mortality (Demling *et al.*, 1988; Torres *et al.*, 1995; Daley *et al.*, 1996; Epstein *et al.*, 1997; Esteban *et al.*, 1997; Epstein & Ciubotaru, 1998; Rady & Ryan, 1999; Meade *et al.*, 2001a, b; Hess, 2002; Whitehead & Slutsky, 2002). Predicting successful extubation presents unique challenges to clinicians. Since mechanical ventilation poses significant risk which increases over time, minimizing the duration of mechanical ventilation as well as the risk of reintubation is crucial in the management of critically ill patients (Cook *et al.*, 2001; MacIntyre *et al.*, 2001).

It is for these reasons that the development of patient assessment and monitoring techniques which easily and safely distinguish those patients ready for discontinuation of ventilatory support from those patients who require continued support is essential (Cook *et al.*, 2001; MacIntyre, *et al.*, 2001).

Advances in technology – capnography

Significant advances in respiratory monitoring technology have occurred over the last decade (Weingarten, 1990). These advances now offer the clinician the ability to monitor and accurately quantify volume of carbon dioxide elimination per unit time ($\dot{V}CO_2$) and dead-space ventilation continuously and non-invasively using volumetric capnography. Additionally, the widespread ability to monitor oxygen consumption is, hopefully, on the horizon. Beyond monitoring gas exchange, these technologic advances provide essential data concerning cardiorespiratory interactions.

Theoretically, the ability to non-invasively monitor these parameters should lead to improvements in patient care, a reduction in length of ventilation, and the resultant reduction in the length of ICU admissions and costs; however, randomized, controlled trials are needed to demonstrate this conclusively. The reduction in hospital costs would occur secondary to a shorter length of mechanical ventilation and a decreased number of arterial blood gas analyses and chest radiographs.

Valuable clinical information can be gained with the use of non-invasive carbon dioxide (CO_2) monitoring. Capnometry (digital display of data) and capnography (graphical display of data) can be either time based or volume based. Specifically, capnography refers to the depiction of exhaled CO_2 during the entire respiratory cycle and provides visual display of the waveforms. Therefore, capnography should be a better marker for dynamic changes in gas exchange than capnometry alone (Breen *et al.*, 1996a; Johnson & Breen, 1999). Proper clinical interpretation of capnographic waveforms are important in optimizing mechanical ventilation. Characteristic waveforms and deviations suggest an abnormality which require recognition and possibly correction (Weingarten, 1990).

Time-based capnometry is best known as end-tidal CO_2 ($ETCO_2$) monitoring. Capnography when used without qualification refers to time-based values. A CO_2 sensor and pneumotachometer are used in combination in volumetric capnography. This permits the calculation of the net quantity of CO_2 expired by the subject (i.e. the difference between expired and inspired CO_2, although normally inspired CO_2 is negligible) and is expressed as a volume of gas rather than a partial pressure or gas fraction.

Although time-based capnography is an effective tool for validating correct placement of the endotracheal tube in the trachea (Birmingham *et al.*, 1986; Holland *et al.*, 1993; Knapp *et al.*, 1999), volumetric capnography may be an even more effective tool for validating appropriate endotracheal tube placement (Sum-Ping *et al.*, 1989). Time-based capnography may provide a false positive reading (i.e., endotracheal tube not in trachea and monitor displays a $ETCO_2$ value) in patients who have

1 antacids or carbonated beverages in the stomach,
2 recently received prolonged bag-valve-mask ventilation prior to intubation,
3 an endotracheal tube tip placed in the pharynx.

A false negative time-based result (i.e., endotracheal tube is in trachea and monitor does not display a $ETCO_2$ value) may occur in patients with severe airway obstruction, poor cardiac output, pulmonary emboli, or pulmonary hypertension.

Both time-based and volume-based capnography display immediate responses to changes in ventilatory strategies and cardiac function. Both $ETCO_2$ and $\dot{V}CO_2$ can be used to determine changes in gas exchange in response to changes in mechanical ventilatory support. Traditionally, it has been taught that the $ETCO_2$ value is useful for managing mechanical ventilation only if a normal plateau is present. However, if physiologic dead-space is not significantly elevated, then the $ETCO_2$ measurement can serve to reliably track changes in partial pressure of CO_2 in arterial blood (P_aCO_2) in many ICU patients.

The correlation between $ETCO_2$ and P_aCO_2 is weakened in patients with significant physiologic dead-space, sepsis, cyanotic heart disease, and impaired cardiac output. Any significant failures in circulation, such as decreased cardiac output, cardiac arrest, or hypotension, will be seen as a decrease in the height of the plateau of the time-based capnogram. Since cardiac output can be reduced by the use of anesthetic agents, hypocapnia, and PEEP, capnography is a valuable tool when attempting to optimize mechanical ventilation. The shape of the time-based capnogram can be very helpful in the management of ventilated patients. For example, there is a delayed upstroke of the expiratory plateau with severe bronchospasm.

Time-based capnography can also be very useful in assessing changes in a patient's cardiovascular status. In the extreme, increases in $ETCO_2$ and $\dot{V}CO_2$ during cardiopulmonary resuscitation signify an increase in cardiac output as spontaneous circulation returns (Isserles & Breen, 1991). This chapter will focus on the use of capnography to minimize the length of mechanical ventilation while optimizing the chances for successful extubation. The use of capnography for assessment of pulmonary perfusion and cardiopulmonary resuscitation is detailed elsewhere in this textbook.

Phases of mechanical ventilation

Mechanical ventilation can be divided into three phases: stabilization, pre-weaning, and weaning. The acute stabilization phase is that phase in which mechanical ventilation is initiated, and the patient is acutely resuscitated and stabilized from a cardiorespiratory standpoint. During this phase, ventilation strategies are geared toward stabilization of the patient with little thought of weaning. The duration of this phase is extremely variable and dependent on both the clinician and the patient. Regardless of the condition necessitating mechanical ventilation, ideally this phase should be extremely short and even non-existent in many patients. Ventilator parameters are often at their maximum during this phase. High mean airway pressures may be necessary to provide adequate oxygenation. Optimal $\dot{V}CO_2$ often requires high alveolar minute ventilation (MV_{alv}). As soon as the patient's condition has been stabilized, the patient is in the pre-wean stage.

The underlying condition that led to the requirement for mechanical ventilation need not be resolved for the patient to move into the pre-wean phase. However, the amount of time the patient spends in this phase will depend greatly on the condition which led to the initiation of ventilation. It is in the pre-wean phase when the goals of ventilation shift from stabilization to lung protection. Ideally, lung protective ventilation should begin immediately from the time of intubation. However, there is a subset of patients who do require acute stabilization and, thus, lung protective strategies may need to be delayed. Once the patient's cardiorespiratory status acutely stabilizes, an emphasis on lung protection must occur. The lung protective strategies which may be employed for an individual patient might include (but not be limited to) any of the following: low tidal volume ventilation (ARDS Network, 2000), high-frequency ventilation (Clark *et al.*, 1992; Arnold *et al.*, 1994; 2000; Froese, 1997; Derdak *et al.*, 2002), prone positioning (Piehl & Brown, 1976; Chatte *et al.*, 1997; Voggenreiter *et al.*, 1999; Gattinoni *et al.*, 2001), and permissive hypercapnia (Hickling *et al.*, 1990; 1994; Hickling, 2002). Once the patient has demonstrated no increase in ventilator settings and hemodynamic stability for approximately 6 h, the active weaning phase is initiated (Cook *et al.*, 1999).

Essentially, weaning begins as soon as the clinician believes the patient can tolerate any reduction, large or small, in ventilatory support (Marini *et al.*, 2001). It is during the weaning phase that the clinician begins to decelerate ventilator settings in an effort to move toward extubation. While it is important to decrease ventilator support as rapidly as possible, doing so too aggressively may have deleterious effects. Inadequate PEEP levels or tidal volumes can lead to atelectasis and resultant deterioration of gas exchange. Weaning too cautiously can result in patients remaining intubated longer than necessary. While capnography is of great assistance during all phases of ventilation, it is especially useful during weaning.

Tidal volume delivery

During positive pressure ventilation, the quantity of CO_2 expired is routinely controlled by adjusting the total minute ventilation (tidal volume and/or respiratory rate). Since lung protective strategies require low tidal volume ventilation, an accurate determination of the tidal volume delivered to a patient's lungs is essential. Although this seems to be an obvious concept, the question really is: are the tidal volumes indicated by mechanical ventilators actually indicative of the volume of gas seen by the lungs? For adult and larger pediatric patients, the answer is 'yes.' But, for infants and small children, the tidal volumes displayed by the ventilators may not accurately represent the volume of gas delivered to the lungs. Many conventional ventilators measure tidal volume at the expiratory valve. However, secondary to multiple circuit variables, such as circuit compliance, heaters, in-line suction devices, secretions, and condensation, tidal volumes measured at the expiratory valve of a ventilator do not accurately measure true tidal volume delivery to the patient's lung (Cannon *et al.*, 2000). Significant differences in expiratory valve determined tidal volumes, pneumotachometer determined tidal volumes at the endotracheal tube, and calculated effective tidal volumes exist (Cannon *et al.*, 2000).

Considering the overall small tidal volumes used in ventilating infants and young children, even relatively small inaccuracies in tidal volume determination may result in significant adverse conditions. For example, a 10 ml discrepancy might be a 33% error for a 3 kg infant.

Tidal volume determination at the endotracheal tube is more likely to accurately represent the actual tidal volume seen by the patient's lungs than is a tidal volume measured at the expiratory valve of the ventilator. When tidal volumes are measured using a pneumotachometer positioned between the ventilator circuit and the endotracheal tube, the ventilator circuit compliance and the confounding circuit variables are no longer pertinent factors.

Many important patient management decisions are based on tidal volume determination (Hatzakis & Davis, 2002; Manthous, 2002; Soo Hoo & Park, 2002). If the decision to wean is based on inaccurate tidal volume measurements, then patients ready to be weaned may be assessed as unable, whereas patients assessed as ready may, in fact, not be. When delivered tidal volumes are inadequate despite an appropriate tidal volume reading on a ventilator (based on an expiratory valve measurement), a compensatory increase in respiratory rate often follows potentially resulting in a false assumption that the patient is not able to be weaned. Again, this is especially true when mechanically ventilating infants and small children. If the actual volume of gas delivered to the lungs is not accurately known, then the patient may be at risk for developing atelectasis, hypoxia, and hypercapnia. The presence of hypercapnia may or may not have clinical implications depending upon the clinical status of the patient. However, the development of atelectasis and hypoxia is likely to be problematic. If inadequate tidal volumes are used and atelectasis develops, then increased airway pressures may be required to re-inflate the collapsed alveoli. This increase in airway pressure may increase the risk for secondary lung injury through the mechanism of shear injury (Meade *et al.*, 1970; Dreyfuss & Saumon, 1998). The inability to maintain appropriate lung volumes may lead the clinician to believe the patient is not ready to be weaned when, in fact, it is the management of weaning, without adequate knowledge, which created the failure.

Alternately, the clinician may attempt to compensate for the expected discrepancy in tidal volume measurements (expiratory valve versus endotracheal tube) by increasing the ventilator's set delivered tidal volume. However, without an accurate determination of the tidal volume at the endotracheal tube, the risk for overcompensation exists. When overcompensation occurs, the patient is at risk for overdistention resulting in volutrauma and secondary lung injury (Dreyfuss *et al.*, 1988; Hickling *et al.*, 1990; ARDS Network, 2000).

Thus, with proximal flow monitoring at the endotracheal tube, a continuous assessment of the tidal volume delivered to the airways is easily achieved. However, these volumes represent the quantity of gas moving in and out of the lungs but do not provide information as to the portion of the total ventilation which actually participates in gas exchange at the alveolar level.

MV_{alv}

The minute ventilation value displayed on mechanical ventilators represents the amount of gas moving in and out of the lungs per minute (respiratory rate times tidal volume). This calculated or measured value is the sum of alveolar and dead-space ventilation. Alveolar ventilation is the volume of air which reaches the alveoli and participates in gas exchange at the capillary level (minute ventilation less dead-space ventilation) (Lawrence, 1987). To determine the quantity of gas which reaches the alveoli and actively participates in gas exchange, it is important to determine the MV_{alv}. MV_{alv} is determined from the volumetric capnogram (Figure 18.2). Phase 3 of the waveform represents the quantity of gas exhaled from the alveoli. Thus, MV_{alv} becomes the volume of this gas per breath summated over 1 min.

In preliminary data from our institution, a linear regression analysis was utilized to compare total minute ventilation with MV_{alv} in a heterogeneous group of 30 ventilated pediatric ICU patients. Data were collected every minute for 24 h (average number of data points per patient equals 1440). A poor correlation, defined as r^2 less than 0.70, was noted in 37% (11/30) of the patients. Thus, the traditional determination of minute ventilation does not accurately represent the volume of gas involved in gas exchange at the alveoli. Volumetric capnography provides clinicians with a continuous determination of MV_{alv} to optimize ventilator management strategies. As dead-space ventilation approaches zero, then MV_{alv} approaches total minute ventilation.

$\dot{V}CO_2$: volumetric capnography

Capnography allows for the continuous monitoring of the volume of $\dot{V}CO_2$. $\dot{V}CO_2$ is the net volume of CO_2 eliminated through the lungs each minute (ml/min). Since $\dot{V}CO_2$ is affected by ventilation, circulation/perfusion, and, to a lesser degree, diffusion, it is a valuable marker for changes in the cardiorespiratory status of a ventilated patient. $\dot{V}CO_2$ signals future changes in P_aCO_2. The volumetric capnogram has been utilized successfully in the measurement of anatomic dead-space, pulmonary capillary perfusion, and effective ventilation (Romero *et al.*, 1997). Monitoring devices which measure $\dot{V}CO_2$ and display volumetric capnograms provide clinicians with a breath-to-breath indicator of patient gas exchange in response to ventilator settings (Taskar *et al.*, 1995) and the effects of cardiorespiratory interactions (as detailed elsewhere in this textbook).

CO_2 production is determined by metabolism. Therefore, the quantity of CO_2 normally produced is dependant on the patient's body weight and level of activity. For a normal, healthy, resting person with a normal respiratory quotient (RQ = 0.8), an estimated minute production can be calculated by using Brody's formula ($\dot{V}CO_2 = 8 \times Wt^{0.75}$). At rest, an average sized adult produces about 200 ml of CO_2 per minute (Lawrence, 1987). However, for a ventilated patient it is difficult to determine the "normal" $\dot{V}CO_2$ as Brody's formula does not apply as a ventilated patient does not represent "a normal, health, resting person." Thus, it is important to stress the usefulness of $\dot{V}CO_2$ in the management of ventilated patients based on changes over time (i.e., trends) more than absolute values. Several conditions do predictably increase or decrease CO_2 production. CO_2 production is decreased with a decrease in metabolic activity and is increased with an increase in metabolic activity. For example, CO_2 production increases with agitation, fever, and shivering and decreases with sedation/sleep and hypothermia (except if shivering occurs).

CO_2 balance (production versus elimination) in the body is dependent upon four main factors: production, transportation (cells to blood and blood to lungs), storage (skeletal muscle, fat, and bone), and elimination. In a normal, healthy individual, the amount of CO_2 produced from metabolism rapidly equilibrates with the amount of CO_2 eliminated by the lungs. Since areas of dead-space (anatomic and physiologic) do not participate in gas exchange, all expired CO_2 are derived from alveolar gas. As with oxygen consumption, CO_2 production and elimination ($\dot{V}CO_2$) is a continuous process. Therefore, $\dot{V}CO_2$ rapidly reflects changes in ventilation and perfusion regardless of the etiology. Additionally, $\dot{V}CO_2$ reflects the body's physiologic response to changes in mechanical ventilator settings. Capnography is a very useful and sensitive clinical tool reflecting changes in the cardiorespiratory status and metabolic state of the patient (Breen *et al.*, 1996a, b).

By analyzing the volumetric capnogram slopes, clinicians can quickly and easily determine clinical issues of concern (Figure 18.2). Phase 1 represents gas exhaled from the upper airways (i.e., gas exhaled from anatomic dead-space) which generally is void of CO_2 (Johnson & Breen, 1999). Therefore, an increase in phase 1 indicates an increase in anatomic dead-space

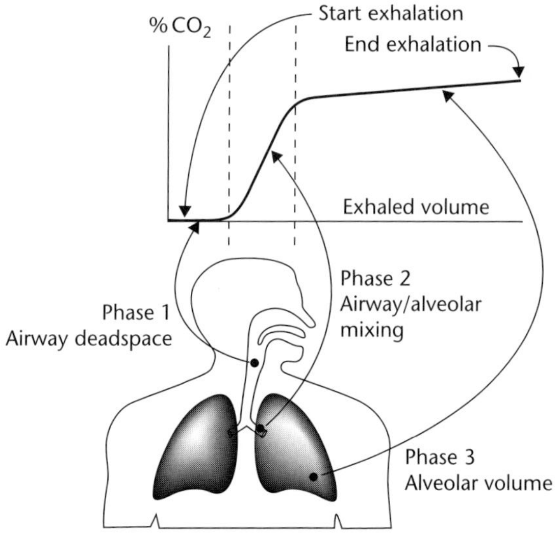

Figure 18.2 *Volumetric capnogram.* The initial portion of the volumetric capnogram (phase 1) represents the quantity of CO_2 eliminated from the large airways. Phase 2 is the transitional zone which represents ventilation from both large and small airways. The phase 3 of the capnogram represents $\dot{V}CO_2$ from the alveoli and, thus, the quantity of gas involved with alveolar ventilation. (Image courtesy of Respironics, Inc., Murrysville, PA.)

ventilation ($V_{d\ ana}$). Phase 2 is the transitional phase from upper to lower airway ventilation and tends to depict changes in perfusion. For example, a decrease in phase 2 slope would be indicative of reducing perfusion. Phase 3 is the area of alveolar gas exchange and represents changes in gas distribution. For example, an increase in the slope of phase 3 is indicative of increased mal-distribution of gas delivery. This topic is discussed in more detail in the chapter on modeling (Chapter 32).

When weaning from mechanical ventilation, it is important to assure that the volume of gas delivered actually participates in gas exchange. Thus, the monitoring of $\dot{V}CO_2$ provides objective data which not only assists in the management of mechanical ventilation but greatly facilitates weaning.

Successful weaning using volumetric capnography is demonstrated in Figure 18.3(a). In the top portion of this figure, MV_{alv} is displayed. Over time spontaneous ventilation (as displayed by the black bars) increases with the total minute ventilation remaining stable. Thus, during this period of time mechanical ventilatory support is being weaned, and the patient assumes the additional work of breathing. In this case of successful weaning, $\dot{V}CO_2$ (as displayed in the bottom portion of the figure) remains stable and then slightly increases. Thus, the patient is tolerating the increased spontaneous respiratory effort and is able to continue to expire CO_2. An arterial blood gas would demonstrate a stable P_aCO_2.

The slight increase in $\dot{V}CO_2$ in Figure 18.3(a) represents an increase in CO_2 production as the patient's work of breathing increases in association with the decrease in ventilator support. This minimal increase in $\dot{V}CO_2$ is typical of successful weaning. A more dramatic increase in $\dot{V}CO_2$ would be consistent with an excessive work of breathing and the potential for impending respiratory decompensation. This scenario would be consistent with a physical assessment of increasing respiratory distress (i.e. retractions, tachypnea, and potentially agitation).

Weaning failure is demonstrated in Figure 18.3(b). In this case, as the ventilator settings are decreased, the patient no longer is able to maintain an adequate degree of spontaneous ventilation and, thus, total minute ventilation falls. This decrease in minute ventilation is associated with a decrease in $\dot{V}CO_2$. An arterial blood gas would reveal an elevated P_aCO_2. Volumetric capnography enables the clinician to notice the weaning failure and to increase the mechanical ventilator support promptly and without the requirement for an arterial blood gas (Boynton & O'Keefe, 1999).

PEEP management

Few clinicians would argue that the determination of appropriate PEEP levels is essential for optimal management of the mechanically ventilated patient with acute lung injury or acute respiratory distress syndrome. However, controversy does exist concerning the best method for achieving the appropriate PEEP level for an individual patient. Ideally, the ideal PEEP level for a specific patient is the value which provides the most optimal lung volume and, thus, the highest oxygenation for the lowest F_IO_2, the greatest pulmonary compliance, and the highest cardiac output. In reality, there is no level of PEEP that achieves all of these goals for a specific patient at a given time. Thus, it is the clinician's responsibility to determine the PEEP level which most optimally balances each of these cardiorespiratory goals.

Maintaining an appropriate level of PEEP may prevent lung derecruitment and the development of atelectasis. On the other hand, the use of excessive PEEP may further exacerbate the presence of overdistention and adversely affect cardiac performance (Cheifetz *et al.*, 1998). Titration of PEEP levels can be effectively achieved by monitoring $\dot{V}CO_2$ and the volumetric capnogram. $\dot{V}CO_2$ is more informative than $ETCO_2$ during changes in PEEP (Breen *et al.*, 1996a; Johnson & Breen, 1999).

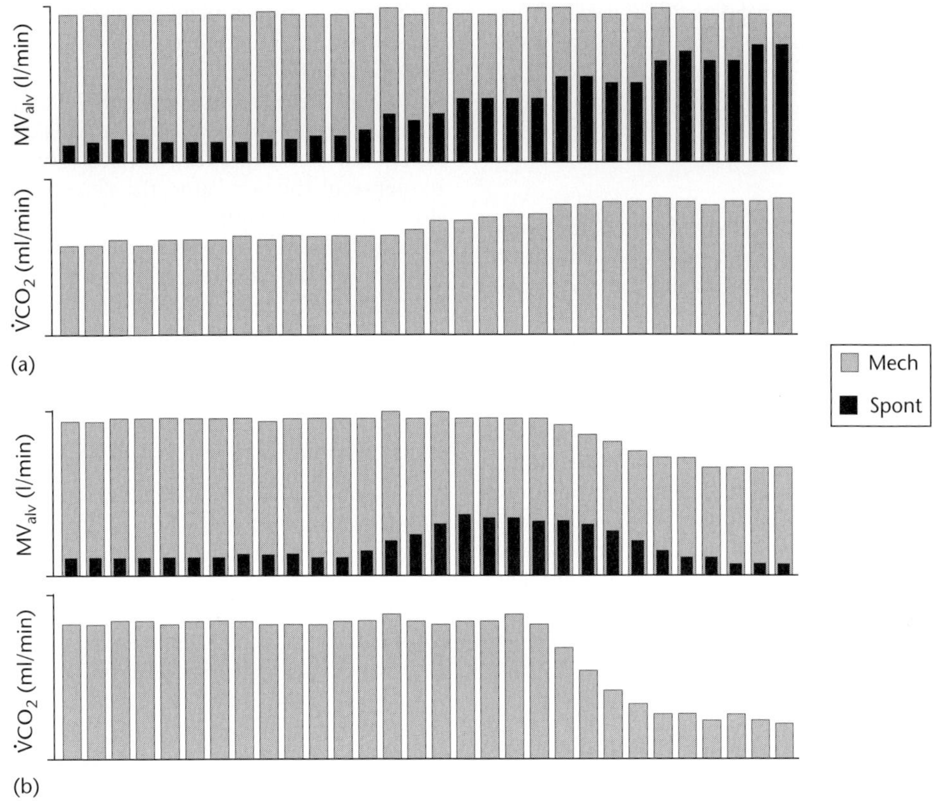

Figure 18.3 Volumetric capnography and weaning from mechanical ventilation. (a) *Successful weaning*. The top panel represents total MV_{alv} as divided between mechanical breaths and spontaneous breaths. In this graph, the patient's spontaneous ventilation (Spont) is increasing as mechanical ventilator (Mech) support (i.e. synchronized intermittent mandatory ventilation, SIMV, rate) is weaned. In the bottom panel, $\dot{V}O_2$ slightly increases over time. Thus, the patient is able to tolerate the transition to spontaneous breathing. The mild increase in $\dot{V}CO_2$ represents increased CO_2 production related to the expected increased work of breathing. (b) *Failure weaning*. The top panel represents total MV_{alv} as divided between mechanical breaths and spontaneous breaths. In this graph, the patient's Spont initially increases as Mech support is weaned. However, over time the patient's respiratory effort deteriorates and minute ventilation falls. In the bottom panel, $\dot{V}CO_2$ decreases over time. Thus, the patient is unable to tolerate the transition to spontaneous breathing. Arterial blood gas analyses would reveal an increasing P_aCO_2. $\dot{V}CO_2$ in ml/min and MV_{alv} in l/min. (Image courtesy of Respironics, Inc., Murrysville, PA.)

Monitoring of $\dot{V}CO_2$ as well as analyzing the slope of the waveform can provide valuable information in the management of PEEP. For example, an increase in $V_{d\ ana}$ is often present when high PEEP levels are applied (Coffey *et al.*, 1983). This increase in $V_{d\ ana}$ is most likely secondary to the restriction of an intact chest wall (Breen *et al.*, 1996b). An increase in $V_{d\ ana}$ can be quickly recognized by an increase in the phase 1 slope of the capnogram. When this condition is present, a reduction in PEEP level should improve MV_{alv}.

Decreased $\dot{V}CO_2$ with a decrease in the phase 2 slope of the waveform is also indicative of excessive PEEP levels. This decrease, however, is caused by decreased pulmonary perfusion (Dueck *et al.*, 1977; Coffey *et al.*, 1983; Nieman *et al.*, 1988). This decrease in perfusion secondary to excessive PEEP levels is generally caused by an increase in intrathoracic pressure creating a decrease in systemic venous return (decreased right ventricular preload) and an increase in pulmonary vascular resistance (increased right ventricular afterload) (Cheifetz *et al.*, 1998). Both of these physiologic changes in loading conditions adversely affect right ventricular function and, thus, global cardiac output. The decrease in pulmonary blood flow reduces CO_2 transport from the tissues to the vasculature of the lung (Johnson, 1999) and subsequently reduces $\dot{V}CO_2$.

Phase 3 of the waveform represents gas distribution at the alveolar level. An increase in the phase 3 slope depicts a mal-distribution of gas. Mal-distribution of gas can be caused by inappropriate PEEP levels. When PEEP levels are inadequate, alveolar collapse can occur resulting in atelectasis.

Extubation

The final stage in mechanical ventilation is the point at which the patient is likely to tolerate discontinuation of mechanical ventilation. Preparing for extubation begins with the assessment of the patient's ability to breathe effectively without the ventilator and the subsequent ability to continue to maintain adequate gas exchange without an artificial airway. Predicting successful extubation remains a daunting challenge for every clinician involved with the care of mechanically ventilated patients, and especially daunting for those working with infants and children. While many measures have been suggested as reliable predictors of successful liberation from mechanical ventilation, few have been proven, and of those few a large percentage require clinicians to perform multiple tests over extended periods of time (Yang & Tobin, 1991; Lee *et al.*, 1994; Ely *et al.*, 2001; Meade *et al.*, 2001a, b).

Many discrepancies still exist when evaluating extubation success. With as many as 20% of recently extubated patients requiring reintubation, great emphasis has been placed on accurately predicting extubation readiness (Epstein, 2002a, b). Due to the increased risks to patients requiring reintubation (Demling *et al.*, 1988; Torres *et al.*, 1995; Daley *et al.*, 1996; Epstein *et al.*, 1997; Esteban *et al.*, 1997; Epstein & Ciubotaru, 1998; Rady & Ryan, 1999; Manthous *et al.*, 1998; Hilbert, 2003), the liberation from mechanical ventilation must be timed carefully. Without objective criteria, variability between clinician thresholds poses a significant clinical problem. A particular strategy may be superior in a setting where clinician threshold for extubation is low, but may fail in a setting where clinician threshold is high. For example, it may appear that clinicians with low extubation failure rates are doing the best job when, in fact, the low rates of extubation failure may come at the cost of prolonged ventilation and its associated complications (Orlowski *et al.*, 1980; Benjamin *et al.*, 1990; Pierson, 1990; Tobias *et al.*, 1994; Manthous *et al.*, 1998; Meade *et al.*, 2001a, b). Extubation failure rates must be assessed in relation to length of ventilation and patient acuity data.

While many extubation failure predictors exist (Khan *et al.*, 1996; Kollef *et al.*, 1997; Venkataraman *et al.*, 2000; Goldstone, 2002), there are a limited number of studies showing effective success indicators. This is especially true in the case of infants and children. In adult patients, the spontaneous breathing trial (SBT) has come into favor recently (Esteban *et al.*, 1995; Kollef *et al.*, 1997; Ely *et al.*, 2001). Using the SBT method, patients are assessed daily on their ability to breathe spontaneously. Once it is determined a patient can maintain effective ventilation without the assistance of the ventilator, the patient is extubated. However, when infants are given a SBT using continuous positive airway pressure (CPAP) through an endotracheal tube, the rate of failure increases (Kim & Boutwell, 1987; Tapia *et al.*, 1995). This is most likely attributed to the increase in work of breathing imposed by resistance through small uncuffed endotracheal tubes. Therefore, many infants who might actually tolerate extubation remain intubated for extended periods of time.

The classic approach to extubation in all age groups is to decrease assisted ventilation to "minimal" settings based more on tradition and subjective assessments than data. With the advent of advanced technology, the clinician has objective data for assessing the ability of patients to be liberated from mechanical ventilation. The physiologic dead-space ratio ($V_d/V_{t\ phys}$) has long been utilized as a marker of lung disease in adult intensive care (Pontoppidan *et al.*, 1965). While V_d/V_t phys greater than 0.60 has been used in the past as an indication for intubation, it was not until recently that $V_d/V_{t\ phys}$ has been studied as a guide for extubation readiness (Hubble *et al.*, 2000). Until the recent improvements in CO_2 monitoring technology, measuring the $V_d/V_{t\ phys}$ ratio was not a simple clinical task. But, with the recent advances in technology, $V_d/V_{t\ phys}$ can now be obtained quickly, accurately, and non-invasively at the bedside. Using a modified Bohr equation, volumetric capnography can rapidly calculate and display V_d/V_t values. Additionally, an increase from baseline of phase 1 slope of the volumetric capnogram can be seen in the presence of an increase in $V_{d\ ana}$ (Figure 18.2).

While there are no studies to date on the effectiveness of V_d/V_t phys as a predictor of extubation success in adults, V_d/V_t less than 0.5 has been shown to be predictive of extubation success in infants and children (Hubble *et al.*, 2000). The SBT used in adults assesses the ratio of frequency to tidal volume (f/V_t) to determine extubation readiness. However, an increase in dead-space would lead to a decrease in effective tidal volume and a compensatory increase in frequency. Thus, the result would be an increased f/V_t. Additionally, alveolar dead-space is increased in the presence of excessive PEEP, intrinsic lung disease, and airway obstruction. Therefore, an increased $V_d/V_{t\ phys}$ warrants investigation prior to an extubation trial.

Summary

With the majority of patients in the ICU setting requiring mechanical ventilation, minimizing the duration of mechanical ventilation while optimizing the potential for successful extubation is crucial in the management of critically ill patients. A number of differing opinions exist as to the best mode for weaning from mechanical ventilation. However, to date, there is little evidence proving one mode is superior than another for weaning. Whatever ventilator mode is utilized, weaning from mechanical ventilation should begin as soon as the patient stabilizes. A clear-cut organized plan based on objective criteria which is adjusted to meet changes in patient status is clearly recommended. Careful consideration must be given to provide optimal weaning and reliable extubation strategies.

Capnography, both time and volumetric, allows for mechanical ventilatory strategies to be designed with clear, precise, objective criteria. With the data provided by capnography, adequate gas delivery, optimal PEEP, and effective ventilation can be established with the least amount of mechanical assistance regardless of clinician or institutional preferences.

References

ARDS Network (2000). Ventilation with lower tidal volumes as compared with traditional tidal volumes for acute lung injury and the acute respiratory distress syndrome. *New. Engl. J. Med.*, **342**: 1301–1308.

Arnold, J.H., Hanson, J.H., Toro-Figuero, L.O., Gutierrez, J., Berens, R.J. & Anglin, D.L. (1994). Prospective, randomized comparison of high-frequency oscillatory ventilation and conventional mechanical ventilation in pediatric respiratory failure. *Crit. Care Med.*, **22**: 1530–1539.

Arnold, J.H., Anas, N.G., Luckett, P., Cheifetz, I.M., *et al.* (2000). High frequency oscillatory ventilation in pediatric respiratory failure: a multicenter experience. *Crit. Care Med.*, **28**: 3913–3919.

Benjamin, P.K., Thompson, J.E. & O'Rourke, P.P. (1990). Complications of mechanical ventilation in a children's hospital multidisciplinary intensive care unit. *Respir. Care*, **35**: 873–878.

Birmingham, P.K., Cheney, F.W. & Ward, R.J. (1986). Esophageal intubation: a review of detection techniques. *Anesth. Analg.*, **65**: 886–891.

Boynton, J.H. & O'Keefe, G. (1999). The use of VCO_2 in predicting successful liberation from mechanical ventilation. *Respir. Care*, **44**: 1243.

Breen, P.H., Serina, E.R. & Barker, S.J. (1996a). Measurements of pulmonary CO_2 elimination must exclude inspired CO_2 measured at the capnometer sampling site. *J. Clin. Monit.*, **12**: 231–236.

Breen, P.H., Mazumdar, B. & Skinner, S.C. (1996b). Comparison of end-tidal PCO_2 and average alveolar expired PCO_2 during positive end-expiratory pressure. *Anesth. Analg.* **82**: 368–373.

Cannon, M.L., Cornell, J., Tripp-Hamel, D.S., Gentile, M.A., Hubble, C.L., Meliones, J.N. & Cheifetz, I.M. (2000). Tidal volumes for ventilated infants should be determined with a pneumotachometer placed at the endotracheal tube. *Am. J. Respir. Crit. Care Med.*, **162**: 2109–2112.

Chatte, G., Sab, J.M., Dubois, J.M., Sirodot, M., Gaussorgues, P. & Robert, D. (1997). Prone position in mechanically ventilated patients with severe acute respiratory failure. *Am. J. Respir. Crit. Care Med.*, **155**: 473–478.

Cheifetz, I.M., Craig, D., Quick, G., *et al.* (1998). Increasing tidal volumes and pulmonary overdistention adversely affect pulmonary vascular mechanics and cardiac output in a pediatric swine model. *Crit. Care Med.*, **26**: 710–716.

Clark, R.H., Gerstmann, D.R., Null Jr, D.M. & deLemos, R.A. (1992). Prospective randomized comparison of high-frequency oscillatory and conventional ventilation in respiratory distress syndrome. *Pediatrics*, **89**: 5–12.

Coffey, R.L., Albert, R.K. & Robertson, H.T. (1983). Mechanisms of physiological dead space response to PEEP after acute oleic acid lung injury. *J. Appl. Physiol.*, **55**: 1550–1557.

Cook, D., Meade, M., Guyatt, G., Griffith, L. & Booker, L. (1999). Criteria for weaning from mechanical ventilation: summary. *AHRQ Publication* no. 01-E010.

Cook, D., Meade, M., Guyatt, G., Butler, R., Aldawood, A. & Epstein, S. (2001). Trials of miscellaneous interventions to wean from mechanical ventilation. *Chest*, **120**: 438S–444S.

Daley, B.J., Garcia-Perez, F. & Ross, S.E. (1996). Reintubation as an outcome predictor in trauma patients. *Chest*, **110**: 1577–1580.

Demling, R.H., Read, T., Lind, L.J. & Flanagan, H.L. (1988). Incidence and morbidity of extubation failure in surgical intensive care patients. *Crit. Care Med.*, **16**: 573–577.

Derdak, S., Mehta, S., Stewart, T.E., *et al.* (2002). Multicenter oscillatory Ventilation For Acute Respiratory Distress Syndrome Trial (MOAT) Study Investigators. High-frequency oscillatory ventilation for acute respiratory distress syndrome in adults: a randomized, controlled trial. *Am. J. Resp. Crit. Care Med.*, **166**: 801–808.

DeRobertis, E.S., Servillo, G., Tufano, R. & Jonson, B. (2001). Aspiration of deadspace allows isocapnic low tidal volume ventilation in acute lung injury. Relationships to gas exchange and mechanics. *Intens. Care Med.*, **27**: 1496–1503.

Dreyfuss, D. & Saumon, G. (1998). Induced lung injury: lessons from experimental studies. *Am. J. Respir. Crit. Care Med.*, **157**: 294–323.

Dreyfuss, D., Soler, P., Basset, G. & Saumon, G. (1988). High inflation pressure pulmonary edema. *Am. Rev. Respir. Dis.*, **137**: 1159–1164.

Dueck, R., Wagner, P.D. & West, J.B. (1977). Effects of positive end-expiratory pressure on gas exchange in dogs with normal and edematous lungs. *Anesthesiology*, **47**: 359–366.

Ely, E.W., Meade, M., Haponik, E.F., Kollef, M., Cook, D.J., Guyatt, G.H. & Stoller, J.K. (2001). Mechanical ventilator weaning protocols driven by non-physician health-care professionals: evidence-based clinical practice guidelines. *Chest*, **121**: 1947–1955.

Epstein, S.K. (2002a). Decision to extubate. *Intens. Care Med.*, **28(5)**: 535–546.

Epstein, S.K. (2002b). Extubation. *Respir. Care*, **47**: 483–492.

Epstein, S.K. & Ciubotaru R.L. (1998). Independent effects of etiology of failure and time to reintubation on outcome for patients failing extubation. *Am. J. Resp. Crit. Care Med.*, **158**: 489–493.

Epstein, S.K., Ciubotaru, R.L. & Wong, J.B. (1997). Effect of failure extubation on the outcome of mechanical ventilation. *Chest*, **112**: 186–192.

Esteban, A.F., Tobin, M.J., Alia, I., *et al.* (1995). The Spanish Lung Failure Collaborative Group. A comparison of four methods of weaning patients from mechanical ventilation. *New. Engl. J. Med.*, **332**: 345–350.

Esteban, A., Alia, I., Gordo, F., *et al.* (1997). The Spanish Lung Failure Collaborative Group. Extubation outcome after spontaneous breathing trials with t-tube or pressure support ventilation. *Am. J. Respir. Crit. Care Med.*, **156**: 459–465.

Froese, A.B. (1997). High-frequency oscillatory ventilation for adult respiratory distress syndrome: let's get it right this time! *Crit. Care Med.*, **25**: 906–908.

Gattinoni, L., Tognoni, G., Pesenti, A., *et al.* (2001). Effect of prone positioning on the survival of patients with acute respiratory failure. *New. Engl. J. Med.*, **345**: 568–573.

Goldstone, J. (2002). The pulmonary physician in critical care – 10: difficult weaning. *Thorax*, **57**: 986–991.

Hatzakis, G.E. & Davis, G.M. (2002). Fuzzy logic controller for weaning neonates from mechanical ventilation. *Proceedings/AMIA Annual Symposium*, pp. 315–319.

Henneman, E., Dracup, K., Ganz, T., Molayeme, O. & Cooper, C. (2001). Effects of a collaborative weaning plan on patient outcome in the critical care setting. *Crit. Care Med.*, **29**: 297–303.

Hess, D.R. (2002). Liberation from mechanical ventilation: weaning the patient or weaning old-fashioned ideas? *Crit. Care Med.*, **30**: 2154–2155.

Hickling, K.G. (2002). Permissive hypercapnia. *Resp. Care Clin. North. Am.*, **8**: 155–169.

Hickling, K.G., Walsh, J., Henderson, S. & Jackson, R. (1990). Low mortality associated with low lung volume pressure limited ventilation with permissive hypercapnia in severe respiratory distress syndrome. *Intens. Care Med.*, **16**: 372–377.

Hickling, K.G., Walsh, J., Henderson, S. & Jackson, R. (1994). Low mortality rate in adult respiratory distress syndrome using low-volume, pressure-limited ventilation with permissive hypercapnia: a prospective study. *Crit. Care Med.*, **22**: 1568–1578.

Hilbert, G. (2003). Difficult to wean chronic obstructive pulmonary disease patients: avoid heat and moisture exchangers. *Crit. Care Med.*, **31**: 1580–1581.

Holland, R., Webb, R.K. & Runciman, W.B. (1993). The Australian Incident Monitoring Study. Oesophageal intubation: an analysis of 2000 incident reports. *Anaesth. Intens. Care*, **21**: 608–610.

Hubble, C.L., Gentile, M.A., Tripp, D.S., Craig, D.M., Meliones, J.N. & Cheifetz, I.M. (2000). Deadspace to tidal volume ratio predicts successful extubation in infants and children. *Crit. Care Med.*, **28**: 2034–2040.

Isserles, S.A. & Breen, P.H. (1991). Can changes in end-tidal PCO_2 measure changes in cardiac output? *Anesth. Analg.*, **73**: 808–814.

Johnson, J.L. & Breen, P.H. (1999). How does positive end-expiratory pressure decrease pulmonary CO_2 elimination in anesthetized patients? *Respir. Physiol.*, **118**: 227–236.

Khan, N., Brown, A. & Venkataraman, S.T. (1996). Predictors of extubation success and failure in mechanically ventilated infants and children. *Crit. Care Med.*, **24**: 1568–1579.

Kim, E.H. & Boutwell, W.C. (1987). Successful direct extubation of very low birth weight infants from low intermittent mandatory ventilation rate. *Pediatrics*, **80**: 409–414.

Knapp, S., Kofler, J., Stoiser, B., *et al.* (1999). The assessment of four different methods to verify endotracheal tube placement in the critical care setting. *Anesth. Analg.* **88**: 766–770.

Kollef, M.H., Shapiro, S.D., Silver, P., *et al.* (1997). A randomized, controlled trial of protocol – directed versus physician – directed weaning from mechanical ventilation. *Crit. Care Med.*, **25**: 567–574.

Lawrence, M. (1987). The essentials for patient care and evaluation. In: *Pulmonary Physiology in Clinical Practice*. St. Louis, C.V. Mosby.

Lee, K.H., Hui, K.P., Chan, T.B., Tan, W.C. & Lim, T.K. (1994). Rapid shallow breathing (frequency–tidal volume ratio) did not predict extubation outcome. *Chest*, **105**: 540–543.

MacIntyre, N.R.M., Cook, D.J. & Guyatt, G.H. (2001). Evidence-based guidelines for weaning and discontinuing ventilatory support. *Chest*, **120**: 375S–395S.

Manthous, C.A.M. (2002). The anarchy of weaning techniques. *Chest*, **121**: 1738–1740.

Manthous, C.A., Schmidt, G.A. & Hall, J.B. (1998). Liberation from mechanical ventilation: a decade of progress. *Chest*, **114**: 886–901.

Margolin, G. & Groeger, J.S. (2002). Ventilator-induced lung injury and its relationship to recruitment maneuvers. *Crit. Care Med.*, **30**: 2161–2162.

Marini, J.J., Tobin, M.J., Guyatt, G., *et al.* (2001). Trials comparing lternative weaning modes and discontinuation assessments. *Chest*, **120**: 425S–437S.

Meade, M., Guyatt, G., Sinuff, T., Griffith, L., Hand, L., Toprani, G. & Cook, D.J. (1970). Stress distribution in lungs: a model of pulmonary elasticity. *J. Appl. Physiol.*, **28**: 596–608.

Meade, M., Guyatt, G., Cook, D., *et al.* (2001a). Predicting success in weaning from mechanical ventilation. *Chest*, **120**: 400S–424S.

Meade, M., Guyatt, G., Sinuff, T., Griffith, L., Hand, L., Toprani, G. & Cook, D. J. (2001b). Trials comparing alternative weaning modes and discontinuation assessments. *Chest*, **120**: 425S–437S.

Nieman, G.F., Paskanik, A.M. & Bredenberg, C.E. (1988). Effect of positive end-expiratory pressure on alveolar capillary perfusion. *J. Thorac. Cardiovasc. Surg.*, **95**: 712–716.

Orlowski, J.P., Ellis, N.G., Amin, N.P. & Crumrine, R.S. (1980). Complications of airway intrusion in 100 consecutive cases in a pediatric ICU. *Crit. Care Med.*, **8**: 324–331.

Piehl, M.A. & Brown, R.S. (1976). Use of extreme position changes in acute respiratory failure. *Crit. Care Med.*, **4**: 13–14.

Pierson, D.J. (1990). Complications of mechanical ventilation. In: Simmons, D.H., (ed.) *Current Pulmonology*, Vol. 9. Yearbook Medical Publishers, Chicago, IL. pp. 19–46.

Pontoppidan, H., Hedley-Whyte, J., Bendizen, H.H., Laver, M. B. & Radford Jr, E.P. (1965). Ventilation and oxygenation requirements during prolonged artificial ventilation in patients with respiratory failure. *New. Engl. J. Med.*, **273**: 401–409.

Rady, M.Y. & Ryan, T. (1999). Perioperative predictors of extubation failure and the effect on clinical outcome after cardiac surgery. *Crit. Care Med.*, **27**: 340–347.

Romero, P.V., Lucangelo, U., Lopez-Aguilar, J., Fernandez, R. & Blanch, L. (1997). Physiologically based indices of volumetric capnography in patients receiving mechanical ventilation. *Eur. Resp. J.*, **10**: 1309–1315.

Sinha, S.K. & Donn, S.M. (2000). Weaning from assisted ventilation: art or science? *Arch. Dis. Child. (Fetal Neonat. Edn)*, **83**: F64–F70.

Soo Hoo, G.W. & Park, L. (2002). Variations in the measurement of weaning parameters – a survey of respiratory therapists. *Chest*, **121**: 1947–1955.

Suematsu, Y., Sato, H., Ohtsuka, T., Kotsuka, Y., Araki, S. & Takamoto, S. (2000). Predictive risk factors for delayed extubation in patients undergoing coronary artery bypass grafting. *Heart Vessels*, **15**: 214–220.

Sum-Ping, S.T., Mehta, M.P. & Anderton, J.M. (1989). A comparative study of methods of detection of esophageal intubation. *Anesth. Analg.*, **69**: 627–632.

Tapia, J.L., Bancalari, A., Gonzalez, A. & Mercado, M.E. (1995). Does continuous positive airways pressure (CPAP) during weaning from intermittent mandatory ventilation in low birth weight infants have risks or benefits? *Pediatr. Pulmonol.*, **19**: 269–274.

Taskar, V., John, J., Larsson, A., Wetterberg, T. & Jonson, B. (1995). Dynamics of carbon dioxide elimination following ventilator resetting. *Chest*, **108**: 196–202.

Tobias, J.D., Deshpande, J.K. & Gregory, D.F. (1994). Outpatient therapy of iatrogenic drug dependency following prolonged sedation in the pediatric intensive care unit. *Intens Care Med.*, **20**: 504–507.

Torres, A., Gatell, J.M., Aznar, E., *et al.* (1995). Re-intubation increases the risk of nosocomial pneumonia in patients needing mechanical ventilation. *Am. J. Respir. Crit. Care Med.*, **152**: 137–141.

Venkataraman, S.T., Khan, N. & Brown, A. (2000). Validation of predictors of extubation success and failure in mechanically ventilated infants and children. *Crit. Care Med.*, **28**: 2991–2996.

Voggenreiter, G., Neudeck, F., Aufmkolk, M. (1999). Intermittent prone positioning in the treatment of severe and moderate posttraumatic lung injury. *Crit. Care Med.*, **27**: 2375–2382.

Weingarten, M. (1990). Respiratory monitoring of carbon dioxide and oxygen a ten year perspective. *J. Clin. Monit.*, **6**: 217–225.

Whitehead, T.S. & Slutsky, A.S. (2002). The pulmonary physician in critical care: ventilator induced lung injury. *Thorax*, **57**: 635–642.

Yang, K.L. & Tobin, M.J. (1991). A prospective study of indexes predicting the outcome of trials of weaning from mechanical ventilation. *New. Engl. J. Med.*, **324**: 1445–1450.

Zhang, H., Downey, G.P., Suter, P.M., Slutsky, A.S., Marco Ranieri, V. (2002). Conventional mechanical ventilation is associated with bronchoalveolar lavage-induced activation of polymorphonuclear leukocytes: a possible mechanism to explain the systemic consequences of VILI in patients with ARDS. *Anesthesiology*, **97**: 1426–1433.

SPECIAL SITUATIONS

SECTION 1e

CAPNOGRAPHY AND ADJUNCTS OF MECHANICAL VENTILATION 19

U. Lucangelo, F. Bernabè, A. Gullo & L. Blanch

Introduction

Mechanical ventilation is a life-saving treatment for patients with acute respiratory failure. The objectives of mechanical ventilation are to correct acute severe hypoxemia and to support or replace the action of the respiratory muscles in situations of acute ventilatory or cardiocirculatory failure. Over the past decade other therapeutic options or adjuncts have been explored. A better understanding of the pathophysiology of respiratory failure can contribute to a better outcome for our patients.

The carbon dioxide (CO_2) tension difference between pulmonary capillary blood and alveolar gas is usually small in normal subjects where end-tidal partial pressure of CO_2 ($P_{et}CO_2$) approximates alveolar and arterial PCO_2 (P_ACO_2 and P_aCO_2, respectively). Physiologic dead-space is the primary determinant of the ΔPCO_2 in patients with normal cardiorespiratory system. Patients with cardiopulmonary diseases have altered ventilation/perfusion ($\dot{V}/\dot{Q}$) ratios producing abnormalities of both dead-space and intrapulmonary shunt, which may also affect the ΔPCO_2. Differences between P_aCO_2 and $P_{et}CO_2$ (ΔPCO_2) beyond 5 mmHg are attributed to abnormalities in physiologic dead-space and/or an increase in venous admixture (the fraction of the cardiac output that passes through the lungs without taken oxygen) (Fowler, 1948; Fletcher *et al.*, 1981; Piiper *et al.*, 1987; Hess, 1990; Feihl, 2003). The advanced technology combination of airway flow monitoring and mainstream capnography allows breath-by-breath bedside calculation of pulmonary dead-space and CO_2 elimination (Fletcher *et al.*, 1981; Romero *et al.*, 1997). Therefore, the use of capnography as a monitoring tool in the course of acute respiratory failure may provide with clinicians important physiologic information.

The purpose of this chapter is to highlight the role of capnography as a monitoring tool at the bedside during the use of different adjuncts to mechanical ventilation in critically ill patients.

Positive end-expiratory pressure

Acute respiratory distress syndrome (ARDS) is characterized by an increased membrane permeability, a decreased oncotic pressure and an augmented transvascular hydrostatic pressure gradients that cause non-cardiogenic pulmonary edema, atelectasis and loss of lung volume. As a result, $\dot{V}/\dot{Q}$ heterogeneity and intrapulmonary shunts increase, and oxygenation becomes severely impaired. Mechanical ventilation is a supportive life-saving therapy but it can further damage the lungs. Importantly, this damage can be indistinguishable from the pulmonary alterations attributable to the ARDS (Amato *et al.*, 1998; The ARDS Network, 2000). It is essential to know the internal mechanism of the heterogeneity distribution of regional atelectasis, lung tissue damage, edema formation and inflammatory response in ARDS patients undergoing mechanical ventilation. Many studies, indeed, have attempted to explain the effects of the ventilator on regional lung structure and mechanical function in ARDS patients. In ARDS, the entire lung volume is considerably reduced and the distribution of regional atelectasis is irregular thus supporting the concept, that areas of an injured lung are excluded from ventilation (Gattinoni *et al.*, 1995; Pelosi *et al.*, 1995, 1996; Puybasset *et al.*, 1998; Vieira *et al.*, 1999).

The application of positive end-expiratory pressure (PEEP) is used to increase lung volume and to improve oxygenation in patients with acute lung injury (ALI) (Suter *et al.*, 1975). Using chest computed tomography (CT) scan during a progressive increase in PEEP from 0 to 20 cmH_2O, Gattinoni *et al.* (1995) reported that tidal volume distribution in the lungs decreased significantly in the upper lung level (non-dependent areas), did not change in the middle levels and increased significantly in the lower levels (dependent areas) in supine patients diagnosed with ARDS. In other words, PEEP reduced the reopening-collapsing tissue, keeping the lung tissue recruited at end-inspiration open. If a moderate/high PEEP level is

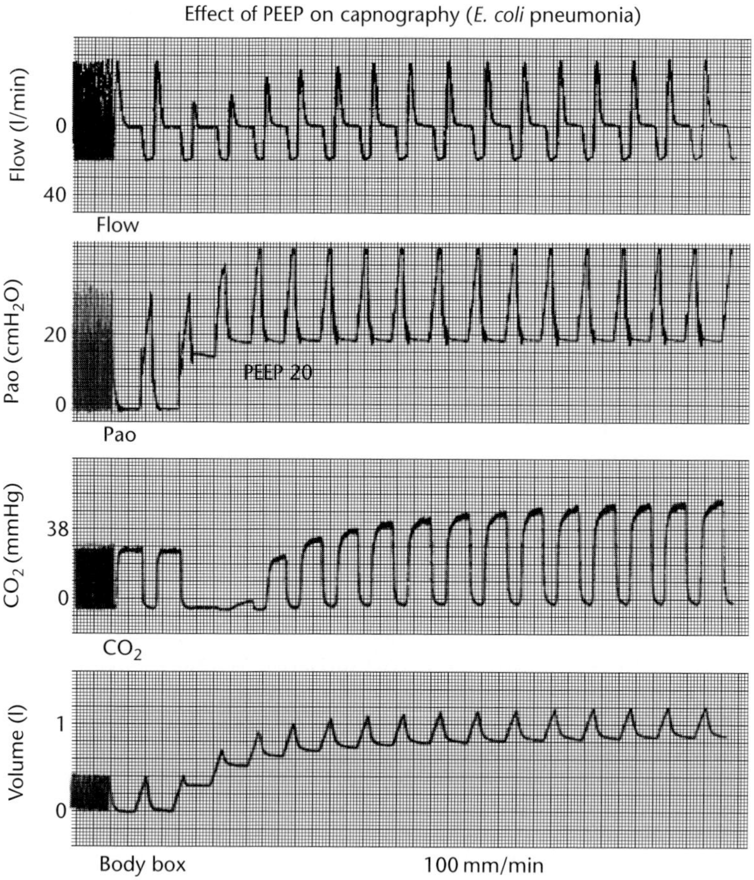

Figure 19.1 Tracings of airflow (Flow), airway pressure (Pao), expired capnograms (CO_2) and tidal volume (Volume) in an experimental animal with ALI due to *Escherichia coli* pneumonia. Increasing PEEP from 0 to 20 cmH_2O induces an increase in lung volume. Absence of the capnogram for several breaths after PEEP indicates absence of expired volume until cumulative tidal volume exceeds lung volume expansion induced by PEEP. (Courtesy of Dr. Avi Nahum, St. Paul, MN.)

used in an attempt to keep all alveoli open, the level of tidal volume should not reach high end-inspiratory plateau pressures (>35 cmH_2O) because little additional lung tissue is recruited and further hyperinflation might be caused, as demonstrated by CT scan (Vieira *et al.*, 1999; Crotti *et al.*, 2001). In summary, alveolar recruitment and overdistension coexist in different parts of the lung after PEEP application in patients with ARDS (Puybasset *et al.*, 2000).

The increase in physiologic dead-space in anesthetized normal patients may be attributed to the introduction of muscle paralysis and positive pressure breathing that causes a reduction of lung volume and alters the normal distribution of $\dot{V}/\dot{Q}$ across the lung (Fletcher *et al.*, 1981). In ALI alveolar dead-space is large and does not vary systematically with PEEP (Blanch *et al.*, 1999; Smith & Fletcher *et al.*, 2000; Beydon *et al.*, 2002). However, when PEEP is used in the hope of recruiting collapsed lung units and thus improving oxygenation, PEEP-induced overdistension may instead increase alveolar dead-space (Coffey *et al.*, 1983; Beydon *et al.*, 2002) (Figure 19.1). In fact, recruitment in ARDS is associated with decreased arterial minus end-tidal CO_2 difference (Blanch *et al.*, 1987).

The relationship between the effects of PEEP on volumetric capnography and in respiratory system mechanics have been studied in a series of patients with normal lungs, moderate ALI and severe ARDS. Blanch *et al.* (1999) found that respiratory system compliance was markedly decreased and total respiratory system resistance increased in ARDS compared with similar measurements in control patients. Total physiologic dead-space and expired CO_2 slope of the phase III were higher and steeper, respectively in ALI patients compared with control patients and, in ARDS patients compared with ALI patients (Figure 19.2). Alveolar ejection volume (VAE) was lowest in ARDS. The almost rectangular shape of the expired capnogram depends on the homogeneity of the gas distribution and alveolar ventilation (Fowler, 1948; Engel, 1985; Ream *et al.*, 1995). Lung heterogeneity creates regional differences in CO_2 concentration and gas from high $\dot{V}/\dot{Q}$ regions first appear in the upper airway during exhalation. This sequential emptying

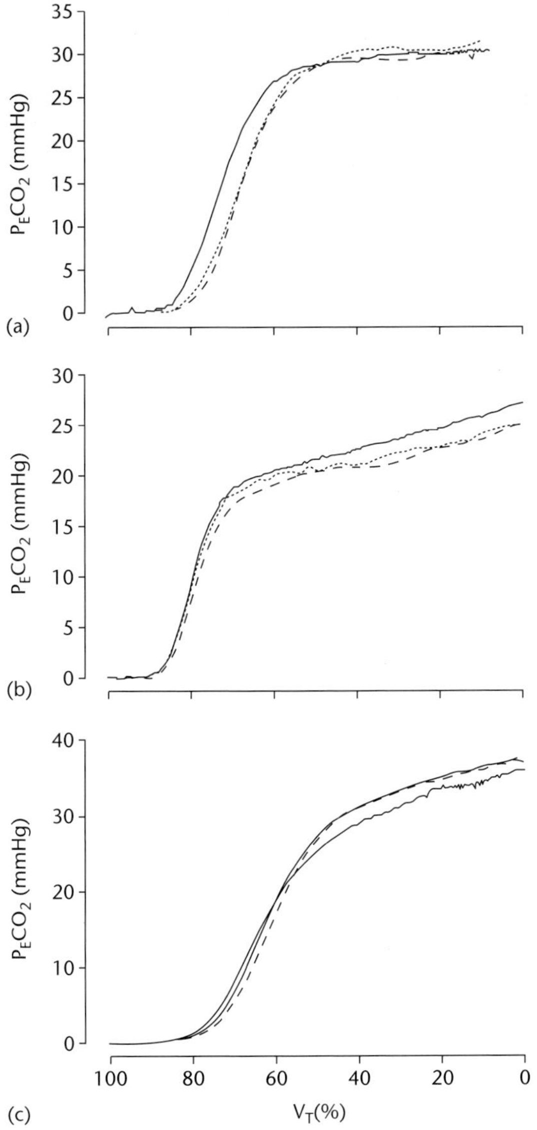

Figure 19.2 Tracings of expiratory CO_2 tension (P_ECO_2) as a function of expired tidal volume (V_T, %) obtained in representative patients at different PEEP 0 (solid line), 10 (short-dashed line) and 15 (long-dashed line) cmH_2O for a normal subject (a), a patient with ALI (b), and a patient with ARDS (c). Application of PEEP had little effect on CO_2 elimination. (Reproduced with permission from Blanch, L., Lucangelo, U., Lopez-Aguilar, J., Fernandez, R. & Romero, P. (1999). Volumetric capnography in patients with acute lung injury: effects of positive end-expiratory pressure. *Eur. Respir. J.*, **13:** 1048–1054.)

contributes to the rise of the alveolar plateau (Engel, 1985; Meyer *et al.*, 1990), the greater the $\dot{V}/\dot{Q}$ heterogeneity, the steeper the expired CO_2 slope of the phase III. Accordingly, the slope of the alveolar plateau

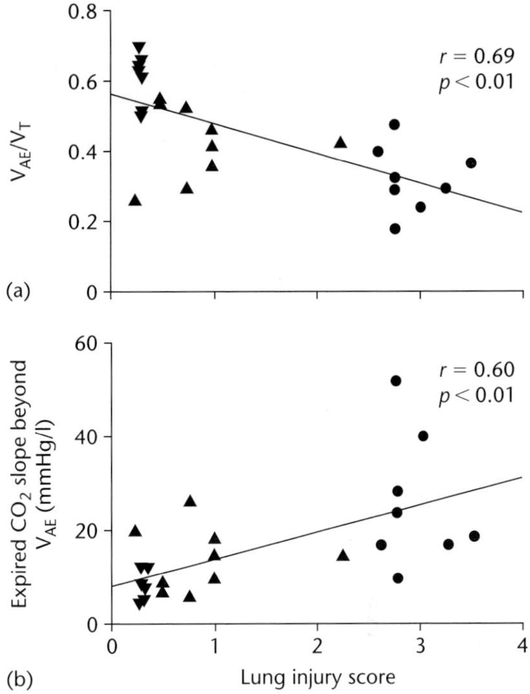

Figure 19.3 Relationship between indices of volumetric capnography (alveolar ejection volume, V_{AE}/V_T and phase III expired CO_2 slope) and lung injury score at zero end-expiratory pressure in different groups of patients (▼: control subjects; ▲: ALI; ●: ARDS). (Reproduced with permission from Blanch, L., Lucangelo, U., Lopez-Aguilar, J., Fernandez, R. & Romero, P. (1999). Volumetric capnography in patients with acute lung injury: effects of positive end-expiratory pressure. *Eur. Respir. J.*, **13:** 1048–1054.)

correlated with the severity of airflow obstruction (Blanch *et al.*, 1991; You *et al.*, 1994).

A significant correlation was found between capnographic indices and lung injury score suggesting that the severity of disease affects volumetric capnographic indices and the mechanical properties of the respiratory system (Blanch *et al.*, 1999) (Figure 19.3). Characteristic features of ALI are alveolar and capillary endothelial cell injuries that result in alterations of pulmonary microcirculation. Consequently, adequate pulmonary ventilation and blood flow across the lungs are compromised and physiologic dead-space increases. Since a high dead-space fraction represents an impaired ability to excrete CO_2 due to any kind of $\dot{V}/\dot{Q}$ mismatch (Feihl, 2003), Nuckton *et al.* (2002) postulated and demonstrated that the measurement of physiologic dead-space in standardized conditions (same tidal volume and PEEP) was independently associated with an increased risk of death in patients diagnosed with ARDS.

PEEP (within physiologic limits) improved respiratory mechanics in normal subjects and worsened lung tissue resistance in patients with respiratory failure, however, it did not affect volumetric capnographic indices (Blanch *et al.*, 1999). The same findings have been reported by other authors. Smith and Fletcher (2000) found that PEEP did not modify CO_2 elimination in patients immediately after heart surgery. Beydon *et al.* (2002) studied the effect of PEEP on dead-space and its partitions in patients with ALI. They found a large alveolar dead-space that remained unchanged after raising PEEP from 0 to 15 cmH_2O although patients in whom oxygenation improved with PEEP showed a concurrent decrease in alveolar dead-space and vice versa. Experimentally, Coffey *et al.* (1983) found in oleic acid induced ARDS, that low PEEP reduced physiologic dead-space and intrapulmonary shunt. Conversely and in the same animals, high PEEP increased the fraction of ventilation derived from areas with high $\dot{V}/\dot{Q}$ resulting in an increased physiologic dead-space. Variations in dead-space and their partitions with application of PEEP largely depend on the type, degree and stage of the lung injury. Moreover, the results of the above-mentioned studies also suggest that the ARDS lung, independently of the location of the lung densities, is globally affected by the disease. At present, capnographic indices in individual patients might enable us to track physiologic changes related to manipulations of the ventilator such as changing the amount of PEEP.

Unilateral lung injury

Studies of unilateral lung injury demonstrate that the consolidated lung regions do not expand fully during inflation to total lung capacity (Craven *et al.*, 1979; Mink *et al.*, 1981). Impaired mechanical properties of the consolidated lung are associated with very poor ventilation. Moreover, hypoxemia is due to both increased shunt and $\dot{V}/\dot{Q}$ mismatch in the injured regions, and local hypoxic vasoconstriction in most instances appears to be ineffective in directing blood flow away from the consolidated lobe. Kanarek *et al.* (1975) and Mink *et al.* (1981) demonstrated these contentions in a case report and a canine model of pneumonia, respectively, showing that PEEP increases fractional perfusion to the infected lobe and may worsen gas exchange. However, the effect of global PEEP on regional lung volume remains controversial. In patients with asymmetric lung injury, tidal volume is unfavorably distributed: healthy lung regions exhibiting normal compliance will tend to hyperinflate, whereas affected lung regions with decreased compliance will tend to remain collapsed. In a canine model of unilateral lung edema Blanch *et al.* (1992) demonstrated that PEEP and tidal volume ventilation can improve oxygenation despite a redistribution of blood flow towards the damaged lung and a decrease in the respiratory system compliance of the healthy lung. An increase in lung volume to near total lung capacity of the healthy lung flattens the pressure–volume relationship, thus decreasing healthy lung compliance and contributing to the redistribution of the tidal volume to the injured lung. Whether PEEP worsens or improves gas exchange depends on the relative magnitude of regional lung mechanical changes (Carlon *et al.*, 1978).

In the setting of unilateral lung injury, measurement of global respiratory system mechanics does not provide clinically useful information for setting ventilator parameters as the mechanical impairment of the injured parts of the lung cannot be specifically assessed (Kanarek & Shannon, 1975; Blanch *et al.*, 1992a, b). In several cases using independent lung ventilation, Carlon *et al.* (1978) showed that selective PEEP was useful to improve respiratory failure when conventional therapy failed. In a canine lobar pneumonia model, Light *et al.* (1981) clearly demonstrated that unilateral PEEP improved oxygenation and intrapulmonary shunt. In patients with unilateral thoracic trauma, Cinella *et al.* (2001) found that the use of independent lung ventilation, setting tidal volume and PEEP to keep plateau airway pressure below 26 cmH_2O in both lungs, improved both oxygenation and $\dot{V}/\dot{Q}$ mismatch. Early in the course of the disease, the diseased lung exhibited a decreased CO_2 elimination compared with the non-affected lung. Equal CO_2 elimination in both lungs was used as a criterion to stop independent lung ventilation and resume conventional mechanical ventilation.

Tracheal gas insufflation

Tracheal gas insufflation (TGI) is an adjunct to mechanical ventilation that allows ventilation with small tidal volumes while CO_2 is satisfactorily cleared. Pioneering studies demonstrated in healthy experimental animals and in humans with respiratory failure that the expiratory flushing of proximal dead-space decreased minute ventilation without change in P_aCO_2. Recent work demonstrates that conventional mechanical ventilation aided by TGI may represent a novel ventilatory strategy that succeeds in limiting both the distending forces acting on the lung and the P_aCO_2 elevation with permissive hypercapnia. Since the anatomic dead-space remains relatively constant as tidal volume is reduced, low tidal volumes are associated with a high dead-space to tidal volume ratio. TGI applied together with conventional mechanical ventilation, effectively reduces the size of the dead-space compartment and improves overall CO_2 elimination by replacing the anatomic dead-space normally laden with CO_2 during expiration with fresh gas. As a consequence, less CO_2 is recycled to the alveoli during the next inspiration and the ventilatory efficiency of each tidal respiration is improved. Therefore, TGI reduces anatomic dead-space and increases alveolar ventilation for a given frequency and tidal volume combination (Nahum *et al.*, 1992a, b; Ravenscraft *et al.*, 1993; Richecoeur *et al.*, 1999; Blanch, 2001; Blanch *et al.*, 2001a, b). The efficacy of TGI on P_aCO_2 diminishes when an enlarged alveolar component dominates the total physiologic dead-space. However, Nahum *et al.* (1995) demonstrated that allowing P_aCO_2 to rise to supranormal levels (a permissive hypercapnia strategy) counteracted the lack of efficacy of TGI to remove CO_2 when increased alveolar dead-space and decreased alveolar ventilation coexist.

The main effect of TGI is to flush the dead-space from the carina to the Y of the ventilator circuit. However, TGI has also a distal effect that contributes to the removal of CO_2. The distal effect consists of a jet area extending from the catheter tip and a turbulent region extending beyond the jet towards the alveoli. The extent of the jet and turbulence regions is related to flow velocity at the catheter tip and velocity is directly related to flow rate and inversely related to the internal diameter of the TGI catheter (Nahum *et al.*, 1992b). Although the distal effect enhances CO_2 removal, the presence of the catheter and the jet effect oppose expiratory flow favouring auto-PEEP (Kalfon *et al.*, 1997; Blanch *et al.*, 2001a).

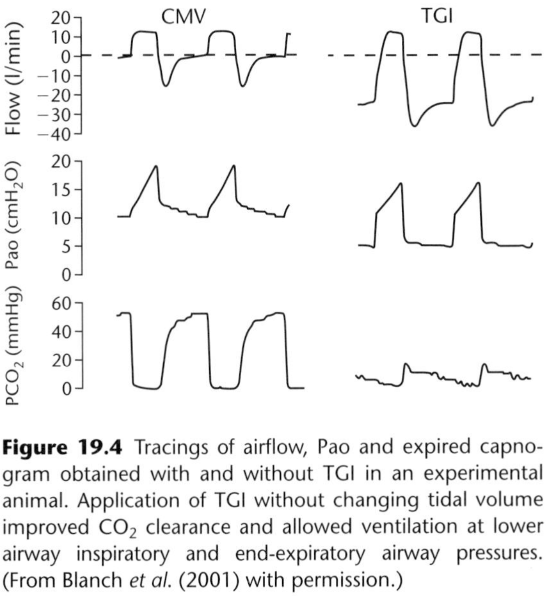

Figure 19.4 Tracings of airflow, Pao and expired capnogram obtained with and without TGI in an experimental animal. Application of TGI without changing tidal volume improved CO_2 clearance and allowed ventilation at lower airway inspiratory and end-expiratory airway pressures. (From Blanch *et al.* (2001) with permission.)

The efficacy of TGI can be monitored by capnography. The observation of capnograms provides an indication of the effect of TGI on the CO_2 concentration of the gas remaining in the proximal anatomic dead-space compartment at the onset of inspiration (Figure 19.4). Although in patients with respiratory failure $P_{et}CO_2$ is a poor estimate of P_aCO_2 (Blanch *et al.*, 1994), changes in $P_{et}CO_2$ induced by TGI correlated significantly with changes in P_aCO_2 justifying routine measurement of $P_{et}CO_2$ during TGI application as a marker of its effectiveness (Ravenscraft, 1993; Kuo *et al.*, 1996; Saura *et al.*, 1996).

High-frequency and percussive ventilation

High-frequency ventilation (HFV) was introduced in clinical practice in the early 1970s, following the experiences by Oberg and Sjostrand (1969). Many HFV techniques have been used since then, all characterized by a breathing frequency higher than 1 Hz (60 breaths/min), tidal volume lower than dead-space volume, and low peak pressure. HFV techniques have three essential elements in common: a high-pressure flow generator, a valve for flow interruption, and a circuit for connection to the patient. Depending on the frequences used, we talk of "high-frequency jet ventilation" (HFJV), and a variant of this high-frequency flow interruption (HFFI), "high-frequency oscillation" (HFO), and "high-frequency positive-pressure ventilation" (HFPPV). Lower pressures (60–300 cycles/min) are normally used in HFPPV, whereas higher values are typical for HFO (60–2400 cycles/min) (Gioia & Rogers, 1985; Branson, 1995).

Two studies (Fort *et al.*, 1997; Mehta *et al.*, 2001) led to a significant improvement in gas exchanges in ARDS patients by using HFO. These studies offered evidence that chances for survival are not only related to the initial disease, but also to early treatment, and that the HFO technique must be considered life-saving in cases that do not respond to conventional mechanical ventilation. Other HFV modes, such as HFJV and HFPPV have been widely used as well, mostly during diagnostic examinations of the upper airways (laryngo- and bronchoscopic imaging, tracheal surgery, etc.) (Borg *et al.*, 1980). The main advantage of these techniques is the limited cyclic displacement of thoracic and pulmonary structures, with a better exposure of the operating region.

Independent of the disease, HFV presented a risk of dynamic lung hyperinflation caused by the decrease in expiration time (Te). The rapid increase in lung volume and intrathoracic pressure is attributed to the high rate of gas flow. This happens mainly with ventilation

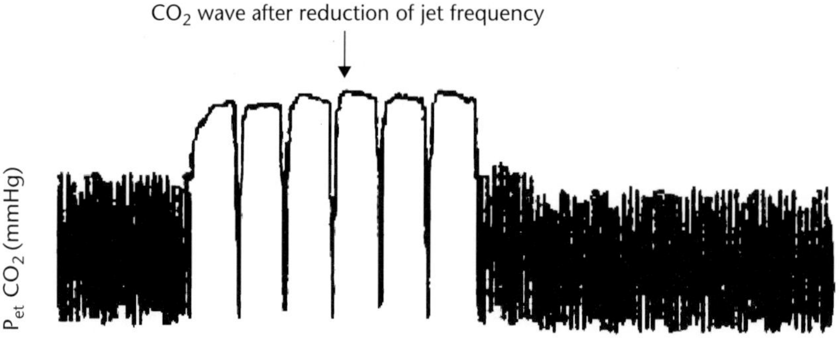

Figure 19.5 Capnography during HFJV. Large single waves indicate the capnograms after suspending jet frequency. (Reproduced with permission from Kil, H.K., Kim, O.W., Choi, H.S. & Nam, Y.T. (2002). Monitoring of $P_{et}CO_2$ during high frequency jet ventilation for laryngomicrosurgery. *Yonsei Med. J.*, **43:** 20–24.)

techniques with passive expiration, such as HFJV and HFPPV, although it has also been reported with HFO, where there is an active expiration. For all these reasons, HFV techniques, and in particular HFJV, should be avoided in patients with airway obstruction or with an increase in airways resistance (Rouby *et al.*, 1985). Furthermore, negative hemodynamic effects have also been observed, neither related to the kind of HFV technique, nor to the high frequencies used, but to the action of the high mean airway pressure in the presence of altered thoracic and pulmonary compliances.

Another important clinical aspect concerning HFV is CO_2 monitoring. All these techniques employ sub-tidal volumes that cannot be directly measured. The difficulty to assess the adequacy of ventilation and CO_2 washout is one of the most important technical problems associated with these techniques. Recently, Kil *et al.* (2002) has measured capnographic curves and $P_{et}CO_2$ during discontinuation from HFJV (100 cycles/min) after 5–6 single breaths of conventional mechanical ventilation. They observed in 40 American Society of Anesthesiologist grade 1 (ASA1) patients undergoing laryngeal microsurgery that $P_{et}CO_2$ could closely reflect P_aCO_2 (Figure 19.5). An alternative way to find adequate ventilator settings during HFV is by using transcutaneous PCO_2 monitoring device (1998). Frietsch *et al.* (2000) found that monitoring of HFJV during prolonged rigid bronchoscopy is easily performed by capnography through the light channel of the rigid bronchoscope although the reliability of capnography was lost with flooded airways. It is of only limited value during endoscopic instrumentation with the concomitant airway obstruction. Therefore, non-invasive CO_2 monitoring represents an useful adjunct to the analysis of arterial blood gases and will probably reduce the number of invasive arterial blood gases during HFJV.

A different HFV technique is the high-frequency percussive ventilation (HFPV), introduced by F.M. Bird[1] as a rhythmic cyclic ventilation with flow regulation, which produces a controlled pressure. HFPV associates the positive aspects of controlled mechanical ventilation (CMV) with those of HFV. HFPV is delivered by a ventilatory circuit with a high-frequency flow supplier. A switch valve represents the real peculiarity of this ventilation technique, being an interface between the device and the simulator: this unit is called "Phasitron®". This device operates on the basis of the Venturi principle and delivers mini-bursts of air, with frequency and duration set by the operator (Branson, 1995; Lucangelo *et al.*, 2003). In the case shown in Figure 19.6, percussive frequency operates at 720 cycles/min, conventional mechanical ventilation frequency is 14 cycles/min, with an inspiration to expiration (I/E) ratio of 1/1. In clinical practice, the expiratory phase may be completely passive (Figure 19.6) or it may include a percussive oscillation (Figure 19.7).

HFPV was initially used for the treatment of acute respiratory diseases caused by burns and smoke inhalation (Loring *et al.*, 1983; Rodeberg *et al.*, 1984; Branson, 1995; Lentz & Peterson, 1997; Mlcak, 1996; Reper *et al.*, 1998), and in the treatment of the newborn affected by hyaline membrane disease or infant respiratory distress syndrome (Campbell *et al.*, 1991). Later on, there was a wider application in cases of severely compromised gas exchange, where conventional mechanical ventilation had failed. To date, the data reported in the literature have proved its effectiveness and safety in several types of disease, either affecting the respiratory system (e.g. ARDS, chest trauma) (Velmahos *et al.*, 1999), or in head- (Hurst *et al.*, 1988) and multiple-trauma patients (Hurst *et al.*, 1987), where the effects of conventional mechanic ventilation might compromise other organ functions. The peculiarity of this hybrid technique is that it allows $P_{et}CO_2$ and CO_2 tracings. However, the presence of

[1] Personal communication.

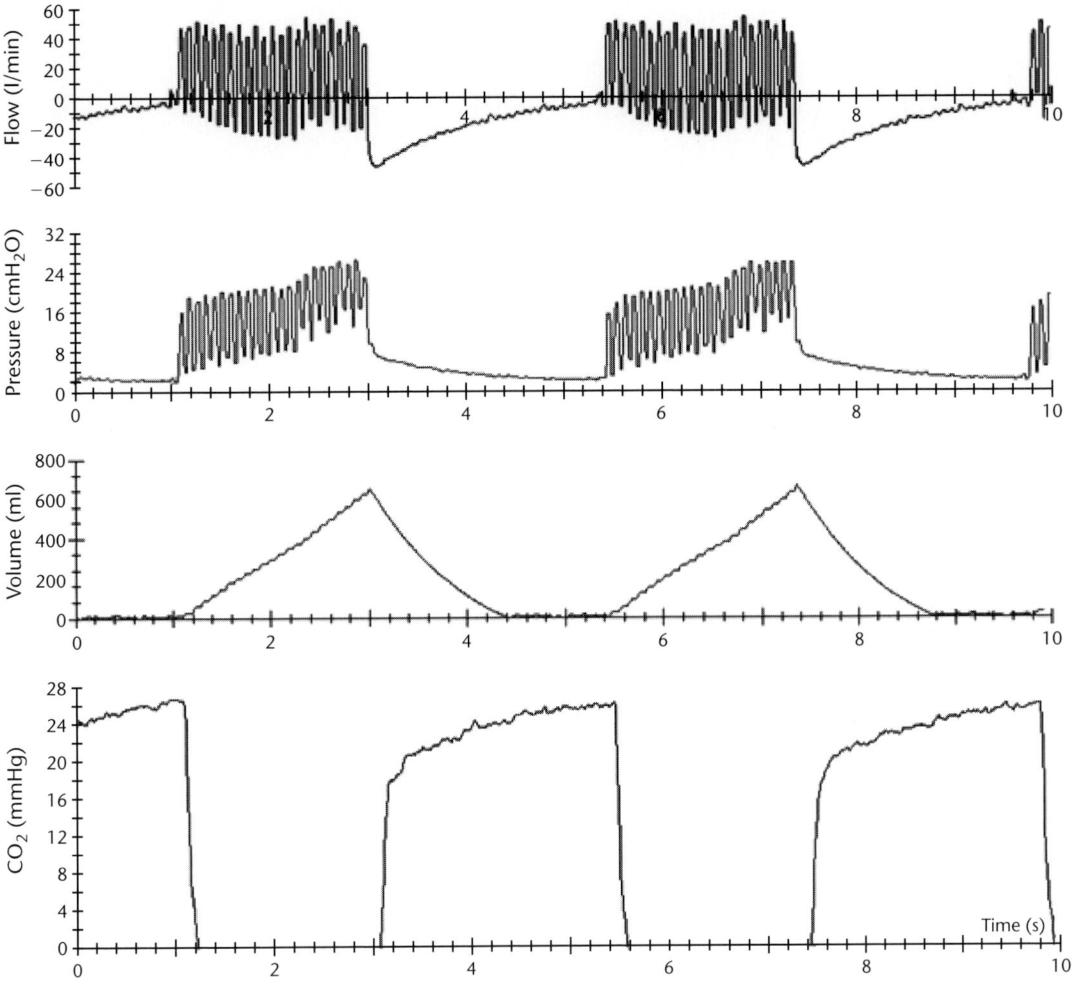

Figure 19.6 Flow, airway pressure, volume and CO_2 tracings during HFPV. Percussions are applied only during inspiratory phase and CO_2 waveform remains unaltered.

expiratory pulsatile flow does not enable a predictive correlation between P_aCO_2 and $P_{et}CO_2$. The capnographic trace stability allows a proper monitoring of HFPV ventilator setting at bedside (Lucangelo *et al.*, 2001, 2003). In this case, a combined transducer (mainstream capnograph plus a pneumotachograph) has been used at a sampling frequency of 100 Hz (CO_2SMO Plus!, Respironics-Novametrix).

Inhalation medication

Drug delivery via airways during mechanical ventilation is a common practice and for some medications is the preferred route. In these patients, several medications with different properties may be given by direct instillation or as an aerosol. Among these therapies are bronchodilators, perfluorocarbons, vasoactive drugs, surfactant, antibiotics, anti-inflammatory drugs, mucolytics, inmunomodulating substances and gene therapy. During mechanical ventilation, inhaled bronchodilator drugs significantly decrease inspiratory airway resistance in patients with chronic obstructive pulmonary disease and in patients with acute asthma (Dhand & Tobin, 1997). Decreased resistance is associated, at a given tidal volume, with a reduced ventilator inspiratory pressure. Moreover, because resistance to expiratory flow might also be reduced, less dynamic hyperinflation favors CO_2 elimination. You *et al.* (1994) demonstrated significant correlations between spirometry and several capnographic indices and concluded that the capnogram shape is a quantitative method for evaluating the severity of bronchospasm. Yaron *et al.* (1996) found

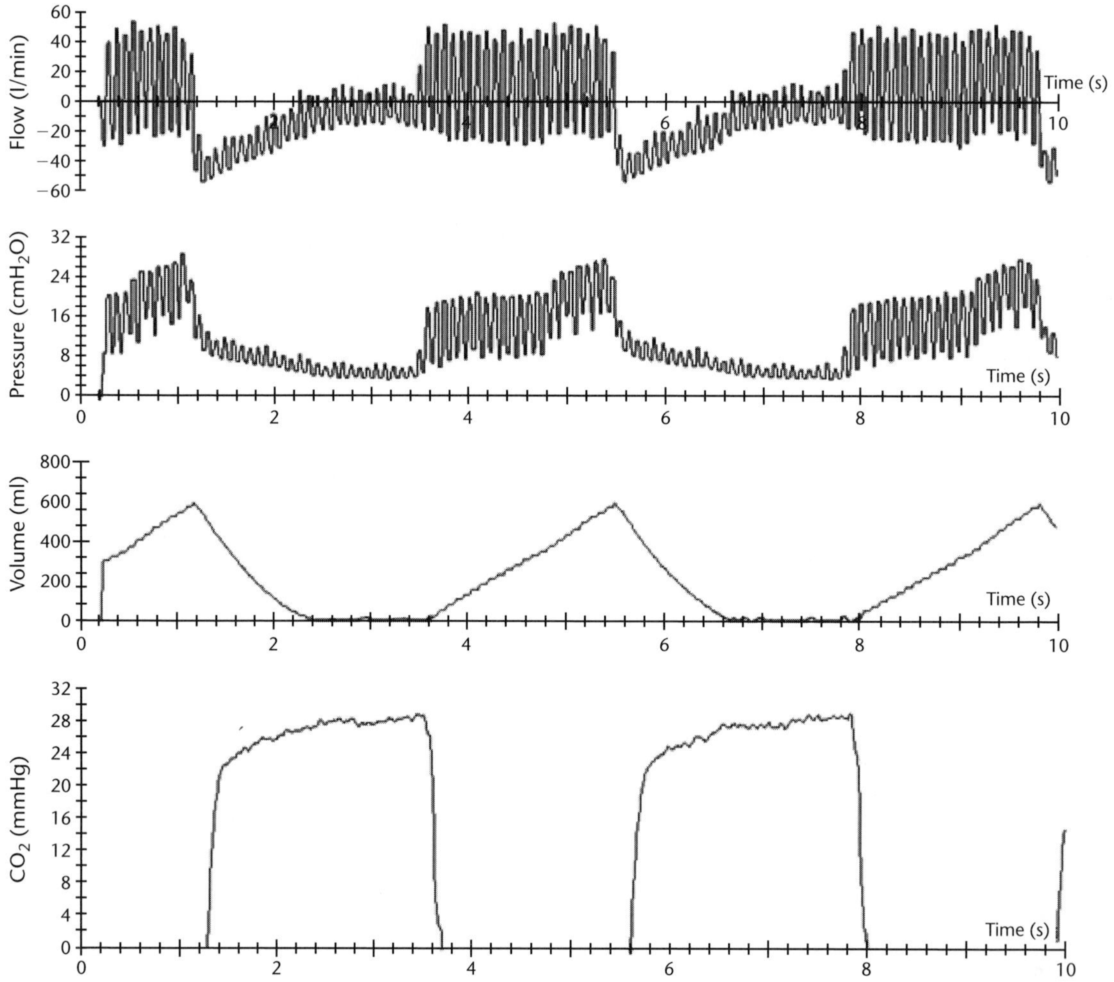

Figure 19.7 Flow, airway pressure, volume and CO_2 tracings during HFPV. Percussions are applied during both inspiratory and expiratory phases. Note that percussion does not affect expired capnogram despite low pressure percussive oscillatory trend.

significant changes in peak expiratory flow rates and in the plateau phase of the expiratory capnogram in asthmatic subjects after inhaled beta-agonist therapy. In fact, a correlation of spirometry or lung mechanics and capnographic indices is usually found as bronchospasm is relieved or when dynamic hyperinflation is improved (Blanch *et al.*, 1994).

Partial liquid ventilation (PLV) with perfluorocarbons (Tutuncü *et al.*, 1993a, b; Hirschl *et al.*, 1996) has been proposed as a new modality to recruit lung units in ALI. Perfluorocabon, due to its low surface tension and high density (1.91 g/cm^3) may facilitate opening of collapsed, non-compliant dependent lung segments. Consequently, perfluorocarbon may function as "liquid PEEP", preventing complete collapse of unstable alveoli even at low airway pressures, thereby improving oxygenation and decreasing shear forces acting on the lung parenchyma. The amount of PEEP needed to optimize gas exchange during PLV in a lung lavage model of ALI has been found to be approximately 10 cmH_2O (Blanch *et al.*, 2001b; Kirmse *et al.*, 1998). The impact of PLV on CO_2 elimination have been recently studied. Mates *et al.* (1996) found that PLV resulted in CO_2 retention and increased aCO_2–ACO_2 difference at similar ventilator settings. Moreover, negative phase III slopes of CO_2 expirograms occurred during PLV when perfluorocarbon was heterogeneously distributed and flooded regions characterized by prolonged emptying times and low P_ACO_2 empty late in expiration (Figure 19.8).

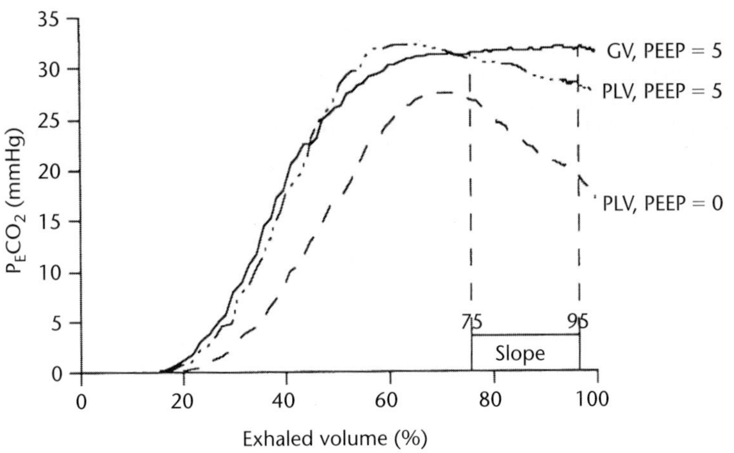

Figure 19.8 P_ECO_2 as a function of exhaled volume (mean of 8 breaths) during gas ventilation (GV) at PEEP of 5 cmH_2O (GV), during PLV at PEEP 0 and 5 cmH_2O. A negative slope of exhaled CO_2 is observed during PLV + PEEP and magnified after PEEP removal. See text for explanation. (Reproduced with permission from Mates, E.A., Tarczy-Hornoch, P., Hildebrandt, J., Jackson, J.C. & Hlastala, M.P. (1996). Negative slope of exhaled CO_2 profile. Implications for ventilation heterogeneity during partial liquid ventilation. *Adv. Exp. Med. Biol.*, **388**: 585–597.)

Conclusions

The advanced technology combination of airway flow monitoring and mainstream capnography allows breath-by-breath calculation of the pulmonary dead-space and CO_2 elimination at the bedside. For these reasons, the use of volumetric capnography is clinically advantageous. Measurement of dead-space fraction early in the course of the acute respiratory failure may provide clinicians important physiologic and prognostic information. Further studies are warranted to assess whether the continuous measurement of different derived capnographic indices is useful for risk identification and stratification, and to track the effect of a therapeutic intervention during the course of the disease in critically ill patients.

References

The Acute Respiratory Distress Syndrome Network (2000). Ventilation with lower tidal volumes compared with traditional tidal volumes for acute lung injury and the acute respiratory distress syndrome. *New Engl. J. Med.*, **342**: 1301–1308.

Amato, M.B., Barbas, C.S., Medeiros, D.M., Magaldi, R.B., *et al.* (1998). Effect of a protective-ventilation strategy on mortality in the acute respiratory distress syndrome. *New Engl. J. Med.*, **338**: 347–354.

Beydon, L., Uttman, L., Rawal, R. & Jonson, B. (2002). Effects of positive end-expiratory pressure on dead space and its partitions in acute lung injury. *Intens. Care Med.*, **28**: 1239–1245.

Biro, P., Eyrich, G. & Rohling, R. (1998). The efficiency of CO_2 elimination during high frequency jet ventilation for laryngeal microsurgery. *Anesth. Analg.*, **87**: 180–184.

Blanch, L., Fernandez, R., Benito, S., Mancebo, J. & Net, A. (1987). Effect of PEEP on the arterial minus end-tidal carbon dioxide gradient. *Chest*, **92**: 451–454.

Blanch, L., Fernandez, R. & Artigas, A. (1991). The effect of autoPEEP on the P_aCO_2–$P_{et}CO_2$ gradient and expired CO_2 slope in critically ill patients during total ventilatory support. *J. Crit. Care*, **6**: 202–210.

Blanch, L., Roussos, C., Brotherton, S., Michel, R.P. & Angle, M.R. (1992a). Effect of tidal volume and PEEP in ethclorvynol-induced asymetric lung injury. *J. Appl. Physiol.*, **73**: 108–116.

Blanch, L., Fernández, R., Baigorri, F., Valles, J. & Artigas, A. (1992b). Efecto del volumen corriente y de la posición sobre la oxigenación y la mecánica pulmonar en pacientes afectos de neumonía unilateral ventilados mecanicamente. *Med. Intens.*, **16**: 318–323.

Blanch, L., Fernandez, R., Saura, P., Baigorri, F. & Artigas, A. (1994). Relationship between expired capnogram and respiratory system resistance in critically ill patients during total ventilatory support. *Chest*, **105**: 219–223.

Blanch, L., Lucangelo, U., Lopez-Aguilar, J., Fernandez, R. & Romero, P. (1999). Volumetric capnography in patients with acute lung injury: effects of positive end-expiratory pressure. *Eur. Respir. J.*, **13**: 1048–1054.

Blanch, L. (2001). Clinical studies of tracheal gas insufflation. *Respir. Care*, **46**: 158–166.

Blanch, L., Van der Kloot, T.E., Youngblood, A.M., Murias, G., *et al.* (2001a). Application of tracheal gas insufflation to acute unilateral lung injury in an experimental model. *Am. J. Respir. Crit. Care Med.*, **164**: 642–647.

Blanch, L., Van der Kloot, T.E., Youngblood, A.M., Adams, A.B., *et al.* (2001b). Selective tracheal gas insufflation during partial liquid ventilation improves lung function in an animal model of unilateral acute lung injury. *Crit. Care Med.*, **29**: 2251–2257.

Borg, U., Eriksson, I. & Sjostrand, U. (1980). High frequency positive-pressure ventilation (HFPPV): a review based upon its use during bronchoscopy and for laryngoscopy and microlaryngeal surgery under anesthesia. *Anesth. Analg.*, **59**: 594–603.

Bowie, J.R., Smith, R.A. & Downs, J.B. (1993). Absence of a capnogram after positive end-expiratory pressure. *J. Clin. Monit.*, **9**: 78–80.

Branson, R.D. (1995). High-frequency ventilators. In: Branson, R.D., Hess, D.R. & Chatburn, R.L. (eds) *Respiratory Care Equipment*. Lippincott; pp. 458–467.

Carlon, G.C., Ray Jr, C., Klein, R., Goldiner, P.L. & Miodownik, S. (1978). Criteria for selective positive end-expiratory pressure and independent synchronized ventilation of each lung. *Chest*, **74**: 501–507.

Craven, K.D., Oppenheimer, L. & Wood, L.D.H. (1979). Effects of contusion and flail chest on pulmonary perfusion and oxygen exchange. *J. Appl. Physiol.*, **47**: 729–737.

Coffey, R.L., Albert, R.K. & Robertson, H.T. (1983). Mechanisms of physiologic dead space response to PEEP after acute oleic acid lung injury. *J. Appl. Physiol.*, **55**: 1550–1557.

Campbell, P.J., Chilton, H.W., Garvey, P.A. & Gupta, J.M. (1991). Volumetric diffusive respirator use in neonatal respiratory failure. *J. Paediatr. Child Health*, **27**: 31–33.

Cinnella, G., Dambrosio, M., Brienza, N., Giuliani, R., Bruno, F., Fiore, T. & Brienza, A. (2001). Independent lung ventilation in patients with unilateral pulmonary contusion. Monitoring with compliance and $ETCO_2$. *Intens. Care Med.*, **27**: 1860–1867.

Crotti, S., Mascheroni, D., Caironi, P., Pelosi, P., *et al.* (2001). Recruitment and derecruitment during acute respiratory failure. A clinical study. *Am. J. Respir. Crit. Care Med.*, **164**: 131–140.

Dhand, R. & Tobin, M.J. (1997). Inhaled bronchodilator therapy in mechanically ventilated patients. *Am. J. Respir. Crit. Care Med.*, **156**: 3–10.

Engel, L.A. (1985). Intraregional gas mixing and distribution. In: Engel, L.A., Paiva, M. (eds) *Gas Mixing and Distribution in the Lung*. Marcel Dekker, Inc., New York. pp. 287–358.

Fowler, W.S. (1948). Lung function studies II: the respiratory dead-space. *Am. J. Physiol.*, **154**: 405–410.

Fletcher, R., Jonson, B., Cumming, G. & Brew, J. (1981). The concept of dead space with special reference to the single breath test for carbon dioxide. *Br. J. Anesth.*, **53**: 77–88.

Fort, P., Farmer, C., Westerman, J., Johannigman, J., Beninati, W., Dolan, S. & Derdak, S. (1997). High frequency oscillatory ventilation for adult respiratory distress syndrome – a pilot study. *Crit. Care Med.*, **25**: 937–947.

Frietsch, T., Krafft, P., Becker, H.D., Buelzebruck, H. & Wiedemann, K. (2000). Intermittent capnography during high-frequency jet ventilation for prolonged rigid bronchoscopy. *Acta Anesthesiol. Scand.*, **44**: 391–397

Feihl, F. (2003). Respiratory dead space and survival in the acute respiratory distress syndrome. In: Gullo, A. (ed.) *Anesthesia Pain Intensive Care and Emergency Medicine*, Vol.1. Springer, Berlin/Heidelberg/New York; pp. 275–287.

Gioia, F.R. & Rogers, M.C. (1985). High-frequency ventilation of the lungs. In: Atkinson, R.S. and Adams, A. (eds) *Recent Advances in Anaesthesia and Analgesia*. Churchill Livingstone, London; pp. 63–78.

Gattinoni, L., Pelosi, P., Crotti, S. & Valenza, F. (1995). Effects of positive end-expiratory pressure on regional distribution of tidal volume and recruitment in adult respiratory distress syndrome. *Am. J. Respir. Crit. Care Med.*, **151**: 1807–1814.

Hurst, J.M., Branson, R.D. & DeHaven, C.B. (1987). The role of high-frequency ventilation in post-traumatic respiratory insufficiency. *J. Trauma*, **27**: 236–241.

Hurst, J.M., Branson, R.D. & Davis, K. (1988). High-frequency percussive ventilation in the management of elevated intracranical pressure. *J. Trauma*, **28**: 1363–1367.

Hess, D. (1990). Capnometry and capnography: technical aspects, physiologic aspects, and clinical applications. *Respir. Care*, **35**: 557–576.

Hirschl, R.B., Pranikoff, T., Wise, C., Overbeck, M.C., *et al.* (1996). Initial experience with partial liquid ventilation in adult patients with the acute respiratory distress syndrome. *J. Am. Med. Assoc.*, **275**: 383–389.

Kanarek, D.J. & Shannon, D.C. (1975). Adverse effect of positive end-expiratory pressure on pulmonary perfusion and arterial oxygenation. *Am. Rev. Respir. Dis.*, **112**: 457–459.

Kalfon, P., Rao, G.S., Gallart, L., Puybasset, L., Coriat, P. & Rouby, J.J. (1997). Permissive hypercapnia with and without expiratory washout in patients with severe acute respiratory distress syndrome. *Anesthesiology*, **87**: 6–17.

Kuo, P.H., Wu, H.D., Yu, C.J., Yang, S.C., Lai, Y.L. & Yang, P.C. (1996). Efficacy of tracheal gas insufflation in acute respiratory distress syndrome with permissive hypercapnia. *Am. J. Respir. Crit. Care Med.*, **154**: 612–616.

Kirmse, M., Fujino, Y., Hess, D. & Kacmarek, R.M. (1998). Positive end-expiratory pressure improves gas exchange and pulmonary mechanics during partial liquid ventilation. *Am. J. Respir. Crit. Care Med.*, **158**:1550–1556.

Kil, H.K., Kim, O.W., Choi, H.S. & Nam, Y.T. (2002). Monitoring of $P_{et}CO_2$ during high frequency jet ventilation for laryngomicrosurgery. *Yonsei Med. J.*, **43**: 20–24.

Light, R.B., Mink, S.N. & Wood, L.D.H. (1981). The effect of unilateral unilateral PEEP on gas exchange and pulmonary perfusion in canine lobar pneumonia. *Anesthesiology*, **55**: 251–255.

Loring, W.R. III, Cioffi. W.G., Mason, A.D., McManus, W.F. & Pruitt, B.A. (1983). Improved survival of burned patients with inhalation injury. *Arch. Surg.*, **128**: 772–780.

Lentz, C.W. & Peterson, H.D. (1997). Smoke Inhalation is a Multilevel Insult to the Pulmonary System. *Curr. Opin. Pulm. Med.*, **3**: 221–226.

Lucangelo, U., Fontanesi, F. & Bird, F.M. (2001). High-frequency percussive ventilation. In: Gullo, A. (ed.) *Anaesthesia, Pain, Intensive Care and Emergency Medicine – APICE*. Springer-Verlag. pp. 163–171.

Lucangelo, U., Fontanesi, L., Antonaglia, V., Antolini, F., Berlot, G., Liguori, G. & Gullo, A. (2003a). High frequency percussive ventilation (HFPV). Case Reports. *Minerva Anestesiol.*, **69**: 853–857, 858–860.

Lucangelo, U., Fontanesi, L., Antonaglia, V., Pellis, T., *et al.* (2003b). High frequency percussive ventilation (HFPV). Principles and techniques. *Minerva Anestesiol.*, **69**: 841-848, 848–851.

Mink, S.N., Light, R.B. & Wood, L.H.D. (1981). Effect of PEEP on gas exchange and pulmonary perfusion in canine lobar pneumonia. *J. Appl. Physiol.*, **50**: 517–523.

Meyer, M., Mohr, M., Schulz, H. & Piiper, J. (1990). Sloping alveolar plateaus of CO_2, O_2, and intravenously infused C_2H_2 and $CHClF_2$ in the dog. *Respir. Physiol.*, **81**: 137–152.

Mates, E.A., Tarczy-Hornoch, P., Hildebrandt, J., Jackson, J.C. & Hlastala, M.P. (1996). Negative slope of exhaled CO_2 profile. Implications for ventilation heterogeneity during partial liquid ventilation. *Adv. Exp. Med. Biol.*, **388**: 585–597.

Mlcak, R.P. (1996). Ventilation Strategies for Smoke Inhalation. *J. Resp. Care Practitioners*, 103–106.

Mehta, S., Lapinsky, S.E., Hallett, D.C., Merker, D., *et al.* (2001). Prospective trial of high frequency oscillation in adult with acute respiratory distress syndrome. *Crit. Care Med.*, **29**: 1360–1369.

Nahum, A., Burke, W.C., Ravenscraft, S.A., Marcy, T.W., Adams, A.B., Crooke, P.S. & Marini, J.J. (1992a). Lung mechanics and gas exchange during pressure-control ventilation in dogs. Augmentation of CO_2 elimination by an intratracheal catheter. *Am. Rev. Respir. Dis.*, **146**: 965–973.

Nahum, A., Ravenscraft, S.A., Nakos, G., Burke, W.C., Adams, A.B., Marcy, T.W. & Marini, J.J. (1992b). Tracheal gas insufflation during pressure-control ventilation. Effect of the catheter position, diameter and flow rate. *Am. Rev. Respir. Dis.*, **146**: 1411–1418.

Nahum, A., Shapiro, R.S., Ravenscraft, S.A., Adams, A.B. & Marini, J.J. (1995). Efficacy of expiratory tracheal gas insufflation in a canine model of lung injury. *Am. J. Respir. Crit. Care Med.*, **152**: 489–495.

Nuckton, T.J., Alonso, J.A., Kallet, R.H., Daniel, B.M., Pittet, J.F., Eisner, M.D. & Matthay, A. (2002). Pulmonary dead-space fraction as a risk factor for death in the acute respiratory distress syndrome. *New Eng. J. Med.*, **346**: 1281–1286.

Oberg, P.A. & Sjostrand, U. (1969). Studies of blood pressure regulation. In: Common carotid artery clamping in studies of the carotid-sinus baroreceptor control of the systemic blood pressure. *Acta. Physiol. Scand.*, **75**: 276–287.

Piiper, J. & Scheid, P. (1987). Diffusion and convection in intrapulmonary gas mixing. In: Fishman, A.P., Farhi, L.E., Tenney, S.M. & Geiger, S.R. (eds) *Handbook of Physiology*, Section 3, *The Respiratory System*, Vol. IV. American Physiological Society, Bethesda, Maryland; pp. 51–69.

Pelosi, P., Cereda, M., Foti, G., Giacomini, M. & Pesenti, A. (1995). Alterations of lung and chest wall mechanics in patients with acute lung injury: effects of positive end-expiratory pressure. *Am. J. Respir. Crit. Care Med.*, **152**: 531–537.

Pelosi, P., Crotti, S., Brazzi, L. & Gattinoni, L. (1996). Computed tomography in adult respiratory distress syndrome: what has it taught us? *Eur. Respir.*, **9**: 1055–1062.

Puybasset, L., Cluzel, P., Chao, N., Slutsky, A.S., Coriat, P. & Rouby, J.J. (1998). A computed tomography scan assessment of regional lung volume in acute lung injury. *Am. J. Respir. Crit. Care Med.*, **158**: 1644–1654.

Puybasset, L., Gusman, P., Muller, J.C., Cluzel, P., Coriat, P. & Rouby, J.J. (2000). Regional distribution of gas and tissue in acute respiratory distress syndrome III. Consequences for the effects of positive end-expiratory pressure. *Intens. Care Med.*, **26**: 1215–1227.

Rodeberg, D.A., Housinger, T.A. & Warden, G.D. (1984). Improved ventilation function in burn patients using volumetric diffuse ventilation. *J. Am. Coll. Surg.*, **179**: 518–522.

Rouby, J.J., Simonneau, G., Benhamou, D. & Sartene, R., *et al.* (1985). Factors influencing pulmonary volumes and CO_2 elimination during high-frequency jet ventilation. *Anesthesiology*, **63**: 473–482.

Ravenscraft, S.A., Burke, W.C., Nahum, A., Adams, A.B., Nakos, G., Marcy, T.W. & Marini, J.J. (1993). Tracheal gas insufflation augments CO_2 clearance during mechanical ventilation. *Am. Rev. Respir. Dis.*, **148**: 345–351.

Ream, R.S., Screiner, M.S., Neff, J.D., McRae, K.M., Jawad, A.F., Scherer, P.W. & Neufeld, G.R. (1995). Volumetric capnography in children. Influence of growth of the alveolar plateau slope. *Anesthesiology*, **82**: 64–73.

Romero, P.V., Lucangelo, U., Lopez-Aguilar, J., Fernandez, R. & Blanch, L. (1997). Physiologically based indices of volumetric capnography in patients receiving mechanical ventilation. *Eur. Respir. J.*, **10**: 1309–1315.

Reper, P., Dankaert, R., van Hille, F., van Laeke, P., Duinslaeger, L. & Vanderkelen, A. (1998). The usefulness of combined high frequency percussive ventilation during acute respiratory failure after smoke inhalation. *Burns*, **24**: 34–38.

Richecoeur, J., Lu, Q., Vieira, S.R., Puybasset, L., Kalfon, P., Coriat, P. & Rouby, J.J. (1999). Expiratory washout versus optimization of mechanical ventilation during permissive hypercapnia in patients with severe acute respiratory distress syndrome. *Am. J. Respir. Crit. Care Med.*, **160**: 77–85.

Suter, P.M., Fairley, H.B. & Isenberg, I. (1975). Optimum end-expiratory pressure in patients with acute pulmonary failure. *New Engl. J. Med.*, **292**: 284–289.

Saura, P., Lucangelo, U., Blanch, L., Artigas, A., Mas, A. & Fernandez, R. (1996). Factores determinantes de la reducción de la P_aCO_2 con la insuflación de gas traqueal en pacientes con lesión pulmonar aguda. *Med. Intens.*, **20**: 246–251.

Smith, R.P.R. & Fletcher, R. (2000). Positive end-expiratory pressure has little effect on carbon dioxide elimination after cardiac surgery. *Anesth. Analg.*, **90**: 85–88.

Tutuncü, A.S., Faithfull, N.S. & Lachmann, B. (1993a). Intratracheal perfluorocarbon administration combined with mechanical ventilation in experimental respiratory distress syndrome: dose-dependent improvement of gas exchange. *Crit. Care Med.*, **21**: 962–969.

Tutuntü, A.S., Faithfull, N.S. & Lachmann, B. (1993b). Comparison of ventilatory support with intratracheal perfluorocarbon administration and conventional mechanical ventilation in animals with acute respiratory failure. *Am. Rev. Respir. Dis.*, **148**: 785–792.

Velmahos, G.C., Chan, L.S., Tatevossian, R., Cornwell, III E.E., Dougherty, W.R., Escudero, J. & Demetriades, D. (1999). High-frequency percussive ventilation improves oxygenation in patients with ARDS. *Chest*, **116**: 440–446.

Vieira, S.R., Puybasset, L., Lu, Q., Richecoeur, J., Cluzel, P., Coriat, P. & Rouby, J.J. (1999). A scanographic assessment of pulmonary morphology in acute lung injury. Significance of the lower inflection point detected on the lung pressure-volume curve. *Am. J. Respir. Crit. Care Med.*, **159**: 1612–1623.

You, B., Peslin, R., Duvivier, C., Vu, V.D. & Grilliat, J.P. (1994). Expiratory capnography in asthma: evaluation of various shape indices. *Eur. Respir. J.*, **7**: 318–323.

Yaron, M., Padyk, P., Hutsinpiller, M. & Cairns, C.B. (1996). Utility of the expiratory capnogram in the assessment of bronchospasm. *Ann. Emerg. Med.*, **28**: 403–407.

CIRCULATION: TRANSPORT OF CARBON DIOXIDE AND PULMONARY BLOOD FLOW

SECTION **1f**

CARDIOPULMONARY RESUSCITATION 20

D.C. Cone, J.C. Cahill & M.A. Wayne

Introduction

Sudden cardiac death accounts for approximately 1000 deaths per day in the US. Sudden cardiac death is not a single clinical entity or disease process; rather, it is a syndrome and the final step in a wide variety of fatal processes. The emergency medical services (EMS) system of the US and of other nations is largely geared toward responding to and attempting to resuscitate victims of out-of-hospital cardiac arrest (OOHCA), despite discouraging statistics indicating that very few of these patients are in fact successfully resuscitated. In most EMS systems, OOHCA survival percentages are in the single digits (Becker *et al.*, 1991; Lombardi *et al.*, 1994; International Guidelines 2000 Conference on Cardiopulmonary Resuscitation and Emergency Cardiac Care, 2000).

One of the key treatment modalities for cardiac arrest of any cause is cardiopulmonary resuscitation (CPR). CPR consists essentially of manual compression of the patient's chest in an effort to create forward blood flow, combined with periodic mouth-to-mouth or mechanically aided ventilation in an effort to deliver oxygen to the lungs. Although having another person attempt to palpate a carotid, femoral, or other pulse during chest compressions may provide some assessment of the success of the compressions (a palpable pulse accompanying each compression suggests reasonable forward blood flow through the circulatory system), there has been no method devised for non-invasively monitoring the effectiveness of CPR in real time. Capnography may provide a means for such monitoring.

In the majority of cases, CPR and other treatment efforts are unsuccessful, and the patient is eventually pronounced dead. A number of clinical indicators can be used to determine when those efforts should be terminated, including degeneration of the electrical rhythm of the heart to asystole, despite electrical and chemical treatment (Bailey *et al.*, 2000), or the absence of any cardiac movement on ultrasonographic imaging (Blaivas & Fox, 2001). The former method requires only a portable electrocardiograph, found on advanced life support rescue vehicles worldwide, while the latter requires an ultrasound machine, a device that has just begun to be employed in the out-of-hospital setting. Capnography can likely provide another clinical indicator of death, guiding decisions to terminate resuscitative efforts. This chapter will discuss two roles for capnography in the assessment and treatment of patients in cardiac arrest: evaluation of the efficacy of CPR and cessation of resuscitation.

Cardiac output, end-tidal carbon dioxide, and CPR

A number of animal studies have shown an excellent correlation between end-tidal carbon dioxide ($ETCO_2$) and cardiac output during states of low flow (Isserles & Breen, 1991; Idris *et al.*, 1994; Jin *et al.*, 2000) and during CPR (Trevino *et al.*, 1985; Weil *et al.*, 1985; Grundler *et al.*, 1986; Gudipati *et al.*, 1988). Human studies have found the same (Falk *et al.*, 1988; Ornato *et al.*, 1990; Shibutani *et al.*, 1994; Blumenthal & Voorhees, 1997b), though one study found this relationship to be logarithmic (Ornato *et al.*, 1990), while others have found it to be linear (Falk *et al.*, 1988; Shibutani *et al.*, 1994). If CO_2 production and ventilation are relatively constant during CPR (Kern *et al.*, 1992), one would expect $ETCO_2$ to reflect the pulmonary blood flow generated by CPR. However, only when ventilation is relatively constant can $ETCO_2$ accurately reflect circulatory status (Kalenda, 1978; Weil *et al.*, 1985; Garnett *et al.*, 1987; Shibutani *et al.*, 1994; Blumenthal & Voorhees, 1997a, b; Jin *et al.*, 2000). The interpretation of $ETCO_2$ in the field must take into account that controlled ventilations may be difficult or impossible when CPR is being interrupted as the patient is being moved or rescuers change positions. It is also not clear whether changes in the ratio of alveolar dead-space to tidal volume (V_{DS}/V_T) can affect the correlation between $ETCO_2$ and cardiac output (Isserles & Breen, 1991; Shibutani *et al.*, 1994).

Several researchers have suggested that the close correlation between cardiac output and $ETCO_2$ readings might be utilized to monitor, in real time, the effectiveness of CPR (Garnett *et al.*, 1987; Lepilin *et al.*, 1987; Gudipati *et al.*, 1988; Ward *et al.*, 1993; Blumenthal & Voorhees, 1997a). The first such suggestion appears to have come in 1978, when Kalenda (1978) calling $ETCO_2$, during constant ventilation, a "precise and constant mirror of lung perfusion and hence of cardiac output", published a series of three patients being monitored with capnography during CPR. This paper reported a decrease in $ETCO_2$ as the person performing CPR fatigued, followed by an increase in $ETCO_2$ as a new rescuer took over, presumably providing better chest compressions. He also demonstrated a gradual diminution then loss of $ETCO_2$ in patients not resuscitated, and a significant rise in $ETCO_2$ in a patient who regained a spontaneous pulse. Kalenda (1978) concludes with a single sentence: "The value of capnography as a guide to the efficacy of cardiac massage is clearly demonstrated."

Other studies have borne out this conclusion. Falk *et al.* (1988) studied 13 cardiac arrests in 10 patients and found that $ETCO_2$ decreased from a mean of 1.4% pre-arrest to 0.4% after the onset of cardiac arrest. It then increased to 1.0% with CPR. Return of spontaneous circulation (ROSC) was heralded with a rapid increase to 3.7% (presumably as forward flow improved abruptly), followed by stabilization at 2.4% 4 min later. In those patients where ROSC was not achieved, $ETCO_2$ remained at an average of 0.7%. The authors suggest that routine monitoring of $ETCO_2$ at the bedside, or in any other location, including the field, would be preferable to palpation of the carotid pulse (Gudipati *et al.*, 1988) in monitoring the effectiveness of CPR.

An animal study tested the feasibility of using the volume of CO_2 excreted[1] (CO_2ex) in the airway as a non-invasive measure of CPR efficacy (Blumenthal & Voorhees, 1997a). It was found that cardiac output accounted for greater than 65% of the variability seen in CO_2ex during CPR. The authors indicate that despite the ability of their method carefully to control alveolar ventilation, other variables, such as tissue perfusion, could not be controlled. Changes in regional blood flow during cardiac arrest and CPR can affect the amount of viable tissue (tissue that is still producing CO_2) and mobile CO_2 stores being perfused. Without a better understanding of changes in the stores of CO_2 in the body during low-flow and no-flow states (Voorhees *et al.*, 1980), the ability to interpret precisely $ETCO_2$ values during CPR will remain limited. Despite this limitation, the authors believe that the monitoring of CO_2 excretion does provide a reasonable overall picture of the level of perfusion achieved by CPR.

It should be noted that at least one study has found the relationship between cardiac output and $ETCO_2$ to be unreliable. In an animal model, using open-chest cardiac massage, delivering a constant cardiac output (as measured by a flow probe in the ascending aorta), $ETCO_2$ decreased over the first 5 min after the induction of ventricular fibrillation, but then gradually, but continuously, increased with CPR, for the 50 min duration of the protocol (Morimoto *et al.*, 1993). This occurred despite a constant cardiac output and was due primarily to an increase in CO_2 excretion, which the authors postulate might be due to an increase in pulmonary capillary blood flow over time, or an increase in CO_2 production, factors not directly measured. The authors believe that $ETCO_2$ readings may change over time during CPR even if cardiac output is constant. These changes may complicate estimating the effectiveness or prognostic value of CPR. A 1989 study by Sanders *et al.* (1989) showed a similar finding of a gradual, but significant, increase in $ETCO_2$, over time, in patients who were unable to be resuscitated. However, there was significantly less control of CPR technique, and thus of cardiac output, in this study.

A recent animal study found an excellent relationship ($r = 0.88$, $P < 0.001$) between $ETCO_2$ and stroke volume as measured with transesophageal echocardiographic (TEE) imaging (Pernat *et al.*, 2003). The authors of this study suggest that indicator dilution techniques generally used to measure cardiac output are less reliable under conditions of very low flow, as with CPR (van Grondelle *et al.*, 1983; Hillis *et al.*, 1986; Tournadre *et al.*, 1997). The TEE approach allowed investigators to confirm that $ETCO_2$ is quantitatively predictive of stroke volume index. The loss of reliability under low-flow conditions may explain some of the inconsistencies mentioned. TEE has yet to be introduced in human studies.

Several studies have used the relationship between $ETCO_2$ and cardiac output to test a third variable. Ward *et al.* (1993) in a series of 15 patients who had failed initial resuscitation attempts, provided either manual CPR or mechanical CPR, delivered by the Thumper® device (Michigan Instruments, Grand Rapids MI), while monitoring $ETCO_2$ to determine which provided a greater cardiac output. The mean $ETCO_2$ seen with manual CPR was 6.9 torr versus a mean of 13.6 torr with mechanical CPR ($P < 0.001$). While noting that the reasons for the apparently better cardiac output with the mechanical device were unclear, the authors suggest that monitoring $ETCO_2$

---

[1]
$$CO_2ex = \left[\frac{PCO_2}{\text{barometric pressure}}\right] \times (\text{tidal volume}) \times (\text{breaths/min})\ \text{ml/min/kg}$$

might help optimize chest compressions during CPR. In another study using the Thumper® device, Ornato *et al.* (1989) tested blood flow delivered by various CPR compression forces. They used radial artery pressure and $ETCO_2$ as determinants of blood flow.

Berg and coworkers used $ETCO_2$ to test audio-prompted rate guidance on the quality of pediatric CPR (Berg *et al.*, 1994). Although a somewhat higher $ETCO_2$ was measured during rate-prompted 100 compression/min CPR as compared to the baseline CPR, the difference was not significant (11 torr versus 4 torr, $P = 0.08$). However, $ETCO_2$ was significantly higher during rate-prompted 140 compression/min CPR than at baseline (12 torr versus 4 torr, $P < 0.05$). A similar study in adults found mean $ETCO_2$ values of 8.7 torr during baseline CPR, versus 14.0 during rate-prompted CPR at either 80 or 120 compressions/min ($P < 0.01$) (Kern *et al.*, 1992).

Coronary and cerebral perfusion pressure during CPR

Using a canine cardiac arrest model, a good correlation ($r = 0.78$, $P < 0.01$) between $ETCO_2$ and coronary perfusion pressure was found (Sanders *et al.*, 1985a). Another study published the same year by the same group, using slightly different techniques, found somewhat better results ($r = 0.91$, $P < 0.01$) (Sanders *et al.*, 1985b). It has been postulated that the higher cerebral perfusion pressure simply reflects better overall vascular tone during CPR, and that better vascular tone results in higher $ETCO_2$ via improved pulmonary blood flow (Asplin & White, 1995). However, the true physiologic relationship between coronary perfusion pressure and $ETCO_2$ remains unclear.

An animal model with ultrasound flow probes and radioactive microspheres was used to examine the relationships between $ETCO_2$ and cardiac output, cerebral perfusion, and renal perfusion (Lewis *et al.*, 1992). The correlation (r value) between $ETCO_2$ and cardiac output was 0.90, consistent with other studies discussed above. The correlation between $ETCO_2$ and cerebral blood flow was lower, but still significant ($r = 0.64$, $P = 0.01$). However, when *partial* correlation coefficients were determined, to ascertain whether $ETCO_2$ primarily correlated with cardiac output or with cerebral blood flow, values were $r = 0.70$ for cardiac output ($P < 0.05$) and $r = 0.30$ for cerebral perfusion ($P > 0.05$). This suggests that during CPR, $ETCO_2$ follows cardiac output and not cerebral blood flow; thus, cardiac output does not necessarily correlate with cerebral flow. The authors believe that this likely limits the usefulness of $ETCO_2$ as a non-invasive measure of cerebral flow during CPR.

Bicarbonate and epinephrine during CPR

It has been noted in a number of studies that $ETCO_2$ values may change transiently after the administration of intravenous epinephrine or sodium bicarbonate. This is not surprising in the case of sodium bicarbonate, which rapidly increases the overall CO_2 difference and thus the $ETCO_2$ reading (Garnett *et al.*, 1987). In general, this increase is not as large as is seen with ROSC, and is transient. In one study, for example, the readings increased from a mean of 0.8% to a mean of 2.1% (roughly 6–16 torr) after sodium bicarbonate was administered into the central circulation, but returned to baseline in 2 min (Falk *et al.*, 1988). Another study mentions a similar observation; the authors noted that $ETCO_2$ increases with the administration of bicarbonate, but then returns to baseline within 5 min. These data were not presented as part of that study, but appear to be observations that prompted them to discard $ETCO_2$ values obtained in the first 5 min after administration of sodium bicarbonate (Sanders *et al.*, 1989).

The case with epinephrine is more complex. Having anecdotally noted a decrease in $ETCO_2$ following epinephrine administration (Callaham & Barton, 1990), and noting similar findings from animal studies (Ralston *et al.*, 1985; Martin *et al.*, 1990) Callaham, Barton & Matthay (1992) prospectively studied this. $ETCO_2$ readings were taken on arrival at the emergency department (ED), and 4 min (or as close to 4 min as possible) after the administration of the largest dose of IV epinephrine. The $ETCO_2$ increased in 28% of the 64 subjects, decreased in 39%, and did not change in 33%. The average change was a decrease of 0.3 torr (not significant).

In a similar study, 20 OOHCA patients were examined (Cantineau *et al.*, 1994). $ETCO_2$ decreased from a mean of 16.7 torr prior to epinephrine administration, to a mean of 12.6 torr 3 min after peripheral IV injection of 2 mg of epinephrine ($P < 0.0001$). $ETCO_2$ decreased in 14 patients, and did not change in six. The authors acknowledge that the mechanism of the observed decrease is not known. And they postulated that the redistribution of blood flow resulting from the vasoconstriction of non-myocardial and non-cerebral vascular beds is associated with an increased afterload, likely altering pulmonary perfusion. A decrease in mixed venous CO_2 concentration may also be involved, though support for this mechanism is not compelling. Redistribution of blood flow within the lungs may also be involved (Tang *et al.*, 1991). Regardless of mechanism, Cantineau *et al.* (1994) recommend caution when interpreting $ETCO_2$ readings collected soon after epinephrine administration.

The most recent study of this phenomenon was conducted by Lindberg *et al.* (2000). In an animal model, the investigators found an *increase* in coronary perfusion pressure after either epinephrine or norepinephrine was administered, but a *decrease* in $ETCO_2$. The authors believe that the increase in coronary perfusion pressure reflects overall vasoconstriction, with redistribution of blood flow away from non-vital organs to selectively perfuse vital organs including the heart. At the same time, they believe that overall cardiac output is reduced due to increased afterload, causing the decrease in $ETCO_2$ they observed. Others have suggested that a decrease in $ETCO_2$ after vasopressor administration may be a marker of vasomotor responsiveness, a good prognostic sign (Callaham *et al.*, 1992).

$ETCO_2$ and prognosis during cardiac arrest

A number of studies, in both animals (Trevino *et al.*, 1985; Sanders *et al.*, 1985b; Gudipati *et al.*, 1988; Blumenthal & Voorhees, 1997b) and humans, have examined the prognostic capabilities of capnography for patients undergoing CPR. The first such study, by Sanders *et al.* (1985b) monitored $ETCO_2$ continuously during resuscitation from an induced cardiac arrest, and the mean $ETCO_2$ for each animal after the resuscitation interval was determined. It was found that this mean $ETCO_2$ was significantly higher for animals that were able to be resuscitated (using high-pressure chest compressions at 80 lb) than for those animals that could not be resuscitated (using low-pressure compressions at 40 lb) (mean of 9.6 torr versus 3.2 torr, $P < 0.01$).

In a particularly interesting animal study, Blumenthal and Voorhees (1997b) examined CO_2 excretion in an animal model, by measuring the partial pressure of CO_2 in the airway, then calculating total CO_2 excretion in ml/min/kg. The study found no differences before CPR (mean 13.81 ml/kg/min for survivors, 13.06 for non-survivors, $P = 0.57$), but a significant difference after 3 min of ventricular fibrillation and 13 min of CPR (mean 6.74 ml/kg/min for survivors, 4.88 for non-survivors, $P < 0.0001$). These values represent calculated CO_2 excretion, not raw $ETCO_2$ values; however, they do seem to support the findings of other studies: better values during CPR suggest a better prognosis. A "cutoff" value for survival of 7.0 ml/min/kg had a positive predictive value of 0.83, and a negative predictive value of 0.73. No animal with a CO_2 excretion rate of less than 5.0 ml/min/kg survived.

Unfortunately, in examining the human studies, it quickly becomes clear that differences in inclusion criteria (pulseless electrical activity versus all arrest rhythms), outcome measure (ROSC versus survival), setting (field versus ED versus in-hospital), and measure of central tendency reported (median versus mean $ETCO_2$ values) limit our ability to draw firm conclusions, or to establish a consensus "cutoff" or threshold value for terminating resuscitation efforts. Differing methodologies in terms of types of $ETCO_2$ readings compound the issue: some studies report the maximum reading obtained, and some report a reading taken after 1 or 2 min of capnographic monitoring. Table 20.1 summarizes the results of several of the human studies that are discussed here.

The first human study to examine the role of capnometry in the prediction of cardiac arrest survival was conducted in 1987. In an observational series of 23 patients who sustained OOHCA and were brought to the ED still in arrest, Garnett *et al.* (1987) calculated the mean of the $ETCO_2$ readings taken on five consecutive ventilator-assisted breaths, 3–5 min after ED arrival. They found no difference between the mean value for the 10 patients who obtained ROSC (1.7%) versus the 13 patients who did not obtain ROSC (1.8%). The authors contrast these findings to those of Sanders *et al.* (1985b) and postulate that the underlying chronic heart and lung disease found in typical OOHCA patients may cause them to differ significantly in terms of arrest physiology from the canines in the Sanders *et al.*, model discussed above.

The next human study of the prognostic value of $ETCO_2$ in cardiac arrest resuscitation involved 35 cardiac arrests in 34 patients (Sanders *et al.*, 1989). The nine patients who survived the resuscitation (defined as having a stable blood pressure when the resuscitation team was dismissed by the physician in charge) had higher average $ETCO_2$ readings during CPR than the 26 who did not, with means of 15 torr versus 7 torr ($P < 0.001$). The initial, final, maximum, and minimum readings were also all higher in the resuscitated patients. No patient with an average $ETCO_2$ reading of less than 10 torr was resuscitated. The three patients who survived to hospital discharge had higher average $ETCO_2$ readings than the 32 who did not leave the hospital, with means of 17 torr versus 8 torr ($P = 0.20$). Perhaps due to the small number of survivors, the initial, final, and maximum $ETCO_2$ values did not differ between these groups, though the minimum was higher in survivors than non-survivors.

Two additional studies confirmed these findings on ED patients (Callaham & Barton, 1990; Steedman & Robertson, 1990). It should be noted, however, that in the former study, while a cutoff of 15 torr yielded the best sensitivity and specificity for survival as determined

Table 20.1 Mean $ETCO_2$ levels for successful and unsuccessful cardiac arrest resuscitation

Study	Setting	*N*	Outcome measure	Reading taken	Success	No success	*P* value	Threshold value proposed	Sensitivity	Specificity	PPV	NPV
Garnett *et al.* (1987)	ED	23	ROSC	Mean of 5 breaths	1.7%	1.8%	Not given					
Voorhees *et al.* (1980)	ED and hosp	35	ROSC	Mean	15	7	<0.001	10	1.00	0.77	0.60	1.00
Callaham & Barton (1990)	ED	55	ROSC	1 min	19	5.2	<0.0001	15	0.71	0.98	0.91	0.91
Steedman & Robertson (1990)	ED	12	ROSC		2.63%	1.64%	<0.001					
Kern *et al.* (1992)	ED and hosp	23	ROSC	Mean	17.9	10.4	<0.01					
Callaham *et al.* (1992)	ED	64	ROSC					5	0.93	0.47	0.36	0.96
								10	0.40	0.87	0.50	0.82
								15	0.07	0.98	0.50	0.77
Asplin & White (1995)	EMS	27	ROSC	1 min	23.0	13.2	0.0002					
				2 min	26.8	15.4	0.0019					
				Max	30.8	22.7	0.0154					
Cantineau *et al.* (1996)	EMS	24	ROSC	Initial	18.4	10.2	<0.01					
				Min	13.9	7.5	<0.01					
				Max	29.9	18.1	<0.01					
	EMS	96						10	1.00	0.67		
Wayne *et al.* (1995)	EMS	90	ROSC	Initial	11.7	10.9	0.672					
				20 min	3.9	31	<0.0001	10	0.973	1.00	1.00	0.889
Levine *et al.* (1997)	EMS	150	adm to hosp	Initial	12.3	12.2	0.93					
				20 min	4.4	32.8	<0.001	10	1.00	1.00	1.00	1.00
Salen *et al.* (2001)	ED	53	adm to hosp	Peak	35*	13.7*	<0.01	16				
Grmec & Klemen (2001)	EMS	139	adm to hosp	Initial				10	1.00	0.90		
Grmec & Kupnik (2003)	EMS	246	adm to hosp	Initial	2.12 kPa	1.09 kPa	0.035	10	1.0	0.74		
			d/c from ICU	Initial	2.63 kPa	1.21 kPa	<0.01	10	1.0	0.80		

*Median value; all others are means. All readings are in torr, except where % or kPa is shown. PPV: positive predictive value; NPV: negative predictive value; EMS: out-of-hospital emergency medical services; ED: emergency department; hosp: hospital; ROSC: return of spontaneous circulation; adm: admission; d/c: discharge; ICU: intensive care unit; Max: maximum; Min: minimum.

with a receiver operating characteristics (ROC) curve, four patients who had both initial and later $ETCO_2$ readings of less than 10 torr were resuscitated. This led the authors to caution that a low $ETCO_2$ value might not be an adequate reason, by itself, to end resuscitative efforts (Callaham & Barton, 1990). The authors further advise that the ROC curve can allow the individual clinician to choose a threshold with levels of sensitivity and specificity that he or she feels are justified. It has been postulated that these data, and similar reports of ROSC after prolonged resuscitative attempts, with low $ETCO_2$ values (Cantineau *et al.*, 1994) may account for the reluctance of the scientific community to incorporate $ETCO_2$ monitoring into life support algorithms (Levine *et al.*, 1997).

One of the studies discussed above, comparing $ETCO_2$ at different chest compression rates, found that patients with ROSC had a mean $ETCO_2$ level of 17.9 torr, compared to a mean of 10.4 torr in those who did not achieve ROSC (Kern *et al.*, 1992). One of the studies examining the role of epinephrine examined several threshold values, using the first recorded $ETCO_2$ value upon the patient's arrival at the ED (Callaham *et al.*, 1992). Values are presented in the table; not surprisingly, sensitivity decreases and specificity increases as higher thresholds are chosen. No actual $ETCO_2$ values were reported.

Following a four-patient feasibility case series (White & Asplin, 1994), a study by Asplin & White (1995) conducted in the Rochester, MN EMS system, examined the role of $ETCO_2$ readings as determined by paramedics on victims of OOHCA, using an early portable capnograph weighing 3.6 kg. Monitoring was begun as soon as possible after endotracheal intubation and, not knowing when the optimal time for taking prognostic $ETCO_2$ readings might be, the authors collected data after 1 and 2 min, and the maximum $ETCO_2$ reading for each patient. The mean 1-, 2-min, and maximum values were all higher in those patients who demonstrated ROSC in the field than those who did not (P values of 0.0002, 0.0019, and 0.0154, respectively). With only three patients surviving to hospital discharge, no attempt was made to compare $ETCO_2$ values for survivors versus non-survivors.

A similar study published by Cantineau *et al.* (1996) found that in a derivation set of 24 patients, mean initial, minimum, and maximum $ETCO_2$ values recorded during the first 20 min of resuscitation were all higher in patients who experienced ROSC than those who did not. In a validation follow-up with 96 patients, the authors' proposed threshold of 10 torr provided 100% sensitivity and 67% specificity for ROSC. This contrasts with a study by Varon *et al.* (1991), which found a level of greater than 2% (roughly 14 torr) in all survivors of both OOHCA and in-hospital cardiac arrests; however, Varon's study involved the use of colorimetric $ETCO_2$ devices, with values based on estimates of color change.

A study by Wayne *et al.* (1995) in Whatcom County, Washington examined 90 patients with OOHCA. There was no difference in the *initial* $ETCO_2$ recorded by the paramedics (mean of 11.7 torr for those did not achieve ROSC in the field, versus 10.9 for those who did, $P = 0.672$), but after 20 min, a significant difference was noted (3.9 versus 31, $P < 0.0001$). Testing a hypothetical threshold of 10 torr for determining inability to resuscitate, no patient with a value below the threshold was resuscitated.

A follow-up study tested the *a priori* hypothesis that an $ETCO_2$ level of 10 torr or less, sustained for 20 min, would predict failure to survive OOHCA of the pulseless electrical activity type (Levine *et al.*, 1997). This study similarly found no difference in the initial $ETCO_2$ (mean of 12.3 for non-survivors versus 12.2 for survivors, $P = 0.93$), but a substantial difference at 20 min (mean of 4.4 versus 32.8, $P < 0.001$). No patient with a 20-min level of 10 torr or less survived; sensitivity, specificity, positive predictive value, and negative predictive value were all 100%, though an upper 99% binomial confidence limit of 3.9% was calculated and reported given the sample size.

One of several studies to examine the active compression/decompression CPR (ACD/CPR) technique used $ETCO_2$ as a marker for cardiac output, to compare the hemodynamics generated by the ACD/CPR method as compared to standard CPR in the out-of-hospital setting (Mauer *et al.*, 1998). The EMS physicians staffing the advanced life support units in this German study measured $ETCO_2$ immediately upon intubation, and every 2 min afterward until either ROSC was achieved, or 10 min had passed. Although no difference was found between the ACD/CPR and standard CPR groups, it was noted that median $ETCO_2$ values were higher at 0, 2, 4, 6, and 10 min in the group of patients who achieved ROSC in the field and were admitted to the hospital, compared to those who were pronounced dead at the scene. No patient who survived at least 6 h had an $ETCO_2$ level of less than 15 torr; however, sensitivity, specificity, and predictive values are not presented for this resuscitation threshold. It is worth noting that, in performing their power and sample size calculations, the authors used a reference value of 12 torr, citing the studies by Callaham & Barton (1990) and Sanders *et al.* (1989). Additionally, a rise in $ETCO_2$ was noted *prior* to a palpable pulse in patients with ROSC.

Salen *et al.* (2001) published a two-center study examining both cardiac ultrasonography and capnography as predictors of survival to hospital admission for patients undergoing ED resuscitation. The median peak $ETCO_2$ of those who ultimately survived the cardiac arrest was either 35 or 39 torr, significantly ($P < 0.01$) higher than those who did not survive (13.7 torr) (Salen *et al.*, 2001). (The paper's abstract, data table, and discussion section report 35 torr, while the results section and the accompanying editorial (Sanders *et al.*, 2001) use 39 torr.) No patient with an $ETCO_2$ of less than 16 torr survived the arrest, though one non-survivor did have an $ETCO_2$ of 48 torr. In multivariate logistic regression, each 1-torr increase in $ETCO_2$ was associated with 16% greater odds of surviving. Further, using a stepwise logistic regression model, the area under an ROC curve was 0.9096, showing excellent prediction of survival. Although not all patients in this study underwent both cardiac ultrasonography and capnography, higher $ETCO_2$ levels were more strongly associated with survival than was ultrasonographic evidence of cardiac movement.

Another study found that initial, final, maximum, minimum, and mean $ETCO_2$ values were all higher in patients who were resuscitated than in those who were not (Grmec & Klemen, 2001). No patient with an initial, mean, and final reading of less than 10 torr survived. A similar study (Grmec & Kupnik, 2003) was published in which capnography was added to the previously described Mainz Emergency Evaluation Scoring System (Grmec & Gasparovic, 2001). Initial and final $ETCO_2$ value were higher in those with ROSC versus those without, and those who survived (defined here as discharge from the intensive care unit) versus those who did not. All patients with ROSC, and all who survived, had initial $ETCO_2$ values of greater than 10 torr. These prehospital data, combined with the findings from Wayne *et al.* (1995), provide strong support for a resuscitation threshold of 10 torr in the field.

Finally, it should be noted that none of the above studies included trauma patients; all involved patients with "medical" cardiac arrest. It appears that only two studies have examined the use of $ETCO_2$ in trauma patients, and both of these were performed in the operating room (OR) (Wilson *et al.*, 1996; Tyburski *et al.*, 2002). In a retrospective study published in 1996, Wilson *et al.* (1996) examined the records of 100 critical trauma patients (40% mortality for the cohort). They found that patients with an initial $ETCO_2$ value of 28 torr or less experienced 57% mortality, compared to 30% mortality in those with readings of 29 torr or greater ($P = 0.016$). Similarly, patients with a final OR reading of 24 torr or lower experienced 59% mortality, compared to 24% mortality for those with a reading of 25 torr or higher ($P < 0.001$). In a prospective study published in 2002, this same group found that the *initial* $ETCO_2$ reading was lower in patients who survived their surgical resuscitation than in those who died (29 torr versus 33 torr, $P = 0.011$). A final reading of 27 torr or greater was associated with 5% mortality, while a reading of 24 torr or lower was associated with 68% mortality (Tyburski *et al.*, 2002). These authors comment on 59 patients with a post-resuscitation systolic blood pressure of greater than 120 mmHg. In this group, the "traditional" measures of trauma resuscitation (blood pressure, pH, HCO_3^-, and base deficit) did not correlate well with survival, but $ETCO_2$ did. This same pattern held when the authors examined systolic blood pressure thresholds of 110 mmHg or 100 mmHg. To date, it appears that no studies have been conducted of the measurement of $ETCO_2$ in critical trauma patients in the out-of-hospital setting.

In summary, it appears that $ETCO_2$ offers an effective tool to assist in evaluating the progress and results of medical resuscitation. We lack data to recommend an extrapolation to trauma patients.

References

Asplin, B.R. & White, R.D. (1995). Prognostic value of end-tidal carbon dioxide pressures during out-of-hospital cardiac arrest. *Ann. Emerg. Med.*, **25**: 756–761.

Bailey, E.D., Wydro, G.C. & Cone, D.C. (2000). Termination of resuscitation in the prehospital setting for adult patients suffering nontraumatic cardiac arrest. National Association of EMS Physicians Standards and Clinical Practice Committee. *Prehosp. Emerg. Care*, **4**: 190–195.

Becker, L.B., Ostrander, M.P., Barrett, J. & Kondos, G.T. (1991). Outcome of CPR in a large metropolitan area–where are the survivors? *Ann. Emerg. Med.*, **20**: 355–361.

Berg, R.A., Sanders, A.B., Milander, M., Tellez, D., Liu, P. & Beyda, D. (1994). Efficacy of audio-prompted rate guidance in improving resuscitator performance of cardiopulmonary resuscitation on children. *Acad. Emerg. Med.*, **1**: 35–40.

Blaivas, M. & Fox, J.C. (2001). Outcome in cardiac arrest patients found to have cardiac standstill on the bedside emergency department echocardiogram. *Acad. Emerg. Med.*, **8**: 616–621.

Blumenthal, S.R. & Voorhees, W.D. (1997a). The relationship between airway carbon dioxide excretion and cardiac output during cardiopulmonary resuscitation. *Resuscitation*, **34**: 263–270.

Blumenthal, S.R. & Voorhees, W.D. (1997b). The relationship of carbon dioxide excretion during cardiopulmonary resuscitation to regional blood flow and survival. *Resuscitation*, **35**: 135–143.

Callaham, M. & Barton, C. (1990). Prediction of outcome of cardiopulmonary resuscitation from end-tidal carbon dioxide concentration. *Crit. Care Med.*, **18**: 358–362.

Callaham, M., Barton, C. & Matthay, M. (1992). Effect of epinephrine on the ability of end-tidal carbon dioxide readings to predict initial resuscitation from cardiac arrest. *Crit. Care Med.*, **20**: 337–343.

Cantineau, J.P., Lambert, Y., Merckx, P., *et al.* (1996). End-tidal carbon dioxide during cardiopulmonary resuscitation in humans presenting mostly with asystole: a predictor of outcome. *Crit. Care Med.*, **24**: 791–796.

Cantineau, J.P., Merckx, P., Lambert, Y., Sorkine, M., Bertrand, C. & Duvaldestin, P. (1994). Effect of epinephrine on end-tidal carbon dioxide pressure during prehospital cardiopulmonary resuscitation. *Am. J. Emerg. Med.*, **12**: 267–270.

Falk, J.L., Rackow, E.C. & Weil, M.H. (1988). End-tidal carbon dioxide concentration during cardiopulmonary resuscitation. *New. Engl. J. Med.*, **318**: 607–611.

Garnett, A.R., Ornato, J.P., Gonzalez, E.R. & Johnson, E.B. (1987). End-tidal carbon dioxide monitoring during cardiopulmonary resuscitation. *J. Am. Assoc.*, **257**: 512–515.

Grmec, S. & Gasparovic, V. (2001). Comparison of APACHE II, MEES and Glasgow Coma Scale in patients with nontraumatic coma for prediction of mortality. Acute physiology and chronic health evaluation. Mainz Emergency Evaluation System. *Crit. Care*, **5**: 19–23.

Grmec, S. & Klemen, P. (2001). Does the end-tidal carbon dioxide ($ETCO_2$) concentration have prognostic value during out-of-hospital cardiac arrest? *Eur. J. Emerg. Med.*, **8**: 263–269.

Grmec, S. & Kupnik, D. (2003). Does the Mainz Emergency Evaluation Scoring (MEES) in combination with capnometry (MEESc) help in the prognosis of outcome from cardiopulmonary resuscitation in a prehospital setting? *Resuscitation*, **58**: 89–96.

Grundler, W., Weil, M.H. & Rackow, E.C. (1986). Arteriovenous carbon dioxide and pH gradients during cardiac arrest. *Circulation*, **74**: 1071–1074.

Gudipati, C.V., Weil, M.H., Bisera, J., Deshmukh, H.G. & Rackow, E.C. (1988). Expired carbon dioxide: a noninvasive monitor of cardiopulmonary resuscitation. *Circulation*, **77**: 234–239.

Hillis, L.D., Firth, B.G. & Winniford, M.D. (1986). Comparison of thermodilution and indocyanine green dye in low cardiac output or left-sided regurgitation. *Am. J. Cardiol.*, **57**: 1201–1202.

Idris, A.H., Staples, E.D., O'Brien, D.J., *et al.* (1994). End-tidal carbon dioxide during extremely low cardiac output. *Ann. Emerg. Med.*, **23**: 568–572.

International Guidelines 2000. Conference on Cardiopulmonary Resuscitation and Emergency Cardiac Care (2000). Part 2: Ethical aspects of CPR and ECC. *Circulation*, **102**: I–I1221.

Isserles, S.A. & Breen, P.H. (1991). Can changes in end-tidal PCO_2 measure changes in cardiac output? *Anesth. Analg.*, **73**: 808–814.

Jin, X., Weil, M.H., Tang, W., *et al.* (2000). End-tidal carbon dioxide as a noninvasive indicator of cardiac index during circulatory shock. *Crit. Care Med.*, **28**: 2415–2419.

Kalenda, Z. (1978). The capnogram as a guide to the efficacy of cardiac massage. *Resuscitation*, **6**: 259–263.

Kern, K.B., Sanders, A.B., Raife, J., Milander, M.M., Otto, C.W. & Ewy, G.A. (1992). A study of chest compression rates during cardiopulmonary resuscitation in humans. The importance of rate-directed chest compressions. *Arch. Intern. Med.*, **152**: 145–149.

Lepilin, M.G., Vasilyev, A.V., Bildinov, O.A. & Rostovtseva, N.A. (1987). End-tidal carbon dioxide as a noninvasive monitor of circulatory status during cardiopulmonary resuscitation: a preliminary clinical study. *Crit. Care Med.*, **15**: 958–959.

Lewis, L.M., Stothert, J., Standeven, J., Chandel, B., Kurtz, M. & Fortney, J. (1992). Correlation of end-tidal CO_2 to cerebral perfusion during CPR. *Ann. Emerg. Med.*, **21**: 1131–1134.

Levine, R.L., Wayne, M.A. & Miller, C.C. (1997). End-tidal carbon dioxide and outcome of out-of-hospital cardiac arrest. *New. Engl. J. Med.*, **337**: 301–306.

Lindberg, L., Liao, Q. & Steen, S. (2000). The effects of epinephrine/norepinephrine on end-tidal carbon dioxide concentration, coronary perfusion pressure and pulmonary arterial blood flow during cardiopulmonary resuscitation. *Resuscitation*, **43**: 129–140.

Lombardi, G., Gallagher, J. & Gennis, P. (1994). Outcome of out-of-hospital cardiac arrest in New York City. The Pre-Hospital Arrest Survival Evaluation (PHASE) Study. *J. Am. Assoc.*, **271**: 678–683.

Martin, G.B., Gentile, N.T., Paradis, N.A., Moeggenberg, J., Appleton, T.J. & Nowak, R.M. (1990). Effect of epinephrine on end-tidal carbon dioxide monitoring during CPR. *Ann. Emerg. Med.*, **19**: 396–398.

Mauer, D., Schneider, T., Elich, D. & Dick, W. (1998). Carbon dioxide levels during pre-hospital active compression–decompression versus standard cardiopulmonary resuscitation. *Resuscitation*, **39**: 67–74.

Morimoto, Y., Kemmotsu, O., Murakami, F., Yamamura, T. & Mayumi, T. (1993). End-tidal CO_2 changes under constant cardiac output during cardiopulmonary resuscitation. *Crit. Care Med.*, **21**: 1572–1576.

Ornato, J.P., Levine, R.L., Young, D.S., Racht, E.M., Garnett, A.R. & Gonzalez, E.R. (1989). The effect of applied chest compression force on systemic arterial pressure and end-tidal carbon dioxide concentration during CPR in human beings. *Ann. Emerg. Med.*, **18**: 732–737.

Ornato, J.P., Garnett, A.R. & Glauser, F.L. (1990). Relationship between cardiac output and the end-tidal carbon dioxide tension. *Ann. Emerg. Med.*, **19**: 1104–1106.

Pernat, A., Weil, M.H., Sun, S. & Tang, W. (2003). Stroke volumes and end-tidal carbon dioxide generated by precordial compression during ventricular fibrillation. *Crit. Care Med.*, **31**: 1819–1823.

Ralston, S.H., Tacker, W.A., Showen, L., Carter, A. & Babbs, C.F. (1985). Endotracheal versus intravenous epinephrine during electromechanical dissociation with CPR in dogs. *Ann. Emerg. Med.*, **14**: 1044–1048.

Salen, P., O'Connor, R., Sierzenski, P., *et al.* (2001). Can cardiac sonography and capnography be used independently and in combination to predict resuscitation outcomes? *Acad. Emerg. Med.*, **8**: 610–615.

Sanders, A.B., Atlas, M., Ewy, G.A., Kern, K.B. & Bragg, S. (1985a). Expired PCO_2 as an index of coronary perfusion pressure. *Am. J. Emerg. Med.*, **3**: 147–149.

Sanders, A.B., Ewy, G.A., Bragg, S., Atlas, M. & Kern, K.B. (1985b). Expired PCO_2 as a prognostic indicator of successful resuscitation from cardiac arrest. *Ann. Emerg. Med.*, **14**: 948–952.

Sanders, A.B., Kern, K.B. & Berg, RA. (2001). Searching for a predictive rule for terminating cardiopulmonary resuscitation. *Acad. Emerg. Med.*, **8**: 654–657.

Sanders, A.B., Kern, K.B., Otto, C.W., Milander, M.M. & Ewy, G.A. (1989). End-tidal carbon dioxide monitoring during cardiopulmonary resuscitation. A prognostic indicator for survival. *J. Am. Assoc.*, **262**: 1347–1351.

Shibutani, K., Muraoka, M., Shirasaki, S., Kubal, K., Sanchala, VT. & Gupte, P. (1994). Do changes in end-tidal PCO_2 quantitatively reflect changes in cardiac output? *Anesth. Analg.*, **79**: 829–833.

Steedman, D.J. & Robertson, C.E. (1990). Measurement of end-tidal carbon dioxide concentration during cardiopulmonary resuscitation. *Arch. Emerg. Med.*, **7**: 129–134.

Tang, W., Weil, M.H., Gazmuri, R.J., Sun, S., Duggal, C. & Bisera, J. (1991). Pulmonary ventilation/perfusion defects induced by epinephrine during cardiopulmonary resuscitation. *Circulation*, **84**: 2101–2107.

Tournadre, J.P., Chassard, D. & Muchada, R. (1997). Overestimation of low cardiac output measured by thermodilution. *Br. J. Anaesth.*, **79**: 514–516.

Trevino, R.P., Bisera, J., Weil, M.H., Rackow, E.C. & Grundler, W.G. (1985). End-tidal CO_2 as a guide to successful cardiopulmonary resuscitation: a preliminary report. *Crit. Care Med.*, **13**: 910–911.

Tyburski, J.G., Collinge, J.D., Wilson, R.F., Carlin, A.M., Albaran, R.G. & Steffes, C.P. (2002). End-tidal CO_2-derived values during emergency trauma surgery correlated with outcome: a prospective study. *J. Trauma*, **53**: 738–743.

van Grondelle, A., Ditchey, R.V., Groves, B.M., Wagner, Jr, W.W. & Reeves, J.T. (1983). Thermodilution method overestimates low cardiac output in humans. *Am. J. Physiol.*, **245**: H690–H692.

Varon, A.J., Morrina, J. & Civetta, J.M. (1991). Clinical utility of a colorimetric end-tidal CO_2 detector in cardiopulmonary resuscitation and emergency intubation. *J. Clin. Monit.*, **7**: 289–293.

Voorhees, W.D., Babbs, C.F. & Tacker, Jr, W.A. (1980). Regional blood flow during cardiopulmonary resuscitation in dogs. *Crit. Care Med.*, **8**: 134–136.

Ward, K.R., Menegazzi, J.J., Zelenak, R.R., Sullivan, R.J. & McSwain, Jr, N.E.. (1993). A comparison of chest compressions between mechanical and manual CPR by monitoring end-tidal PCO_2 during human cardiac arrest. *Ann. Emerg. Med.*, **22**: 669–674.

Wayne, M.A., Levine, R.L. & Miller, C.C. (1995). Use of end-tidal carbon dioxide to predict outcome in prehospital cardiac arrest. *Ann. Emerg. Med.*, **25**: 762–767.

Weil, M.H., Bisera, J., Trevino, R.P. & Rackow, E.C. (1985). Cardiac output and end-tidal carbon dioxide. *Crit. Care Med.*, **13**: 907–909.

White, R.D. & Asplin, B.R. (1994). Out-of-hospital quantitative monitoring of end-tidal carbon dioxide pressure during CPR. *Ann. Emerg. Med.*, **23**: 25–30.

Wilson, R.F., Tyburski, J.G., Kubinec, S.M., *et al.* (1996). Intraoperative end-tidal carbon dioxide levels and derived calculations correlated with outcome in trauma patients. *J. Trauma*, **41**: 606–611.

EMBOLISM 21

J.T. Anderson

Introduction

Pulmonary embolism presents a clinical diagnostic dilemma. About 650,000 patients are diagnosed with pulmonary embolism each year in the US and approximately 50,000–200,000 die as a result of pulmonary embolism (Olin, 2002; Wood, 2002). The majority of deaths from pulmonary embolism occur within the first hour. Appropriate therapy of patients surviving beyond the first hour decreases the death rate from 30% down to a rate between 2.5% and 10% (Capan & Miller, 2001; Olin, 2002). Prompt identification of patients with pulmonary embolism allows institution of appropriate therapy.

Most commonly, pulmonary embolism is due to blood clots, which travel through the venous system to lodge in the pulmonary arterial tree. Alternatively, embolism may be due to gas (i.e. air or carbon dioxide (CO_2) gas) (Souders, 2000), tumor, fat, or even bone cement (Fabbri *et al.*, 1996).

Parameters derived from capnography have been utilized for a number of decades to detect the presence of pulmonary emboli. Advances in technology have brought capnography to the bedside; this chapter describes the pathophysiologic basis and use of capnography in the detection of pulmonary embolism from a variety of causes.

Background

The true challenge in the management of pulmonary embolism is the prompt and accurate recognition of the presence of pulmonary embolism. Reliable and timely diagnosis of pulmonary embolism continues to challenge the clinician. Large autopsy studies show that up to 70% of patients who die as a direct result of pulmonary embolism were not identified prior to death (Goldhaber *et al.*, 1982; Karwinski & Svendsen, 1989; Olin, 2002; Wood, 2002). Presenting symptoms such as tachypnea and shortness of breath (Bell *et al.*, 1977), or alterations in arterial oxygen content (Stein *et al.*, 1995; 1996) are non-specific; indeed, such abnormalities are more commonly due to conditions such as postoperative atelectasis or pneumonia. Early and appropriate therapy decreases the mortality rate of pulmonary embolism substantially (Capan & Miller, 2001; Olin, 2002). Conversely, since only about 20–40% of patients with clinically suspect pulmonary embolism actually have pulmonary embolism; empiric treatment may unnecessarily expose patients to a risk of bleeding. Unfortunately, common diagnostic techniques including ventilation/perfusion ($\dot{V}/\dot{Q}$) scanning, pulmonary angiography, or computerized tomographic (CT) angiography are cumbersome, invasive, and require transportation of potentially critically ill patients, or involve the use of radiation or nephrotoxic agents. A simple, rapid bedside method to screen for, or more importantly, diagnose pulmonary embolism would prove useful. To this end, several investigators have pursued parameters derived from capnography to detect and diagnose pulmonary embolism. In general these parameters reflect changes in respiratory deadspace associated with the pulmonary embolism.

Respiratory deadspace

Appropriate appreciation of the use of parameters derived from time or volumetric capnography to evaluate for the presence of pulmonary emboli requires a thorough understanding of respiratory deadspace. Pulmonary embolism results in an increase in respiratory deadspace, specifically alveolar deadspace that can be evaluated with parameters obtained with capnography.

Respiratory deadspace represents the extent to which the exhaled tidal volume contains alveolar gas. Mathematically, this was expressed by Bohr (1891) as:

$$\frac{V_d}{V_t} = 1 - \frac{F_ECO_2}{F_ACO_2},$$

where V_d is the deadspace, V_t the tidal volume, and F_ECO_2 and F_ACO_2 are the fractions of CO_2 in mixed exhaled gas and alveolar gas, respectively. Due to difficulties with measurement of alveolar CO_2,

Enghoff (1938) utilized the partial pressure of CO_2 in arterial blood (P_aCO_2) in the place of F_ACO_2. The P_aCO_2 represented a "physiologic integrator of the CO_2 pressures existing in all parts of the lung" (Riley *et al.*, 1946). Expressed mathematically as:

$$\frac{V_d}{V_t} = 1 - \frac{P_ECO_2}{P_aCO_2}.$$

This latter equation represents the total or physiologic deadspace. In general, the respiratory system can be thought of as being comprised of two components, namely a component involved with transport of respiratory gases and a component associated with the exchange of respiratory gases. Inefficiencies in either of these components result in "wasted ventilation" and contribute to overall deadspace. *Airway deadspace* (or convective deadspace) is the portion of total deadspace due to inefficiencies in the transport component and *alveolar deadspace* is the portion due to inefficiencies in the component involved in the exchange of gases.

Airway deadspace is sometimes referred to as anatomic deadspace. The term anatomic deadspace implies a fixed interface and therefore a fixed volume. However, the location of the interface, and therefore the volume of the airway deadspace, is altered by factors such as inspiratory rate or breath holding. Generally, factors that favor diffusion or improve convection will shift the interface and decrease airway deadspace. For instance, a prolonged inspiratory phase and an end-inspiratory pause will decrease the deadspace (Fletcher *et al.*, 1981).

The alveolar deadspace represents inefficiencies in exchange of CO_2 and O_2. Specifically, alveolar deadspace represents inefficiencies distal to the interface of inspired gas and alveolar gas – the interface between where convection is important and where diffusion is important (Fletcher *et al.*, 1981). Pulmonary embolism alters deadspace primarily as a result of an increased alveolar deadspace. Unfortunately, a number of alternative pulmonary conditions such as asthma and chronic obstructive pulmonary disease (COPD) also alter alveolar deadspace. Differences in the effects of pulmonary embolism on the capnographic waveforms can be exploited to improve specificity of pulmonary embolism detection. Understanding of these differences requires knowledge of the various forms of alveolar deadspace.

Four general mechanisms can lead to an elevated alveolar deadspace. An elevation in alveolar deadspace can result from alterations either within (Figure 21.1) or between respiratory units (Figures 21.2 and 21.3). Further, though use of P_aCO_2 is a practical representation of the alveolar PCO_2 (P_ACO_2), venous admixture can result in an apparently elevated alveolar deadspace (Figure 21.4). Last, differences in flow of gases and blood as a function of time may cause a temporal mismatching thereby resulting in inefficient gas exchange and increased alveolar deadspace. Of note, an individual patient may have increased alveolar deadspace from any or all of the above mechanisms – the mechanisms are not mutually exclusive.

Incomplete mixing of gases *within* the respiratory units results in an increased alveolar deadspace (Figure 21.1). This type of alveolar deadspace is decreased by factors that favor more complete mixing or allow increased time for diffusion. For example, a decelerating flow waveform and an end-expiratory pause would decrease alveolar deadspace. Differences in the degree of mixing as one moves axially toward the periphery results in increased variability in the $\dot{V}/\dot{Q}$ ratios in terminal respiratory units. Distal respiratory units with low $\dot{V}/\dot{Q}$ ratios empty late in exhalation and increase the slope of the resultant capnogram.

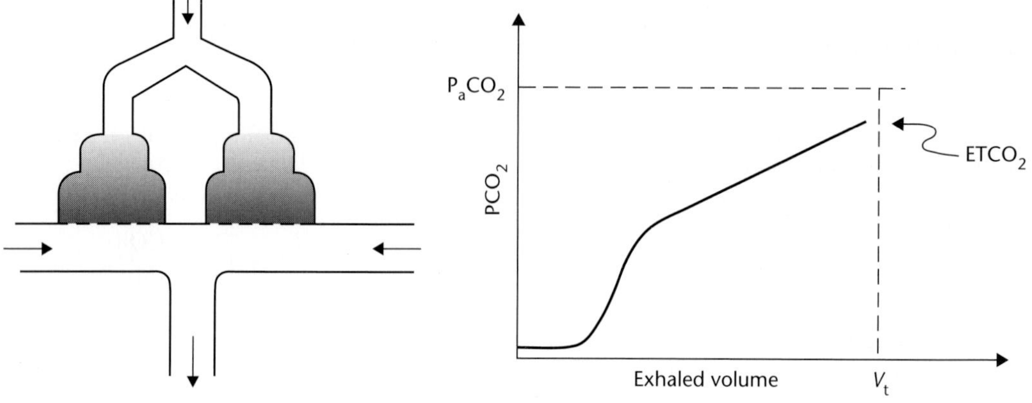

Figure 21.1 *Mechanism for elevated alveolar deadspace.* Two respiratory units with alterations in $\dot{V}/\dot{Q}$ matching within respiratory units and the resulting capnogram.

Mismatching *between* respiratory units results from two basic pathophysiologic mechanisms that can be differentiated with capnography. Spatial differences in gas or blood flow between respiratory units in the lung cause inefficiency in gas exchange reflected as an elevated alveolar deadspace (Figures 21.2 and 21.3). First, differences in the mechanical properties of the respiratory units, as may occur in chronic bronchitis, increase the alveolar deadspace (Figure 21.2). Due to differences in the time constants of the respiratory units, the P_ACO_2 will vary between respiratory units. In this situation, individual respiratory units will empty sequentially at differing rates/times dependent upon mechanical properties. Respiratory units with prolonged time constants will empty later in the expiratory cycle; these units have an increased PCO_2 and therefore increase the slope of the resultant capnogram. This mechanism also is ameliorated by factors that favor improved diffusion such as a prolonged breath or end-inspiratory. Second, spatial differences between respiratory units may result from spatial differences in blood flow as occurs with pulmonary embolism (Figure 21.3). Occlusion of the pulmonary vasculature by an embolism will result in a lack of CO_2 flux to the alveolus in the effected vascular distribution. Because ventilation to the effected alveoli continues unabated, PCO_2 in these alveoli decreases. The mechanical properties may not be affected to a great extent. As a result, these alveoli will empty in parallel with other respiratory units with similar time constants. Increased alveolar deadspace from this mechanism is not affected to any great extent with respiratory maneuvers in contrast to the preceding mechanisms. Differences in the emptying of respiratory units will later be shown to be of importance to differentiate increased alveolar

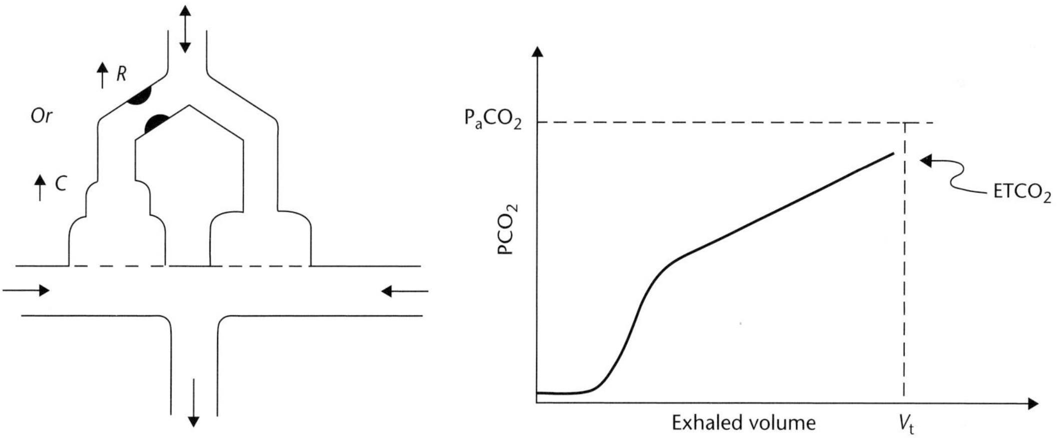

Figure 21.2 *Mechanism for elevated alveolar deadspace.* Two respiratory units with different emptying rates due to differences in airway resistance (*R*) and compliance (*C*) and the resulting capnogram. Note increased *R* or *C* will result in a longer time constant or a slower emptying rate.

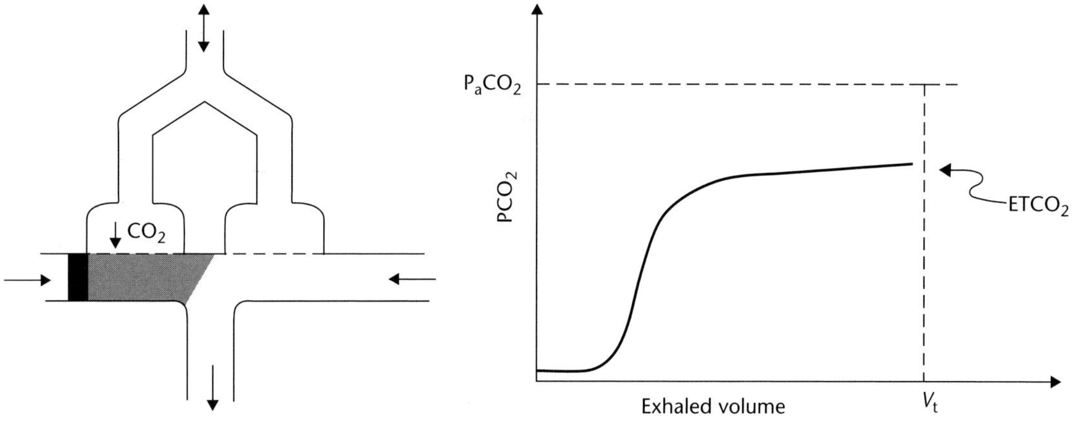

Figure 21.3 *Mechanism for elevated alveolar deadspace.* Two respiratory units with occlusion of pulmonary vasculature with the resulting decrease in the end-tidal value and the resulting volumetric capnogram.

deadspace from pulmonary embolism from that due to alternative diagnoses.

The third mechanism for an elevated alveolar deadspace is a byproduct of the method used to calculate deadspace. P_aCO_2 is taken as a physiologic integrator of the P_ACO_2 present throughout the lung. As such, it is a practical representation of "P_ACO_2" that was substituted into the Bohr equation to calculate deadspace. However, venous admixture may result in an increased P_aCO_2 as CO_2 rich mixed venous blood effectively bypasses the lung. Usually, this effect is minor and can be disregarded. However, in the presence of a large shunt, the alveolar deadspace may appear elevated (Figure 21.4). This mechanism is unaffected by temporal alterations.

Lastly, temporal mismatching of the flow of gases and blood will result in increased alveolar deadspace. This mechanism is seen with controlled ventilation (Fletcher, 1981). During normal spontaneous breathing, expiratory flow as a function of time approximates a square wave. However, the flow of passive exhalation during controlled mechanical ventilation follows an exponential curve. Most of the exhaled breath leaves early during exhalation. In contrast, with positive pressure ventilation, pulmonary blood flow as a function of time during exhalation differs from that of exhaled breath flow – flow is maximal at end-exhalation. This last mechanism can be ameliorated by alterations in ventilator settings. Maintaining an adequate FRC will minimize the effects of temporal mismatching by providing a buffer to significant changes in alveolar gas composition (Fletcher, 1981).

Principles of pulmonary embolism detection

Distinguishing pulmonary embolism from alternative diagnoses can be accomplished by exploiting differences in the shape of the volumetric capnogram

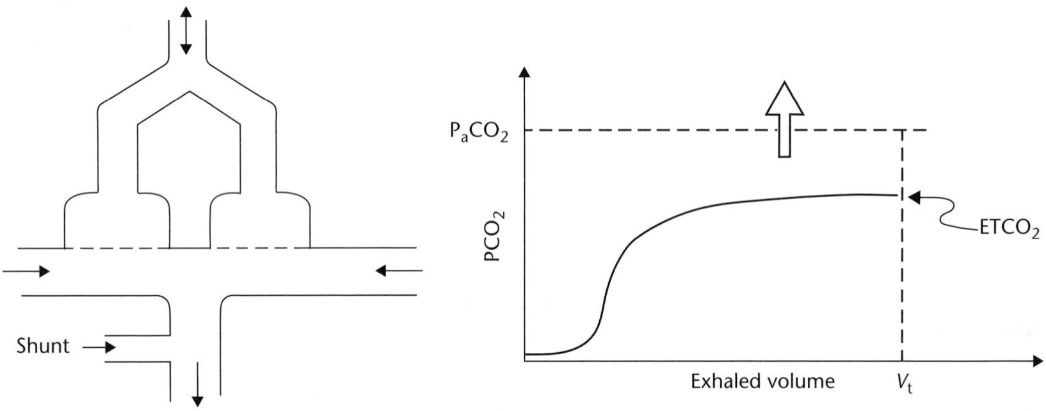

Figure 21.4 *Mechanism for elevated alveolar deadspace.* Two respiratory units with a large shunt and the resulting volumetric capnogram.

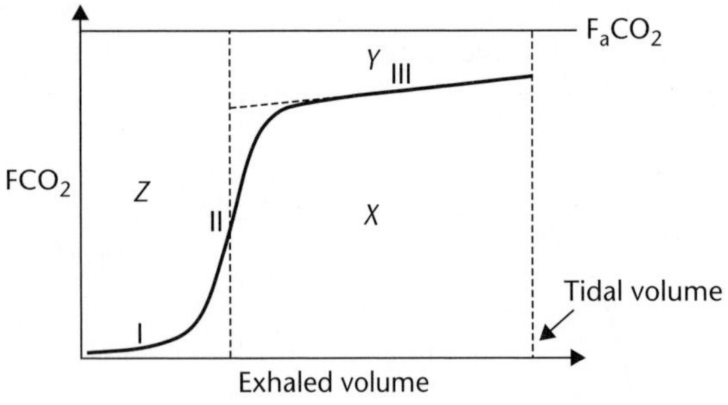

Physiologic deadspace: $$\frac{V_{d\,phys}}{V_T} = \frac{Y+Z}{X+Y+Z}$$

Alveolar deadspace: $$\frac{V_{d\,alv}}{V_T} = \frac{Y}{X+Y+Z}$$

Anatomic deadspace: $$\frac{V_{d\,anat}}{V_T} = \frac{Z}{X+Y+Z}$$

Figure 21.5 *Volumetric capnogram.* Lines are drawn to divide the curve into three large areas – labeled *X*, *Y*, and *Z*. The vertical line dividing phase II is placed such that the area under the curve equals the area labeled *X*. By substituting fractional CO_2 values for partial pressure values, calculated areas of the curve correspond to volumes of gas. The total area ($X + Y + Z$) represents the theoretical volume of CO_2, which could be eliminated with an exhaled breath equilibrated with the CO_2 in arterial blood. The area *X* represents the actual volume of exhaled CO_2 per breath (fractional $CO_2 \times$ volume exhaled breath).

(Figures 21.5 & 21.6), specifically the slope of phase III, and/or by employing various respiratory maneuvers including forced exhalations.

In general, the slope of phase III may be essentially horizontal or sloping. Pulmonary embolism will decrease the slope of phase III towards horizontal (Figure 21.6(a)). Alternatively, lung disease such as COPD will generally result in an increased slope of phase III (Figure 21.6(b)). Pulmonary embolism results in an occlusion or limitation of flow in the pulmonary vasculature to respiratory units. The alveoli within these affected respiratory units are cut off from the supply of CO_2 carried in the pulmonary arterial vessels. Because ventilation continues, the P_ACO_2 will decrease below that value within similarly ventilated alveoli in normally perfused respiratory units. Perfusion to peripheral alveoli appears to be especially effected. These alveoli tend to empty later and contribute to the latter part of phase III. As a result, the latter part of phase III is depressed out of proportion to the rest of phase III thereby resulting in a horizontal phase III (Figure 21.6(a)). In contrast, in the presence of COPD, the peripheral alveoli continue to have a supply of CO_2 due to intact perfusion; however, ventilation is impaired. The P_ACO_2 in these peripheral alveoli will increase towards the PCO_2 level in mixed venous blood. Because these alveoli tend to empty during the latter part of phase III, the slope is increased (Figure 21.6(b)).

Methods of pulmonary embolism detection

Physiologic deadspace

Physiologic deadspace is generally assessed using the Enghoff (1938) modification of the Bohr equation,

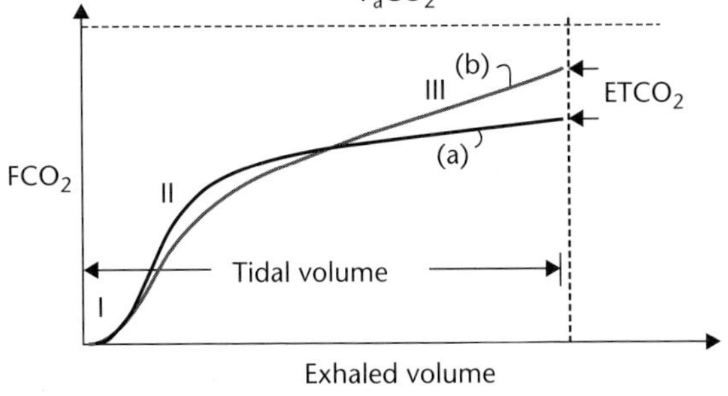

Figure 21.6 Volumetric capnograms with (a) near horizontal phase III slope but significant end-tidal–arterial gradient (pulmonary embolism) and (b) increased phase III slope (e.g. COPD).

which substitutes a P_aCO_2 value for P_ACO_2. Multiple exhaled breaths are collected in a large bag. The PCO_2 of the collected gas represents the mixed exhaled gas. A simultaneous blood gas is obtained to determine the P_aCO_2 and physiologic deadspace is calculated. Alternatively, the physiologic deadspace can be determined from volumetric capnography (Figure 21.5). Pulmonary embolism leads to an increase in the physiologic deadspace by virtue of an increase in alveolar deadspace – a component of the physiologic deadspace. Burki (1986) evaluated the utility of physiologic deadspace to diagnose pulmonary embolism. They used a cutoff of 40% as indicative of a pulmonary embolism. With this cutoff alone, they reported a sensitivity of 100% though specificity was only 55%. They found some improvement with the use of spirometry. Eriksson *et al.* (1985), however, found considerable overlap in the values of physiologic deadspace between patients with and without pulmonary embolism. This was particularly notable in patients with underlying pulmonary disease (Eriksson *et al.*, 1985; 1989). Further, Anderson *et al.* (1999), in a small group of surgical patients, found the physiologic deadspace to have a sensitivity of only 60%. This was confirmed in a larger surgical group (Anderson *et al.*, submitted).

Time capnography

Arterial – End-tidal PCO_2 gradient

Time capnography is essentially ubiquitous. It holds great appeal by virtue of its availability. In the presence of pulmonary emboli, the PCO_2 in alveoli within the distribution of the occluded pulmonary vessels decreased (Figure 21.7). This alveolar gas mixes with the exhaled gas of perfused alveoli and results in a decreased end-tidal PCO_2 ($P_{et}CO_2$). Even small clots seem capable of changing the end-tidal CO_2 ($ETCO_2$). Carroll (1992) simulated a 1-ml embolism by inflation of a pulmonary artery catheter. A change in $P_{et}CO_2$ was readily apparent in 20 of 24 patients. Several investigators have used this finding to non-invasively detect pulmonary embolism either by measurement of the arterial–alveolar CO_2 difference, or by calculation of the difference as a fraction of the P_aCO_2.

Robins *et al.* (1959) reported that the difference between CO_2 tension and arterial blood and that within the end-tidal exhaled breath was inncreased in patients with pulmonary embolism. He demonstrated an increased difference in seven of 10 patients with clinically suspected pulmonary embolism. The normal arterial–$ETCO_2$ difference was considered to be less than 5 mmHg. Despite the simplicity of measurement

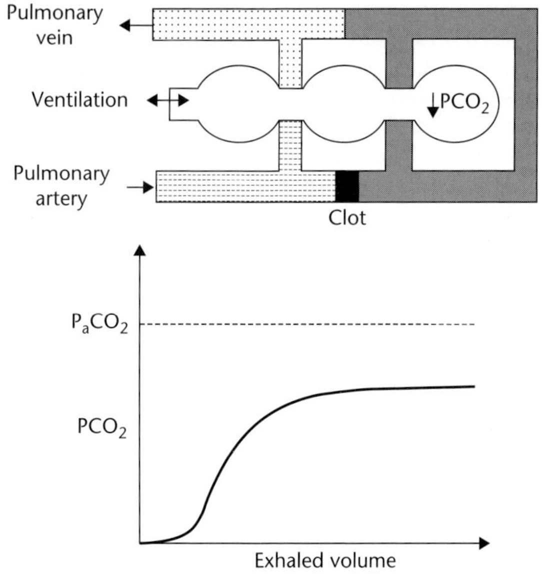

Figure 21.7 Effect of clot (i.e. pulmonary embolus) on ventilated but not perfused peripheral alveoli and resulting capnogram.

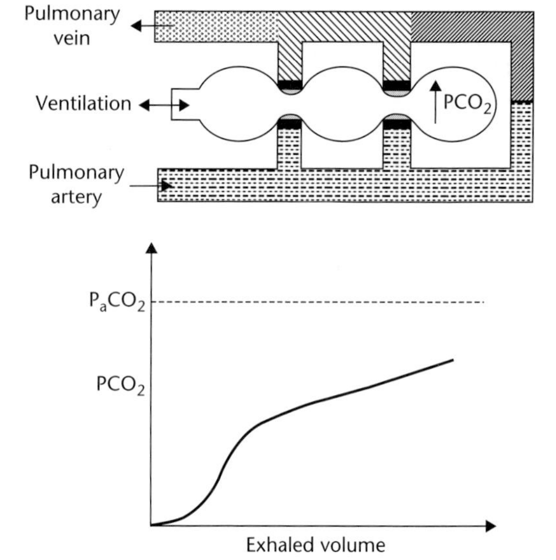

Figure 21.8 Effect of increased ventilation/perfusion mismatching (i.e. COPD) and the resulting capnogram.

of the arterial–ETCO_2 difference, multiple researchers have questioned its utility in real practice. Colp and Williams (1962) demonstrated an elevated arterial–end-tidal CO_2 difference in only three of seven patients with clinically suspected pulmonary embolism. Hatle and Rokseth (1974) evaluated the utility of the arterial–end-tidal CO_2 difference in several groups of patient with differing diagnoses. Nineteen healthy subjects did have a difference less than 5 mmHg. Further, all but one of their patients with large pulmonary emboli had difference exceeding 5 mmHg. However, 10 of 17 patients with small pulmonary emboli had a normal difference. Additionally, the difference was elevated in several patients with various diagnoses including chronic bronchitis, emphysema, myocardial infarction, primary pulmonary hypertension, and shock. Eriksson *et al.* (1989) also demonstrated significant overlap of the difference in patients with angiographically demonstrated pulmonary emboli and patients with an obstructive lung disease, interstitial lung disease, and even patients with clinically suspected pulmonary emboli who had a negative pulmonary angiogram. More recently, Anderson *et al.* (1999), in a group of postoperative surgical patients, found measurement of the arterial–alveolar CO_2 difference to have a sensitivity of 70% and a specificity of 71.8% using a cutoff value of 0.2. Sensitivity was improved to 90% if a cutoff value of 0.05 was used, though at the expense of specificity that was decreased to 38.5%.

Alveolar deadspace fraction

Nunn and Hill (1960) described a parameter that they called alveolar deadspace fraction expressed mathematically as:

$$\text{Alveolar deadspace fraction} = \frac{P_aCO_2 - ETCO_2}{P_aCO_2}.$$

Fletcher *et al.* (1981) pointed out that alveolar deadspace fraction as a measure of alveolar deadspace is incorrect in concept and may result in large errors in the estimation of true alveolar deadspace. Inspection of the volumetric capnogram demonstrates that with a sloping phase III, the ETCO_2 changes significantly depending on the tidal volume. In the presence of a steeply sloping phase III, as may occur with COPD, the true alveolar deadspace (represented by area *Y* divided by the total area encompassed by areas *X*, *Y*, and *Z*; Figure 21.5) would be underestimated by alveolar deadspace fraction. Nonetheless, the alveolar deadspace fraction is readily obtained, generally elevated in the presence of increased alveolar deadspace, and can be used as a surrogate to measure changes in alveolar deadspace – though with these limitations (Figure 21.8).

Multiple investigators have used the alveolar deadspace fraction to non-invasively screen for the presence of pulmonary embolism. Kline *et al.* (1997) evaluated the use of the alveolar deadspace fraction in 170 ambulatory emergency room patients with suspected pulmonary embolism. Fifteen percent of patients were diagnosed with pulmonary embolism. Using a cutoff value of 0.2

the overall sensitivity of the test for the detection of pulmonary embolism was 88.5% and the specificity was 66%. Further, they found the test had a negative predictive value of 96.9%. They found a combination of alveolar deadspace fraction and D-dimer measurement to have a sensitivity of 100%. Johanning *et al.* (1999) in a group of intensive care unit (ICU) patients, found all patients with pulmonary embolism to have an alveolar deadspace fraction that exceeded 0.2. However, eight of 14 patients without pulmonary embolism had alveolar deadspace fraction exceeding 0.2, though several of their patients were ventilated. More recently, Rodger *et al.* (2001) used a lower cutoff value of 0.15 to evaluate inpatients and outpatients at Ottawa hospital suspected of having pulmonary embolism. They specifically excluded patients on mechanical ventilation. Using this lower cutoff value, they reported a sensitivity of 79.5%, a specificity of 70.3%, and a negative predictive value of 90.7%. Anderson *et al.* (1999) in a group of surgical patients including patients who were mechanically ventilated, reported a sensitivity of 60%, a specificity 76.9%, and a negative predictive value of 88.2% when using a cutoff of 0.2.

The accuracy of the both the arterial–$ETCO_2$ difference and alveolar deadspace fraction can be improved with a forced maximal expiration. Inspection of the volumetric capnogram demonstrates that in the presence of a steep phase III slope (as results with COPD or interstitial lung disease) (Figure 21.6(a)) the $ETCO_2$ level will vary depending on the depth of exhalation. Following a maximal exhalation, the arterial–$ETCO_2$ difference and alveolar deadspace fraction will be less than with a normal exhalation. Conversely, in the presence of pulmonary embolism the slope of phase III is more horizontal (Figure 21.6(b)). In this case, the difference and alveolar deadspace fraction is not significantly altered.

In the presence of lung disease, such as COPD, the decrease in the arterial–$ETCO_2$ difference and alveolar deadspace fraction with a maximal exhalation maneuver results from several mechanisms. For one, maximal exhalation results in more complete emptying of the lungs including peripheral alveoli that have a higher PCO_2 level. Further, maximal exhalation is generally preceded with a maximal inhalation, often with a brief inspiratory hold. This results in more even distribution of gases within the alveoli and decreased alveolar deadspace. Emphysema and chronic bronchitis cause increased alveolar deadspace as a result of incomplete mixing within respiratory units, or regional ventilatory inequalities due to differences in mechanical properties in separate regions of the lung. Both of these mechanisms are ameliorated with prolonged inspiration and an end-inspiratory pause. In contrast, pulmonary embolism is associated with a horizontal phase III. In this case, the $ETCO_2$ level does not vary much with alterations in exhaled volume. Pulmonary embolism results in an elevated alveolar deadspace as a result of regional variations in perfusion to respiratory units without significant change in mechanical properties. This mechanism of increased alveolar deadspace is not significantly altered with the respiratory maneuvers above.

Multiple investigators have reported on the utility of forced exhalation to improve the accuracy of measurements based upon time capnography (Chopin *et al.*, 1990; Kline *et al.*, 1997; Johanning *et al.*, 1999). Chopin *et al.* (1990) evaluated the ability of a forced exhalation to differentiate patients with an increased deadspace due to COPD from patients with an elevated deadspace due to a pulmonary embolism. They derived a value R, which corresponded to the alveolar deadspace fraction calculated at the end of a maximal exhalation. Using a cutoff value of 5% they achieved a sensitivity and negative predictive value of 100%, a specificity of 65%, and positive predictive value of 74%.

Volumetric capnography

Alveolar deadspace

Alveolar deadspace is increased by pulmonary embolism. Alveolar deadspace is readily measured by evaluation of the volumetric capnogram using the method of Fowler (1948) (Figure 21.5). In a multi-institutional study involving six urban emergency rooms, Kline *et al.* (2001) evaluated the use of alveolar deadspace as a means to rapidly exclude the diagnosis of pulmonary embolism. They evaluated a total of 380 patients in whom 64 (16.8%) had pulmonary embolism. Patients were evaluated with a respiratory profile monitor (CO_2SMO Plus!, Respironics-Novametrix, LLC) and had the alveolar deadspace determined. Physiologic and airway deadspace were measured directly; alveolar deadspace was calculated as the difference between physiologic and airway deadspace. Using a cutoff value of 20%, they reported a sensitivity of 67% and a specificity of 76%. When combined with measurement of D-dimer, the sensitivity was improved to 98.4%. Of note, they excluded patients who had clinical evidence of shock or were unable to breathe room air or be cooperative during the measurement. Anderson *et al.* (1999) in a consecutive series of surgical patients, without exclusion criteria, demonstrated an overall sensitivity of 80% and a specificity of 61.5%. Alveolar deadspace was directly measured utilizing the method of Fowler (Figure 21.5) on a Ventrak Respiratory Monitoring System (Respironics-Novametrix, LLC).

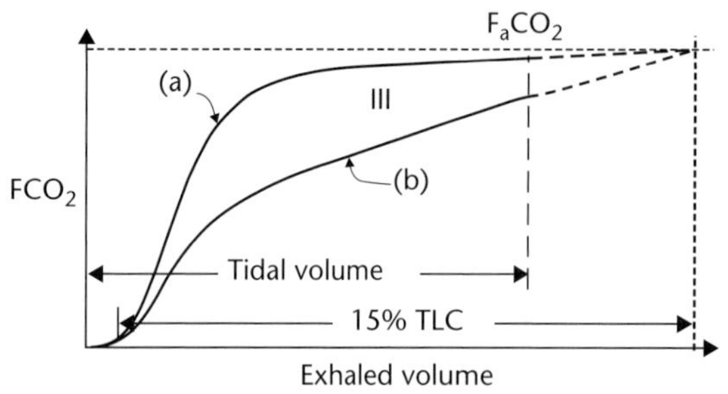

Figure 21.9 Volumetric capnogram illustrating extrapolated phase III slope for (a) normal patients (b) patients with obstructive and interstitial pulmonary disease.

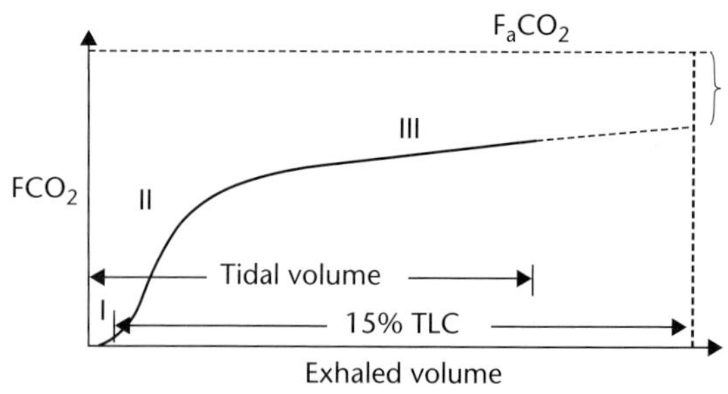

Figure 21.10 Volumetric capnogram illustrating extrapolated phase III slope for patient with pulmonary embolus. Difference between arterial CO_2 value and extrapolated CO_2 value indicated.

Late deadspace fraction

Bedside screening of pulmonary embolism suffers from two major limitations. First, the patient's baseline respiratory deadspace is generally unknown. Second, respiratory maneuvers such as forced exhalations require patient cooperation that may be limited or inconsistent. Eriksson *et al.* (1985; 1989) described a derived parameter, late deadspace fraction ($F_d$late), which attempts to compensate for these limitations. This method takes advantage of differences in the phase III slope between patients with pulmonary embolism and patients with other pulmonary diseases. Further, because the value is extrapolated, patient cooperation is less important than methods dependent upon forced exhalation.

$F_d$late is determined by fitting to the phase III slope a logarithmic curve of the form:

$$FCO_2 = a + b \times \ln(V_E),$$

where FCO_2 is the fractional CO_2 in the exhaled breath; V_E, the exhaled volume (beginning at the start of phase II); and a and b are constants.

Eriksson *et al.* (1989) found that the FCO_2 value of the extrapolated phase III curve reached fractional concentration of CO_2 in arterial blood (F_aCO_2) levels at a V_E of approximately 15% predicted total lung capacity (TLC) in normal patients and patients with obstructive and interstitial pulmonary disease (Figure 21.9). However, in patients with pulmonary emboli, the FCO_2 value of the extrapolated phase III curve failed to reach F_aCO_2 levels at 15% TLC (Figure 21.10). The authors expressed this "late deadspace fraction" as:

$$F_d\text{late} = \frac{F_aCO_2 - F_{15\%\ TLC}CO_2}{F_aCO_2}.$$

Table 21.1 Receiver operating characteristic (ROC) plots: area under the curve for various studies

$F_d$late	
Overall	0.96 ± 0.05
Spontaneous breathing	0.99 ± 0.03
Mechanically ventilated	0.85 ± 0.18
Physiologic deadspace	0.73 ± 0.10
Alveolar deadspace	0.84 ± 0.08
Arterial–$ETCO_2$ difference	0.86 ± 0.08
$ETCO_2$ deadspace	0.83 ± 0.08

The area under the ROC curve represents the ability of a test to accurately discriminate between groups i.e. positive or negative for the presence of pulmonary embolism. A value of 1.0 would reflect perfect discrimination; a value of 0.50 would be no better than "tossing a coin". A value of greater than 0.90 would reflect excellent discrimination.

Eriksson *et al.* (1989) found $F_d$late effective in the detection and diagnosis of pulmonary embolism. All 39 patients with pulmonary embolism had an elevated $F_d$late value. Additionally, the $F_d$late was normal in patients with alternative pulmonary diseases or in normal patients. In a small pilot study, Anderson *et al.* (1999) also found that $F_d$late was able to identify pulmonary embolism in a group of surgical patients. In a follow-up of a consecutive series of surgical patients with suspected pulmonary embolism, Anderson *et al.* (submitted) again found the $F_d$late effective in the detection of pulmonary embolism in surgical patients. When compared to alternative methods based upon deadspace, $F_d$late proved to be superior (Table 21.1). Overall, using pulmonary angiography as a gold standard, $F_d$late was found to have a sensitivity of 100%, a specificity of 87.2%, a negative predictive value of 100%, and a positive predictive value of 66.7%. In spontaneous breathing patients (which made up the majority of patients), the sensitivity again was 100%, specificity was 96.6%, negative predictive value 100%, and positive predictive value 88.9%. $F_d$late performed less well in ventilated patients with a sensitivity of 100%, a specificity of 60%, a negative predictive value of 100%, and a positive predictive value of 33.3%. Further, in this consecutive group of patients, following a screening algorithm using $F_d$late and D-dimer would have eliminated the need for pulmonary angiography or chest CT angiography in 70% of patients with clinically suspected pulmonary embolism.

Limitations of capnographic detection of pulmonary embolism

Bedside tests based on capnography have immense appeal in the evaluation of possible pulmonary embolism. The necessary equipment is readily available and portable. It is unnecessary to transport the patient; screening can be done at the patient's bedside. Further, ongoing measurements can be readily repeated; in fact, patients can be continuously monitored. Two major hurdles exist: the baseline deadspace is generally unknown, and a variety of alternative pathologic states other than pulmonary embolism can result in an elevated alveolar deadspace.

More liberal use of time and volumetric capnography would allow measurement of baseline deadspace as well as allow real-time detection of changes in respiratory deadspace. The utility of ongoing capnographic monitoring was evaluated by Johanning *et al.* (1999) in a group of ICU patients with suspected pulmonary embolism. In this small cohort, all patients later shown to have a pulmonary embolism had an increase in deadspace compared to baseline. Patients who did not have pulmonary embolism had a decrease in deadspace.

Increased deadspace due to common pulmonary diseases, such as COPD and interstitial lung disease, can be differentiated from pulmonary embolism by the methods above that exploit differences in the slope of phase III with or without respiratory maneuvers. In contrast, alternative pathologic states such as pulmonary hypotension or large right to left shunt result in phase III slopes that resembled those with pulmonary embolism. Similar to pulmonary embolism, pulmonary arterial hypotension may leave some alveoli under- or non-perfused thereby leading to increased alveolar deadspace. A variety of clinical situations may lead to pulmonary arterial hypotension including hemorrhage, septic, or cardiogenic shock. Mechanical ventilation with positive pressure exacerbates the effect of pulmonary arterial hypotension on alveolar deadspace. These factors largely explain the decreased specificity noted in mechanically ventilated ICU patients. Fortunately, in clinical practice, most patients with pulmonary embolism are neither in shock nor mechanically ventilated. In a consecutive series of patients with suspected pulmonary embolism (Anderson et al., submitted), the majority of the patients were hemodynamically stable and spontaneously breathing. Future refinements and research in the future will likely deal with these limitations. In the series reported by Hatle and Rokseth (1974) one patient with shock resulting in an elevated arterial–end-tidal difference had a decrease with a maximal exhalation. Courtney *et al.* (2002) in an animal model demonstrated that shock due to pulmonary embolism resulted in a greater deadspace increase than hemorrhagic shock of an equivalent extent.

Special

Detection of air or CO_2 embolism

Gas embolism, generally air or CO_2, can arise from a variety of clinical conditions though two basic mechanisms are primarily responsible. Air may be entrained into the venous system when the venous pressure falls below atmospheric pressure such as may occur during neurosurgical procedures in the upright position. Alternatively, during laparoscopic procedures, CO_2 under pressure may gain access to the venous system. In either case, massive air or CO_2 embolism can result in obstruction of the pulmonary vascular tree, and impairment of right ventricular and pulmonary function. Interestingly, as compared with blood clot, gas embolism can cross the capillary system and embolize into the systemic arterial system.

The incidence of gas embolism reported in the literature is variable. Using precordial Doppler measurements (sensitive to as little as 0.05 ml/kg), air embolism has been noted in as many as 58% of patients undergoing craniotomy in the upright position and 25% of patients undergoing craniotomy in the supine or prone position. In other procedures at risk for air embolism, the incidence of embolism ranged from 7% for cervical spine surgery to 65% in patients undergoing Cesarean section (Souders, 2000). Reports of the incidence of CO_2 embolism is likewise variable. Clinically significant CO_2 embolism is uncommon. One report of 113,253 gynecologic laparoscopies reported only 15 embolisms resulting from CO_2 insufflation (Phillips *et al.*, 1976). More recent studies, using echocardiography, have been able to demonstrate sub-clinical CO_2 embolism in 11 of 16 patients undergoing laparoscopic cholecystectomy (Derouin *et al.*, 1996).

The tolerated dose of gas depends upon the solubility of the gas. A portion of the gas will be excreted in the

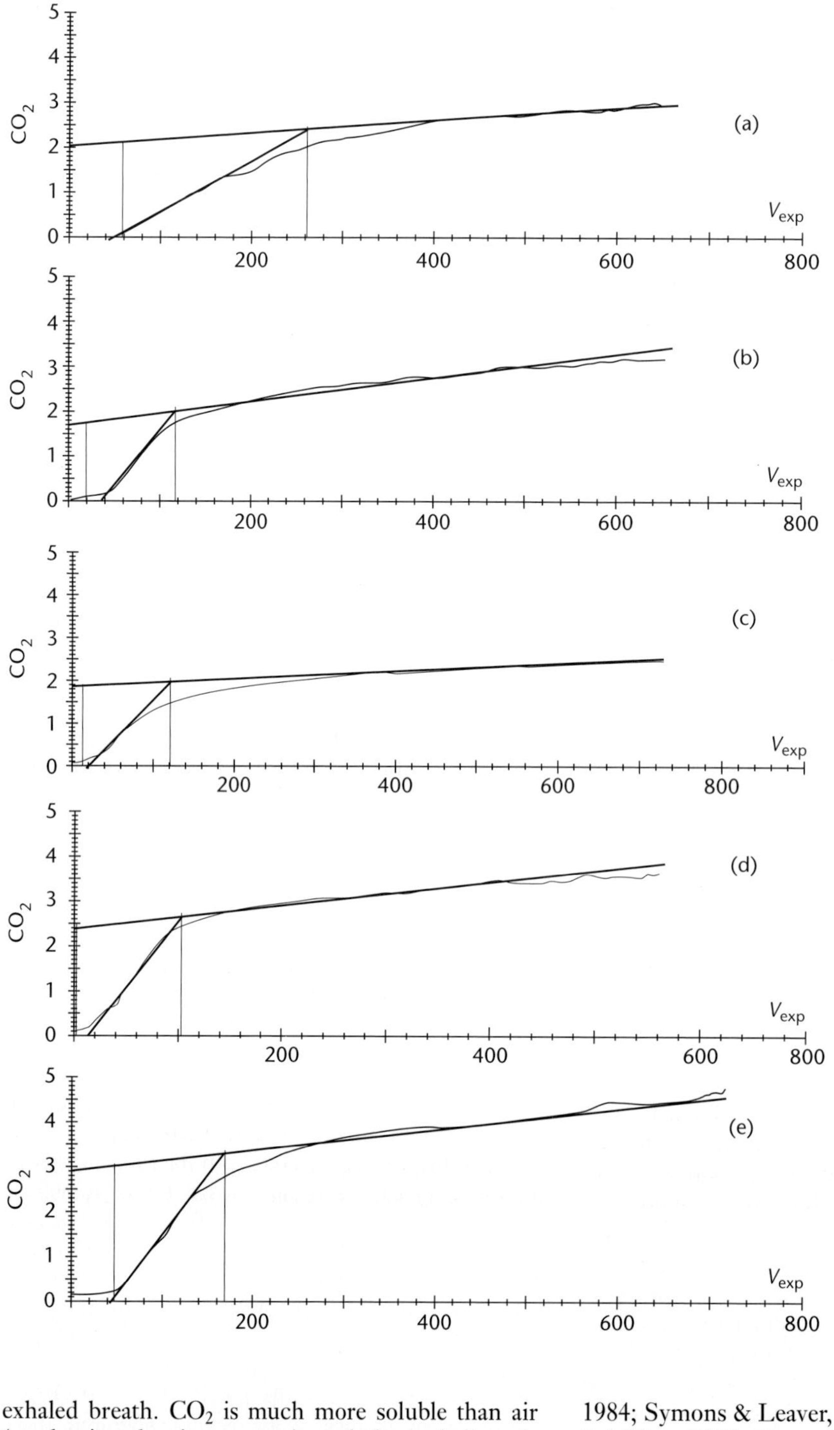

Figure 21.11 (a) A patient who presented in shock as a result of massive pulmonary emboli had a physiologic deadspace of 70% and alveolar deadspace of 60%. (b) After treatment with urokinase and heparin for a period of 12 h, the patient's physiologic and alveolar deadspaces decreased to 54% and 47%, respectively. (c) Shortly thereafter, the patient had a recurrent pulmonary embolism confirmed by pulmonary angiography. Likewise, the physiologic deadspace had increased to 61% and the alveolar deadspace had increased to 55%. (d) After 24 h of treatment with urokinase administered at a higher dose, the physiologic and alveolar deadspaces had decreased to 47% and 40%, respectively. (e) After 48 h of treatment the physiologic and alveolar deadspaces decreased further to 41% and 30%, respectively. Note the best-fit lines for phases II and III are overlaid on the curves and vertical lines mark the transition between phases I and II, and II and III.

exhaled breath. CO_2 is much more soluble than air (predominately nitrogen gas), and the embolic volume required for a given clinical manifestation is higher with CO_2 embolism. Rapid embolism of air of approximately 1 ml/kg will result in early symptoms of a gasp and hypotension. Larger volumes of 4–7 ml/kg result in death (Shulman & Aronson, 1984; Symons & Leaver, 1985; Souders, 2000; Capan & Miller, 2001). Generally, the limiting factor for survival is the ability of the right ventricle to pump against the added load. In contrast to air embolism, Mann *et al.* (1997) found in pigs that embolization of approximately 4 ml CO_2/kg was required to cause hypotension. Nonetheless, it should be realized that the rate of CO_2 insufflation to maintain pneumoperitoneum is often at rates of 1–8 ml/s – suggesting significant potential for the development of a massive CO_2 embolism (Capan & Miller, 2001).

Various methods exist to assess patients for the presence of gas embolism during surgery. Precordial Doppler ultrasound is frequently chosen due to its availability and high sensitivity (Souders, 2000; Capan & Miller, 2001). In the presence of air embolism, a sound like a "washing machine" is readily appreciated. Disadvantages of Doppler ultrasound include difficulty with positioning secondary to body habitus or due to patient positioning at the time of surgery. Transesophageal echocardiography is also associated with a high sensitivity; however, it is both less available and much more invasive (Souders, 2000; Capan & Miller, 2001). Though less sensitive to the presence of small amounts of air or CO_2 embolism, monitoring of capnography has the advantage of being readily available, reliable, and reproducible (Souders, 2000; Capan & Miller, 2001). Capnographic evaluation is more sensitive than monitoring of oxygen saturation or direct visual observation of the patient.

Both air embolism and CO_2 embolism result in an increase in alveolar deadspace as a result of an "airlock" in the vessels in which the gas bubbles lodge. Additionally, the partial pressures of individual gases will differ from that normally present in the blood. In the case of air embolism – an initial increase in end-tidal nitrogen may be identified due to the increased supply of nitrogen to the alveolus and subsequently into the expired breath (Souders, 2000; Capan & Miller, 2001). Generally, CO_2 embolism is manifested acutely with a sudden increase in $ETCO_2$ (Shulman & Aronson, 1984). Oppenheimer *et al.* (1956) demonstrated a biphasic change in $ETCO_2$ in dogs undergoing CO_2 embolization. Initially, there was an increase in the $ETCO_2$ as a result of increased excretion of CO_2. As additional bubbles accumulated in the pulmonary arterial, the alveolar deadspace was increased resulting in a decreased $ETCO_2$ level. In both air embolism and CO_2 embolism there is a "washout curve" during which the $ETCO_2$ returns to normal as the gases are excreted or dissipated.

Resolution of pulmonary embolism/thrombolytic therapy

Occasionally, thrombolytic therapy is used to dissolve large pulmonary emboli, particularly in the presence of compromised right ventricular function. As the pulmonary emboli are broken up and previously non-perfused alveoli are perfused, the alveolar deadspace decreases. This is reflected by changes in the capnographically derived parameters mentioned earlier. Numerous investigators have demonstrated the ability to track changes in the pulmonary embolic burden with the use of capnography. Wiegand *et al.* (2000) in a small group of 12 patients with massive pulmonary embolism requiring mechanical ventilation analyzed the $ETCO_2$ before and after thrombolytic therapy. The 10 surviving patients were noted to have a decrease in their arterial–$ETCO_2$ difference to a mean of 9.8–2.8 mmHg. Recurrent embolism was detected in two patients manifested as a sudden reduction in $ETCO_2$. Recently, the ability of volumetric capnography to track the resolution of pulmonary emboli with thrombolytic therapy was evaluated (Anderson, personal communication) (Figure 21.11). Additional investigators have also reported on the utility of parameters to derive from capnography to evaluate response to thrombolytic therapy.

Summary/conclusion

Diagnosis of embolism, and in particular of pulmonary embolism, continues to plague the clinician. Early detection and prompt initiation of therapy has been shown to decrease morbidity and mortality. Evaluation of patients with various parameters derived from capnography holds promise for the early bedside non-invasive detection of embolism thereby allowing prompt and appropriate therapy.

References

Anderson, J.T., Owings, J.T. & Goodnight, J.E. (1999). Bedside noninvasive detection of acute pulmonary embolism in critically ill surgical patients. *Arch. Surg.*, **134**: 869–874; discussion 874–875.

Anderson, J.T., Owings, J.T., Perlstein, J., *et al.* A noninvasive bedside algorithm to exclude pulmonary embolism in surgical patients. *J. Trauma*, [abstract] (submitted).

Bell, W.R., Simon, T.L. & DeMets, D.L. (1977). The clinical features of submassive and massive pulmonary emboli. *Am. J. Med.*, **62**: 355–360.

Bohr, C. (1891). Über die Lungenathmung. *Skand. Archiv. Physiol.*, **2**: 236.

Burki, N.K. (1986). The dead space to tidal volume ratio in the diagnosis of pulmonary embolism. *Am. Rev. Respir. Dis.*, **133**: 679–685.

Capan, L.M. & Miller, S.M. (2001). Monitoring for suspected pulmonary embolism. *Anesthesiol. Clin. N. Am.*, **19**: 673–703.

Carroll, G.C. (1992). Capnographic trend curve monitoring can detect 1-ml pulmonary emboli in humans. *J. Clin. Monit.*, **8**: 101–106.

Chopin, C., Fesard, P., Mangalaboyi, J., Lestavel, P., Chambrin, M.C., Fourrier, F. & Rime, A. (1990). Use of capnography in diagnosis of pulmonary embolism during acute respiratory failure of chronic obstructive pulmonary disease [published erratum appears in *Crit. Care Med.*, 1991; 19: 450–451] *Crit. Care Med.*, **18**: 353–357.

Colp, C.R. & Williams Jr, M.H. (1962). Pulmonary function following pulmonary embolization. *Am. Rev. Respir. Dis.*, **85**: 799–807.

Courtney, D.M., Watts, J.A. & Kline, J.A. (2002). End tidal CO_2 is reduced during hypotension and cardiac arrest in a rat model of massive pulmonary embolism. *Resuscitation*, **53**: 83–91.

Derouin, M., Couture, P., Boudreault, D., Girard, D. & Gravel, D. (1996). Detection of gas embolism by transesophageal echocardiography during laparoscopic cholecystectomy. *Anesth. Analg.*, **82**: 119–124.

Enghoff, H. (1938). Volumen inefficax. *Uppsala Lakaref. Forhand.*, **44**: 191–218.

Eriksson, L., Wollmer, P., Jonson, B., Fletcher, R., Albrechtsson, U., Larusdottir, H. & Olsson, C.G. (1985). SBT-CO_2: a new method for the diagnosis of pulmonary embolism? *Clin. Physiol.*, **5**: 111–115.

Eriksson, L., Wollmer, P., Olsson, C.G., *et al.* (1989). Diagnosis of pulmonary embolism based upon alveolar dead space analysis. *Chest*, **96**: 357–362.

Fabbri, G., Perin, S., Coli, A. & Lari, S. (1996). Pulmonary embolism associated with use of bone cement during hip arthroplasty. *Chir. Organ. Mov.*, **81**: 347–349.

Fletcher, R., Jonson, B., Cumming, G. & Brew, J. (1981). The concept of deadspace with special reference to the single breath test for carbon dioxide. *Br. J. Anaesth.*, **53**: 77–88.

Fowler, W. (1948). Lung function studies. II. The respiratory dead space. *Am. J. Physiol.*, **154**: 405.

Goldhaber, S.Z., Hennekens, C.H., Evans, D.A., Newton, E.C. & Godleski, J.J. (1982). Factors associated with correct antemortem diagnosis of major pulmonary embolism. *Am. J. Med.*, **73**: 822–826.

Hatle, L. & Rokseth, R. (1974). The arterial to end-expiratory carbon dioxide tension difference in acute pulmonary embolism and other cardiopulmonary diseases. *Chest*, **66**: 352–357.

Johanning, J.M., Veverka, T.J., Bays, R.A., Tong, G.K. & Schmiege, S.K. (1999). Evaluation of suspected pulmonary embolism utilizing end-tidal CO_2 and D-dimer. *Am. J. Surg.*, **78**: 98–102.

Karwinski, B. & Svendsen, E. (1989). Comparison of clinical and postmortem diagnosis of pulmonary embolism. *J. Clin. Pathol.*, **42**: 135–139.

Kline, J.A., Meek, S., Boudrow, D., Warner, D. & Colucciello, S. (1997). Use of the alveolar dead space fraction (Vd/Vt) and plasma D-dimers to exclude acute pulmonary embolism in ambulatory patients. *Acad. Emerg. Med.*, **4**: 856–863.

Kline, J.A., Israel, E.G., Michelson, E.A., O'Neil, B.J., Plewa, M.C. & Portelli, D.C. (2001). Diagnostic accuracy of a bedside D-dimer assay and alveolar dead-space measurement for rapid exclusion of pulmonary embolism: a multicenter study. *J. Am. Med. Assoc.*, **285**: 761–768.

Mann, C., Boccara, G., Fabre, J.M., Grevy, V. & Colson, P. (1997). The detection of carbon dioxide embolism during laparoscopy in pigs: a comparison of transesophageal Doppler and end-tidal carbon dioxide monitoring. *Acta Anaesthesiol. Scand.*, **41**: 281–286.

Nunn, J.F. & Hill, H.W. (1960). Respiratory dead space and arterial to end-tidal CO_2 tension difference in anesthetized man. *J. Appl. Physiol.*, **15**: 383–389.

Olin, J.W. (2002). Pulmonary embolism. *Rev. Cardiovasc. Med.*, **3**: S68–S75.

Oppenheimer, M.J., Durant, T.M., Stauffer, H.M., Steward, G.H., Lynch, P.R. & Barrera, F. (1956). In vivo visualization of intracardiac structures with gaseous carbon dioxide. *Am. J. Physiol.*, **186**: 325–334 [abstract].

Phillips, J., Keith, D., Hulka, J., Hulka, B. & Keith, L. (1976). Gynecologic laparoscopy in 1975. *J. Reprod. Med.*, **16**: 105–117.

Riley, R.L., Lilienthal, J.L.J., Proemmel, D.D. & Frank, R.E. (1946). On the determination of the physiologically effective pressures of oxygen and carbon dioxide in alveolar air. *Am. J. Physiol.*, **147**: 191.

Robins, E.D., Julian, D.G., Travis, D.M. & Grump, C.H. (1959). A physiologic approach to the diagnosis of acute pulmonary embolism. *New Engl. J. Med.*, **260**: 586–591.

Rodger, M.A., Jones, G., Rasuli, P., Raymond, F., Djunaedi, H., Bredeson, C.N. & Wells, P.S. (2001). Steady-state end-tidal alveolar dead space fraction and D-dimer: bedside tests to exclude pulmonary embolism. *Chest*, **120**: 115–119.

Shulman, D. & Aronson, H.B. (1984). Capnography in the early diagnosis of carbon dioxide embolism during laparoscopy. *Can. Anaesth. Soc. J.*, **31**: 455–459.

Souders, J.E. (2000). Pulmonary air embolism. *J. Clin. Monit. Comput.*, **16**: 375–383.

Stein, P.D., Goldhaber, S.Z. & Henry, J.W. (1995). Alveolar–arterial oxygen difference in the assessment of acute pulmonary embolism. *Chest*, **107**: 139–143.

Stein, P.D., Goldhaber, S.Z., Henry, J.W. & Miller, A.C. (1996). Arterial blood gas analysis in the assessment of suspected acute pulmonary embolism. *Chest*, **109**: 78–81.

Symons, N.L. & Leaver, H.K. (1985). Air embolism during craniotomy in the seated position: a comparison of methods for detection. *Can. Anaesth. Soc. J.*, **32**: 174–177.

Wiegand, U.K., Kurowski, V., Giannitsis, E., Katus, H.A. & Djonlagic, H. (2000). Effectiveness of end-tidal carbon dioxide tension for monitoring thrombolytic therapy in acute pulmonary embolism. *Crit. Care Med.*, **28**: 3588–3592.

Wood, K.E. (2002). Major pulmonary embolism: review of a pathophysiologic approach to the golden hour of hemodynamically significant pulmonary embolism. *Chest*, **121**: 877–905.

PULMONARY BLOOD FLOW MONITORING: NONINVASIVE CARDIAC OUTPUT

22

R. Dueck

Introduction

The need for a noninvasive measurement of cardiac performance has been appreciated for more than a 100 years (Vandam & Fox, 1998). Routine history and physical examination can readily distinguish patients with a normal heart versus someone in heart failure. However, differentiation of mild versus moderately impaired cardiac function, or compensated versus compromised diastolic left ventricular dysfunction, requires considerable expertise. Most of the special cardiac tests are not well suited for measuring cardiac performance after trauma, during anesthesia and surgery or during respiratory failure and/or sepsis. The 1970 introduction of the pulmonary artery (PA) catheter for central venous pressure (CVP), PA and PA wedge pressure (PAP and PAWP, respectively), followed by the addition of thermal dilution cardiac output (Q_{TD}), was heralded as a welcome solution. However, the rising concern over PA catheter risks has renewed consideration of noninvasive cardiac output (Q_T) monitoring via the Fick principle from pulmonary blood flow. Intermittent or continuous Q_T can be used to determine the cause of hypotension, for example, from hypovolemia (low Q_T and high systemic vascular resistance (SVR)) versus sepsis (high Q_T and low SVR), or from a failing left ventricle. Clinical research and experience have confirmed that noninvasive Q_T monitoring via the Fick principle provides this information as effectively as PA catheter-based thermal dilution Q_T measurement.

This chapter will first review the background and theory of Fick principle Q_T measurements for both the complete and partial carbon dioxide (CO_2) rebreathing methods, followed by end-tidal partial pressure of CO_2 ($P_{et}CO_2$) and volumetric capnography shortcuts for breath-to-breath pulmonary blood flow assessment, and finally some clinical examples of Q_T monitoring via the partial CO_2 rebreathing method.

Background and theory

The classic Fick principle provides an estimate of pulmonary capillary blood flow (Q_C), which comprises 98% of total cardiac output (Q_T) in subjects with little or no intrapulmonary or intracardiac shunting (Fick, 1870; Vandam & Fox, 1998). Historically, clinical application of the Fick method has employed both oxygen (O_2) and CO_2 as the physiologic tracer, as shown in Equations (22.1) and (22.2) below. Both O_2 consumption ($V'O_2$) and CO_2 elimination ($V'CO_2$) rate can be measured noninvasively. However, when O_2 is the physiologic tracer, both arterial and mixed venous samples are required, via indwelling arterial and PA catheters. Arterial and mixed venous O_2 content (C_aO_2 and C_vO_2, respectively) are then used to derive Q_C as:

$$Q_C = \frac{V'O_2}{C_aO_2 - C_vO_2}. \tag{22.1}$$

When CO_2 is the tracer, the Fick equation becomes:

$$Q_C = \frac{V'CO_2}{C_vCO_2 - C_aCO_2}. \tag{22.2}$$

A major advantage with CO_2 as the physiologic tracer is that in subjects with normal lungs both arterial and mixed venous CO_2 (C_aCO_2 and C_vCO_2, respectively) content can be estimated or derived via noninvasive methods, as shown below.

However, technical limitations with the Fick CO_2 method during the 1950s and 1960s gave way to the predominant use of indocyanine green dye dilution for Q_T measurement, as this required only a CVP injection port and continuous arterial sampling for dye densitometry. When the balloon-tipped PA catheter was introduced in 1970, it led to the development of thermal dilution Q_T measurement with a thermistor placed at the distal end of the PA catheter. The convenience and utility associated with obtaining CVP, PA, PAWP and repetitive Q_T measurements in critical care, trauma and major operative procedures produced rapid acceptance of thermal dilution Q_T as the "gold standard".

Nevertheless, critical review of the risk/benefit profile for placement and continuous use of a PA catheter has greatly heightened concern over this invasive monitoring technology.

Complete rebreathing CO_2 Fick Q_C method

These pressing concerns stimulated a renewed look at the inherently less invasive CO_2 rebreathing application of the Fick principle shown in Equation (22.2). The earlier methodology was designed for "complete rebreathing" to estimate mixed venous PCO_2, (P_vCO_2) along with inspired, mixed expired and arterial PCO_2 (via $P_{et}CO_2$) values. More specifically, when a satisfactory sample of alveolar PCO_2 (P_ACO_2) was obtained, as in a large breath $P_{et}CO_2$ from normal breathing or complete rebreathing, C_aCO_2 and C_v CO_2 content, respectively, could be derived:

$$C_cCO_2 = (6.957[\text{Hgb}] + 94.864) \times \log(1.0 + 0.1933P_ACO_2), \qquad (22.3)$$

where C_cCO_2, pulmonary capillary CO_2 content (whether arterial or mixed venous from normal or rebreathing $P_{et}CO_2$, respectively); Hgb, hemoglobin concentration; P_ACO_2 assumed equal to $P_{et}CO_2$. Mixed expired PCO_2 measurement required a one-way valve to separate inspired from expired air and an expired air collection bag.

However, it was learned as long ago as the 1920s that equilibration of alveolar with mixed venous blood during complete rebreathing is not achieved before mixed venous PCO_2 (P_vCO_2) starts increasing from recirculation of the elevated P_ACO_2 (Hamilton *et al.*, 1928). Collier, therefore, developed a rapid infrared analyzer end-tidal gas "equilibrium" method to estimate P_vCO_2 from a brief (<18 s) period of rebreathing into a 1 l bag charged with CO_2 at approximately 7 mmHg higher than $P_{et}CO_2$ (Collier, 1956). This provided a P_vCO_2 estimate that was an average 0.1 mmHg higher than P_vCO_2 measured by the Van Slyke apparatus. It is noteworthy that Collier concluded the 3.1 mmHg standard deviation (SD) was too high for estimating Q_C, because the average P_aCO_2–P_vCO_2 difference is only 6 mmHg. Meanwhile, Defares (1958) developed an "exponential" method by measuring PCO_2 from end-tidal expired gas samples taken after each of six 1000–2000 ml exhalations into a rebreathing bag. This exponential PCO_2 regression back to time zero provided an average -0.1 ± 0.2 mmHg less P_vCO_2 compared to Haldane analysis of the P_vCO_2 blood sample obtained just prior to rebreathing. Dubois and colleagues (1952) also learned that the period of rebreathing leads to significant lung tissue uptake of CO_2, requiring a correction of the P_vCO_2 estimate.

In spite of these technical issues and concerns, updated applications of the "equilibrium" and "exponential" methods have persisted in the literature. Vanhees *et al.* (2000) recently compared the Collier equilibrium and Defares exponential approaches to estimate P_vCO_2 in healthy volunteers at rest and during exercise, using fully automated devices replete with computer software for deriving the P_vCO_2 estimate, thereby minimizing observer bias. The "equilibrium" method was employed with high rebreathing bag CO_2 (from 6 to 15%) to assure a rapid equilibration with P_vCO_2 and a high O_2 concentration. With their modified version of the Defares "exponential" method, 2% CO_2 was placed in the rebreathing bag for rest and 4% CO_2 for exercise conditions. (Even with this modest CO_2 charge in the rebreathing bag, a true equilibration is still not reached before recirculation raises P_vCO_2, thus the need for an exponential equation to estimate P_vCO_2.) Estimated Q_T was higher at rest with the exponential versus equilibrium method (average Q_C 9.8 versus 8.4 l/min, respectively, $P < 0.001$), although subjects were more likely to request an end to the exercise study during the equilibrium method. This trend was related to the high CO_2 content in the rebreathing bag for the equilibrium method under exercise conditions, up to 15%, for speeding up equilibration during high Q_T conditions. However, the Q_C difference between these two methods disappeared with exercise, and both the methods showed excellent correlation between Q_C and $V'O_2$, ranging from $r^2 = 0.79$ to 0.88. Thus the complete CO_2 rebreathing method for obtaining a noninvasive Q_C estimate may be best suited for studying exercise in subjects with healthy lungs.

One innovative approach to avoid the effect of rising C_vCO_2 during rebreathing was to introduce a nonphysiologic tracer for estimating Q_C, such as acetylene (C_2H_2) or nitrous oxide (N_2O), because early body uptake of C_2H_2 or N_2O essentially removes them from mixed venous blood during brief rebreathing periods, even during the higher Q_T conditions associated with exercise. However, this method also required correction for lung tissue uptake of the tracer gas, and sophisticated and expensive mass spectrometry technology was needed to make high precision breath-to-breath C_2H_2 or N_2O measurements (Sackner *et al.*, 1975). Here again, this noninvasive methodology required healthy lungs for accurate Q_C estimates.

Meanwhile, the limitations of the complete CO_2 rebreathing method led to a series of mathematical and analytical innovations. There was a single breath CO_2 rebreathing method, which was shown to have a level of variability that was too high (Hlastala *et al.*, 1972). Then came the "one-step" rebreathing method by Farhi *et al.* (1976) that avoided the need for estimating C_vCO_2 content. In addition, it eliminated the concern for lung tissue uptake of CO_2 during rebreathing, and could be used for exercise conditions. However, there were a number of sophisticated technical elements, such as inducing the subject to provide the perfect tidal volume and frequency, and determining the appropriate size rebreathing bag and CO_2 charge in the bag for deriving $V'CO_2$ precisely at the time P_ACO_2 recovered back to time zero; that is, prior to the induced increase in minute ventilation. This noninvasive method was clearly unreliable for patients with lung disease because of the need to obtain perfectly timed P_aCO_2 measurements to determine their P_aCO_2–$P_{et}CO_2$ difference during normal and complete rebreathing conditions. In addition, the compliant rebreathing bag and the need for patient cooperation made it technically unsuitable for patients requiring assisted mechanical ventilation.

Partial rebreathing CO_2 Fick Q_C method

Gedeon *et al.* (1980) were concerned about the Q_C error induced by estimates of P_vCO_2 in the denominator of the CO_2 rebreathing method ($C_vCO_2 - C_aCO_2$, (see Equation (22.2)), because this difference is small compared to Q_C. They therefore presented theory and evidence to show that C_vCO_2 could remain an unknown and be removed from the equation by adding a second Fick equation, for example, by increasing or decreasing $V'CO_2$ for a short period with an increase or decrease in dead-space (V_D). In contrast to complete rebreathing estimates of C_vCO_2, the relatively modest P_aCO_2 alteration with a brief V_D change allowed assumption of a linear CO_2 dissociation curve and decreased the lung tissue PCO_2 effects. They demonstrated that their estimate of Q_C could be repeated every 15 min. This method was best suited for subjects whose lungs were mechanically ventilated, and thus provided a practical noninvasive Q_C option for respiratory care and anesthetized patients. Capek and Roy (1988) found that when such a "partial rebreathing" period was limited to 30 s, C_vCO_2 did not increase significantly, so the partial rebreathing method could provide Q_C estimates continuously at 3.5-min intervals. In normal lungs, $P_{et}CO_2$ could be used to estimate P_aCO_2, thereby making the Q_C estimate entirely noninvasive. However, Capek and Roy concluded that this method was sensitive to significant changes in Hgb, for example, a 30% change in Hgb led to a 15% Q_C error, although it was less sensitive to changes in V_D or shunting. This approach has now been formally designated the "partial CO_2 rebreathing" Q_C method.

De Abreu *et al.* (1997) compared the partial CO_2 rebreathing Q_C method to thermal dilution total Q_T (Q_{TD}) using a PA catheter in sheep with normal lungs versus lungs with oleic acid induced pulmonary edema. They found that the overall correlation of non-shunted pulmonary capillary blood flow between methods was good, $r^2 = 0.73$, $P < 0.0001$. However, the difference between the two methods, $Q_{TD} - Q_C$, was significantly improved with an intrapulmonary shunt correction during pulmonary edema. In a follow-up sheep study where hyper- and hypodynamic conditions were induced, and increased alveolar dead-space and shunting, the $P_aCO_2 - P_{et}CO_2$ difference contributed significantly to $Q_{TD} - Q_C$ (De Abreu *et al.*, 2003). They therefore recommended using measured P_aCO_2 for more accurate Q_C estimates, especially for large V_D and low Q_T states. At high Q_T conditions they suspected that P_aCO_2 measurement error contributed significantly to Q_C, probably due, in part, to the inherently decreased P_vCO_2–P_aCO_2 differences (and possibly also, in part, due to P_vCO_2 elevation from recirculation with an increased Q_T. A differential form of the Fick equation is used to accommodate the change in alveolar ventilation with increased V_D that provides the second equation to solve for the two unknowns, $Q_{C,pr}$ and C_vCO_2:

$$Q_{C,pr} = \frac{V'CO_{2,1}}{C_{v,1}CO_2 - C_{a,1}CO_2} = \frac{V'CO_{2,2}}{C_{v,2}CO_2 - C_{a,2}CO_2}, \tag{22.4}$$

where sample subscripts 1 and 2 ($C_{v,1}$ and $C_{v,2}$) indicate mixed venous values during normal and partial rebreathing, respectively, while ($C_{a,1}CO_2$, $C_{a,2}CO_2$) represent the corresponding arterial values. Equation (22.4) requires an assumption of constant $Q_{C,pr}$ and constant C_vCO_2 between normal and partial rebreathing periods. From basic algebra ($X = A/B - C/D = (A - C)/(B - D)$, this differential equation can then be rewritten as:

$$Q_{C,pr} = \frac{V'CO_{2,1} - V'CO_{2,2}}{(C_{v,1}CO_2 - C_{a,1}CO_2) - (C_{v,2}CO_2 - C_{a,2}CO_2)}. \tag{22.5}$$

The terms in the denominator of Equation (22.5) can be rearranged as:

$$Q_{C,pr} = \frac{V'CO_{2,1} - V'CO_{2,2}}{(C_{v,1}CO_2 - C_{v,2}CO_2) - (C_{a,1}CO_2 - C_{a,2}CO_2)}. \tag{22.6}$$

If the assumptions ($Q_{C,pr}$ and C_vCO_2 do not change) are met, then $C_{v,1}CO_2 - C_{v,2}CO_2 = 0$, and Equation (22.6) collapses to:

$$Q_{C,pr} = \frac{(V'CO_{2,1} - V'CO_{2,2})}{(C_{a,1}CO_2 - C_{a,2}CO_2)}$$

or

$$Q_{C,pr} = \frac{\Delta V'CO_2}{\Delta C_aCO_2}, \tag{22.7}$$

where $\Delta V'CO_2 = V'CO_{2,1} - V'CO_{2,2}$ and $\Delta C_aCO_2 = C_{a,1}CO_2 - C_{a,2}CO_2$. Inspired and expired tidal volume, along with inspired and expired PCO_2, are measured continuously to derive $V'CO_2$ with each breath. A mainstream CO_2 sensor is used for breath-to-breath PCO_2 and $V'CO_2$ measurements (shown in Figure 22.1) as a means of avoiding the errors associated with PCO_2 delay and rise/decay times from a gas sampling line and sensor chamber. $P_{et}CO_2$ values and CO_2 solubility are used to measure $C_{a,1}CO_2 - C_{a,2}CO_2$ as ΔC_aCO_2 according to the method shown in Equation (22.3).

A convenient way of changing ventilation for normal versus partial rebreathing is to introduce a variable size serial dead-space, especially one that can be automatically included and excluded in the circuit by a pneumatic valve via computer data acquisition and monitor control software, also shown in Figure 22.1. The partial rebreathing circuit shown is expandable and retractable, thus readily adjustable for different tidal volumes. The size of the serial dead-space should also be adjusted for conditions of relatively high dead-space, such as those seen with positive end-expiratory pressure (PEEP), or with low tidal volume and added mask dead-space, to avoid lowering $V'CO_2$ too close to zero during partial rebreathing.

An example of breath-to-breath serial non-rebreathing/partial rebreathing measurements for deriving $\Delta V'CO_2/\Delta C_aCO_2$ is shown in Figure 22.2. During normal breathing (baseline and recovery period) the partial rebreathing valve is turned off, while the valve is turned *on* for partial rebreathing. Thus $V'CO_2$ decreases abruptly and $P_{et}CO_2$ increases rapidly during valve *on* and then $V'CO_2$ recovers rapidly (with a brief overshoot) while $P_{et}CO_2$ decreases back to normal during recovery and baseline periods.

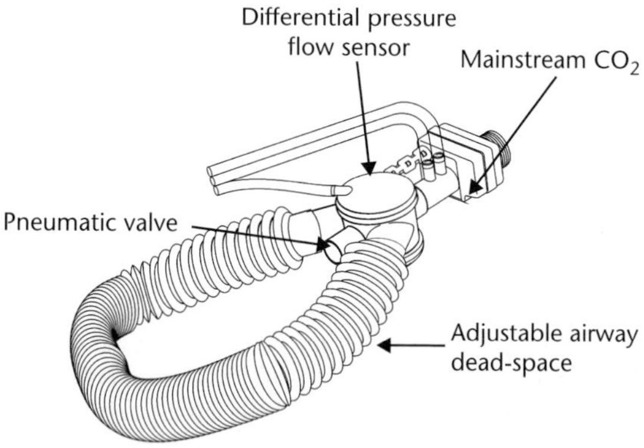

Figure 22.1 The disposable NICO® sensor for single patient use is a combination of an on-airway flow sensor, on-airway/mainstream CO_2 sensor, adjustable dead-space tubing and pneumatic valve. It is connected in-between the endotracheal tube of the patient and the Y-piece of the breathing circuit. (Image courtesy of Respironics, Inc., Murrysville, PA.)

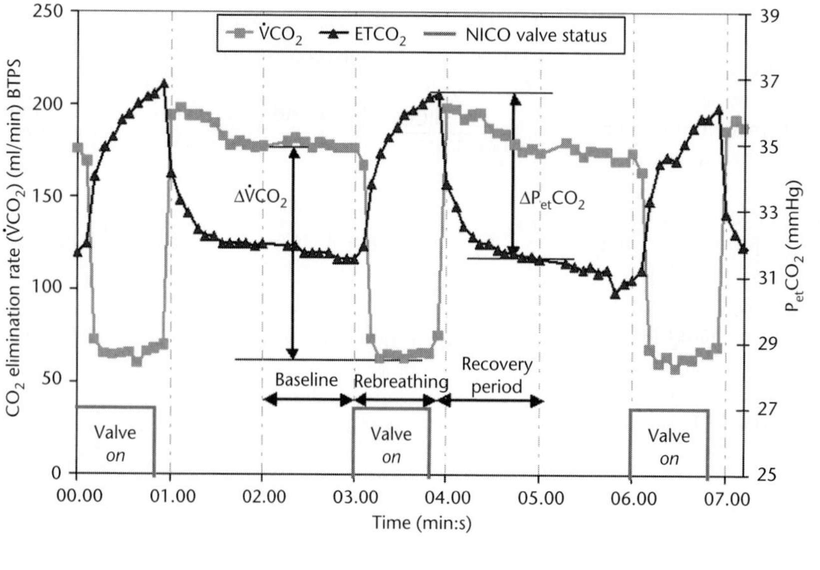

Figure 22.2 Typical $Q_{C,pr}$ waveforms: The $\dot{V}CO_2$ and $ETCO_2$ recording shows breath-to-breath measurements of $V'CO_2$ and $P_{et}CO_2$ during periods of baseline or normal ventilation (60 s), rebreathing (valve *on*, 50 s) and recovery periods (70 s). (Image courtesy of Respironics, Inc., Murrysville, PA.)

De Abreu *et al.* (1997) recommended that the Q_T estimates obtained from $Q_{C,pr}$ measurements should incorporate a correction for intrapulmonary shunt or venous admixture. They measured intrapulmonary shunt from C_aO_2 and C_vO_2 content via arterial and PA catheters in animal studies. However, when the intent is to avoid placing a PA catheter for mixed venous samples, a less invasive method is needed. Haryadi *et al.* (2000) used the iso-hunt lines described by Benator and colleagues (1973) to derive a shunt estimate from inspired O_2 fraction (F_IO_2) and arterial partial pressure of O_2 (P_aO_2). These shunt isopleths are a series of continuous curves representing the relationship between P_aO_2 and F_IO_2 for different shunt values, whose mathematical derivations are readily applied online with known F_IO_2 and P_aO_2. This enabled Haryadi *et al.* (2000) to introduce their shunt correction with the following equation:

$$Q_T = \frac{Q\,Q_{C,pr}}{(1 - Q_s/Q_T)}, \tag{22.8}$$

where Q_s is the shunted pulmonary blood flow.

A measured P_aO_2 value is needed for estimating shunt when high F_IO_2 leads to P_aO_2 values >100 mmHg. When P_aO_2 is <100 mmHg, arterial O_2 saturation via pulse oximetry (S_pO_2) may be used to estimate shunt via these isopleths.

Haryadi *et al.* (2000) also recommend correcting for $P_aCO_2 - P_{et}CO_2$ differences in patients with lung disease, using measured P_aCO_2 values. In addition, they recommend correcting for alveolar dead-space effects during partial rebreathing because unperfused alveoli ($P_ACO_2 = 0$) delay the equilibration of P_aCO_2 and $P_{et}CO_2$ during partial rebreathing (see the Appendix in Haryadi *et al.*, 2000). This contrasts with complete rebreathing, where $P_{et}CO_2$ elevation is considerably greater.

Partial rebreathing pulmonary blood flow findings

An animal study comparing partial CO_2 rebreathing ($Q_{C,pr}$) with thermal dilution Q_T (Q_{TD}) was performed by Haryadi *et al.* (2000), where Q_T was raised with dobutamine infusion (2.5–15 µg/kg/min) and lowered with halothane (0.5–4.0%) inhalation and/or inferior vena cava clamping. The continuous Q_T trend in Figure 22.3 shows a satisfactory level of agreement between the two methods for direction of change, while abrupt changes show a brief phase lag by NICO ($Q_{C,pr}$). This phase lag with abrupt changes may be related to two kinds of buffering for $V'CO_2$ and $P_{et}CO_2$. First, there is a large CO_2 storage capacity in body tissues. This may produce a modest obligatory phase lag, especially in the ratio of an increasing $\Delta V'CO_2/\Delta P_{et}CO_2$, that is, increasing $Q_{C,pr}$. Second, continued CO_2 elimination from the lung with constant (controlled) ventilation during a decrease in CO_2 delivery to the lungs with a decrease in Q_C may produce a factitiously high $\Delta V'CO_2/\Delta P_{et}CO_2$ ratio, as suggested especially during the first falling Q_T cycle in Figure 22.3. Thus the response time of changing $Q_{C,pr}$ based on the Fick principle for CO_2 is inherently limited by the need for stable CO_2 elimination conditions. In spite of these changing boundary conditions, it is clear that the agreement between $Q_{C,pr}$ and Q_{TD} is very good, as indicated by the weighted correlation coefficient, $r = 0.93$ and by Bland Altman

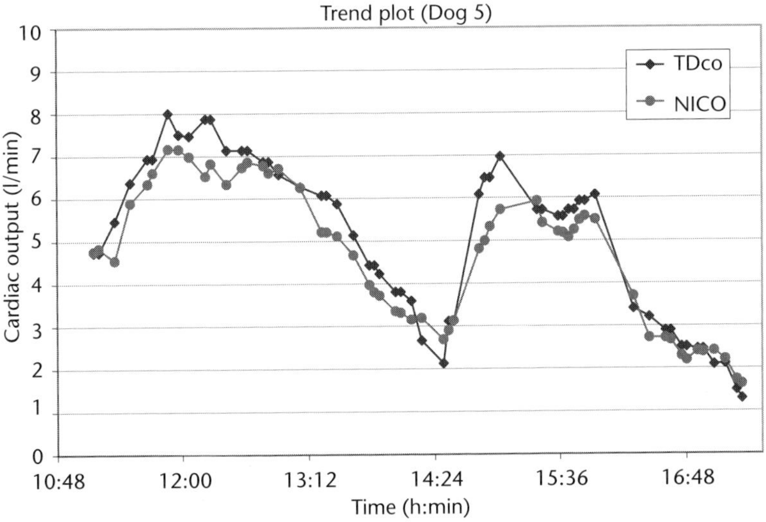

Figure 22.3 This trend plot shows $Q_{C,pr}$ (NICO) and bolus thermodilution (TDco) Q_T measurements when cardiac output was raised with dobutamine infusion and lowered with halothane inhalation. The weighted correlation coefficient showed $r = 0.93$. (Image courtesy of Respironics, Inc., Murrysville, PA.)

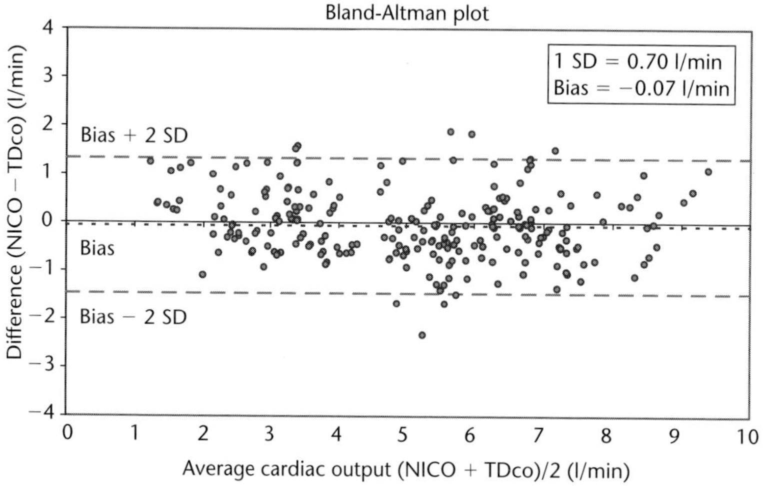

Figure 22.4 Bland Altman plot: Differences between NICO ($Q_{C,pr}$) and TDco (Q_{TD}) are plotted against the average of the two. Bias = Average difference (NICO − TDco) was −0.07 l/min, as shown by the dotted line. The precision (SD of the difference) was 0.70 l/min. The dashed lines indicate ±2 SDs from the bias. (Image courtesy of Respironics, Inc., Murrysville, PA.)

statistics. The precision (SD of the difference) was 0.70 l/min and bias (mean difference) was −0.07 l/min, as illustrated in the Bland Altman plot shown in Figure 22.4. The Bland Altman plot also shows no systematic difference for high or low cardiac output values.

Numerous clinical studies in coronary artery bypass graft (CABG) surgery patients comparing partial CO_2 rebreathing with thermal dilution cardiac output have shown a similar level of agreement between the two methods (Haryadi *et al.*, 2000).

Tachibana *et al.* (2002) recently assessed the accuracy of $Q_{C,pr}$ (NICO monitor) compared with Q_{TD} (PA catheter) methods when tidal volume was reduced from 12 to 6 ml/kg in ICU patients after CABG surgery. The 50% tidal volume reduction was associated with a significant negative bias for $Q_{C,pr}$, that is, lower than Q_{TD} values. A follow-up study suggested that it was the decreased minute volume, rather than the decreased tidal volume, that affected accuracy of the NICO versus Q_{TD} (Tachibana *et al.*, 2003). A major concern with both of these studies is the insufficient time allowed for P_vCO_2 to stabilize after the large minute volume reduction. The lengthy period needed to raise the high capacity body stores of CO_2 before tissue PCO_2 (the CO_2 source) became high enough to drive $V'CO_2$ back to control values was almost certainly responsible for the significant negative $Q_{C,pr}$ bias. Indeed, Taskar *et al.* (1995) reported that the time constant for $V'CO_2$ recovery (to control) was 17.1 ± 9.9 min for a 10% minute volume (V'_E) increase and 35 ± 10.7 min for a 10% reduction in V'_E. This contrasts with Tachibana's 50% V'_E reduction and a 15 min interval $Q_{C,pr}/Q_{TD}$ measurement, almost certainly too brief an interval for an abrupt V'_E reduction.

An interesting clinical analogy is seen with rapid red blood cell (RBC) transfusion. It is associated with a large, abrupt $Q_{C,pr}$ reduction because of the high PCO_2 in stored blood. This scenario, however, is distinctly different from an abrupt ventilation reduction, because rapid infusion of stored RBCs is accompanied by a rapid increase in $V'CO_2$ as the RBCs traverse the ventilated lung, preventing the CO_2 bolus from being stored in the body. Within a few (3–6) minutes, $P_{et}CO_2$, $V'CO_2$ and the $Q_{C,pr}$ estimate recover to control, while $Q_{C,pr}$ usually increases above pre-transfusion values with the improved blood volume (BV) and Hgb.

Odenstedt *et al.* (2002) performed another critical analysis of $Q_{C,pr}$ (NICO) versus Q_{TD} (PA catheter) in 15 operating room (OR) and ICU patients. They found a high overall correlation between the two measurements: $Q_{TD} = 0.99Q_{c,pr}$, where $r = 0.96$ over a Q_{TD} range of 2.3–15.7 l/min and $Q_{C,pr}$ range of 2.3–18.1 l/min. The within-subject correlation was also excellent; $r = 0.88$. There was no significant overall bias ($Q_{TD} - Q_{C,pr}$ was 0.04 l/min) and the limits of agreement (bias ± 2 SD) were: − 1.68 and 1.76 l/min, although there was a small trend towards overestimation by $Q_{C,pr}$ at higher values. Independent assessment of $V'CO_2$ using CO_2 insufflation into a lung model showed a 2–9% underestimation (by the NICO) at a respiratory frequency of 10 and a 5–13% underestimation at a frequency of 15–20. The authors speculate that a high correlation combined with minimal bias for $Q_{TD} - Q_{C,pr}$ could be due to a small $P_{et}CO_2$ error balancing a $V'CO_2$ bias, thus canceling out the error. Intrapulmonary shunt estimates with the Nunn shunt isopleths were on an average, 11% lower compared with shunt values derived from mixed venous and

Table 22.1 Bias, precision and relative error of NICO and CCO against BCO at four operative stages

	Postindution	Aorta cross-clamp	Iliac reperfusion	Peritoneal closure
Bias ± precision (l/min)				
NICO	−0.1 ± 0.61	−0.52 ± 0.95	−0.99 ± 0.86*	−0.72 ± 0.97*
CCO	0.23 ± 0.81	0.37 ± 1.05	0.2 ± 1.12	0.72 ± 1.57*
Relative error (%)				
NICO	−1.2 ± 18.3	−11.1 ± 23.9	−19.1 ± 15.1	−14.9 ± 15.2
CCO	6.7 ± 23.4	10.9 ± 26.2	3.5 ± 19.6	12.1 ± 22.7

Data by Kotake *et al.* were collected from 28 patients and expressed as bias ± precision (1 SD of bias). Differences against BCO (Bolus Q_{TD}) were statistically analyzed with repeated measures ANOVA. Relative error (%) is defined as [either (NICO or CCO) − BCO]/BCO and expressed in mean ± SD, thus not subject to statistical analysis.
*$P < 0.05$ vs. after anesthetic induction. BCO, CCO and NICO = bolus thermodilution, continuous thermodilution and noninvasive cardiac output, respectively. (Reproduced with permission from Kotake, Y., Moriyama, K., Innami, Y., Shimizu, H., Ueda, T., Morisaki, H. & Takeda, J. (2003). Performance of noninvasive partial CO_2 rebreathing cardiac output and continuous thermodilution cardiac output in patients undergoing aortic reconstruction surgery. *Anesthesiology*, **99**: 283–288.)

arterial blood O_2 content differences. However, this shunt difference was clearly inconsistent with the high level of agreement between the two total cardiac output measurements. The authors postulate a difference in "effective pulmonary blood flow" based on low ventilation/perfusion ($\dot{V}_A/\dot{Q}$) ratio. Presumably the authors meant that the shunt estimates from the Q_{TD} measurements were too high because of the effect of low $\dot{V}_A/\dot{Q}$ areas on shunt measurements. However, in the presence of elevated inspired O_2 ($F_IO_2 > 0.21$), the effect of areas with low $\dot{V}_A/\dot{Q}$ on O_2 uptake is minimized. Thus a more likely explanation would be errors in blood gas-derived (rather than direct (co-oximeter)) O_2 content values for calculating the shunt (Johnson *et al.*, 1993).

The question of a predictable clinical source bias was addressed in an abdominal aortic reconstruction case study by Kotake *et al.* (2003). They measured bolus Q_{TD} via PA catheter, compared with continuous Q_{TD} (CCO) and with $Q_{C,pr}$ (NICO), during four distinct periods of surgery: (1) after anesthetic induction, (2) during aortic cross-clamp, (3) after reperfusion of the iliac artery and (4) during peritoneal closure. Overall bias and precision was -0.58 ± 0.91 l/min for the NICO and 0.38 ± 1.17 l/min for the CCO. The NICO bias increased after iliac reperfusion, while the CCO bias increased during peritoneal closure, as shown in Table 22.1. Kotake *et al.* (2003) did not determine the reason for the "reperfusion" NICO bias change, but speculated there may have been modest changes in $V'CO_2$ and dead-space that were not statistically significant. (It is not clear whether their $Q_{C,pr}$ values were corrected for potential $P_aCO_2-P_{et}CO_2$ difference changes after reperfusion.) They then proposed that $Q_{C,pr}$ with the NICO may be valuable for identifying significant hemodynamic abnormalities, but additional PA catheter data on left ventricular filling pressures and intrapulmonary shunting may be needed when patients have serious cardiac and pulmonary disease. This concern would be most relevant in patients at risk for fluid overload because of congestive heart failure (CHF) or acute lung injury (ALI) leading to adult respiratory distress syndrome (ARDS).

Finally, a computer model study of $Q_{C,pr}$ measurements by Yem *et al.* (2003) suggested that the period of rebreathing may be a cause of systematic error. They concluded that for $Q_{C,pr} < 3$ l/min a rebreathing period of 50 s was needed, although for $Q_{C,pr} > 6$ l/min a rebreathing period of 50 s was excessive. They suggested that a time constant for CO_2 in an alveolar compartment was inversely proportional to the product of the solubility of CO_2 in blood and the $Q_{C,pr}$. This led to their recommendation of applying either a variable period of rebreathing, depending on the latest $Q_{C,pr}$ value, or a proportional correction factor. These suggested modifications obviously need to be tested in animal and/or human subjects.

Shortcuts to pulmonary blood flow assessment

Clinical experience with $P_{et}CO_2$ has repeatedly demonstrated that severe acute reduction in pulmonary blood flow during constant ventilation is accompanied by a major $P_{et}CO_2$ reduction, while rapid cardiac output recovery produces $P_{et}CO_2$ recovery. This observation was first reported by Leigh *et al.* (1957). They assumed acute Q_T reduction based on sudden profound hypotension with PA clamping during intrathoracic surgery, while it was obvious during ventricular fibrillation. They also observed dramatic improvement in $P_{et}CO_2$ with unclamping of the PA and with effective open cardiac massage. More recently, Barton *et al.* (1988) found that 14 emergency department patients with cardiac arrest who developed a palpable pulse during resuscitation had a significantly higher $P_{et}CO_2$ than those who did not ($P_{et}CO_2$ 19 versus 5 mmHg, respectively). Thus capnometry has potential as a prognostic indicator of lung perfusion and Q_T during CPR, and has been used to assess the efficacy of different CPR compression rates for improving lung perfusion (Ornato *et al.*, 1988). Similarly though less dramatic changes are observed during periods of rapid surgical bleeding, fluid resuscitation and transfusion. It should be remembered that the reliability of $P_{et}CO_2$ as an indicator of pulmonary blood flow may be briefly confounded by the high PCO_2 of stored RBCs. Furthermore, gradual, moderate changes in Q_T are not so readily discerned by $P_{et}CO_2$ monitoring.

Availability of volumetric capnometry has also facilitated breath-to-breath online CO_2 production ($V'CO_2$) measurement. Obviously, an abrupt reduction in Q_C will be accompanied by a reduction in $V'CO_2$. However, it is inherent in constant ventilation that reduction in $V'CO_2$ will be more gradual as $P_{et}CO_2$ falls, because the high solubility of CO_2 in blood enables continued CO_2 elimination despite the falling P_ACO_2 associated with falling pulmonary blood flow. This implies that neither $V'CO_2$ nor $Q_{C,pr}$ provide immediately accurate reflections of the change in Q_C during a period when $P_{et}CO_2$ and $V'CO_2$ are changing rapidly. Thus reliable estimates of Q_C with $Q_{c,pr}$ measurement are based on assumption of stable or steady state gas exchange (Q_C, ventilation and $V'CO_2$) conditions. However, rapidly falling $P_{et}CO_2$ and $V'CO_2$ are immediate indicators of inadequate tissue perfusion due to falling Q_T. These indicators, in turn, provide an instantaneous indication for rapid intravenous (i.v.) fluid infusion, blood transfusion, vasopressor or inotropic intervention for the immediate circulatory challenge, as shown in the following section.

Clinical experience with noninvasive pulmonary blood flow monitoring

Hypotension due to vasodilation

There are many kinds of clinical scenarios where noninvasive Q_T monitoring provides valuable insight and guidance. A simple, clear example is an elderly patient without a known history of cardiovascular disease who develops unusually severe hypotension with i.v. propofol anesthesia that persists in spite of generous i.v. fluid administration. This can be especially troublesome when the surgical stimulus is not intense, as is common, for example, during middle ear surgery. Personal experience has included several such instances where the patient had an excellent Q_T determined by $Q_{C,pr}$, yielding a cardiac index (CI, which is measured by cardiac output/body surface area) of 3 l/min/m^2, while SVR was in the 750 dynes s/cm^5 range. A continuous i.v. phenylephrine infusion was then provided to raise SVR and maintain blood pressure (BP) in a satisfactory range with only a minor reduction in CI from the increased afterload.

A "thready pulse"

A previously healthy 40-year-old obese woman arrived at our OR for an emergency exploratory laparotomy with "air under the diaphragm", thus a presumptive diagnosis of perforated duodenal ulcer. She was tachycardic with a heart rate of 110. Placing a large bore i.v. proved difficult. So the emergency surgery was expedited by inducing general anesthesia with etomidate and phenylephrine, after which the second i.v. was started successfully for fluid resuscitation with Pentastarch 1000 and 3000 ml lactated Ringers solution. Repeated i.v. phenylephrine boluses were needed in spite of the fluids, while arterial catheter (A-line) placement attempts were unsuccessful. Indeed, the radial artery pulse "felt feeble" at the outset, and soon both radial artery pulses became completely non-palpable! The ulnar artery pulse could only be felt during inspiration and even then it was "thready". The surgeons reported that the abdomen had gross pus from a ruptured appendix, removed it and washed out the abdomen, then quickly closed the abdomen in hope of starting their next emergency case in a timely manner. However, because there was no urine output from the indwelling catheter, this "thready" pulse could mean she was still hypovolemic; so noninvasive Q_T measurements were obtained with the NICO monitor (Respironics-Novametrix, Inc.). Surprisingly, Q_T was 7.9 l/min, mean arterial BP was 58 mmHg (cuff) and SVR was estimated at 465 dynes s/cm^5 (with a CVP estimate of 10 mmHg). The high Q_T and low SVR with pus in the abdomen from a ruptured appendix were consistent with a "sepsis" picture, so i.v. dopamine infusion was started at 3 μg/kg/min. BP responded remarkably well, now making it easier to place the radial artery catheter. This proved critical during a stormy night of treating the fulminant sepsis with high dose vasopressor infusion and intensive fluid resuscitation.

In reviewing the earlier situation in the OR, the anesthesiologists were unable to differentiate between a hypovolemic (vasoconstricted) "thready pulse" versus a septic (vasodilated) "weak pulse". Once the diagnosis of sepsis became apparent, it was clear that this shock-like state demanded immediate vasopressor and fluid therapy! Such a dramatic example of clinical uncertainty from routine clinical assessment greatly strengthened the case for obtaining an expedient cardiac output measurement. This led to the appropriate therapy (i.v. dopamine infusion plus rapid crystalloid and colloid fluid infusion).

Hypovolemia

Significant preoperative hypovolemia also remains an unexpected though surprisingly common cause of intraoperative hypotension. BV may be reduced as a consequence of inadequate antihypertensive therapy, dehydration from fasting and/or a bowel preparation for colon resection or from fluid restriction in a patient with impaired renal function. CI can be remarkably low in such patients, but usually responds well to i.v. fluid loading with crystalloid and/or colloid solutions. A clinical correlate of this scenario is that hematocrit will fall precipitously after fluid resuscitation, leaving very little margin for further reduction from surgical blood loss. Thus, if the CI falls to 2.0 or below with general anesthesia, recovers significantly from fluid therapy but then falls below 2.0 again with surgical blood loss, it is likely that such a patient will need blood transfusion. Serious consideration should be given to the possibility that the persistent hemodynamic instability may be from insufficient cardiac reserve to compensate for acute anemia. Myocardial O_2 supply may be inadequate to meet the increased demand because of the reduced O_2 carrying capacity of the anemic blood and/or persistent hypovolemia. Hypotension will exacerbate the supply/demand imbalance, especially if there is significant coronary artery disease. However, vasopressor therapy may not improve cardiac performance if BV remains too low or Hgb falls to a critical level.

Continuous CI monitoring for the combined effects of BV reduction and acute anemia should therefore be considered in patients with limited cardiovascular reserve during moderate to high risk surgical procedures. Such procedures include major bowel resection, radical retropubic prostatectomy (RRP), radical cystectomy with ileal diversion, total hip replacement, aortofemoral bypass and abdominal aortic aneurysm repair. Similar considerations should be given to patients scheduled for multiple segment spine surgery with metal fixation.

Radical retropubic prostatectomy

We proposed that intraoperative changes in CI during RRP would reflect BV changes from surgical bleeding, especially when hematocrit (Hct) fell to the 23–28% range. We recorded the lowest systolic BP, CI, Hct and BV associated with 500 ml increments of estimated blood loss (EBL) up to the decision to transfuse (by an anesthesiologist not directly involved with the study, but having full access to all the data except BV (determined after surgery)). The contribution of Hct, BP and CI to the decision to transfuse was compared for: (1) all 36 subjects and (2) subjects whose Hct fell to 23–28%, using receiver operator curve (ROC) analysis. For 21 of the 36 subjects (58%) who were transfused, the decision to transfuse was based primarily on Hct, as shown by: (1) ROC area: Hct, 0.98; BP, 0.78; CI, 0.74 and by (2) data shown in Table 22.2. When Hct fell to the 23–28% range, ROC area changed to: Hct, 0.94; CI, 0.92; BP, 0.74. A CI of $<2.5\,l/min/m^2$ in the Hct 23–28% subgroup was associated with significantly reduced BV (46.6 ± 6.7 ml/kg lean body mass, $P = 0.0003$), higher Hct and NS difference in BP, as shown in Table 22.3. Regression of CI and BV showed higher correlation for the 24 subject subgroup with Hct 23–28%: $r^2 = 0.65$, $P = 0.0001$ (Figure 22.5; Dueck *et al.*, 2003), compared with: $r^2 = 0.34$, $P = 0.0003$, for all 36 subjects (Figure 22.6).

Noninvasive CI monitoring therefore reflected an average 22.9% BV reduction when CI was $<2.5\,l/min/m^2$ for subjects with Hct 23–28% during surgical bleeding. This suggests that CI was a hypovolemia indicator during acute hemodilution with surgical blood

Table 22.2 Blood transfusion findings in 36 radical retropubic prostatectomy patients

All subjects	*N*	EBL (ml)	BV (ml/kg)	Hct (%)	CI (l/min/m²)	BP (mmHg)
No transfusion	15	1177 ± 515	57.8 ± 12.1	29 ± 3	2.74 ± 0.45	109 ± 16
Transfusion	21	1390 ± 471	51.7 ± 9.5	24 ± 2	2.39 ± 0.59	91 ± 15
Significance		NS	NS	$P < 0.0001$	NS	$P = 0.0016$

EBL, BV and CI were NS different for the 21 patients who were transfused, while Hct and systolic arterial BP were significantly lower compared with the 15 subjects who were not transfused. (From Dueck, R., *et al.* (2003) with permission.)

Table 22.3 Radical retropubic prostatectomy patients with hematocrit 23–28%

	N	BV (ml/kg)	Hct (%)	CI (l/min/m^2)	BP (mmHg)
Low CI < 2.5	12	46.6 ± 6.7	27 ± 2	2.03 ± 0.23	91 ± 16
Low CI > 2.5	12	62.6 ± 10.5	25 ± 1	2.97 ± 0.38	102 ± 18
Significance		$P = 0.0003$	$P = 0.0034$	$P < 0.0001$	NS

The 24 subjects whose Hct fell to the 23–28% range during surgical bleeding had a significantly lower BV if CI was <2.5 l/min/m^2, even though their Hct was higher and systolic BP was NS different. (From Dueck, R., *et al.* (2003) with permission.)

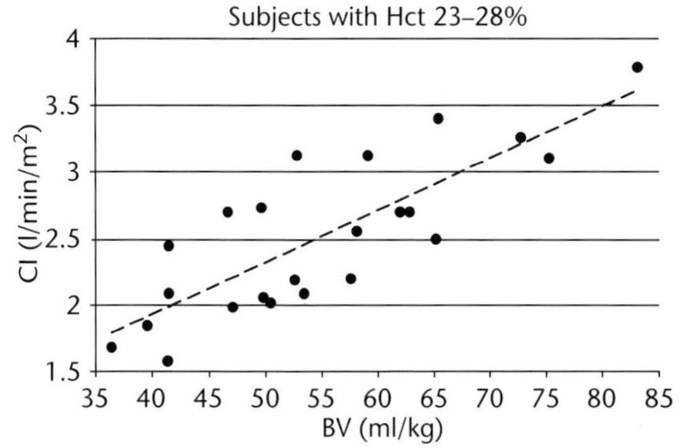

Figure 22.5 The CI and BV relationship for the 24 subject subgroup with Hct 23–28% showed a correlation coefficient, $r^2 = 0.65$, $P = 0.0001$. This was probably the basis for a ROC area of 0.92 at the time of decision to either give or avoid a RBC transfusion during RRP.

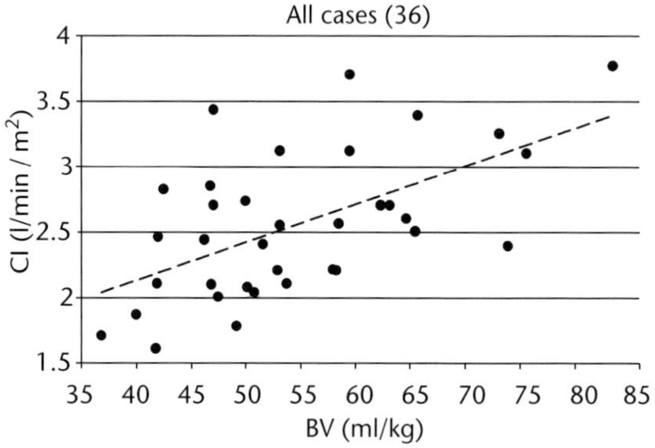

Figure 22.6 The CI and BV relationship for all 36 subjects showed a correlation coefficient, $r^2 = 0.34$, $P = 0.0003$. The lower correlation was consistent with a ROC Area of 0.74 at the time the decision was made to either give or avoid a blood transfusion. Presumably there were other reasons for CI variation in subjects whose Hct was >28 and did not require a transfusion.

loss. The high ROC area ($R = 0.92$) for CI in this subgroup supports the value of CI as a monitor to help with the transfusion decision during RRP. This may be related to the importance of BV for enabling the heart to compensate for acute anemia during surgical blood loss.

Abdominal aortic cross-clamp

Figure 22.7 presents an example of the effects of abdominal aortic cross-clamping on CI during aorto-femoral bypass surgery. At the beginning of surgery the CI trend showed a compromised CI in the 2.0 l/min/m^2 range. Five minutes after the 9:53 aortic cross-clamp there was a 50% CI reduction to the 1.0 l/min/m^2 range, indicating inability of the heart to compensate for the acute afterload increase. In spite of the large CI drop, systolic arterial BP climbed progressively to 180 mmHg. This period of stress was relieved by the surgeon releasing the aortic cross-clamp at 10:17. An i.v. nitroprusside infusion was then started, providing a CI around 3.0 l/min/m^2. This allowed the surgeon to resume aortic cross-clamp at 11:04, with CI stabilizing in the 2.0–2.5 l/min/m^2 range.

Figure 22.8 provides an expanded view of the changes induced by the aortic cross-clamp at 9:53, and the recovery after release of the cross-clamp at 10:17. (a) Breath-to-breath changes in CO_2 elimination rate ($\dot{V}CO_2$) during normal and partial rebreathing periods. (b) The corresponding changes in $P_{et}CO_2$. (c) The 3-min cycle CI values derived from $Q_{C,pr}$. Note that both $V'CO_2$ and $P_{et}CO_2$ recordings show dramatic reduction soon after 9:53 and an apparent CO_2 bolus into the lungs soon after release of the aortic cross-clamp at 10:17 and a fluctuating CI recovery. The CI from $Q_{C,pr}$ monitoring may not have provided precise measurements during the most unsteady pulmonary gas exchange conditions. However, the acute directional changes appropriately reflected critical hemodynamic responses to aortic cross-clamp and unclamping. Fortunately, the surgeon's decision to remove the cross-clamp was followed by rapid cardiac improvement. The further CI recovery with nitroprusside infusion (started at 10:25) represented

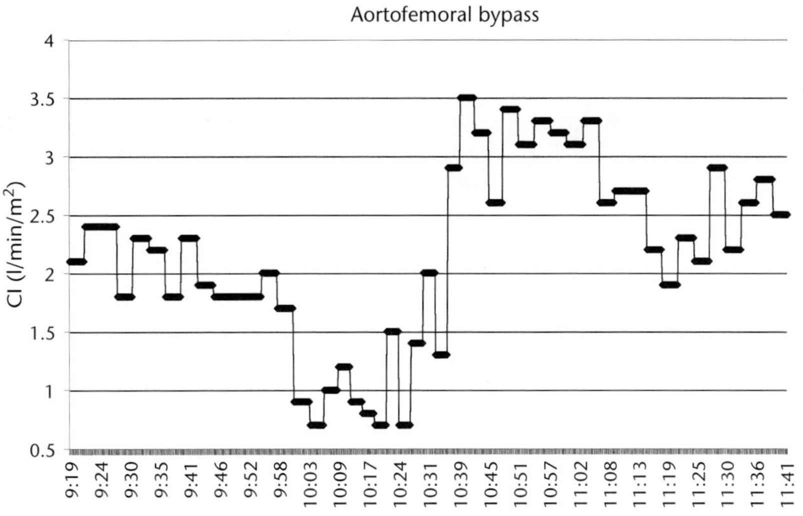

Figure 22.7 A continuous trend of CI versus time is presented from a patient with severe peripheral vascular disease during general anesthesia and surgery for aortofemoral bypass. Note that CI was only in the 2.0 l/min/m^2 range prior to infrarenal aortic cross-clamp, then fell to less than 1.0 l/min/m^2 after aortic cross-clamp after 9:53. (The delayed CI changes are in part related to the 3-min $Q_{C,pr}$ cycle.) CI recovered after release of the aortic cross-clamp at 10:17 and improved to the 3.0 l/min/m^2 range with nitroprusside infusion, enabling aortic cross-clamp to resume at around 11:04.

effective therapy for this patient's compromised heart during the stress of abdominal aortic cross-clamp.

Congestive heart failure

Preoperative echocardiographic evaluation of a patient scheduled for RRP showed mild aortic stenosis, moderate concentric left ventricular (LV) hypertrophy and abnormal diastolic function. An adenosine-sestamibi technetium cardiac stress test showed hypokinesis of the inferobasal wall and decreased inferior wall uptake. Perioperative metoprolol therapy for coronary disease was started 3 days preoperatively according to the cardiology consultant's recommendations. In addition, the cardiology consultant recommended that invasive monitoring with a PA catheter was not needed.

General anesthesia for RRP was provided with direct radial artery BP and NICO noninvasive Q_T monitoring. CI was predominantly in the 1.5 l/min/m^2 range, although frequent i.v. bolus doses of ephedrine and phenylephrine ensured adequate arterial BP. In addition, vigorous i.v. crystalloid and colloid infusion, as well as rapid RBC transfusion, provided two periods where CI temporarily improved into the 2.0 l/min/m^2 range, prior to the sustained improvement near the end of surgery, as shown in Figure 22.9. These fluids accumulated to a total of 6 units of RBCs, 1000 ml Hetastarch, 3000 ml Ringers solution and 1000 ml saline for a total EBL of 3000 ml. A base deficit was present on arterial blood gases, which progressed to a nadir of −7. During the last hour of surgery repeated sighs were needed for low O_2 saturation, so fiberoptic bronchoscopy was performed; which showed the endotracheal tube was 3 cm above the carina. There were no bronchial mucous plugs, but the airway epithelium appeared suspicious for tracheobronchial edema. A chest radiograph showed pulmonary congestion, even though a PA catheter was placed and indicated a PAWP of 10 mmHg. Thermal dilution CI was consistent with the 3.5 l/min/m^2 determined by the NICO monitor. The patient received modest dose i.v. diuretic therapy and mechanical ventilation overnight and was then weaned and extubated successfully.

Review of this patient's unusually poor tolerance of anesthesia and surgical blood loss suggests that his diastolic dysfunction was more severe than appreciated during preoperative cardiology evaluation. The initial appropriate response to i.v. fluids before significant surgical bleeding, followed by persistently low CI in spite of rapid i.v. fluid and blood transfusion during two periods of significant blood loss, suggest that he may have required a relatively high LV filling pressure to develop an adequate CI. This raises the possibility that his prophylactic beta blockade therapy may have compromised his response to acute surgical anemia. The improved cardiac performance when blood transfusion caught up with blood loss near the

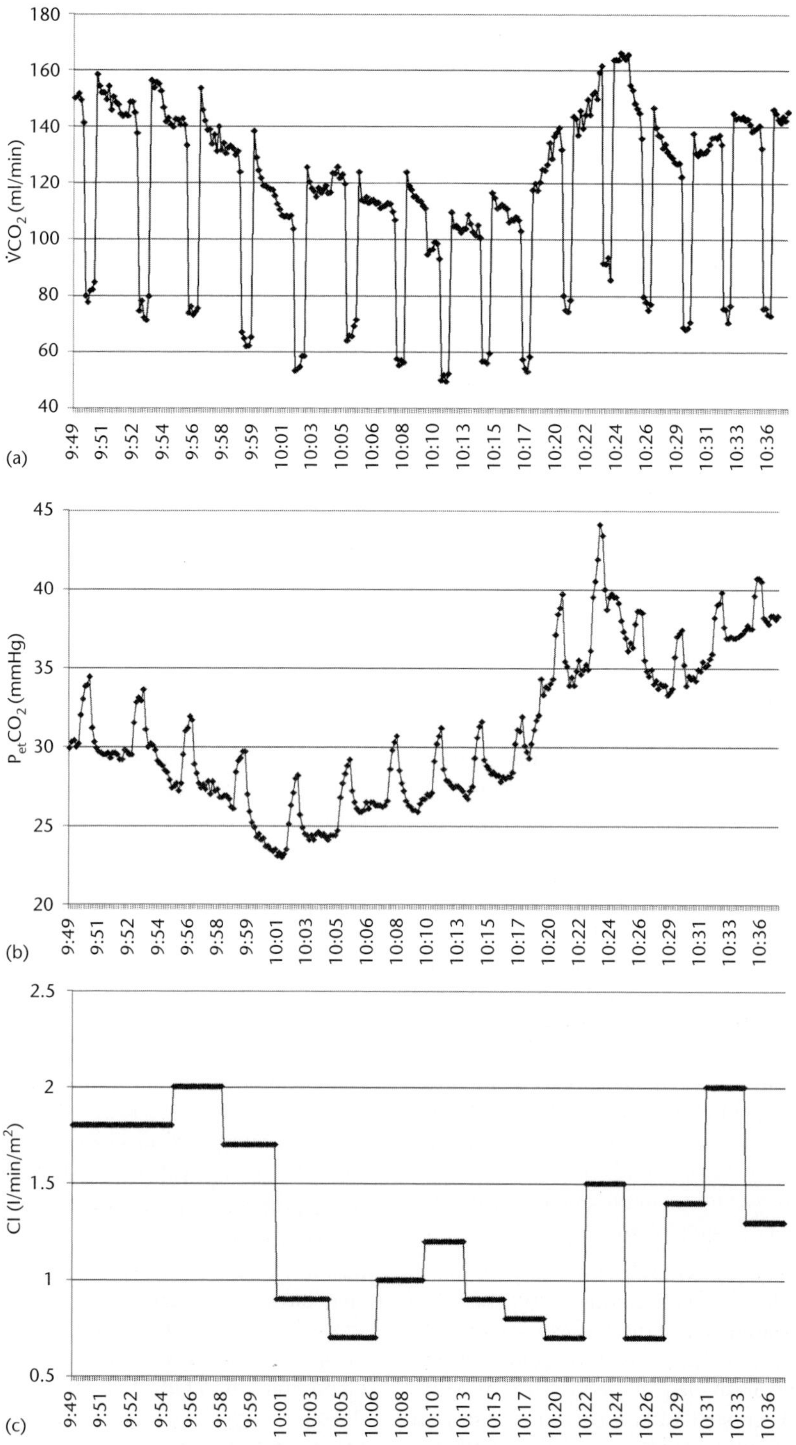

Figure 22.8 An expanded breath-to-breath CO_2 elimination rate ($\dot{V}CO_2$) and $P_{et}CO_2$ trend is presented for the 3-min normal and partial rebreathing ($Q_{C,pr}$) cycles, during the period in which aortic cross-clamp was first applied at 9:53 and then released at 10:17 in the CI trend plot shown in Figure 22.7. Note that both $\dot{V}CO_2$ and $P_{et}CO_2$ trends demonstrate a rapid fall in CO_2 elimination from the lung after aortic cross-clamp and a bolus CO_2 delivery after release of the aortic cross-clamp. These acute changes are reflected by fluctuating CI changes (lower panel), indicative of the unstable hemodynamic conditions associated with the major afterload effects on this patient's heart.

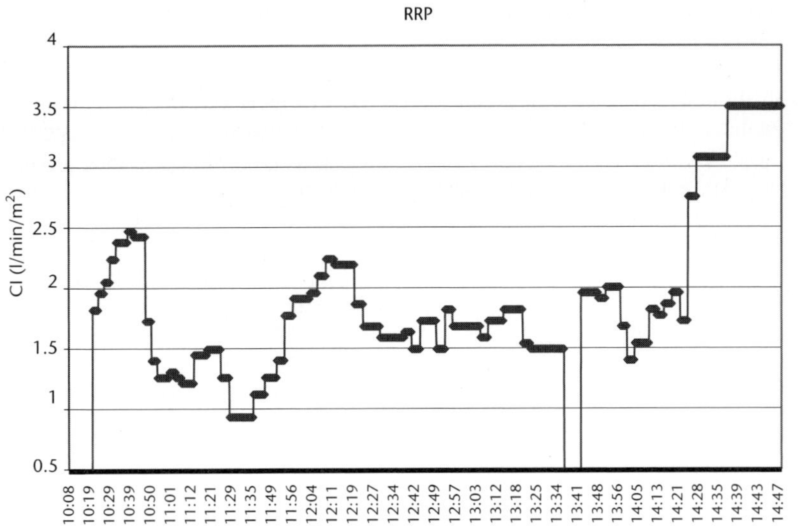

Figure 22.9 The CI trend for this patient during RRP shows significant periods of heart failure (CI $< 2.0\,l/min/m^2$) in spite of vigorous i.v. fluids and blood transfusion for a total 3000 ml blood loss. A postoperative chest X-ray showed pulmonary congestion, which was treated with i.v. lasix and overnight assisted mechanical ventilation.

end of surgery supports this general assessment. However, by this time the falling pulmonary gas exchange represented CHF, as demonstrated by the postoperative chest radiograph. It is therefore reasonable to suggest that the low CI and metabolic acidosis during rapid bleeding might have responded more favorably to i.v. dopamine or dobutamine infusion than the repeated bolus doses of phenylephrine and ephedrine. A more effective direct-acting inotropic agonist might have reduced the pulmonary congestion and improved tissue perfusion. A patient whose CI shows poor tolerance of rapid blood loss and acute anemia may therefore require more intensive inotropic vasoactive therapy to assure an adequate cardiac output response to i.v. fluids and blood transfusion.

Summary

Noninvasive cardiac output measurement via the Fick principle for CO_2 has evolved from a theoretical concept in 1870 to an effective clinical application in 2003. There is clear evidence that reliable, meaningful pulmonary blood flow (Q_C) estimates can be derived from CO_2 elimination and $P_{et}CO_2$ measurements. This technology is well suited to replace invasive PA catheter and thermal dilution Q_T measurements during trauma, surgery and critical care, thereby reducing the inherent risks associated with invasive methods. A recent prospective study demonstrated that CI falling below the $2.5\,l/min/m^2$ range during surgical bleeding was associated with hypovolemia when hematocrit was 23–28%. Such evidence of cardiac compromise supports the decision to transfuse with RBCs. Clinical experience has also provided dramatic hemodynamic profiles of vasodilation, hypovolemia, sepsis and acute heart failure, for example, from cross-clamping the abdominal aorta. Continuous noninvasive Q_T monitoring can therefore provide critical cardiovascular information during everyday clinical practice.

References

Barton, C.W. & Callaham, M.L. (1988). Successful prediction by capnometry of resuscitation from cardiac arrest. *Ann. Emerg. Med.*, **17**: 393 [abstract].

Benator, S.R., Hewlett, A.M. & Nunn, J.F. (1973). The use of iso-shunt lines for control of oxygen therapy. *Br. J. Anaesth.*, **45**: 711–718.

Capek, J.M. & Roy, R.J. (1988). Noninvasive measurement of cardiac output using partial CO_2 rebreathing. *IEEE Trans. Biomed. Eng.*, **35**: 653–661.

Collier, C.R. (1956). Determination of mixed venous CO_2 tensions by rebreathing. *J. Appl. Physiol.*, **9**: 25–29.

De Abreu, M.G., Quintel, M., Ragaller, M. & Albrecht, D.M. (1997). Partial carbon dioxide rebreathing: a reliable technique for noninvasive measurement of nonshunted pulmonary capillary blood flow. *Crit. Care Med.*, **25**: 675–683.

De Abreu, M.G., Winkler, T., Pahlitzsch, T., Weismann, D. & Albrecht, D.M. (2003). Performance of the partial CO_2

rebreathing technique under different hemodynamic and ventilation/perfusion matching conditions. *Crit. Care Med.*, **31**: 543–551.

Defares, J.G. (1958). Determination of P_VCO_2 from the exponential CO_2 rise during rebreathing. *J. Appl. Physiol.*, **13**: 159–164.

Dueck, R., Mitchell, M., Albo, M. & Yi, K. (2003). Noninvasive cardiac index as a blood volume surrogate to assess the need for transfusion during radical retropubic prostatectomy. *ASA Meeting Abstracts*, A-180.

Dubois, A.B., Britt, A.G. & Fenn, W.O. (1952). Alveolar CO_2 during the respiratory cycle. *J. Appl. Physiol.*, **4**: 535–548.

Farhi, L.E., Nesarajah, M.S., Olszowka, A.J., Metildi, L.A. & Ellis, A.K. (1976). Cardiac output determination by simple one-step rebreathing technique. *Resp. Physiol.*, **28**: 141–159.

Fick, A. Über die Messung des Blutquantums in den Herzventrikeln. In: *Sitzungsberichte der Phys.-Med. Ges. zu Würzburg. XIV. Sitzung am 9 Juli*, 1870, p. 16.

Gedeon, A., Forslund, L., Hedenstierna, G. & Romano, E. (1980). A new method for noninvasive bedside determination of pulmonary blood flow. *Med. Biol. Eng. Comput.*, **18**: 411–418.

Hamilton, W.F., Moore, J.W. & Kinsman, J.M. (1928). Delay of blood in passing through the lungs as an obstacle to the determination of the CO_2 tension of the mixed venous blood. *Am. J. Physiol.*, **82**: 656–664.

Haryadi, D.G., Orr, J.A., Kuck, K., McJames, S. & Westenskow, D.R. (2000). Partial CO_2 rebreathing indirect Fick technique for noninvasive measurement of cardiac output. *J. Clin. Monit.*, **16**: 361–374.

Hlastala, M.P., Wranne, B. & Lenfant, C.J. (1972). Single-breath method of measuring cardiac output – a reevaluation. *J. Appl. Physiol.*, **33**: 846–848.

Johnson, P.A., Bihari, D.J., Raper, R.F., Haughton, M.A., Fisher, M.M. & Herkes, R.G. (1993). A comparison between direct and calculated oxygen saturation in intensive care. *Anaesth. Intens. Care*, **21**: 72–75.

Kotake, Y., Moriyama, K., Innami, Y., Shimizu, H., Ueda, T., Morisaki, H. & Takeda, J. (2003). Performance of noninvasive partial CO_2 rebreathing cardiac output and continuous thermodilution cardiac output in patients undergoing aortic reconstruction surgery. *Anesthesiology*, **99**: 283–288.

Leigh, M.D., Jenkins, L.C., Belton, M.K. & Lewis, G.B. (1957). Continuous alveolar carbon dioxide analysis as a monitor of pulmonary blood flow. *Anesthesiology*, **18**: 878–882.

Odenstedt, H., Stenqvist, O. & Lundin, S. (2002). Clinical evaluation of a partial CO_2 rebreathing technique for cardiac output monitoring in critically patients. *Acta Anaesth. Scand.*, **46**: 152–159.

Ornato, J.P., Gonzalez, E.R, Garnett, A.R., *et al.* (1988). Effect of cardiopulmonary resuscitation compression rate on end-tidal carbon dioxide concentration and arterial pressure in man. *Crit. Care Med.*, **16**: 241–245.

Sackner, M.A., Greeneltch, D., Heiman, M.S., Epstein, S. & Atkins, N. (1975). Diffusing capacity, membrane diffusing capacity, capillary blood volume, pulmonary tissue volume, and cardiac output measured by a rebreathing technique. *Am. Rev. Resp. Dis.*, **111**: 157–165.

Tachibana, K., Imanaka, H., Miyano, H., Takeuchi, M., Kumon, K. & Nishimura, M. (2002). Effect of ventilatory settings on accuracy of cardiac output measurement using partial CO_2 rebreathing. *Anesthesiology*, **96**: 96–102.

Tachibana, K., Imanaka, H., Takeuchi, M., Takauchi, Y. & Miyano, H. (2003). Noninvasive cardiac output measurement using partial rebreathing carbon dioxide rebreathing is less accurate at settings of reduced minute ventilation and when spontaneous breathing is present. *Anesthesiology*, **98**: 830–837.

Taskar, V., John, J., Larsson, A., Wetterberg, T. & Jonson, B. (1995). Dynamics of carbon dioxide elimination following ventilator resetting. *Chest*, **108**: 196–202.

Vandam, L.D. & Fox, J.A. (1998). Adolf Fick (1829–1901), Physiologist. A heritage for anesthesiology and critical care medicine. *Anesthesiology*, **88**: 514–518.

Vanhees, L., Defoor, J., Schepers, D., Bruselle, S., Reybrouck, T. & Fagard, R. (2000). Comparison of cardiac output measured by two automated methods of CO_2 rebreathing. *Med. Sci. Sport. Exer.*, **32**: 1028–1034.

Yem, J.S., Yongquan, T., Turner, M.J. & Baker, A.B. (2003). Sources of error in noninvasive pulmonary blood flow measurements by partial rebreathing. *Anesthesiology*, **98**: 881–887.

PARTIAL PRESSURE END-TIDAL CARBON DIOXIDE MONITORING FOR PATIENTS WITH ACUTE RESPIRATORY DISTRESS SYNDROME: EFFECTS OF PHYSIOLOGIC DEAD-SPACE VOLUME

23

M.J. Banner

Introduction

Monitoring the *partial pressure of end-tidal carbon dioxide* ($P_{et}CO_2$) is essential for assessing the appropriateness of ventilation for patients in the operating room. However, this type of monitoring is not widely used in the intensive care unit (ICU) for critically sick adults with compromised pulmonary function and related organ dysfunction. It is ironic that exhaled CO_2 monitoring is not applied routinely to these patients, for their situation is far more tenuous than those with normal pulmonary function in the operating room. A reason for this irony may be a belief that exhaled CO_2 data are spurious due to abnormal alveolar minute ventilation-to-perfusion ($\dot{V}_A/\dot{Q}$) matching conditions across the lungs of patients with acute respiratory distress syndrome (ARDS). In a few situations this may be true, but not for most patients with ARDS attached to life-support ventilators. Exhaled CO_2 monitoring in the ICU may offer considerable insight for assessment and treatment.

The themes of this chapter are the physiology of CO_2 elimination in the lungs, operational theory and use of *volume-based* capnography, dead-space volume (V_D) conditions affecting the accuracy of $P_{et}CO_2$ for predicting arterial blood CO_2, and practical reasons for routinely using volume-based capnography for patients with ARDS.

CO_2 is generated during oxidative metabolism within the cells. Catabolism of one glucose molecule in the tricarboxylic acid cycle (TCA) yields six molecules of CO_2. As it is a non-polar molecule, CO_2 is highly lipid soluble and can diffuse easily across cell membranes from the cells into the blood for transport to the lungs. CO_2 is transported in the blood in three forms: (1) dissolved in the plasma and measured as the PCO_2, approximately 7% is transported in this form; (2) bound to hemoglobin and known as carbamino hemoglobin ($HbCO_2$), approximately 23% is transported in this form; and as (3) bicarbonate ion (HCO_3^-) in the plasma, approximately 70% is transported in this form (Guyton, 1981).

When mixed venous blood from the right ventricle enters the lungs, CO_2 diffuses out of the alveoli and is then exhaled, where it can be measured by capnometry. $P_{et}CO_2$, measured at end-exhalation, is essentially the same as the alveolar PCO_2 (P_ACO_2). Phase III of a capnogram (Figure. 23.1) reaches a peak, usually during the final phase of exhalation, and is referred to as the $P_{et}CO_2$. In normal individuals, $P_{et}CO_2$ is approximately 2–3 mmHg lower than arterial blood PCO_2 (P_aCO_2) (Moon & Camporesi, 2000). Chronic pulmonary disease and acute disturbances in $\dot{V}_A/\dot{Q}$ usually widen this difference. At times, $P_{et}CO_2$ may be greater than P_aCO_2 (Fletcher & Veintemilla, 1989; Russell *et al.*, 1990; Russell & Graybeal, 1995). Other than a possible calibration error, causes for this may be slow respiratory rate or an increased in mixed venous PCO_2. For such situations, cyclic variations in P_ACO_2 (rapidly changing between mixed venous and arterial values) may be large, resulting in $P_{et}CO_2$ to be larger than P_aCO_2 (Moon & Camporesi, 2000).

The measured $P_{et}CO_2$ (or P_ACO_2) depends on the interaction effects of two physiologic variables acting simultaneously in the presence of each other; that is, CO_2 output per minute from the lungs ($\dot{V}CO_2$) and V_A. Mathematically, these variables may be expressed in the following proportionality:

$$P_{et}CO_2 \propto \frac{\dot{V}CO_2}{V_A}\ .$$

As indicated, $P_{et}CO_2$, and thus P_ACO_2, varies directly with $\dot{V}CO_2$ and inversely with V_A. $\dot{V}CO_2$ is affected by both systemic cellular production of CO_2 and pulmonary blood flow. Decreased $P_{et}CO_2$ values are associated with acute increases in V_A, assuming no changes in $\dot{V}CO_2$. An acute decrease in pulmonary

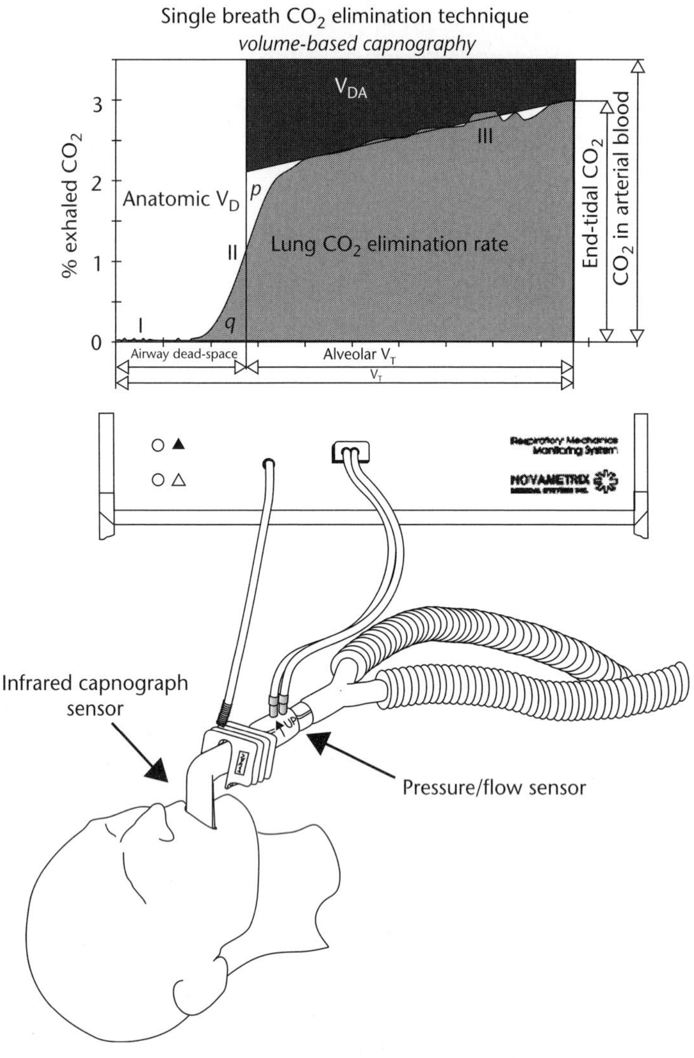

Figure 23.1 The single breath CO_2 elimination technique using volume-based capnography has used in a commercially available monitor (Novametrix-Respironics) is shown. CO_2, pressure, and flow sensors, combined and positioned between the endotracheal tube and Y-piece of the ventilator breathing circuit, direct data to the computerized monitor to construct a plot of exhaled CO_2 over exhaled V_T. Three phases to this plot are: Phase I, the beginning of exhalation, a transient phase, where no CO_2 is detected; Phase II, there is a rapid upslope of CO_2 which comprises gas in the upper airways mixing with alveolar gas; and Phase III, the flat upper portion of the plot, is essentially alveolar gas. This phase reaches a peak usually at the final phase of exhalation and is called the end-tidal CO_2 value. By plotting the CO_2 pressure in mmHg on the vertical axis, then this value would be referred to as the $P_{et}CO_2$. After entering the patient's P_aCO_2 value, physiologic and V_{DA} are calculated. Anatomic V_D, lung CO_2 elimination rate, $P_{et}CO_2$, tidal and minute volume, and peak, mean airway, and PEEP are displayed in real time (see text).

blood flow (e.g. precipitous decrease in cardiac output) decreases $\dot{V}CO_2$ from the lungs, thus, $P_{et}CO_2$ decreases, assuming V_A is unchanged. In this manner, $P_{et}CO_2$ is a reflection of pulmonary blood flow. $P_{et}CO_2$ decreases proportionately for a subject whose metabolic rate decreases and cells are producing less CO_2, assuming no changes in V_A.

Stated another way, $P_{et}CO_2$ allows a global assessment of essential physiologic parameters: $\dot{V}CO_2$, which is affected by cellular metabolism and blood flow, and V_A which is affected by respiratory muscle function and $\dot{V}_A/\dot{Q}$ distribution throughout the lungs (Trillo *et al.*, 1994; Idris, 1995). In clinical practice, additional monitoring is used to differentiate exact mechanisms for a change in $P_{et}CO_2$. Real-time monitoring of $P_{et}CO_2$ can be enhanced through the monitoring of the $\dot{V}CO_2$, arterial perfusion pressure, exhaled ventilation per minute (V_E), alveolar V_D (V_{DA}), and physiologic V_D to tidal volume (V_T) ratio (V_D/V_T).

The later is important for assessing V_A, which, per breath, is calculated by subtracting physiologic V_D from exhaled V_T; that is, $V_A = V_T - V_D$ (West, 2000). For example, V_A is 350 ml if V_T is 500 ml and V_D is 150 ml. Physiologic V_D is the sum of anatomic V_D and V_{DA}. The former is the volume of gas in the conducting airway (nose, mouth, pharynx, larynx, trachea, and main stem bronchi to the terminal bronchioles), and the later is the volume of gas in non-perfused alveoli, both of which do not participate in pulmonary gas exchange. Anatomic V_D is fairly constant, while V_{DA} can increase either chronically, as a result of longstanding pulmonary diseases like emphysema, or acutely, secondary to pulmonary emboli or substantial decreases cardiac output and pulmonary perfusion pressure, for example.

The following equation (Roussos & MacKlem, 1982; West, 1995) demonstrates the importance of knowing physiologic V_D when assessing P_aCO_2:

$$P_aCO_2 = \frac{\dot{V}CO_2}{V_E(1 - V_D / V_T)} \times K$$

where $V_E = V_T \times$ breaths/min, K is a proportionality constant = 760 mmHg, and the denominator term, $V_E\,(1 - V_D/V_T)$, is a method of determining V_A.

For example, consider an adult under normal conditions with a *normal* V_D/V_T ratio of 0.30:

$$P_aCO_2 = \frac{200\ \text{ml/min}}{(500\ \text{ml/breath} \times 12\ \text{breath/min})(1 - 0.30)} \times 760\ \text{mmHg} = 36\ \text{mmHg}$$

Under these conditions, one would expect a $P_{et}CO_2$ value of approximately 30 mmHg. Now, consider the same patient whose V_D/V_T ratio has increased acutely to 0.50 due to over zealous application of positive end-expiratory pressure (PEEP) for example, and whose $\dot{V}CO_2$ and V_E are unchanged:

$$P_aCO_2 = \frac{200\ \text{ml/min}}{(500\ \text{ml/breath} \times 12\ \text{breath/min})(1 - 0.50)} \times 760\ \text{mmHg} = 51\ \text{mmHg}$$

Under the later conditions $P_{et}CO_2$ may be increased above normal because the patient is hypercapnic as a result of increased V_{DA}.

The above example illustrates the importance of garnering *all* requisite physiologic data to determine *specific causes* for anomalies in P_aCO_2, P_ACO_2, and thus $P_{et}CO_2$. Without such data, a naïve clinician may unwittingly believe that the hypercapnia is the result of an acute decrease in V_T and/or breathing frequency only. However, as the data reveals the hypercapnia was *not* the result of diminished V_T, slowing of the breathing rate (decreased minute ventilation), or an acute increase in the cellular production of CO_2 per minute. It was the result of increased V_{DA}, a factor that heretofore has been relegated to theoretical and not practical clinical discussions. This may be due in part because of the difficulty in measuring V_{DA}, as well as the other components in the above equation in an easy, practical manner. Modern, portable bedside respiratory monitoring equipment and techniques allow a more comprehensive assessment of related physiologic variables affecting $P_{et}CO_2$ permitting more appropriate diagnoses (Arnold *et al.*, 1996).

Volume-based capnography – operational theory

The above discussion reveals the complexity of assessing $P_{et}CO_2$ in clinical practice. Time-based capnography, that is plot of exhaled CO_2 over time, is *limited* for it provides a CO_2 waveform, $P_{et}CO_2$ value, and breathing frequency only. More data are needed.

Volume-based capnography plots exhaled CO_2 over *exhaled volume* per breath (Figures 23.1 and 23.2) and offers additional insight vis-à-vis the physiologic concepts discussed above (Nunn, 1977; Arnold *et al.*, 1996). In addition to those data displayed using time-based capnography, volume-based capnography provides: inhaled and exhaled V_T, useful for assessing leakage of gas at the endotracheal cuff site or through a bronchopleural cutaneous fistula, for example; V_E; V_A; peak inflation, mean airway, and PEEP; physiologic, V_{DA}, and anatomic V_D; V_D/V_T ratio; and $\dot{V}CO_2$.

Figure 23.2 illustrates the general operational theory a single exhalation using volume-based capnography (Nunn, 1977). Percent exhaled CO_2 is plotted on the vertical axis with exhaled V_T on the horizontal axis. The first part of exhalation is from the anatomic V_D in the conducting airway. It is devoid of CO_2 (clear, unshaded area). Thereafter, gas is exhaled from the alveoli, for purposes of simplicity only two ventilated alveoli are illustrated. One is perfused, permitting CO_2 diffusion from the blood to the alveolus and up the airway for exhalation, the other is not perfused, precluding CO_2 diffusion and exhalation. The non-perfused alveolus, which may be the result of an embolus occluding local blood flow, for example, represents V_{DA}.

This volume is depicted as the dotted area bounded by the exhaled CO_2 waveform on the bottom (dashed line area), the arterial blood CO_2 on top, the anatomic V_D on the left (clear, unshaded area), and the total exhaled V_T on the right. Physiologic V_D is the sum of anatomic and V_{DA}. The CO_2 value at end-exhalation, a mixture of "ideal" alveolar gas containing CO_2 and V_{DA} gas, is the end-tidal CO_2.

Figure 23.2 is a theoretical depiction, it should not be inferred that all alveoli fall into two discrete compartments – perfused and non-perfused. There exists an infinite range of alveoli where blood flow may be greater than normal, normal, and those with little to no blood flow (Nunn, 1977). Thus, a considerable wide variation in $\dot{V}_A/\dot{Q}$ conditions may exist throughout the lungs. The figure is helpful from a qualitative standpoint in understanding the concepts of measurement of physiologic V_D when using volume-based capnography.

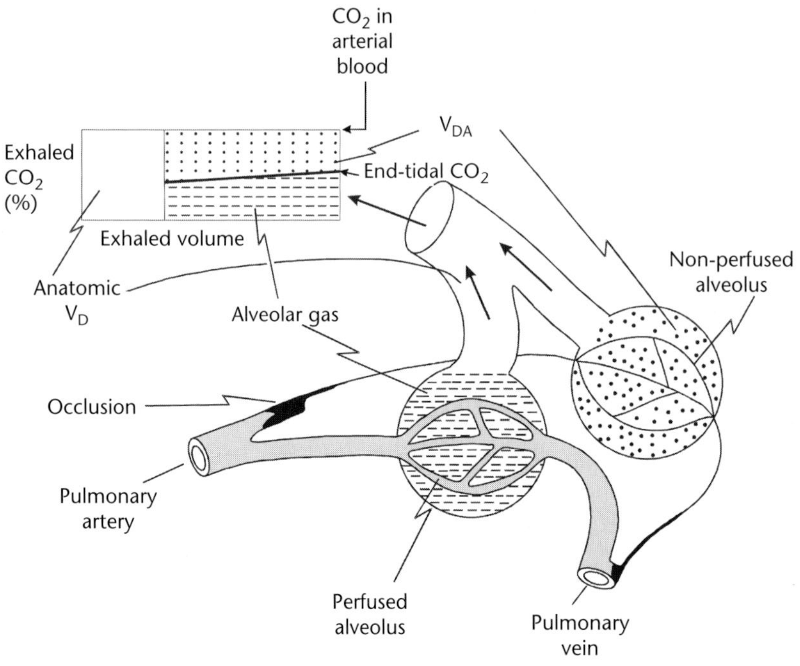

Figure 23.2 Model depicting a normally ventilated and perfused alveolus on the left and a ventilated, non-perfused alveolus on the right, the latter is defined as V_{DA}. No CO_2 is exhaled from the alveolus on the right, predisposing to increases in arterial blood CO_2 as well as decreases in arterial blood O_2. The figure in the rectangle is an idealized representation of a single exhalation plotting exhaled CO_2 over exhaled V_T. Physiologic V_D is the sum of anatomic and V_{DA} components (see text). (Reproduced with permission from Nunn, J.F. (1977). *Applied Respiratory Physiology*, 2nd edition. Butterworths, Boston; pp. 213–245.)

Commercially available technology using a portable, computerized bedside monitor is available for performing volume-based capnography (Novametrix-Respironics) (Figure 23.1) (Arnold *et al.*, 1996; Skimming *et al.*, 2001). This monitor was developed based on the following research. Aitken and Clark-Kennedy (1928) described a method to estimate V_D by plotting exhaled CO_2 over exhaled V_T. Subsequently, Fowler (1948) described a method of assessing V_D by using nitrogen washout in conjuction with a rapid-response nitrogen analyzer. Although he used nitrogen rather than CO_2 as an indicator gas, the plot is similar to that described by Aitken and Clark-Kennedy. Fowler's major contribution was to revise the algorithm for choosing the transition point that separates airway gas measurements from alveolar gas measurements. The areas designated "*p*" and "*q*" as shown in Figure 23.1 are equal. This method determines the site to plot a line perpendicular to the *X*- or exhaled V_T-axis. The point at which the perpendicular line intersects the *X*-axis defines the end of exhaled airway gas and the beginning of exhaled alveolar gas. Thus, this method allows exhaled V_T to be divided into two components: anatomic dead-space V_T and alveolar V_T. Fletcher *et al.* (1981) suggested adding the arterial blood CO_2 fraction to the plot so the V_{DA} area could be defined. Further, he contended that the area labeled "lung CO_2 elimination rate" was equal to the area under the exhaled CO_2–V_T curve. (To determine the rate of CO_2 elimination from the lungs per minute requires multiplying the number of breaths per minute by the volume of CO_2 exhaled per breath.) Under conditions of equilibrium; that is, the rate of the lungs to eliminate and the rate of the cells to produce CO_2 per minute is essentially the same under normal conditions. Thus, the lung CO_2 elimination rate may be thought of as proportional to $\dot{V}CO_2$. Arnold *et al.* (1996) reported favorable results from validation studies performed by using the above described volume-based capnograph monitor (Figure 23.1) to estimate V_D.

Volume-based capnography in the ICU

Areas of *both* low and high $\dot{V}_A/\dot{Q}$ ratios are prevalent in patients with ARDS (West, 2000). This concept is appreciated by reviewing the oxygen (O_2)–CO_2 diagram as described by West. Secondary to decreased alveolar ventilation from a myriad of causes, it is easy to understand the evolution of areas of low $\dot{V}_A/\dot{Q}$ in ARDS; that is relative and absolute right-to-left intrapulmonary shunting of blood. For the former condition, functional residual capacity and V_A are decreased below normal relative to pulmonary perfusion. The later condition may be characterized by the absolute cessation of alveolar ventilation while pulmonary perfusion is unchanged, for example atelectasis. These low $\dot{V}_A/\dot{Q}$ conditions predispose to hypoxemia and hypercapnia.

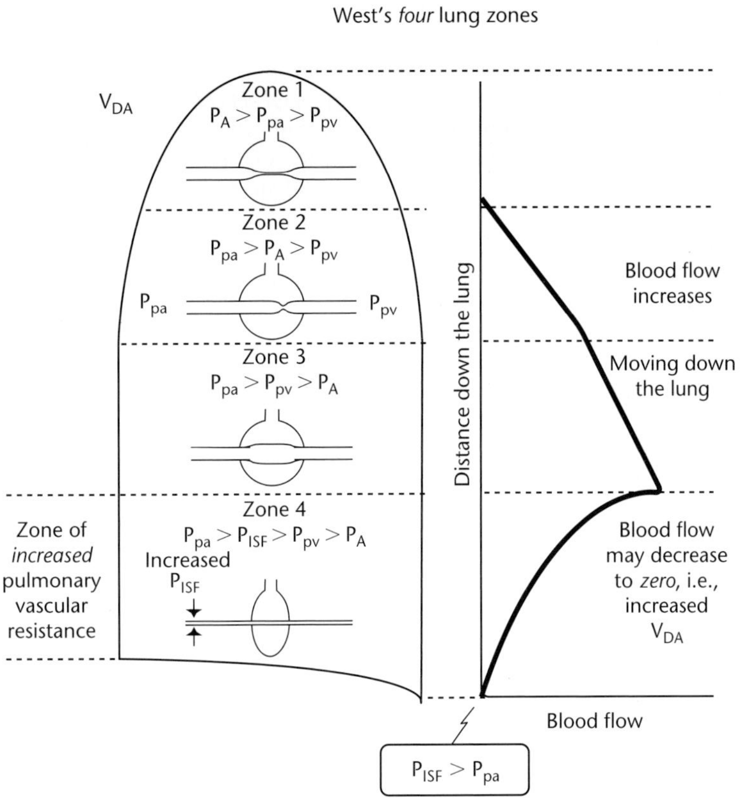

Figure 23.3 Model illustrating four lung zones in an upright lung as described by West (Benumof, 2000). Zone 1 refers to ventilated, non-perfused alveoli (V_{DA}). In Zone 2, blood is flowing to ventilated alveoli since P_{pa} can be greater than alveolar gas pressure (P_A). However, increases in P_A (as may happen when applying inappropriately high levels of PEEP for example (West, 1995)) and/or decreases in P_{pa} (as during shock) predispose to collapse of the pulmonary capillaries, resulting in no perfusion, leading to formation of Zone 1 like units. In Zone 3, P_{pa} exceeds P_{pv} and P_A. Zone 4 is a region characterized by *increased vascular resistance to the pulmonary capillaries.* In this zone, a large amount of fluid has transuded into the pulmonary interstitial compartment from leaky capillaries and/or the lung is at abnormally low volume; both are characteristics of ARDS. (Note the smaller size of alveolus in this zone.) Both circumstances produce increased pulmonary interstitial pressure (P_{ISF}) causing extra-alveolar vessel compression, resulting in increased vascular resistance and decreased regional blood flow predisposing to the development of V_{DA}; that is, when P_{ISF} is greater than P_{pa} blood flow is absent (see text). (Reproduced with permission from Benumof, J.L. (2000). Respiratory physiology and respiratory function during anesthesia. In: Miller, R.D. (ed.) *Anesthesia*, 5th edition. Churchill Livingstone, Philadelphia, PA; pp. 578–618.)

Areas of high $\dot{V}_A/\dot{Q}$ are present with ARDS, that is V_{DA} and alveolar dead-space-like volume units (West, 2000). For the former condition, alveolar ventilation is present while pulmonary perfusion is absent (see right side alveolus in Figure 23.2). For the later condition, alveolar ventilation is present while pulmonary perfusion is decreased below normal. This implies that an infinite range of alveolar dead-space-like volume units may exist (Skimming *et al.*, 2001). For example, perfusion may be decreased by 25% in some alveolar/capillary units, 75% in others, and 90% in still other units. Significant increases in high $\dot{V}_A/\dot{Q}$ units are as *lethal* as relative and absolute right-to-left intrapulmonary shunting of blood, that is arterial blood gas exchange is compromised predisposing to hypoxemia and hypercapnia. A question arises as to what are the physiologic causes for the development of areas of high $\dot{V}_A/\dot{Q}$ for patients with ARDS having no previous pulmonary history?

To address the question, a brief review West's *four* zones or regions of the lungs is useful (Benumof, 2000). These zones describe the interaction effects of pulmonary hydrostatic and alveolar gas pressures governing the distribution of blood flow in the lungs (Figure 23.3). At some height above the heart in the lungs pulmonary artery pressure (P_{pa}) becomes zero. In this region alveolar pressure (P_A) exceeds P_{pa} and pulmonary venous pressure (P_{pv}). As the pressure outside the vessels is greater than the pressure inside the vessels, the vessels are collapsed, there is no blood flow. This region is referred to as Zone 1: $P_A > P_{pa} > P_{pv}$. Since alveolar ventilation is present and pulmonary perfusion is absent, this is defined as V_{DA}, no gas exchange is possible. Further down the lungs P_{pa} increases; when P_{pa} exceeds P_A blood flow begins. This defines Zone 2 where: $P_{pa} > P_A > P_{pv}$. The rate of pulmonary blood flow through this zone is proportional to the difference between the upstream and downstream pressures ($P_{pa} - P_A$). In some areas within this zone where this pressure difference is *minimal* and alveolar ventilation exceeds perfusion, high $\dot{V}_A/\dot{Q}$ matching occurs (alveolar dead-space-like volume effect). Inappropriately high levels of PEEP directed to these areas may be sufficient to increase $P_A > P_{pa}$, thus, converting a previous Zone 2 to a Zone 1 area (V_{DA}) (West, 1995).

Lower in the lungs is a level where P_{pv} exceeds P_A. In this region blood flow is governed by the pulmonary arteriovenous pressure difference ($P_{pa} - P_{pv}$). This defines Zone 3 where: $P_{pa} > P_{pv} > P_A$.

Zone 4 regions of the lungs are characterized by inappropriately high pulmonary hydrostatic pressures, for example patients with severe volume overload or congestive heart failure. During these conditions, fluid may transude out of the pulmonary vessels into the pulmonary interstitial compartment. Leaky capillaries, as in sepsis and ARDS, for example, are additional predisposing factors for fluid transudation into the pulmonary interstitial compartment. Increased pulmonary interstitial hydrostatic pressure (P_{ISF}) resulting from the transdated pulmonary interstitial fluid may significantly affect the distribution of pulmonary blood flow. Inappropriate accumulation of fluid in the pulmonary interstitial space causes P_{ISF} to become positive, exceeding P_{pv}. In this region blood flow is governed by the arterio-interstitial pressure difference ($P_{pa} - P_{ISF}$), which is less than the $P_{pa} - P_{pv}$ difference. Therefore, in this Zone 4 of the lungs where: $P_{pa} > P_{ISF} > P_{pv} > P_A$, blood flow is *less* than in Zone 3.

In addition, loss of lung volume, a hallmark of ARDS due to a decrease in functional residual capacity, is associated with increased vascular resistance of extra-alveolar vessels (West, 2000). Under conditions of decreased lung volume, the tethering action of the pulmonary tissue on the vessels is lost predisposing further increases in P_{ISF}.

Summarizing, Zone 4 is the result of large amounts of fluid transuded into the pulmonary interstitial compartment and/or is possible at low lung volumes, as in ARDS. *Both conditions lead to increased P_{ISF}, causing extra-alveolar vessel compression, increased extra-alveolar vascular resistance, and decreased regional blood flow.* Acute formation of Zone 4 areas in patients with ARDS may explain, in part, the observance of increased physiologic V_D or areas of *high* $\dot{V}_A/\dot{Q}$ in general. Increased local vascular resistance, causing decreased to no blood flow to ventilated alveoli, defines alveolar dead-space-like volume areas and V_{DA}, respectively.

Critical physiologic V_D for $P_{et}CO_2$ to predict P_aCO_2

Significant $\dot{V}_A/\dot{Q}$ abnormalities predispose to large discrepancies between $P_{et}CO_2$ and P_aCO_2. Due to this potential, $P_{et}CO_2$ may be a spurious predictor of P_aCO_2. To address this issue, we performed a clinical study on adults diagnosed with ARDS. *It was hypothesized that at some critical physiologic V_D, $P_{et}CO_2$ fails to predict P_aCO_2 accurately.*

Following institutional review board (IRB) approval, 31 intubated adults (age 39 ± 19 years; weight 84 ± 18 kg; gender 22 males, 9 females) with ARDS receiving ventilatory support were studied. Causes of ARDS resulted from various degrees of pneumonia, trauma, sepsis, congestive heart failure, and multi-organ system failure. There was no previous medical history of chronic respiratory diseases for the study patients. Various combinations of intermittent mandatory ventilation (IMV), PEEP, pressure support ventilation (PSV), and pressure control ventilation (PCV) were applied. The ranges were: ventilator rates from 2 to 22 per min, PEEP levels from 5 to 18 cmH_2O, PSV levels from 5 to 35 cmH_2O, and PCV levels from 20 to 40 cmH_2O. Data from a combined pressure/flow/CO_2 sensor, attached between the endotracheal tube and Y-piece of the ventilator breathing circuit, were directed to a respiratory monitor (Novametrix-Respironics, Figure 23.1). The following measurements were obtained: P_aO_2, P_aCO_2, $P_{et}CO_2$, V_D/V_T ratio, F_IO_2, V_T, V_E, airway pressures, and ventilator rate. The Enghoff equation (Nunn, 1977; West, 1995) programmed into the monitor, was used for the calculation of the V_D/V_T ratio:

$$\frac{V_D}{V_T} = \frac{P_aCO_2 - P_ECO_2}{P_aCO_2},$$

where P_ECO_2 is the *mean* partial pressure of exhaled CO_2 (normally about 28 mmHg in adults). This is not to be confused with $P_{et}CO_2$. Data were analyzed with regression analysis and Wilcoxon Rank Sum test; alpha was set at 0.05 for statistical significance.

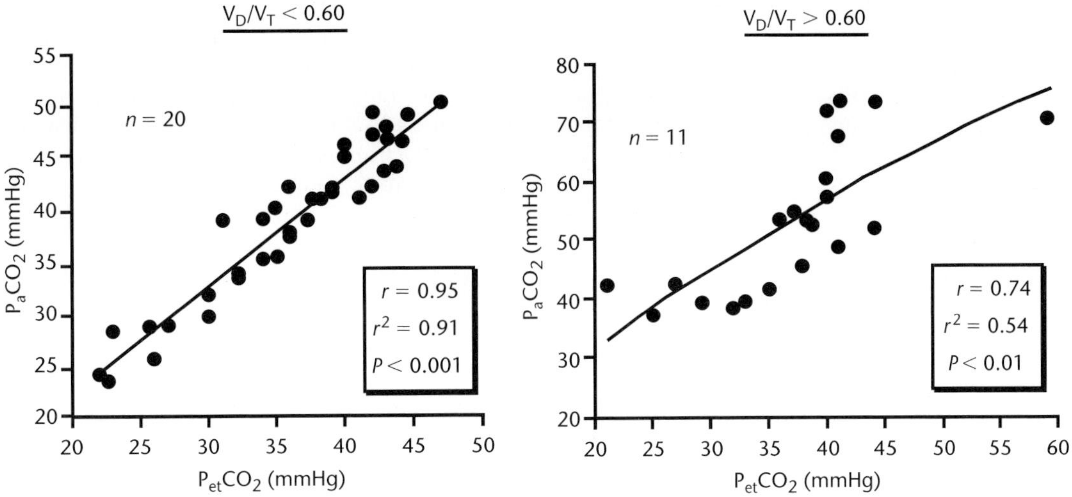

Figure 23.4 Patients with ARDS are differentiated into two groups on the basis of the physiologic V_D/V_T being less than 0.60 (left) and greater than 0.60 (right). Those with V_D/V_T ratios greater than 0.60 had more severe forms of ARDS with grossly abnormal $\dot{V}_A/\dot{Q}$ conditions. The plots show the relationships between the P_aCO_2 on the vertical axes and $P_{et}CO_2$ on the horizontal axes. $P_{et}CO_2$ is an excellent predictor of P_aCO_2 for subjects with V_D/V_T ratios less than 0.60 ($r^2 = 0.91$). While $P_{et}CO_2$ is a poor predictor of P_aCO_2 for subjects with excessively high V_D/V_T ratios greater than 0.60 ($r^2 = 0.54$).

Table 23.1 Ventilation and blood gas data ($n = 31$, adults)

	$V_D/V_T < 0.60$ ($n = 20$)	$V_D/V_T > 0.60$ ($n = 11$)
PIP (cmH_2O)	33 ± 11	44 ± 9*
Ventilator rate (min^{-1})	3 ± 2	12 ± 7*
P_aCO_2 (mmHg)	39 ± 7	53 ± 11*
P_aO_2/F_IO_2 ratio	260 ± 75	180 ± 60*

*$P < 0.05$.

The findings were as follows. Patients were divided into two groups on the basis of their V_D/V_T ratio; that is, $V_D/V_T < 0.60$ and $V_D/V_T > 0.60$. $P_{et}CO_2$ was a very good predictor of P_aCO_2 for patients with a $V_D/V_T < 0.60$ ($r^2 = 0.91$, Figure 23.4). For those with a $V_D/V_T > 0.60$, $P_{et}CO_2$ poorly predicted P_aCO_2 ($r^2 = 0.54$, Figure 23.4). Patients in the higher V_D/V_T ratio group had significantly higher peak inflation pressures (PIP), ventilator rates, P_aCO_2 values, and lower P_aO_2/F_IO_2 ratios than those in the lower V_D/V_T ratio group (Table 23.1).

$P_{et}CO_2$ accurately predicted P_aCO_2 for the majority of patients in the study (65% or 20 of 31) with mild to moderately severe forms of ARDS. $P_{et}CO_2$ did not accurately predict P_aCO_2 for patients with more severe form of ARDS (35%) requiring higher levels of ventilatory support and more compromised arterial blood gas exchange (Table 23.1). These findings reveal that up to a *critical V_D/V_T ratio of approximately 0.60, $P_{et}CO_2$ is an accurate predictor of P_aCO_2 in adults diagnosed with ARDS*. Moreover, we observed that for some with V_D/V_T ratios as high as 0.65, $P_{et}CO_2$ was approximately 5–6 mmHg less than P_aCO_2 providing an accurate prediction of P_aCO_2.

These findings are reaffirmed by other studies. Hubble *et al.* (2000) reported $P_{et}CO_2$ accurately predicted P_aCO_2 with a V_D/V_T ratio up to approximately 0.65, and a V_D/V_T ratio less than 0.50 accurately predicted successful extubation in pediatric patients with ARDS. Takano *et al.* (2003) reported a close correlation ($r = 0.88$) between $P_{et}CO_2$ (measured using a vital capacity maneuver) and P_aCO_2 for patients with compromised pulmonary function, that is those with abnormally high and low $\dot{V}_A/\dot{Q}$ disturbances. In asthmatic patients treated for an exacerbation, Lahn *et al.* (2003) reported a strong, positive correlation ($r = 0.94$) between $P_{et}CO_2$ and P_aCO_2. Although not reported, it is well known that increases in physiologic V_D are commonly associated for patients with chronic respiratory diseases. It is speculated that the V_D/V_T ratios in these subjects were below some critical level so that $P_{et}CO_2$ correlated with P_aCO_2. Weinger & Brimm (1997) reported on 25 adults following coronary artery bypass graft surgery who had mild to moderate $\dot{V}_A/\dot{Q}$ abnormalities and were ventilated using IMV.

Table 23.2 $P_{et}CO_2$ as a predictor of P_aCO_2 in adults with respiratory failure

	Good predictor	Poor predictor
V_D/V_T ratio	0.20–0.60	>0.65
PIP (cmH_2O)	<35	>40
Ventilator rate (breaths/min)	<8	>10–15
P_aCO_2 (mmHg)	<50	>50
P_aO_2/F_IO_2 ratio	250–300	<200

It was found that the $P_{a-et}CO_2$ gradient was 4.24 ± 4.4 mmHg. It was concluded that monitoring the maximal $P_{et}CO_2$, independent of the breathing pattern (spontaneous or mandatory breaths), provided a clinically useful indicator of P_aCO_2.

Considering these data, it may be prudent to re-evaluate using $P_{et}CO_2$ for estimating P_aCO_2, thereby evaluating the appropriateness of ventilation for patients with ARDS. An old belief that $\dot{V}_A/\dot{Q}$ abnormalities associated with ARDS predisposes to inaccurate estimations of P_aCO_2 when using $P_{et}CO_2$ needs to be qualified. It appears that $P_{et}CO_2$ accurately predicts P_aCO_2 for *many* of these patients, and that $P_{et}CO_2$ underestimates P_aCO_2 for only those with the severest forms of ARDS, that is grossly abnormal $\dot{V}_A/\dot{Q}$ changes and significantly increased V_{DA}. Note the right side of Figure 23.4, in subjects with V_D/V_T ratios greater than 0.60, $P_{et}CO_2$ may be substantially less than P_aCO_2. In the author's experience, this form of ARDS is the exception. Generally, patients with V_D/V_T ratios less than 0.60 seem to be much more prevalent.

Table 23.2 provides some suggested guidelines when considering using $P_{et}CO_2$ monitoring for patients with ARDS. In general, $P_{et}CO_2$ appears to be a good predictor of P_aCO_2 when V_D/V_T ratios up to about 0.60–0.65, PIP are low or less than 35 cmH_2O, and using IMV or ventilator rates are less than 8/min. Conversely, $P_{et}CO_2$ may not be a good predictor of P_aCO_2 when V_D/V_T ratios are greater than 0.65, PIP are in excess of 40 cmH_2O, and using IMV rates greater than 10–15/min.

Physiologic V_D and $P_{et}CO_2$ monitoring using volume-based capnography may be useful for titrating PEEP to patients with ARDS. Appropriate application of PEEP restores lung volume and may decrease Zone 4 regions, and thus physiologic V_D across the lung (Rose & Banner, 2000; Schweiger *et al.*, 2003). This may be a dominant effect of PEEP. In an animal model of acute lung injury, Schweiger *et al.* (2003) demonstrated significant decreases in V_D following application of PEEP. A reduction in physiologic V_D may be a good indicator of alveolar recruitment. Conversely, inappropriately high levels of PEEP and ventilator rates potentiates the already increased physiologic V_D in ARDS, further exacerbating the high $\dot{V}_A/\dot{Q}$ disorder in these patients (Froese & Bryan, 1974; Downs & Mitchell, 1976; West, 1995).

References

Aitken, R.S. & Clark-Kennedy, A.E. (1928). On the fluctuation in the composition of alveolar air during the respiratory cycle in muscular exercise. *J. Physiol. (Lond.)* **65**: 389–411.

Arnold, J.H., Thompson, J.E. & Arnold, L.W. (1996). Single breath CO_2 analysis: description and validation of a method. *Crit. Care Med.*, **24**: 96–102.

Benumof, J.L. (2000). Respiratory physiology and respiratory function during anesthesia. In: Miller, R.D. (ed.) *Anesthesia*, 5th edition. Churchill Livingstone, Philadelphia, PA; pp. 578–618.

Downs, J.B. & Mitchell, L.A. (1976). Pulmonary effects of ventilatory pattern following cardiopulmonary bypass. *Crit. Care Med.*, **4**: 295–299.

Fletcher, R. & Veintemilla, F. (1989). Changes in arterial to end-tidal PCO_2 differences during coronary artery bypass grafting. *Acta Anaesth. Scand.*, **33**: 656–658.

Fletcher, R., Jonson, B. & Cumming, G. (1981). The concept of deadspace with special reference to the single breath test for carbon dioxide. *Br. J. Anaesth.*, **53**: 77–81.

Fowler, W.S. (1948). Lung function studies II: the respiratory deadspace. *Am. J. Physiol.*, **154**: 405–416.

Froese, A.B. & Bryan, A.C. (1974). Effects of anesthesia and paralysis on diaphragmatic mechanics in man. *Anesthesiology*, **41**: 242–255.

Guyton, A.C. (1981). *Textbook of Medical Physiology*, 6th edition. W.B. Saunders Co., Philadelphia, PA, pp. 512–513.

Hubble, C.L., Gentile, M.A., Tripp, D.S., Craig, D.M., Meliones, J.N. & Cheifetz, I.M. (2000). Deadspace to tidal volume ratio predicts successful extubation in infants and children. *Crit. Care Med.*, **28**: 2034–2040.

Idris, A. (1995). End-tidal carbon dioxide physiology and monitoring during resuscitation: current concepts in cardiac resuscitation. *Anesth. Clin. North Am.*, **13**: 785–798.

Lahn, M., Gallagher, E., Bijur, P. & Abrams, S. (2003). End-tidal CO_2 determination to predict P_aCO_2 in emergency department asthmatics. *Acad. Emerg. Med.*, **10**: 566.

Moon, R.E. & Camporesi, E.M. (2000). Respiratory monitoring. In: Miller, R.D (ed.) *Anesthesia*, 5th edition. Churchill Livingstone, Philadelphia, PA; pp. 1255–1295.

Nunn, J.F. (1977). *Applied Respiratory Physiology*, 2nd edition. Butterworths, Boston; pp. 213–245.

Rose, J.T. & Banner, M.J. (2000). Effects of positive end expiratory pressure (PEEP) on physiologic deadspace volume to tidal volume ratio (V_D/V_T). *Crit. Care Med.*, **28**: A86.

Roussos, C. & MacKlem, P.T. (1982). The respiratory muscles. *New Engl. J. Med.*, **301**: 786–797.

Russell, G.B. & Graybeal, J.M. (1994). Reliability of end-tidal carbon dioxide gradient in mechanically ventilated patients with multi-system trauma. *J. Trauma*, **36**: 317–320.

Russell, G.B. & Graybeal, J.M. (1995). The arterial to end-tidal carbon dioxide difference in neurosurgical patients during craniotomy. *Anesth. Analg.*, **81**: 806–809.

Russell, G.B., Graybeal, J.M. & Strout, J.C. (1990). Stability of arterial to end-tidal carbon dioxide gradients during postoperative cardiorespiratory support. *Can. J. Anaesth.*, **37**: 560–562.

Schweiger, J.W., Downs, J.B. & Smith, R.A. (2003). Chest wall disruption with and without acute lung injury: effect of continuous positive airway pressure therapy on ventilation and perfusion relationships. *Crit. Care Med.*, **31**: 2364–2370.

Skimming, J.W., Banner, M.J., Spalding, H.K., Jaeger, M.J., Burchfield, D.J. & Davenport, P.W. (2001). Nitric oxide inhalation increases alveolar gas exchange by decreasing deadspace volume. *Crit. Care Med.*, **29**: 1195–1200.

Takano, Y., Sakamoto, O., Kiyofuji, C. & Ito, K. (2003). A comparison of the end-tidal CO_2 measured by portable capnometer and the arterial PCO_2 in spontaneously breathing patients. *Respir. Med.* **97**: 476–481.

Trillo, G., von Planta, M. & Keete, F. (1994). $EtCO_2$ monitoring during low flow states: clinical aims and limits. *Resuscitation*, **27**: 1–8.

Weinger, M.B. & Brimm, J.E. (1997). End-tidal carbon dioxide as a measure of arterial carbon dioxide during intermittent mandatory ventilation. *J. Clin. Monit.*, **3**: 73–79.

West, J.B. (1995). *Pulmonary Pathophysiology*, 5th edition. In: West, J.B. (ed.) Lippincott Williams & Wilkins, Philadelphia, PA; pp. 162–164.

West, J.B. (2000). *Respiratory Physiology*, 6th edition. In: West, J.B. (ed.) Lippincott Williams & Wilkins, Philadelphia, PA; pp. 11–19, 131–142.

THE BASIS FOR CAPNOMETRIC MONITORING IN SHOCK

24

K.R. Ward

Introduction

Shock is a complex entity traditionally defined as a state in which the oxygen utilization or consumption needs of tissues are not matched by sufficient delivery of oxygen. This mismatch commonly results from states of altered tissue perfusion. Common clinical situations that lead to alterations in tissue perfusion include hemorrhage, myocardial infarction and failure, trauma, sepsis, cardiac arrest and others. In many cases mixed etiologies can cause tissue perfusion abnormalities. Regardless of the cause, clinicians will better be able to treat shock if they understand the underlying mechanisms, shared mechanisms and physiologic events.

Figure 24.1 represents the basic relationship between oxygen consumption ($\dot{V}O_2$) (Abraham *et al.*, 1984) and oxygen delivery (DO_2) that is pertinent to individual organs and to the whole body (Schumacker & Cain, 1987; Chittock *et al.*, 1998; Vincent, 1998). $\dot{V}O_2$ can remain constant over a wide range of DO_2. This is possible because most tissue beds are capable of efficiently increasing the ratio of extracted oxygen (OER). This will be reflected by decreasing venous oxygen saturation from each organ. However, when DO_2 reaches a critical threshold, tissue extraction of oxygen cannot be further increased to meet tissue demands. It is at this point that $\dot{V}O_2$ becomes directly dependent on critical DO_2 (DO_2crit) and cells begin to convert to greater levels of anaerobic metabolism as manifested by increases in certain metabolic products such as lactate, nicotinamide adenine dinucleotide, reduced (NADH) and reduced cytochrome oxidase (CtOx). The point of DO_2 crit is the point of dysoxia or ischemia where tissue DO_2 cannot meet tissue oxygen demand (Schumacker & Cain, 1987). Oxygen debt can be defined as the cumulative difference of $\dot{V}O_2$ between baseline and that spent below DO_2 crit. The level of accumulated oxygen debt in shock states is critically linked with both survival and morbidities such as multisystem organ failure (Shoemaker *et al.*, 1988, 1992). Each individual organ system has its own biphasic DO_2–$\dot{V}O_2$ relationship, thus whole body measurement of these factors including surrogates such as systemic lactate are aggregate measures of all organ systems. Obviously the more catastrophic the event (e.g. massive hemorrhage or cardiac arrest) the more likely multiple organs will simultaneously reach DO_2crit.

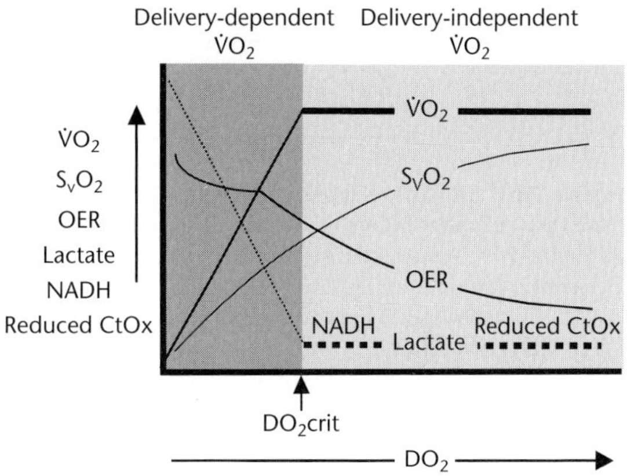

$DO_2 = CO \times C_aO_2$ (normal range: 460–650 ml/min/m^2);
$\dot{V}O_2 = CO \times (C_aO_2 - C_vO_2)$
(normal range: 96–170 ml/min/m^2);
$C_aO_2 = (Hb \times 1.39 \times S_aO_2) + (0.003 \times P_aO_2)$;
$C_vO_2 = (Hb \times 1.39 \times S_vO_2) + (0.003 \times P_vO_2)$.
CO: cardiac output; P_aO_2, arterial oxygen tension;
Hb: Hemoglobin; S_vO_2 normal range 70–80%.

Figure 24.1 Biphasic relationship between DO_2 and $\dot{V}O_2$. OER increases and mixed venous oxygen saturation (S_vO_2) decreases in response to decreased DO_2. Below a DO_2crit, $\dot{V}O_2$ becomes delivery dependent. DO_2 below DO_2crit results in the beginning of anaerobic metabolism as noted by an increase in a variety of cellular products including lactate, NADH, and reduced CtOx. The DO_2crit of various organ systems can occur at points either above or below whole body DO_2crit depending on the metabolic and blood flow regulatory characteristics of the organ system and the rapidity of the reductions in DO_2.

The basis for capnometric monitoring in shock

It is the relationship between $\dot{V}O_2$ and carbon dioxide (CO_2) production ($\dot{V}CO_2$) that forms the general

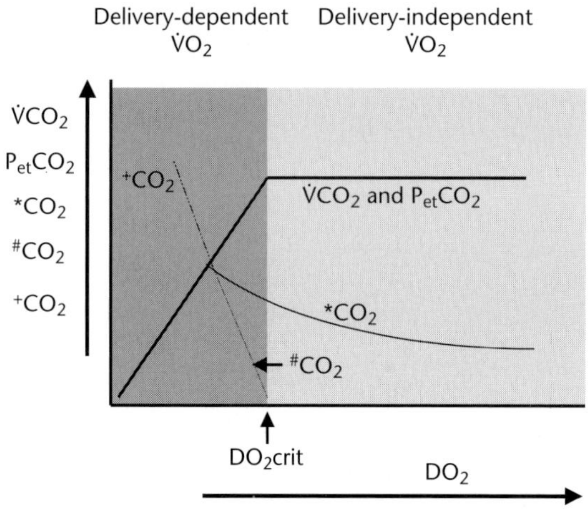

Figure 24.2 Biphasic relationship between DO_2 and $\dot{V}CO_2$. Note the similarities between the relationships as compared to Figure 24.1. When minute ventilation is held constant, DO_2crit can be determined by reductions in $\dot{V}CO_2$ and thus $P_{et}CO_2$. This corresponds to the point of delivery-dependent $\dot{V}O_2$. *CO_2 represents CO_2 that accumulates as a result of decreased removal of aerobically produced CO_2 secondary to decreases in flow (respiratory acidosis). #CO_2 represents additional tissue CO_2 production and accumulation due to buffering of metabolic acids produced by anaerobic metabolism after DO_2crit is reached and would correspond to the production of lactate at the point of DO_2crit (see Figure 24.1). +CO_2 represents the combination of aerobically and aerobically derived CO_2. Overall $\dot{V}CO_2$ is decreased due to drops in $\dot{V}O_2$. Quantities of CO_2 as depicted on the *Y*-axis are not drawn to scale but instead are depicted to demonstrate their temporal relationship to each other in reference to changes in DO_2.

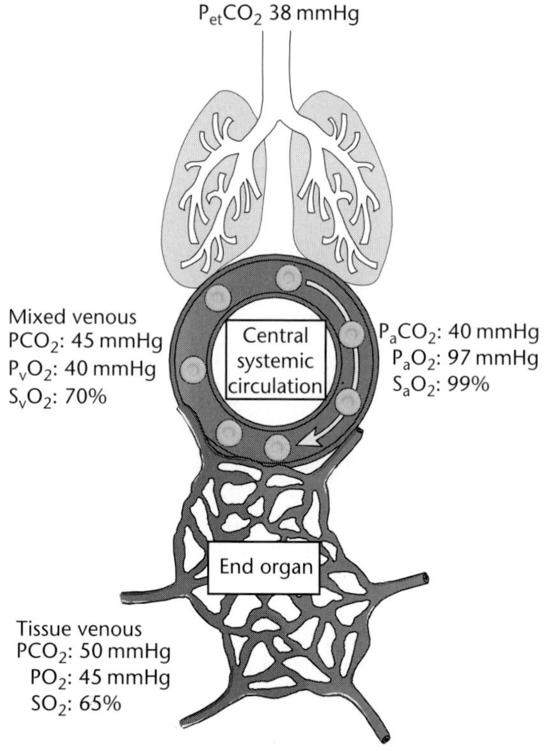

Figure 24.3 Representative blood and tissue gas levels of the normal circulation. Mixed venous values represent aggregate values from all organ systems. Thus tissue venous values are not necessarily identical to mixed venous values but can be higher or lower depending on the individual organ system's level of metabolic activity. The majority of blood volume at the level of the tissue is contained in the venous compartment.

foundation for the value of $\dot{V}CO_2$ and end-tidal PCO_2 ($P_{et}CO_2$) monitoring in shock states. Aerobic metabolism generates CO_2 and water through its consumption of glucose and other substrates. For the most part $\dot{V}O_2$ and $\dot{V}CO_2$ are very tightly coupled and thus parallel to each other. The respiratory quotient (RQ), which represents $\dot{V}CO_2/\dot{V}O_2$, is on average 0.85. This is of course an aggregate measure of the RQ of various organ systems, some of which use mainly glucose such as the brain, and others like the liver, which use combinations of substrates such as glucose, protein and fat.

The ability of $P_{et}CO_2$ monitoring to reflect tissue perfusion lies in its ability to closely reflect alveolar CO_2. Alveolar CO_2 is determined mainly by the combination of $\dot{V}CO_2$, pulmonary capillary blood flow (i.e. cardiac output (CO) minus right-to-left shunt), and alveolar ventilation. As such, alveolar CO_2 and $P_{et}CO_2$ are linearly related to $\dot{V}CO_2$. $\dot{V}CO_2$ in turn depends on two different factors: metabolic production and pulmonary excretion of CO_2. In low flow states with steady-state ventilation, $\dot{V}CO_2$ declines secondary to decreased metabolism, decreased delivery of CO_2 to the lungs, and to ventilation/perfusion ($\dot{V}/\dot{Q}$) mismatches in the lung. These $\dot{V}/\dot{Q}$ mismatches result in an enormous increase in deadspace (up to 0.7 in severe shock such as in cardiac arrest and during cardiopulmonary resuscitation (CPR) (Hindman, 1990). This results in a widening of the arterial PCO_2 (P_aCO_2) to $P_{et}CO_2$ difference and is further reflected by mixed venous hypercarbia (Figures 24.3–24.5). $\dot{V}CO_2$, which is difficult to measure, also declines secondary to reductions in actual CO_2 production, from decreases in DO_2 (Weil *et al.*, 1986; Relman, 1986; Dubin *et al.*, 2000). Although sometimes described as a logarithmic relationship, $\dot{V}CO_2$ and thus $P_{et}CO_2$ have almost the same biphasic relationship with DO_2 as does $\dot{V}O_2$ (Figure 24.2). As such, DO_2crit has been determined by following changes in $\dot{V}CO_2$ and $P_{et}CO_2$. DO_2crit as

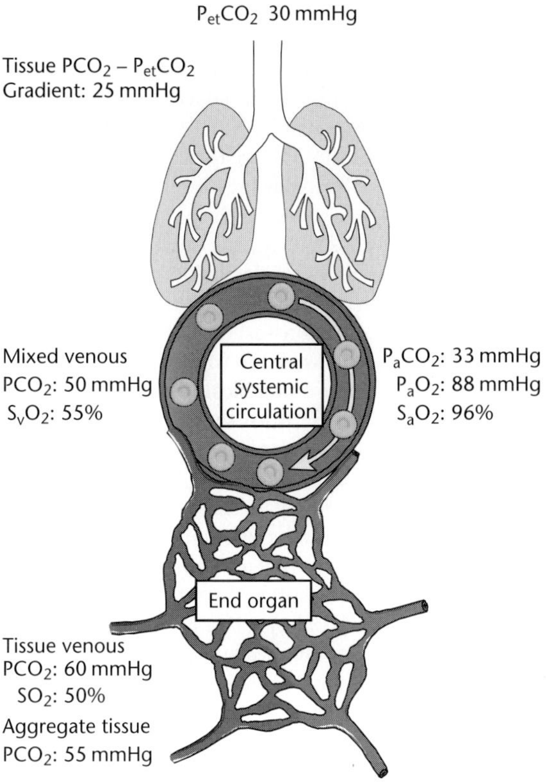

Figure 24.4 Representative blood and tissue gas levels of compensated or early shock states. Note that $P_{et}CO_2$ and arterial gas levels are not significantly altered despite abnormal values as the level of the tissues. Examination of the $P_{et}CO_2$ to tissue PCO_2 gradient of a sensitive tissue bed has been demonstrated to be capable of detecting early shock states as well as to ensure adequate resuscitation and prevents misinterpretation of the tissue PCO_2 due to alterations in minute ventilation. See text for potential tissue PCO_2 measurements. Gradients greater than 11 mmHg are believed to be abnormal.

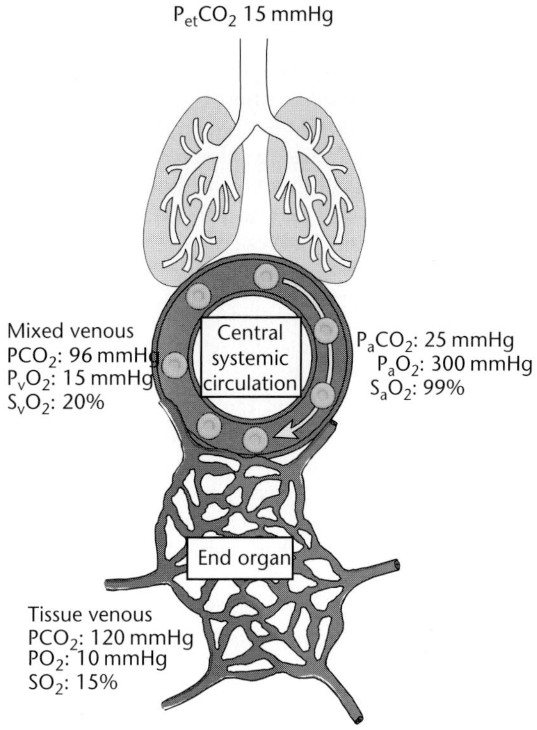

Figure 24.5 Representative blood and tissue gas levels of severe uncompensated shock states such as cardiac arrest or massive hemorrhage. Due to the tremendous reductions in blood flow produced large deadspace in the lungs is created thus producing gaps between mixed venous PCO_2, $P_{et}CO_2$, and P_aCO_2. The severe reductions in DO_2 to each organ system results in very high oxygen extraction at the level of the tissue which produces very low tissue venous PO_2 and thus SO_2 levels. The very high venous PCO_2 levels are due to both decreased removal of aerobically and anaerobically produced CO_2 (see Figure 24.5). As with Figure 24.3, the mixed venous values represent aggregate values of all organ systems.

determined by inflective changes of $P_{et}CO_2$ and $\dot{V}CO_2$ during steady-state ventilation does not significantly differ compared to determination using changes in $\dot{V}O_2$ or lactate production (Guzman *et al.*, 1997; Dubin *et al.*, 2000).

Although $\dot{V}CO_2$ and $P_{et}CO_2$ decrease upon reaching DO_2crit, tissue PCO_2 increases (Figures 24.3–24.5). Concomitant with decreases in DO_2 (prior to DO_2crit), increases in tissue CO_2 will occur because decreased blood flow will reduce the amount of aerobically produced CO_2 removed from tissue, creating a tissue respiratory acidosis (Schlichtig *et al.*, 1996; Jin *et al.*, 1998; Sato *et al.*, 1998). $\dot{V}O_2$ at the tissue prior to reaching DO_2crit remains constant due to increases in OER and again are reflected by decreases in hemoglobin (Hb) oxygen saturation of venous blood from the tissue. Additional tissue CO_2 will be produced after DO_2crit is reached when metabolic acids, such as lactic acid, are produced and then buffered by tissue bicarbonate (Schlichtig & Bowles, 1994).

Due to these links $\dot{V}CO_2$ and thus $P_{et}CO_2$ are linearly related to DO_2 during states of oxygen supply dependent metabolism. In shock states as severe as cardiac arrest, where oxygen content does not significantly change, the major component of DO_2, tracked by $\dot{V}CO_2$ or $P_{et}CO_2$, is pulmonary blood flow ($\approx$CO). This is, of course, advantageous during CPR because almost without exception, CPR is only capable of producing a flow state in which $\dot{V}O_2$ is directly dependent upon DO_2. In other shock states such as hemorrhage, $\dot{V}CO_2$ and $P_{et}CO_2$ will still track DO_2 in states of oxygen supply dependent metabolism, however, it will not be possible in real time to know to what degree, each component of DO_2 (CO or oxygen content) is most responsible for the change. However, at this stage DO_2crit, regardless of the type of shock, CO is likely to be significantly reduced, in part because the heart itself is falling below its DO_2crit resulting in significant global myocardial dysfunction.

In practical application, neither $\dot{V}O_2$ nor $\dot{V}CO_2$ is commonly monitored in the acute setting for several reasons (Chittock *et al.*, 1998). To do so would require use of a metabolic cart and the technique of indirect calorimetry, or the insertion and use of a pulmonary artery catheter and the use of derivatives of the Fick method. Both are not currently practical especially in the pre-hospital setting or emergency department. However, as indicated earlier, the relationship between $P_{et}CO_2$ and $\dot{V}CO_2$, and hence $\dot{V}O_2$, is sufficiently coupled to allow $P_{et}CO_2$ to be used as a monitoring tool in shock. To do this, both alveolar ventilation (minute ventilation) and $\dot{V}CO_2$ must be relatively constant. If they are, then changes in $P_{et}CO_2$ will reflect changes in the pulmonary capillary blood flow ($\approx$CO) and hence the major component of DO_2.

Although $\dot{V}CO_2$ production during shock is difficult to measure, there are not likely to be wide swings in the RQ to affect the general coupling between $\dot{V}O_2$ and $\dot{V}CO_2$. The tissue hypercarbia that occurs during shock states is reflected in venous blood including the pulmonary artery (Figures 24.3–24.5). The elevated concentrations of CO_2 in the mixed venous blood pool and the increases in alveolar deadspace that routinely occur in severe shock states will ensure that small changes in $\dot{V}CO_2$ do not cause appreciable changes in $P_{et}CO_2$ (Weil *et al.*, 1986). Only greatly enhanced DO_2 will result in a dramatic and sustained increase in $\dot{V}CO_2$ and hence $P_{et}CO_2$. Minute ventilation should thus be held relatively constant if $P_{et}CO_2$ is used as an indicator of CO.

Sudden drops in $P_{et}CO_2$ when no changes in ventilation have been made can be interpreted as significant deterioration in CO consistent with returning to a state below DO_2crit (Guzman *et al.*, 1997; Dubin *et al.*, 2000). In these instances a state of profound shock is developing and the patient is accumulating significant levels of oxygen debt.

Tissue specific monitoring

Figures 24.1 and 24.2 demonstrate the biphasic relationship between $\dot{V}O_2$ and $\dot{V}CO_2$ with DO_2 not only for the whole body but also for individual organ systems, which may have DO_2crit values that differ from whole body DO_2crit. Studies have demonstrated, for example in hemorrhagic and septic shock, that the DO_2crit of the splanchnic bed occurs at a higher global DO_2 than the DO_2crit of the whole body (Schlichtig *et al.*, 1991; Bowles *et al.*, 1992; Schlichtig & Bowles, 1994). Because of this, evidence of alterations in DO_2 to an organ system, such as the splanchnic bed or even skin or muscle, would be detected even earlier by monitoring the venous effluent for decreases in Hb oxygen saturation (as OER increases) or for increases in partial pressure of carbon dioxide in venous blood (P_vCO_2) because aerobically produced CO_2 is removed less efficiently. In severe and sudden shock states, such as massive hemorrhage or cardiac arrest, profound delivery-dependent $\dot{V}O_2$ is reached so that all organ systems rapidly pass their DO_2crit values. As such, each would demonstrate evidence of profound tissue hypoxia and flow stagnation as represented by very low venous Hb oxygen saturations and elevated venous or tissue CO_2 levels. The advantage of monitoring one tissue over another in this setting is difficult to defend and likely has no advantage to monitoring $P_{et}CO_2$ alone. However, in compensated or early states of shock, it is unlikely that $P_{et}CO_2$ monitoring will be capable of detecting changes. The same situation will exist when patients are resuscitated past their whole body DO_2crit while individual tissue beds still suffer oxygen deficits. Upon increasing CO to levels that restore DO_2 above DO_2crit, $P_{et}CO_2$ levels will usually transiently increase above baseline levels (35–45 mmHg) sometimes to levels greater the 80 mmHg, as CO_2 from the tissues is removed and aerobic metabolism is restored. However, simply because $P_{et}CO_2$ has normalized does not mean that tissues are adequately oxygenated. $P_{et}CO_2$ monitoring in compensated and post-resuscitation states can, however, be helpful when combined with a tissue PCO_2 measurement.

$P_{et}CO_2$ and tissue perfusion

Several options to monitor tissue CO_2 have been studied in various shock states. These include transcutaneous CO_2 ($PtcCO_2$) skin monitoring, interstitial fiberoptic PCO_2, gastric mucosal CO_2 via gastric tonometry ($PgCO_2$), and most recently sublingual tonometry ($PslCO_2$) (Tremper *et al.*, 1980; 1981; Ivatury *et al.*, 1996; McKinley *et al.*, 1998a, b; Nakagawa *et al.*, 1998; Weil *et al.*, 1999; Hurley *et al.*, 2000; Ward *et al.*, 2001). $PtcCO_2$, $PgCO_2$ and $PslCO_2$ are non-invasive while interstitial PCO_2 monitoring requires insertion of a probe into tissue parenchyma. Details of these techniques has been well described (Ward *et al.*, 2001). The methods are based on the diffusion of CO_2 from tissue and present the balance between supply of CO_2 to the tissue, CO_2 production by the tissue, and CO_2 removal from the tissue. This balance does not mean all tissue compartments contribute equally. Values will be a composite of vascular and interstitial levels in the immediate environment of the sensor. As approximately 70% of blood in tissues are venous [the tissue CO_2 concentrations will mainly reflect venous PCO_2 (Guyton, 1981; Shepherd, 1983)]. The majority of CO_2 accumulation in each tissue will be secondary to inability to remove aerobically produced CO_2 that was being produced prior to the actual onset of tissue dysoxia or ischemia (Figure 24.2). As mentioned previously, additional CO_2 will be produced in response to metabolic acids (mainly lactate). Animal and human studies have demonstrated tissue CO_2 levels well over 100 mmHg (von Planta *et al.*, 1989; McKinley *et al.*, 1998a, b). Widening of mixed venous to arterial PCO_2 differences have been known for some time to reflect changes in tissue DO_2 (Weil *et al.*, 1986; Rackow *et al.*, 1994). However access to the mixed venous pool is not always practical and in fact may not be as sensitive as properly selected "peripheral" tissue beds.

All of the above methods of tissue PCO_2 monitoring have been demonstrated to be sensitive to microcirculatory changes in blood flow not reflected in global DO_2 and $\dot{V}O_2$. However, because the goal of these measurements is to detect changes in tissue CO_2 as a reflection of changes in DO_2, care must be taken not to misinterpret the values influenced by minute ventilation on tissue PCO_2 (Guzman & Kruse, 1999; Pernat *et al.*, 1999). As normocapnia cannot be ensured in the initial stages of evaluation and resuscitation (especially if the patient is not intubated), use of the tissue CO_2-to-P_aCO_2 gap has been shown to be a more sensitive DO_2 measurement related to changes in tissue CO_2 because hypo- or hyperventilation, while effecting tissue CO_2, will not affect the gap (Bowles *et al.*, 1992; Hurley *et al.*, 2000). Given that the arterial-to-alveolar PCO_2 gap is approximately 4 mmHg, an abnormal tissue-to-$P_{et}CO_2$ gap of 11 mmHg to 14 mmHg suggests perfusion abnormalities (Hurley *et al.*, 2000). Continued elevation of tissue CO_2 resulting from decreases in tissue DO_2 as measured by these methods have been associated with an increased mortality (Tremper *et al.*, 1980; McKinley *et al.*, 1998a, b; McKinley & Butler, 1999; Tatevossian *et al.*, 2000). Normalization of the tissue CO_2-to-$P_{et}CO_2$ gap will help ensure that occult tissue hypoxia is not present, thus helping to avoid further accumulation of oxygen debt and its associated complications. The major problem with using this strategy may be in patients who have rapidly evolving acute lung injury or who are experiencing significant bronchospasm.

Summary

In shock DO_2 to tissue falls behind oxygen demand and CO_2 production decreases in lockstep. Eventually, metabolic acidosis liberates CO_2. These processes differ in magnitude in different organs and vascular beds, thus complicating the interpretation of global CO_2 data. Nevertheless, monitoring end-tidal carbon dioxide ($ETCO_2$) tensions in shock and during resuscitation can prove helpful to the clinician to be aware of the complexity of the pathophysiology of shock.

References

Abraham, E., Bland, R.D., Cobo, J.C. & Shoemaker, W.C. (1984). Sequential cardiorespiratory patterns associated with outcome in septic shock. *Chest*, **85**: 75–80.

Bowles, S.A., Schlichtig, R., Kramer, D.J. & Klions, H.A. (1992). Arteriovenous pH and partial pressure of carbon dioxide detect critical oxygen delivery during progressive hemorrhage in dogs. *J. Crit. Care*, **7**: 95–105.

Chittock, D.R., Ronco, J.J. & Russell, J.A. (1998). Monitoring of oxygen transport and oxygen consumption. In: Tobin, M.J. ed. *Principles and Practice of Intensive Care Monitoring*. McGraw-Hill, New York, pp. 317–343.

Dubin, A., Murias, G., Estenssoro, E., *et al.* (2000). End-tidal CO_2 pressure determinants during hemorrhagic shock. *Intens. Care Med.*, **26**: 1619–1623.

Guyton, A.C. (1981). The systemic circulation. In: Guyton, A.C. ed. *Textbook of Medical Physiology*. 6th edition. W.B. Saunders, Philadelphia, pp. 219.

Guzman, J.A., Lacoma, F.J., Najar, A. & Kruse, J.A. (1997). End-tidal partial pressure of carbon dioxide as a noninvasive indicator of systemic oxygen supply dependency during hemorrhagic shock and resuscitation. *Shock*, **8**: 427–431.

Guzman, J.A. & Kruse, J.A. (1999). Gut mucosal-arterial PCO_2 gradient as an indicator of splanchnic perfusion during systemic hypo- and hypercapnia. *Crit. Care Med.*, **27**: 2760–2765.

Hindman, B.J. (1990). Sodium bicarbonate in the treatment of subtypes of acute lactic acidosis: physiologic considerations. *Anesthesiology*, **72**: 1064–1076.

Hurley, R., Chapman, M.V. & Mythen, M.G. (2000) Current status of gastrointestinal tonometry. *Curr. Opin. Crit. Care*, **6**: 130–135.

Ivatury, R.R., Simon, R.J., Islam, S., Fueg, A., Rohman, M. & Stahl, W.M. (1996). A prospective randomized study of end points of resuscitation after major trauma: global oxygen transport indices versus organ-specific gastric mucosal pH. *J. Am. Coll. Surg.*, **183**: 145–154.

Jin, X., Weil, M.H., Sun, S., Tang, W., Bisera, J. & Mason, E.J. (1998). Decreases in organ blood flows associated with increases in sublingual PCO_2 during hemorrhagic shock. *J. Appl. Physiol.*, **85**: 2360–2364.

McKinley, B.A., Parmley, C.L. & Butler, B.D. (1998a). Skeletal muscle PO_2, PCO_2, and pH in hemorrhage, shock, and resuscitation in dogs. *J. Trauma*, **44**: 119–127.

McKinley, B.A., Ware, D.N., Marvin, R.G. & Moore, F.A. (1998b). Skeletal muscle pH, $P(CO_2)$, and $P(O_2)$ during resuscitation of severe hemorrhagic shock. *J. Trauma*, **45(3)**: 633–636.

McKinley, B.A. & Butler, B.D. (1999). Comparison of skeletal muscle PO_2, PCO_2, and pH with gastric tonometric $P(CO_2)$ and pH in hemorrhagic shock. *Crit. Care Med.*, **27** 1869–1877.

Nakagawa, Y., Weil, M.H., Tang, W., *et al.* (1998). Sublingual capnometry for diagnosis and quantitation of circulatory shock. *Am. J. Respir. Crit. Care Med.*, **157(6 Pt 1)**: 1838–1843.

Pernat, A., Weil, M.H., Tang, W., *et al.* (1999). Effects of hyper- and hypoventilation on gastric and sublingual PCO_2. *J. Appl. Physiol.*, **87**: 933–937.

Rackow, E.C., Astiz, M.E., Mecher, C.E. & Weil, M.H. (1994). Increased venous-arterial carbon dioxide tension difference during severe sepsis in rats (see comments). *Crit. Care Med.*, **22**: 121–125.

Relman, A.S. (1986). Letter. *New Engl. J. Med.*, **315**: 1618.

Sato, Y., Weil, M.H. & Tang, W. (1998). Tissue hypercarbic acidosis as a marker of acute circulatory failure (shock). *Chest*, **114**: 263–274.

Schlichtig, R., Kramer, D.J. & Pinsky, M.R. (1991). Flow redistribution during progressive hemorrhage is a determinant of critical O_2 delivery. *J. Appl. Physiol.*, **70**: 169–178.

Schlichtig, R. & Bowles, S.A. (1994). Distinguishing between aerobic and anaerobic appearance of dissolved CO_2 in intestine during low flow. *J. Appl. Physiol.*, **76**: 2443–2451.

Schlichtig, R., Mehta, N. & Gayowski, T.J. (1996). Tissue-arterial PCO_2 difference is a better marker of ischemia than intramural pH (pHi) or arterial pH–pHi difference. *J. Crit. Care*, **11**: 51–56.

Schumacker, P.T. & Cain, S.M. (1987). The concept of a critical oxygen delivery. *Intens. Care Med.*, **13**: 223–229.

Shepherd, J.T. (1983). Circulation to skeletal muscle. In: Shepherd, J.T., Abboud, F.M., Geiger, S.R., (eds) *Handbook of Physiology*, Vol 3. Bethesda, MD: American Physiology Society, pp. 319–370.

Shoemaker, W.C., Appel, P.L. & Kram, H.B. (1988). Tissue oxygen debt as a determinant of lethal and nonlethal postoperative organ failure. *Crit. Care Med.*, **16**: 1117–1120.

Shoemaker, W.C., Appel, P.L. & Kram, H.B. (1992). Role of oxygen debt in the development of organ failure sepsis, and death in high-risk surgical patients. *Chest*, **102**: 208–215.

Shoemaker, W.C., Thangathurai, D., Wo, C.C., *et al.* (1999). Intraoperative evaluation of tissue perfusion in high-risk patients by invasive and noninvasive hemodynamic monitoring. *Crit. Care Med.*, **27**: 2147–2152.

Tatevossian, R.G., Wo, C.C., Velmahos, G.C., Demetriades, D. & Shoemaker, W.C. (2000). Transcutaneous oxygen and CO_2 as early warning of tissue hypoxia and hemodynamic shock in critically ill emergency patients (see comments). *Crit. Care Med.*, **28**: 2248–2253.

Tremper, K.K., Mentelos, R.A. & Shoemaker, W.C. (1980). Effect of hypercarbia and shock on transcutaneous carbon dioxide at different electrode temperatures. *Crit. Care Med.* **8**: 608–612.

Tremper K.K., Shoemaker W.C., Shippy C.R. & Nolan L.S. (1981). Transcutaneous PCO_2 monitoring on adult patients in the ICU and the operating room. *Crit. Care Med.*, **9**: 752–755.

Vincent, J.L. (1998). Lactate and biochemical indexes of oxygenation. In: Tobin, M.J. ed. *Principles and Practice of Intensive Care Monitoring,* McGraw-Hill, New York; pp 369–376.

von Planta, M., Weil, M.H., Gazmuri, R.J., Bisera, J. & Rackow, E.C. (1989). Myocardial acidosis associated with CO_2 production during cardiac arrest and resuscitation. *Circulation*, **80**: 684–692.

Ward, K.R., Ivatury, R.R., Barbee, R.W. (2001). Endpoints of resuscitation for the victim of trauma. *J. Intens. Care Med.*, **16**: 55–75.

Weil, M.H., Rackow, E.C., Trevino, R., Grundler, W., Falk, J.L. & Griffel, M.I. (1986). Difference in acid–base state between venous and arterial blood during cardiopulmonary resuscitation. *New Engl. J. Med.*, **315**: 153–156.

Weil, M.H., Nakagawa, Y., Tang, W., *et al.* (1999). Sublingual capnometry: a new noninvasive measurement for diagnosis and quantitation of severity of circulatory shock. *Crit. Care Med.*, **27**: 1225–1229.

METABOLISM: CARBON DIOXIDE PRODUCTION

SECTION 1g

CARBON DIOXIDE PRODUCTION AND ANESTHESIA

25

D. Wilner & C. Weissman

The human body is fueled by nutrients and oxygen (O_2) that are metabolized to energy, carbon dioxide (CO_2), and waste products (see Figure 25.3). The amounts of O_2 consumed and CO_2 produced reflect the rate of body metabolism and the types of nutrients metabolized. The tasks of the respiratory and cardiovascular systems are to ensure that the cells of the body receive sufficient O_2 and that adequate amounts of CO_2 are removed. This results in tight coupling between the functioning of the respiratory, cardiovascular, and metabolic systems. Therefore, when interpreting measurements of CO_2 production and O_2 consumption it is important to consider the interaction of these three systems.

CO_2 production*/elimination**

$\dot{V}CO_2 = (VE \times \bar{F}_eCO_2) - (VI \times \bar{F}_ICO_2)$

$\dot{V}CO_2 = VE\,(\bar{F}_eCO_2 - \bar{F}_ICO_2)$ (assuming that VI = VE)

where
VE: expired minute ventilation
VI: inspired minute ventilation
$\bar{F}_eCO_2$: mixed expired CO_2 concentration
$\bar{F}_ICO_2$: mixed inspired CO_2 concentration

O_2 consumption*/uptake**

$\dot{V}O_2 = (VI \times \bar{F}_IO_2) - (VE \times \bar{F}_eO_2)$

$\dot{V}O_2 = VE\,(\bar{F}_IO_2 - \bar{F}_eO_2)$ (assuming that VI = VE)

where
$\bar{F}_IO_2$: mixed inspired O_2 concentration
$\bar{F}_eO_2$: mixed expired O_2 concentration

Respiratory Quotient (RQ)*/respiratory exchange ratio (R)**

$$\frac{RQ}{R} = \frac{\dot{V}CO_2}{\dot{V}O_2}$$

* Steady-state measurement
** Non-steady-state measurement

Figure 25.1 Formulae for metabolic calculations.

CO_2 production and O_2 consumption

Biochemistry and physiology

The overall amount of O_2 consumed and CO_2 produced by the human body is dependent on the rate of metabolism, while the proportion of O_2 consumed to CO_2 produced is dependent on the type of nutrients being metabolized or synthesized. Each cell type and organ system has a different metabolic function and, as a result, has different metabolic rates and nutrient requirements. Therefore, measurements of *whole-body* O_2 consumption and CO_2 production reflect the sum of the quantity and types of O_2-consuming and CO_2-producing activities of the various cell and organ systems of the body.

Nutrient metabolism: oxidation

The cells of the body metabolize carbohydrates, lipids, and proteins to produce energy in the form of high-energy phosphates (adenosine triphosphate, ATP). This is accomplished through both anaerobic and aerobic metabolism. The latter consumes O_2 and produces CO_2, while the former only produces CO_2. The oxidation of each of these nutrients is unique, resulting in the consumption of different amounts of O_2, the production of differing amounts of CO_2 and an assortment of waste products. The process of producing ATP is called oxidative phosphorylation and involves the conversion of these nutrients into acetyl-coenzyme A (acetyl-CoA). Acetyl-CoA then enters the citric acid cycle, which consumes O_2, liberates free energy as ATP and produces H_2O and CO_2 as waste products.

Ingested carbohydrates are converted to glucose. Glucose oxidation consumes and produces equal numbers of O_2 and CO_2 molecules, respectively:

$$C_6H_{12}O_6 + 6O_2 \rightarrow 6CO_2 + 6H_2O + \text{energy}. \quad (25.1)$$

Fats are stored in the body as triglycerides (three fatty acids attached to a glycerol backbone). Triglycerides are hydrolyzed by the enzyme lipoprotein lipase to free fatty acids and glycerol. The glycerol is converted to glucose and metabolized as a carbohydrate. The free fatty acids undergo beta-oxidation in the mitochondria. Unlike glucose oxidation, fatty acid beta-oxidation results in the consumption of more molecules of O_2 than molecules of CO_2 produced (Equation (25.2)). The ratio of O_2 consumed to CO_2 produced during long chain fatty acid oxidation is 0.71. This reaction also produces more than twice the energy (9 kcal/g) produced by the oxidation of either glucose or amino acids (4 kcal/g):

$$\text{Palmitate} + 23O_2 + 129\text{ADP} + 129\text{P}i \rightarrow 16CO_2 + 145H_2O + 129\text{ATP}. \quad (25.2)$$

Amino acids, the basic components of proteins, can also be used as energy substrates. They undergo deamination resulting in amino nitrogen being removed and metabolized to urea. The remaining carbon skeletons are oxidized by the citric acid cycle to CO_2 and H_2O. The oxidation of 1 g of protein consumes 0.965 l of O_2 and produces 0.781 l of CO_2 leading to a ratio of CO_2 produced to O_2 consumed of 0.8.

Lipogenesis

De novo synthesis of fatty acids from carbohydrate is called lipogenesis and occurs in humans ingesting carbohydrates in excess of their daily energy expenditure (EE). Glucose is converted to acetyl-CoA and then synthesized to fatty acids. The ratio of CO_2 produced to O_2 consumed is 8.0–8.7 depending on the fatty acid synthesized. Equation approximates lipogenesis:

$$13C_6H_{12}O_6 + 3O_2 \rightarrow C_{55}H_{104}O_6 + 26CO_2 + 29H_2O \quad . \quad (25.3)$$

CO_2 stores

The body stores CO_2, but not O_2. Consequently, it is necessary to continuously breathe to provide O_2 to the cells. The body stores about 12–14 l (~210 ml CO_2/kg) of CO_2 in a number of locations and forms (Armon *et al.*, 1990). A large pool exists as bicarbonate in the extracellular fluid; each liter of aqueous body fluid contains the equivalent of 500 ml of CO_2. CO_2 is also stored as carbonates in bone (Nunn, 1997, pp. 354–355).

CO_2 production versus CO_2 elimination

In humans, the lungs excrete almost all the CO_2 produced; only a miniscule amount is excreted through the skin (Carlson *et al.*, 1992). Therefore, it is possible to calculate the amount of CO_2 excreted by measuring the difference between the inspired and expired CO_2 contents (see Figure 25.1). Such measurements reflect body CO_2 production only if the subject is in a steady state. In non-steady-state situations these measurements reflect the pulmonary elimination of CO_2 at that point in time. The eliminated CO_2 may originate from CO_2 produced by metabolism, released from the CO_2 stores of the body and from the CO_2 in the blood (dissolved or carried by hemoglobin).

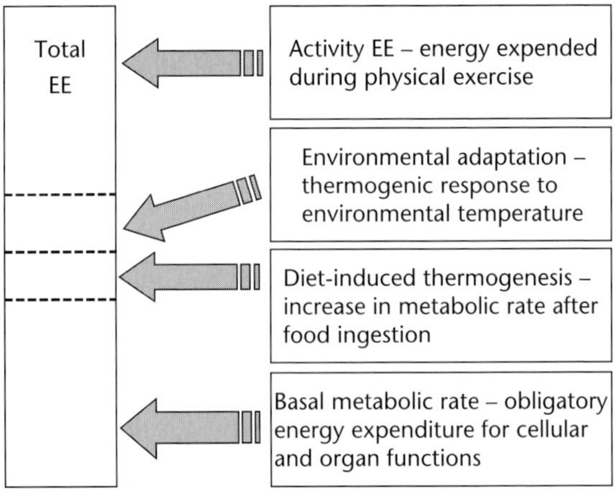

Figure 25.2 Total EE and its components.

To measure true resting/basal CO_2 production, i.e. the amount of CO_2 produced by metabolism, requires that the human subject be in a steady state (Weissman *et al.*, 1984). A steady state is a condition where the outputs of the metabolic, cardiovascular, and respiratory systems are stable so that O_2 uptake and CO_2 excretion by the lungs reflect metabolic activity. To achieve a steady state, a subject should be lying motionless and awake in a comfortable, quiet, thermo-neutral (25°C) environment while not actively digesting food. Thermoneutrality is an environmental temperature where heat production is not stimulated above baseline values (Lowell & Speigleman, 2000). Measurements are considered steady-state values once the CO_2 excretion and O_2 uptake values are stable, that is, they change <10% over a period of at least 5 consecutive minutes (McClave *et al.*, 2003).

Non-steady-state conditions frequently occur while performing measurements of CO_2 excretion and O_2 uptake (Anderson & Breen, 2000). In such cases, measurements of CO_2 output do not reflect metabolism but reflect the amount of CO_2 being eliminated through the lungs. A classic example is acute hyperventilation caused by anxiety or discomfort, which results in a

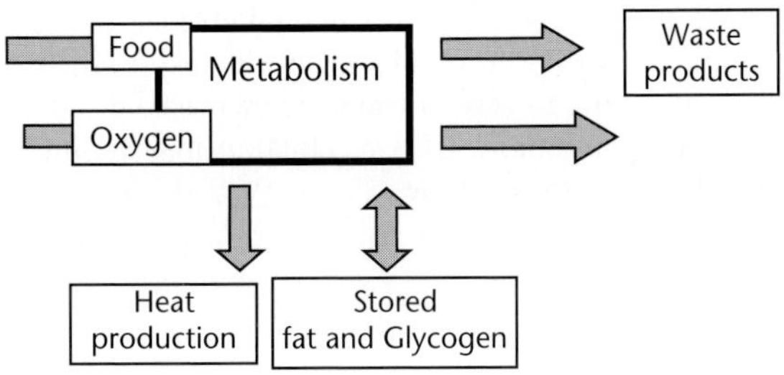

Figure 25.3 Total body metabolism.

transient increase in pulmonary CO_2 excretion and decrease in P_aCO_2 (Nunn, 1977, p. 349; Tobin *et al.*, 1986). Alternately, with the onset of hypoventilation, there is a transient decrease in CO_2 elimination, which reverses once the alveolar CO_2 concentration rises to a new steady state. Similarly, a decrease in cardiac output transiently decreases the pulmonary elimination of CO_2, which remains low until the CO_2 concentration in the mixed venous blood rises to a new steady state. Changes in mechanical ventilator settings resulting in increases or decreases in minute ventilation in paralyzed and sedated mechanically ventilated patients caused unstable CO_2 excretion measurements for at least 120 min (Brandi *et al.*, 1999).

Human metabolism normally operates as a system of supply and demand. Changes in metabolic demand, for example, exercise, require an increase in the supply of O_2 to the tissues and the amount of CO_2 removed from them. Therefore, when interpreting measurements of CO_2 production and O_2 consumption it is imperative that the activity state, and environment and health states be considered (Figure 25.3). During all types of exercise, O_2 consumption and CO_2 production increase as the result of increased intramuscular activity. As exercise loads increase, CO_2 production and O_2 consumption increase in parallel until the anaerobic threshold is reached. Above this threshold there is a continued increase in CO_2 production, but not O_2 consumption. Even simple exercise, such as elevating arms to shoulder level in seated subjects increases CO_2 production by >35% (Courser *et al.*, 1992). Therefore, it is important to observe the activity state of the subjects when measuring CO_2 production and O_2 consumption (Weissman *et al.*, 1986; Weissman & Kemper, 1991). Similarly, subjects in a cold environment will increase metabolic rate in order to maintain body heat, initially by tensing muscles and then by overt shivering. The latter can increase metabolic rate by up to 400%.

A number of additional factors must be considered when measuring and interpreting CO_2 production/elimination measurements. Another source of CO_2 eliminated through the lungs is that produced by colonic bacterial fermentation in the presence of lactulose and similar substances (Ritz *et al.*, 1993; Heresbach *et al.*, 1995). Bicarbonate ions are also produced during the catabolism of glutamine. These ions may then be converted to CO_2 and eliminated by lungs. The absolute contribution of this CO_2 to the overall CO_2 production is still unclear (Wiklund, 1996). Gas leaks around endotracheal tubes, such as those used in the pediatric population render measurements inaccurate because of loss of expiratory minute ventilation (Dietrich *et al.*, 1990). Leaks in ventilator tubing and its connections cause similar losses of minute ventilation.

Metabolism and CO_2 production

Direct versus indirect calorimetry

A subject's metabolic (caloric) expenditure can be directly quantified by measuring whole-body heat loss. Alternately, it can be measured indirectly by measuring O_2 consumption and CO_2 production:

$$\left.\begin{matrix}A\\B\\C\end{matrix}\right\} + O_2 + ADP \rightarrow \text{Heat} + CO_2 + H_2O + ATP. \qquad (25.4)$$

A = Lipids; B = Carbohydrates; C = Proteins.

Direct calorimetry involves measuring body heat loss by placing the subject in a closed chamber around which water of a known temperature flows. Body heat production is calculated from the increase in water temperature caused by the heat produced by the subject. This method is not practical for clinical use. Consequently, an indirect approach to measuring body energy expenditure (EE) was developed. The amount of energy used to consume a specific amount of O_2 and produce a given amount of CO_2 was calculated and validated by simultaneous direct and indirect calorimetry. These simultaneous measurements led Weir (1949) to develop an Equation (25.5) to calculate EE from measurements of O_2 consumption and CO_2 production:

$$EE\ (\text{kcal/day}) = 1.44(3.9 \times \dot{V}O_2 + 1.1 \times \dot{V}CO_2). \qquad (25.5)$$

Simultaneous measurements of nitrogen losses (mainly from the urine and feces) when combined with O_2 consumption and CO_2 production measurements allow for the calculation of substrate utilization. Specifically, calculation of the amounts of protein, lipid, and carbohydrates oxidized.

Energy (caloric) expenditure

EE is labeled as basal, resting, total, activity, or sleeping depending upon when the measurements are made. The classic research measurement, the basal metabolic rate, is made at basal steady-state conditions. Basal conditions are defined as lying awake and motionless in a thermo-neutral environment, immediately upon awakening in the morning, i.e. before breakfast. Such measurements are practical only in research environments and not in the clinical arena. Therefore, most clinical measurements are made at resting conditions: lying in a comfortable (24–26°C) and quiet environment, 3–4 h after a meal. The exception to the latter are patients receiving continuous enteral or parenteral nutrition where resting measurements are made once the nutritional intake has been stable for at least 12 h. Resting EE is about 10% higher than basal expenditure (CO_2 production is about 2–3 ml/kg and O_2 consumption is about 3–4 ml/kg). The measurement for resting EE is done 3–4 h after meals due to the phenomenon of diet-induced thermogenesis. After ingesting foodstuffs, O_2 consumption and CO_2 production increase by 15–20% for 1–3 h. This increase is caused by the oxidation of the food and by other factors. The magnitude of the diet-induced thermogenesis after a protein meal is greater than that after a fat or carbohydrate one.

Total EE is determined by an individual's basal EE, physical activities, dietary intake, and environment (Lowell & Speigleman, 2000) (see Figure 25.2). Sleep, which occupies a third or more of a normal subject's day, decreases EE by 10–15% from basal values for much of the night. EE then begins to increase towards morning. Some, but not all (White *et al.*, 1985), investigators have reported that O_2 consumption and CO_2 production increase during rapid eye movement (REM) sleep. The degree and type of physical activity performed during the waking hours is a major factor influencing the total daily EE. Individuals with sedentary lifestyles expend much less energy than do physical laborers.

Anesthesia and CO_2 production

Anesthesia and surgery greatly affect body homeostasis and consequently alter the functioning of the respiratory, cardiovascular, and metabolic systems, which influence the elimination of CO_2 from the human body. This section will review the many situations during surgery and anesthesiology that affect the excretion of CO_2 from anesthetized patients.

During anesthesia the principle factors influencing blood CO_2 concentrations are the inspired CO_2 concentration, CO_2 production, and alveolar ventilation. The concentration of CO_2 in the inspired gas is normally close to zero but may be increased accidentally or intentionally. CO_2 production may be influenced by anesthesia, type of surgery, and underlying pathologic state.

Minute volume varies widely during anesthesia and surgery. Lower minute volumes occur during spontaneous breathing during either deep anesthesia or partial neuromuscular blockade. Alternately, during mechanical ventilation, very high minute volumes may be attained. In anesthetized spontaneously breathing patients, surgical stimulation can increase ventilation. At various concentrations of inhalational anesthetics, Eger *et al.* (1972) demonstrated that the stimulation of surgical incision caused an increase in alveolar ventilation resulting in a decrease in resting P_aCO_2 by as much as 10 mmHg. In addition, the duration of anesthesia has a role in CO_2 homeostasis. Anesthesia, like sleep, reduces the total-body metabolic rate causing CO_2 production to diminish (Hickey & Severinghaus, 1981). Fourcade *et al.* (1972) observed that during halothane and enflurane anesthesia the resting P_aCO_2 after 6 h was lower than after both anesthesia induction and 3 h of anesthesia. More direct indication that CO_2 production is decreased during anesthesia comes from the work of others (Carli & Elia, 1991; Carli *et al.*, 1993). They found that enflurane caused a 9% decrease in CO_2 production during anesthesia and surgery, which returned to preoperative values after surgery. Similarly, O_2 consumption and CO_2 production decreased 12–15% during halothane and isoflurane anesthesia (with or without surgery). It thus appears that anesthesia produced by inhalational agents depresses CO_2 production. Others observed the influence of age, weight, operation, premedication, caudal anesthesia, and different inhalation anesthetics on CO_2 production. Infants weighing <5 kg had decreased CO_2 productions per kilogram during anesthesia. Increased CO_2 productions per kilogram were measured up to a body weight of 10 kg. Above a 10 kg body weight the amount of CO_2 production per kilogram was decreased and continued to decrease with increasing age (Lindahl *et al.*, 1989a). These findings were supported by other investigators who also observed that children in their teens, although they may have attained adult body weight, had a greater CO_2 production per kilogram body weight than adults during anesthesia (Bain & Spoerel, 1997).

The proposed mechanism for the age-dependent variation in CO_2 production per kilogram might result from partial inhibition by halothane of lipolysis in brown adipose tissue (Lindahl, 1989b). There is greater brown adipose tissue in younger than older infants. Brown tissue is rich in blood vessels and consumes more O_2 than other tissues. Lipolysis and fat mobilization result in CO_2 production and, therefore, halothane inhibition of lipolysis can explain the decrease in CO_2 production observed in young infants.

There are few data on the influence of anesthesia and anesthetic drugs on metabolic gas exchange during surgery. Lind (1995) examined the influence of different surgical procedures on O_2 consumption and CO_2 production. He compared emergency laparotomy, elective laparotomy, knee arthroscopy, and gynecological laparoscopy (a propofol infusion was used to maintain anesthesia), and found a significant increase in O_2 consumption from preskin incision to 5 min after skin incision. The greatest increase in O_2 consumption was seen during elective laparotomy. CO_2 production increased both in the laparoscopy group and, transiently, in the elective laparotomy group, but decreased in the other two groups. In the laparoscopy group the elevated CO_2 production likely represented CO_2 absorption from CO_2 insufflation of the peritoneal cavity. Pestana *et al.* (1996) compared the metabolic gas exchange pattern in patients receiving propofol and midazo-lam for induction and maintenance of anesthesia. Interestingly, he also compared values in patients anesthetized with midazolam but who were receiving a 10% intralipid infusion (the vehicle for propofol) during the anesthesia to evaluate the direct effect of propofol. O_2 consumption increased significantly in all groups at 45 min in respect to basal measurements and remained elevated throughout the study. This is possibly due to surgical stress. CO_2 production decreased gradually during anesthesia. There was a significant decrease in $\dot{V}CO_2$ in all the groups but largest in the groups receiving propofol or midazolam with intralipid. This could be explained by a greater lipid oxidation because fat oxidation is related to lower CO_2 production than the oxidation of proteins or carbohydrates.

A number of studies examined the effects of clonidine, an alpha-2 adrenergic agonist, and midazolam premedication during ketamine anesthesia. Preoperative O_2 consumption and CO_2 production decreased more with clonidine and midazolam premedication than with placebo (Kirvela & Kanto, 1991; Taittonen *et al.*, 1997; 1998). Surprisingly, intraoperative $\dot{V}O_2$ and $\dot{V}CO_2$ values were increased more in the midazolam group than in the clonidine and placebo groups. Midazolam did not prevent a ketamine-induced increase in catecholamines nor did it attenuate the catecholamine response to surgery, which probably contributed to the higher observed intraoperative $\dot{V}O_2$ and $\dot{V}CO_2$. Others observed that clonidine was associated with an attenuation of the increase in $\dot{V}O_2$ and $\dot{V}CO_2$ commonly observed during recovery from anesthesia (Delaunay *et al.*, 1991). The results regarding midazolam appear to conflict with Harding *et al.* (1994) who observed attenuated metabolic, hemodynamic, and ventilatory responses to chest physical therapy after midazolam administration.

Only a few studies have examined the effects of regional and general anesthesia on O_2 consumption and CO_2 production. Watters *et al.* (1993) compared the effects on EE of general anesthesia plus epidural anesthesia with general anesthesia alone and found that O_2 consumption and CO_2 production increased following surgery in both groups for the first 2 postoperative days. This was despite visual analogue pain scale scores being clearly lower in the patients receiving epidural anesthesia. Similar results were obtained by Tulla *et al.* (1992) who found no significant differences in postoperative $\dot{V}CO_2$ and $\dot{V}O_2$ whether hip surgery was performed with general or spinal anesthesia. Diebel *et al.* (1987) reported less increase in O_2 consumption after major thoracic surgery with epidural plus general anesthesia compared to general anesthesia alone. Viale *et al.* (1990) reported only a transient postoperative reduction in O_2 consumption in patients receiving epidural analgesia after major abdominal surgery. These studies seem to indicate that the addition of epidural anesthesia to general anesthesia does not influence CO_2 production.

The hemodynamic effects of epinephrine added to local epidural anesthetics are well documented. However, little is known about the influence of epinephrine on respiratory gas exchange. Steinbrook and Concepcion (2000) observed that the addition of epinephrine, 5 μg/ml, to the epidural injection of 2% lidocaine was associated with a 22% increase in $\dot{V}CO_2$ without a change in $\dot{V}O_2$, despite increases in heart rate and cardiac index. Epidural anesthesia without added epinephrine did not change $\dot{V}O_2$ or $\dot{V}CO_2$.

Neuromuscular blockade

A single dose of succinylcholine, a depolarizing muscle relaxant, significantly increased CO_2 production both 1 and 5 min after succinylcholine-induced fasciculations but caused no demonstrable changes in O_2 consumption (Erbguth & Berguan, 1973). This is interesting because fasciculations produced by succinylcholine presumably increase EE resulting in O_2 consumption by skeletal muscle. Also, a continuous infusion of succinylcholine in dogs has been shown to cause increased O_2 consumption due to increased skeletal activity (Muldoon & Theye, 1969). Christensen *et al.* (1985)

observed an increase in $\dot{V}CO_2$ whether succinylcholine was administered as a bolus or as a continuous infusion. However, in patients pretreated with pancuronium, which prevents fasciculations, no increase in $\dot{V}CO_2$ was observed. Similarly, pretreatment with diazepam has been shown to reduce the increase in CO_2 production observed with succinylcholine (Schon-Olesen *et al.*, 1986). It appears that the increase in CO_2 production is a result of succinylcholine-induced muscle fasciculations and not the direct metabolic effect of the drug.

Vernon and Witte (2000) studied sedated, mechanically ventilated children and observed that, neuromuscular blockade with non-depolarizing drugs caused a significant reduction in O_2 consumption (8.7 ± 1.7%) and EE (10.3 ± 1.8%) and, hence, CO_2 production. The patients in this study were sedated and there was no control group, so it was difficult to assess the exact influence of neuromuscular blockade on $\dot{V}O_2$ and $\dot{V}CO_2$.

CO_2 production and intraoperative events during anesthesia

Laparoscopy

During laparoscopy the abdomen is insufflated, often with CO_2. Therefore, the pulmonary CO_2 output is composed of metabolically produced plus exogenously introduced CO_2 absorbed from the peritoneal cavity. The CO_2 insufflated into the peritoneal cavity diffuses into the abdominal organs and abdominal wall and is then carried by the blood to the lungs. Kasama *et al.* (1996) observed that minute volume during pneumoperitoneum had to be increased by 1.54 times that of the prepneumoperitoneum phase to maintain a constant P_aCO_2. Compared with preinduction values, CO_2 production and O_2 consumption decreased during the period of anesthesia until skin incision. However, with the insufflation of CO_2 into the abdominal cavity, a marked (49%) increase in CO_2 output was observed, while $\dot{V}O_2$ remained stable. These variables returned to preinduction levels during the recovery period. O_2 consumption increased during both gynecologic laparotomy and laparoscopy, while CO_2 production decreased in the laparotomy group and CO_2 output increased during laparoscopy (Lind, 1995). Others (Mullet *et al.*, 1993) reported similar results, with $\dot{V}O_2$ remaining stable but noticed $\dot{V}CO_2$ values increased more during extraperitoneal than during intraperitoneal CO_2 insufflation. Additionally, Liang *et al.* (2002) suggested that intravenous propofol combined with epidural anesthesia for laparoscopic procedures can attenuate the increase in $\dot{V}CO_2$ caused by CO_2 insufflation.

Tourniquet release

Tourniquets are frequently used to provide a bloodless field during orthopedic surgery. Girardis *et al.* (2000) examined the effect of tourniquet inflation duration on gas exchange during general anesthesia. During tourniquet inflation $\dot{V}CO_2$ decreased slightly and $\dot{V}O_2$ remained stable compared to pretourniquet values. This can be attributed to lack of arterial blood flow to the limb. Following tourniquet deflation, $\dot{V}O_2$ and $\dot{V}CO_2$ increased, with peak values occurring after 5 min. Fifteen minutes after tourniquet deflation $\dot{V}CO_2$ returned to basal values, but $\dot{V}O_2$ continued to be increased. O_2 is not supplied to the limb during tourniquet inflation and, therefore, the energy for cellular metabolism is provided by anaerobic metabolism. Tourniquet release results in an increase in $\dot{V}O_2$ to replenish cellular O_2 supplies depleted during limb ischemia. These investigators observed that the magnitude of the increase in $\dot{V}O_2$ after deflation was dependent on the duration of tourniquet inflation. Other studies (Lee *et al.*, 1992; Takahashi *et al.*, 1998) seem to contradict these findings claiming that the increase in $\dot{V}O_2$ and $\dot{V}CO_2$ seen after tourniquet release is related to muscle mass and not the duration of tourniquet inflation. Takahashi *et al.*, (1998) studied the effects of tourniquet application in patients breathing spontaneously under epidural anesthesia. Their findings indicate that the changes in metabolic variables with tourniquet release are dependent on body size i.e., muscle mass, and not the duration of tourniquet application. $\dot{V}O_2$ and $\dot{V}CO_2$ increased after tourniquet release returning to base line values 7–10 min after deflation. The increase in $\dot{V}CO_2$ lasted longer than that of $\dot{V}O_2$. Furthermore, men showed a greater increase in $\dot{V}CO_2$ than women, due to their greater muscle mass. The increase in $\dot{V}CO_2$ was attributed to the release during limb reperfusion of accumulated metabolites, e.g. lactate, and their subsequent metabolism. Spontaneously breathing patients increased their minute ventilation to compensate for the increased $\dot{V}O_2$ and $\dot{V}CO_2$.

Vascular cross-clamping

Clamping and unclamping of the abdominal aorta during major vascular surgery is associated with major hemodynamic and metabolic consequences. Damask *et al.* (1984) examined the metabolic effects of cross-clamping and the effects of narcotic administration during aortic surgery. Three groups of patients were studied:

- Group 1: abdominal aortic aneurysm resection receiving low dose morphine,
- Group 2: aorto-iliac bypass grafts receiving low dose morphine, and

- Group 3: abdominal aortic aneurysm resection receiving high-dose morphine.

Only Group 1 showed a significant decrease in $\dot{V}O_2$ and $\dot{V}CO_2$ upon aortic cross-clamping and a significant increase in $\dot{V}O_2$ and $\dot{V}CO_2$ after aortic unclamping. The decrease in $\dot{V}O_2$ and $\dot{V}CO_2$ upon cross-clamping appeared to be directly related to the reduction in blood flow to the lower extremities. High-dose morphine did not seem to influence the metabolic rate. The large increases in $\dot{V}O_2$ and $\dot{V}CO_2$ observed in Groups 1 and 3 after unclamping reflect an overall increase in total-body metabolism resulting from renewed flow to the extremities and replenishing of O_2 stores depleted during cross-clamp (O_2 debt). Serum lactate levels increased after unclamping in all the groups. Subsequent lactate metabolism can partially explain the increase observed in $\dot{V}CO_2$. The $\dot{V}O_2$ remained elevated until the O_2 debt was repaid. The patients in Group 2 had smaller decreases in $\dot{V}O_2$, $\dot{V}CO_2$, and lactate upon cross-clamping and after unclamping. This was attributed to the presence of chronic collateral circulation thereby minimizing the O_2 debt and lactate production. A similar study compared $\dot{V}O_2$ and $\dot{V}CO_2$ in the early postoperative period in patients after coronary artery bypass graft (CABG) surgery and abdominal aortic surgery (AAS) (Hess *et al.*, 1997). They observed significantly increased $\dot{V}O_2$ and $\dot{V}CO_2$ values in the early postoperative period in patients after AAS most likely because of an O_2 debt that was incurred during aortic clamping. The increases in $\dot{V}O_2$ and $\dot{V}CO_2$ extended into the postoperative period because of thermoregulatory vasoconstriction.

Cardiopulmonary bypass

The use of hypothermic cardiopulmonary bypass (CPB) during open-heart surgery causes many changes in body homeostasis. The effect of changes in core body temperature during and after CPB have major influences on O_2 consumption and CO_2 production. Boschetti *et al.* (1998) observed positive linear correlations between $\dot{V}O_2$ and $\dot{V}CO_2$, and body temperature and blood flow rate during CPB. Starr (1959) also found a direct relationship between CPB flow rate and O_2 consumption. Damask *et al.* (1987) noted a sharp decrease in $\dot{V}O_2$ and $\dot{V}CO_2$ upon initiation of CPB. $\dot{V}O_2$ and $\dot{V}CO_2$ were lowest during core body temperatures of 21–27°C. During rewarming and the immediate postCPB period increases in $\dot{V}O_2$ and $\dot{V}CO_2$ were observed. Similar results have been described by other investigators (Ishitoya *et al.*, 1977; Abbott *et al.*, 1980; Hanhela *et al.*, 1999). The increase in $\dot{V}O_2$ and $\dot{V}CO_2$ after bypass is ascribed to increased total-body metabolism, repayment of the O_2 debt incurred during CPB, and metabolism of anaerobic metabolites accumulated during CPB. Hanhela *et al.* (1999) reported less increase in O_2 consumption and CO_2 production when patients were rewarmed at the end of CPB to a bladder temperature of over 37°C, while also being warmed by external passive techniques.

Temperature and CO_2 production

Hypothermia is common during and after surgery (Sessler, 1994). It usually results from exposure to a cold operating room environment and anesthetic-impaired thermoregulation. Almost all the general anesthetics in clinical use impair autonomic thermoregulatory control and are direct vasodilators. Bacher *et al.* (1997) has shown that intraoperative hypothermia decreases O_2 consumption and CO_2 production. However, recovery from general anesthesia is very often characterized by shivering, which increases O_2 consumption and CO_2 production and also produces untoward hemodynamic and metabolic changes, such as increased heart rate and cardiac output (Ralley *et al.*, 1988). Shivering also occurs without hypothermia, likely caused by emergence from anesthesia. Shivering in response to hypothermia can increase O_2 consumption by as much as 400–500% (Horvath *et al.*, 1956). Ralley *et al.* (1988) showed markedly increased $\dot{V}O_2$ and $\dot{V}CO_2$ in patients shivering after rewarming from CPB. If ventilation is inadequate to match these increases in $\dot{V}CO_2$, hypercarbia and acidosis can result (Sladen, 1985).

Suppression of the shivering response can minimize increases in O_2 consumption and CO_2 production and improve hemodynamic stability (Rodriguez *et al.*, 1983; Zwischenberger *et al.*, 1987). Meperidine can suppress visible shivering and significantly attenuate, but not abolish, the increases in O_2 consumption and CO_2 production (Macintyre *et al.*, 1987). Similar results have been observed when pancuronium and metocurine are administered during postoperative rewarming following coronary revascularization (Zwischenberger *et al.*, 1987). In a comparison study (Cruise *et al.*, 1992), pancuronium was found to be more effective in suppressing the clinical and metabolic effects of shivering after cardiac surgery than meperidine. Clonidine has also been reported to decreased postoperative metabolic demands (Delaunay *et al.*, 1991).

Hyperthermia is associated with increased O_2 consumption and CO_2 production. De las Alas *et al.* (1990) demonstrated in a canine model that CO_2 production and O_2 consumption were early indicators of approaching hyperthermia. Malignant hyperthermia (MH) is an uncommon, potentially fatal autosomal-dominant inherited disorder of skeletal muscle tissue that is triggered by halogenated volatile anesthetics and depolarizing muscle relaxants and is characterized by a hypermetabolic state (Wappler, 2001). Abnormal Ca^{2+} metabolism within the sarcoplasmic reticulum of skeletal muscle cells causes a hypermetabolic response resulting in increased heat production. The clinical picture includes tachycardia, generalized muscle rigidity, myoglobinuria, and increased end-expiratory CO_2 concentrations. The increase in end-expiratory CO_2 concentrations is the result of increased CO_2 production. Neuroleptic malignant syndrome is a syndrome with a clinical picture similar to MH that is induced by chronic use of phenothiazines, butyrophenones, lithium, and other psychoactive drugs. Little is known regarding O_2 consumption and CO_2 production in this syndrome, but because of a clinical picture comparable to MH it is safe to assume that CO_2 production is increased.

References

Abbott, T.R., Goodwin, B., Clark, G., *et al.* (1980). Mass spectrometer measurement of oxygen uptake and carbon dioxide exchange during CPB. *Br. J. Anaesth.*, **52**: 29–40.

Anderson, C.T. & Breen, P.H. (2000). Carbon dioxide kinetics and capnography during critical care. *Crit. Care*, **4**: 207–215.

Armon, Y., Cooper, D.M., Springer, C., Barstow, T.J., Rahimizadeh, H., Landaw, E. & Epstein, S. (1990). Oral [13C] bicarbonate measurement of CO_2 stores and dynamics in children and adults. *J. Appl. Phys.*, **69**: 1754–1760.

Bacher, A., Illievich, U.M., Fitzgerald, R., *et al.* (1997). Changes in oxygen variables during progressive hypothermia in anesthetized patients. *J. Neurosurg. Anesth.*, **9**: 205–210.

Bain, J.A. & Spoerel, W.E. (1997). Carbon dioxide output and elimination in children under anaesthesia. *Can. Anaesth. Soc. J.*, **24**: 533–539.

Boschetti, F., Perinati, G. & Montevecchi, F.M. (1998). Factors affecting the respiratory ratio during cardiopulmonary bypass. *Int. J. Artif. Organs*, **21**: 802–808.

Brandi, L.S., Bertolini, R., Santini, L. & Cavani, S. (1999). Effects of ventilator resetting on indirect calorimetry measurements in the critically ill surgical patient. *Crit. Care Med.*, **27**: 531–539.

Carli, F. & Elia, M. (1991). The independent metabolic effects of enflurane anaesthesia and surgery. *Acta Anaesthiol. Scand.*, **35**: 329–332.

Carli, F., Ronzoni, G., Webster, J., *et al.* (1993). The independent metabolic effects of halothane and isoflurane anaesthesia. *Acta Anaesthiol. Scand.*, **37**: 672–678.

Carlson, D.A., Schreck, C.E. & Brenner, R.J. (1992). Carbon dioxide released from human skin: effect of temperature and insect repellents. *J. Med. Entomol.*, **29**: 165–170.

Christensen, K.J., Olsen, A.S. & Jorgensen, S. (1985). Effects of suxamethoniumon CO_2 production. *Acta Anaesthiol. Scand.*, **29**: 424–426.

Courser, Jr, J.I., Martinez, F.J. & Celli, B.R. (1992). Respiratory response and ventilatory muscle recruitment during arm elevation in normal subjects. *Chest*, **101**: 336–340.

Cruise, C., MacKinnon, J., Tough, J., *et al.* (1992). Comparison of meperidine and pancuronium for the treatment of shivering after cardiac surgery. *Can. J. Anaesth.*, **39**: 563–568.

Damask, M., Weissman, C., Rodriguez, J., *et al.* (1984). Abdominal aortic cross-clamping. Metabolic and hemodynamic consequences. *Arch. Surg.*, **119**: 1132–1137.

Damask, M., Weissman, C., Ashkanazi, J. & Kinney, J.M. (1987). Do oxygen consumption and carbon dioxide production affect cardiac output after cardiopulmonary bypass? *Arch. Surg.*, **122**: 1026–1031.

De las Alas, V., Voorhees, W.P. & Geddes, L.A. (1990). End tidal carbon dioxide concentration, carbon dioxide production, heart rate and blood pressure as indicators of induced hyperthermia. *J. Clin. Monit.*, **6**: 183–185.

Delaunay, L., Bonnet, F. & Duvaldestin, P. (1991). Clonidine decreases postoperative oxygen consumption in patients recovery from general anaesthesia. *Br. J. Anaesth.*, **67**: 397–401.

Diebel, L.N., Lange, M., Schneider, F., *et al.* (1987). Cardiopulmonary complications after major surgery: a role for epidural analgesia. *Surgery*, **102**: 660–666.

Dietrich, K.A., Romero, M.D. & Conrad, S.A. (1990). Effect of gas leak around endotracheal tubes on indirect calorimetry measurements. *J. Parenteral and Enteral Nutr.*, **12**: 408–413.

Eger, E.I., Dolan, W. & Steven, W.C. (1972). Surgical stimulation antagonizes the respiratory depression produced by forane. *Anesthesiology*, **36**: 544.

Erbguth, P. & Berguan, N. (1973). The effect of a single dose of succinylcholine on oxygen consumption and carbon dioxide production in man. *Anesthesiology*, **39**: 447–449.

Fourcade, F., Larson, C., Hickey, R., *et al.* (1972). Effects of time on ventilation during halothane and cyclopropane anesthesia. *Anesthesiology*, **36**: 83.

Girardis, M., Milesi, S., Donato, S., *et al.* (2000). The hemodynamic and metabolic effects of tourniquet application during knee surgery. *Anesth. Analg.*, **91**: 727–731.

Hanhela R, Mustonen A, Korhonen I., *et al.* (1999). The effects of two rewarming strategies on heat balance and metabolism after coronary artery bypass surgery with moderate hypothermia. *Acta Anaesthiol. Scand.*, **43**: 979–988.

Harding, J., Kemper, M. & Weissman, C. (1994). Midazolam attenuates the metabolic and cardiopulmonary responses to an increase in oxygen demand. *Chest*, **106**: 194–200.

Heresbach, D., Flourie, B., Briet, F.D., Achour, L., Rambaud, J.C. & Messing, B. (1995). Effect of colonic fermentation on respiratory gas exchanges measured in the postabsorptive state. *Am. J. Clin. Nutr.*, **62**: 973–978.

Hess, W., Frank, C., Hornburg, B. (1997). Prolonged oxygen debt after abdominal aortic surgery. *J. Cardiothorac. Vasc. Anesth.*, **11**: 149–154.

Hickey, R.F. & Severinghaus, J.W. (1981). Anesthesia and ventilation. In: Horabein, R.F. (ed.) *Regulation of Breathing. Lung Biology in Health and Disease*, part 2 edition. vol. 17. Marcel Dekker, New York.

Horvath, S.M., Spurr, J.B., Hutt, B.K., *et al.* (1956). Metabolic cost of shivering. *J. Appl. Phys.*, **8**: 595–602.

Ishitoya, T., Sato, S., DiBaredetto, G., *et al.* (1977). Oxygen consumption during surface-induced hypothermia under halothane anesthesia. *Ann. Thoracic Surg.*, **23**: 52–57.

Kasama, T., Ikeda, K., Kato, T., *et al.* (1996). Carbon dioxide output in laparoscopic cholecystectomy. *Br. J. Anaesth.*, **76**: 530–535.

Kirvela, O. & Kanto, J. (1991). Clinical and metabolic responses to different types of premedication. *Anesth. Analg.*, **73**: 49–53.

Lee, T., Tweed, W. & Singh, B. (1992). Oxygen consumption and carbon dioxide elimination after release of unilateral lower limb pneumatic tourniquet. *Anesth. Analg.*, **75**: 113–117.

Liang, S.W., Lin, C.S. & Xiao, J. (2002). Effect of intraperitoneal carbon dioxide insufflation on hemodynamics of oxygen consumption during intravenous propofol anesthesia combined with epidural block. *Di Yi Jun Yi Da Xue Xue Bao*, **22**: 166–167.

Lind, L. (1995). Metabolic gas exchange during different surgical procedures. *Anaesthesia*, **50**: 304–307.

Lindahl, S.G., Offord, K.P., Johannesson, G.P., *et al.* (1989a). Carbon dioxide elimination in anaesthetized children. *Can. J. Anaesth.*, **36**: 113–119.

Lindahl, S.G. (1989b). Oxygen consumption and carbon dioxide elimination in infants and children during anaesthesia and surgery. *Br. J. Anaesth.*, **62**: 70–76.

Lowell, B.B. & Speigleman, B.M. (2000). Towards a molecular understanding of adaptive thermogenesis. *Nature*, **404**: 652–660.

Macintyre, P., Pavlin, E. & Duersteg, J. (1987). Effect of meperidine on oxygen consumption, carbon dioxide production and respiratory gas exchange in postanesthesia shivering. *Anesth. Analg.*, **66**: 751–755.

McClave, S.A., Spain, D.A., Skolnock, J.L., *et al.* (2003). Achievement of a steady state optimizes results when performing indirect calorimetry. *J. Parenteral and Enteral Nutr.*, **27**: 16–20.

Muldoon, S.M. & Theye, R.A. (1969). The effects of succinylcholine and d-tubocurarine on oxygen consumption. *Anesthesiology*, **31**: 437–442.

Mullett, C.E., Viale, J., Sagnard, P., *et al.* (1993). Pulmonary carbon dioxide elimination during surgical procedures using intra- or extra-peritoneal carbon dioxide insufflation. *Anaest. Analg.*, **76**: 622–626.

Nunn, J.F. (1977). *Applied Respiratory Physiology*, 2nd edition. Butterworths, London.

Pestana, D., Garcia-de Lorenzo, A. & Madero, R. (1996). Metabolic pattern and lipid oxidation during abdominal surgery – midazolam versus propofol. *Anesth. Analg.*, **83**: 837–843.

Ralley, F., Wynauds, E., Ramsay, J., *et al.* (1988). The effects of shivering on oxygen consumption and carbon dioxide production in patients rewarming from hypothermic cardiopulmonary bypass. *Can. J. Anaesth.*, **35**: 332–337.

Ritz, P., Cloarec, D., Beylot, M., Champ, M., Charbonnel, B., Normand, S. & Krempf, M. (1993). Effects of colonic fermentation on respiratory gas exchanges following a glucose load in man. *Metabolism*, **42**: 347–352.

Rodriguez, J., Weissman, C., Damask, M.C., Askanazi, J., Hyman, A.I. & Kinney, J.M. (1983). Physiologic requirements during rewarming: suppression of shivering response. *Crit. Care Med.*, **11**: 490–497.

Schon-Olesen, A., Christensen, K.J., Hartmann-Anderson, F., *et al.* (1986). CO_2 production after suxamethonium and diazepam. *Acta Anaesthiol. Scand.*, **30**: 625–628.

Sessler, D. (1994).Temperature monitoring in anesthesia. In: Miller, R. (ed.) *Anesthesia*, 4th edition, Churchill Livingstone, Miller Philadelphia; pp. 1363–1382.

Sladen, R.N. (1985). Temperature and ventilation after hypothermic cardiopulmonary bypass. *Anesth. Analg.*, **64**: 816–821.

Starr, A. (1959). Oxygen consumption during cardiopulmonary bypass. *J. Thorac. Cardiovasc. Surg.*, **38**: 46–56.

Steinbrook, R. & Concepcion, M. (2000). Respiratory gas exchange and hemodynamics during lumbar epidural anesthesia: effects of lidocaine with and without epinephrine. *Reg. Anesth. Pain Med.*, **25**: 380–384.

Taittonen, M., Kirvela, O., Aantaa, R., *et al.* (1997). Cardiovascular and metabolic responses to clonidine and midazolam premedication. *Eur. J. Anaesth.*, **14**: 190–196.

Taittonen, M., Kirvela, O., Aantaa, R., *et al.* (1998). The effect of clonidine or midazolam pre-medication on perioperative responses during ketamine anesthesia. *Anesth. Analg.*, **87**: 161–167.

Takahashi, S., Mizutani, T. & Sato, S. (1998). Changes in oxygen consumption and carbon dioxide elimination after tourniquet release in patients breathing spontaneously under epidural anesthesia. *Anesth. Analg.*, **86**: 90–94.

Tobin, M.J., Perez, T., Guenther, S.M., D'Alonzo, G. & Dantzker, R. (1986). Breathing pattern and metabolic behavior during anticipation of exercise. *J. Appl. Phys.*, **60**: 1306–1312.

Tulla, H., Takal, J., Alhava, E., *et al.* (1992). Does the anesthetic method influence the postoperative breathing pattern and gas exchange in hip surgery? A comparison between general and spinal anesthesia. *Acta Anaesth. Scand.*, **30**: 101–105.

Vernon, D.D. & Witte, M.K. (2000). Effect of neuromuscular blockade on oxygen consumption and energy expenditure in sedated, mechanically ventilated children. *Crit. Care Med.*, **28**: 1569–1571.

Viale, J., Annat, G., Tissot, S., *et al.* (1990). Mass spectrometric measurements of oxygen uptake during epidural analgesia combined with general anesthesia. *Anesth. Analg.*, **70**: 589–593.

Wappler, F. (2001). Malignant hyperthermia. *Eur. J. Anaesth.*, **18**: 632–652.

Watters, J., March, R., Desai, D. *et al.* (1993). Epidural anaesthesia and analgesia do not affect energy expenditure after major abdominal surgery. *Can. J. Anaesth.*, **40**: 314–319.

Weir, J.B. (1949). New methods for calculating metabolic rate with special reference to protein metabolic rate with special reference to protein metabolism. *J. Physiol.*, **109**: 1–9.

Weissman, C., Kemper, M., Damask, M.C., Askanazi, J., Hyman, A.I. & Kinney, J.M. (1984). The effect of routine intensive care interactions on metabolic rate. *Chest*, **86**: 815–818.

Weissman, C., Kemper, M., Elwyn, D.H., Askanazi, J., Hyman, A.I. & Kinney, J.M. (1986). The energy expenditure of the mechanically ventilated critically ill patient: an analysis. *Chest*, **89**: 254–259.

Weissman, C. & Kemper, M. (1991). The oxygen uptake-oxygen delivery relationship during ICU interventions. *Chest*, **99**: 430–435.

White, D.P., Weil, J.V. & Zwillich, C.W (1985). Metabolic rate and breathing during sleep. *J. Appl. Phys.*, **59**: 384–391.

Wiklund, L. (1996). Carbon dioxide formation and elimination in man. Recent theories and possible consequences. *Ups. J. Med. Sci.*, **101**: 35–67.

Zwischenberger, J.B., Kirsh, M., Dechert, R.E., *et al.* (1987). Suppression of shivering decreases oxygen consumption and improves hemodynamic stability during postoperative rewarming. *Ann. Thorac. Surg.*, **43**: 428–431.

ORGAN EFFECTS

SECTION

1h

HYPOCAPNIA AND HYPERCAPNIA: TISSUE- AND ORGAN-SPECIFIC EFFECTS 26

O. Akça

Background

Clinically, hypocapnia[1] is induced to treat increased intracranial pressure, diabetic ketoacidosis, near-drowning, congenital diaphragmatic hernia, and pulmonary hypertension in newborns (Laffey & Kavanagh, 2002). Conversely, hypercapnia is induced during the insufflation of the abdomen in laparoscopic surgery, to reverse carbon monoxide poisoning, to augment cerebral perfusion, and as an emergency treatment for central retinal artery occlusion (Laffey & Kavanagh, 1999; Laffey & Kavanagh, 2000). It has been used during emergence from anesthesia in order to enable hyperventilation and thus the rapid elimination of inhalation anesthetics without lowering the patient's partial pressure of carbon dioxide (PCO_2) in arterial blood (P_aCO_2). Patients often develop hypo- or hypercapnia unintentionally from various causes including early asthma, high altitude pulmonary edema, acute lung injury, excessive mechanical ventilation, cardiopulmonary bypass, extracorporeal membrane oxygenation, and high frequency ventilation.

Hypocapnia is normally well tolerated, although it may cause paresthesias, palpitations, myalgic cramps, and seizures (Gluck, 1998). The most important suggested indication is intracranial hypertension with or without neurologic deterioration (Bullock *et al.*, 2000). Despite recommended guidelines against it, hyperventilation to induce hypocapnia continues to be widely practiced (Huizenga *et al.*, 2000; Marion & Spiegel, 2000; Laffey & Kavanagh, 2002). In the US, more than one-third of board-certified neurosurgeons (Marion & Spiegel, 2000) and about half of emergency physicians (Huizenga *et al.*, 2000) routinely use prophylactic hyperventilation in patients with severe traumatic brain injury regardless of possible consequences. Before applying hypocapnia in clinical routine, one needs to consider the full range of effects on patients (Laffey & Kavanagh, 2002).

Hypercapnia is highly protective in experimental models of acute ischemic myocardial, lung, and brain injury (Nomura *et al.*, 1994; Vannucci *et al.*, 1995; Shibata *et al.*, 1998; Laffey & Kavanagh, 1999; Laffey & Kavanagh 2000). Potential mechanisms of this protection include alteration of organ oxygen supply-and-demand kinetics, attenuation of free-radical activity, and prevention of ischemia–reperfusion injury. However, because of insufficient human data, hypercapnia is not yet used clinically to treat organ injuries.

The focus of this chapter will be on the effects of hypo- and hypercapnia at the organ and tissue level.

Effects of CO_2 on the physiology of tissue oxygenation and perfusion

Primary determinants of tissue oxygen availability are arterial oxygen tension, cardiac output, and local perfusion. Core temperature, post-operative pain level, smoking, hypovolemia, and supplemental oxygen and fluid regimen also alter tissue oxygenation in the perioperative setting (Jensen *et al.*, 1991; Kurz *et al.*, 1996; Sheffield *et al.*, 1997; Akça *et al.*, 1999; Greif *et al.*, 2000; Arkilic *et al.*, 2003). An additional factor known to influence peripheral tissue perfusion and oxygenation is P_aCO_2. Hypocapnia decreases the oxygen supply and increases the oxygen demand of tissue, thereby, causing tissue ischemia. In contrast, hypercapnia increases tissue oxygenation and perfusion (Akça *et al.*, 2002; 2003a, b). The correlation of subcutaneous tissue oxygenation and P_aCO_2 appears to be linear in the range of 20–60 mmHg P_aCO_2 (Table 26.1 and Figure 26.1) (Akça *et al.*, 2002). Although hyperventilation-induced hypocapnia may increase alveolar oxygen tension, the other important pulmonary effects of hypocapnic alkalosis such as attenuation of hypoxic pulmonary vasoconstriction

[1] Hypo- and hypercapnia indicate lower or higher than normal CO_2 levels in arterial blood. As long as the gas is in equilibrium with tissue, the terms can also indicate low or high tissue CO_2 levels. The terms do not refer to end-tidal CO_2 values, which often do not reflect arterial values.

Table 26.1 Global hemodynamics and tissue oxygenation as a function of target arterial PCO_2

Target P_aCO_2 (mmHg)	20	30	40	50	60	*P*
Cardiac index (l/min/m^2)	2.7 ± 0.4	2.9 ± 0.4	3.2 ± 0.5	3.6 ± 0.7	3.9 ± 0.2	0.0001
Muscle tissue oxygen saturation (%)*	84.4 ± 7.4	85.8 ± 9.6	86.6 ± 8.1	87.2 ± 8.9	89.0 ± 8.6	0.0004
Laser Doppler flow velocity (U)*	13.6 ± 6.3	13.7 ± 7.7	16.7 ± 6.8	16.2 ± 9.3	17.8 ± 8.5	0.2169
Cerebral oximeter saturation (%)	68.1 ± 10.8	69.1 ± 14.0	78.6 ± 8.6	82.5 ± 10.1	85.4 ± 7.5	<0.0001
Subcutaneous tissue oxygen tension (mmHg)	51.9 ± 9.9	57.8 ± 11.2	65.2 ± 14.5	74.0 ± 12.3	82.4 ± 18.6	<0.0001

Data presented as mean ±SD. See Figure 26.1 for regression analysis. Repeated measure ANOVA was used to analyze normally distributed data. Asterisks (*) indicate non-normally distributed data sets analyzed by Friedman test. (Reproduced with permission from Akça, O., Doufas, A., Morioka, N., Iscoe, S., Fisher, J. & Sessler, D. (2002). Hypercapnia improves tissue oxygenation. *Anesthesiology*, **97**: 801–806.)

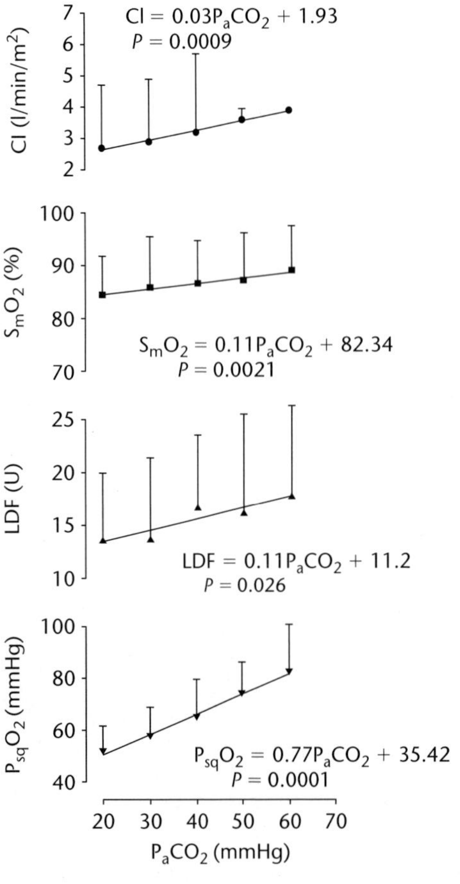

Figure 26.1 Cardiac index (CI), muscle tissue oxygen saturation (S_mO_2), skin blood flow (laser Doppler flow velocity, LDF), and subcutaneous tissue oxygen tension ($P_{sq}O_2$) all increased as a linear function of P_aCO_2. *P* values were obtained from linear regression formula. (Reproduced with permission from Akça, O., Doufas, A., Morioka, N., Iscoe, S., Fisher, J. & Sessler, D. (2002). Hypercapnia improves tissue oxygenation. *Anesthesiology*, **97**: 801–806.)

and increased intrapulmonary shunting result in a net decrease in the partial pressure of arterial oxygen (P_aO_2) (Domino *et al.*, 1993).

Additionally, hypocapnia and alkalosis cause a leftward shift of the oxyhemoglobin dissociation curve. Therefore, oxygen off-loading at the tissue level is restricted. Hypocapnia also causes systemic arterial vasoconstriction, decreasing the global and regional oxygen supply, and compounding the reduction in the delivery of oxygen to tissue (Guzman & Kruse, 1999). Hypercapnia causes a rightward shift of the oxyhemoglobin dissociation curve, increases cardiac output, decreases systemic vascular resistance and oxygen extraction, and thus, overall, increases oxygen availability to tissue (Mas *et al.*, 2000).

Okazaki *et al.* (1989) investigated the effects of CO_2 on the splanchnic visceral organs (liver and kidney) and skeletal muscle in the anesthetized dog. They showed that hyperventilation resulted in a significant decrease in hepatic artery and portal vein blood flow, liver surface partial pressure of oxygen (PO_2), and kidney surface PO_2 in parallel with the decreased P_aCO_2, but these parameters increased dose dependently when CO_2 was added to the inspired gas (hypercapnic hyperventilation). In contrast, skeletal muscle-surface PO_2 was increased by hypocapnia and decreased by hypercapnia. P_aCO_2 corresponded to changes in tissue oxygenation and appeared to exert significant effects on both splanchnic and skeletal muscle perfusion. Thus, injudicious and prolonged hypocapnic hyperventilation may seriously compromise splanchnic organ perfusion and oxygenation (Okazaki *et al.*, 1989). In another study by the same investigative team, Hashimoto *et al.* (1990) studied the effect of CO_2 on the myocardial oxygenation during hemorrhagic shock under normocapnic, hypo- and hypercapnic conditions. Hypocapnia decreased coronary flow and myocardial oxygen tension in the outer and inner layers of the myocardium. In contrast, hypercapnia increased them. Hypocapnia might, therefore, compromise the oxygenation of the myocardium during hemorrhagic shock.

Specific organ and tissue effects of CO_2

Central nervous system and brain

Owing to the skull's bony structure, the cranial cavity is a fixed space, and when the volume of any of its contents increases regardless of cause – hematoma, edema, inflammation or mass – it causes an increase in intracranial pressure. Increased intracranial pressure may result in impaired cerebral perfusion and risk of brain-stem herniation. To reduce intracranial pressure, the volume of the cranial contents must be reduced. Hypocapnic alkalosis decreases the cerebral blood volume owing to its potent cerebral vasoconstriction effect, and thereby, lowers intracranial pressure.

The beneficial effects of hypocapnia on intracranial pressure may be outweighed, however, by the reduced oxygen supply (Weckesser *et al.*, 1999). In the past the phenomenon of *inverse steal* during hypocapnia was postulated to increase regional perfusion to ischemic parts of the brain by stealing perfusion from the uninjured brain tissue; this theory has been rejected (Ruta *et al.*, 1993). Hypocapnia can increase cerebral oxygen demand by increasing neuronal excitability and seizure activity (Huttunen *et al.*, 1999). Additionally, hypocapnia during cardiopulmonary resuscitation may worsen brain injury (Safar *et al.*, 1996).

During prolonged hypocapnia, extracellular fluid bicarbonate decreases, which results in the gradual return of extracellular fluid pH toward normal. In brain tissue, this normalization of local pH also normalizes cerebral blood flow. Therefore, prolonged hypocapnia eventually causes tolerance and might even cause a rebound effect in intracranial pressure and lead to neuronal ischemia. Once the P_aCO_2 returns to normal, rebound hyperperfusion, which triggers an increase in intracranial pressure, may also aggravate reperfusion injury (Gleason *et al.*, 1989).

Cerebral blood flow is preserved better during hypercapnia than during normo- or hypocapnia. Hypercapnia causes greater oxygen delivery, which in turn promotes cerebral glucose utilization, and oxidative metabolism for optimal maintenance of tissue high energy phosphate reserves (Vannucci *et al.*, 1997). Increasing PCO_2 increases oxygenation in the tissues, including brain (Manley *et al.*, 2000; Akça *et al.*, 2002; Akça *et al.*, 2003) and doubles cerebral blood flow without causing a major change in cerebral metabolism (Alberti *et al.*, 1975). Most of the effects of CO_2 on cerebroarterial blood flow are maintained by regulating extracellular fluid pH (Kontos *et al.*, 1977).

Vannucci *et al.* (1995) studied whether hypercapnia protects against and hypocapnia potentiates hypoxic–ischemic brain damage in the immature rat brain. The investigators caused the animals to breathe incremental concentrations of CO_2 (F_ICO_2 0–3–6–9%) for 2 h during the reperfusion phase after 3–4 h of ischemia. They found that hypocapnia was deleterious and increasing levels of CO_2 were protective. However, the protective effect was saturated around an F_ICO_2 of 6% (P_aCO_2 ~54 mmHg), and further increases appeared to abolish the protection (Vannucci *et al.*, 1995). In a follow-up study, the same group showed that during hypercapnia cerebral blood flow was better preserved and the greater oxygen delivery promoted cerebral glucose utilization and oxidative metabolism for optimal maintenance of tissue high energy phosphate reserves (Vannucci *et al.*, 1997). Additionally, the concentration of glutamate was decreased in the cerebrospinal fluid during hypercapnia. The reduction of this excitatory neurotransmitter might offer additional protection for the central nervous system. In a recent *in vitro* study, hypercapnia preconditioning reduced the damage caused by ischemia–reperfusion in rat brain slices (Akça *et al.*, 2003).

A possible mediator responsible for the increase in cerebroarterial blood flow and vasodilation during hypercapnia is nitric oxide (NO) (Faraci *et al.*, 1994; Iadecola *et al.*, 1994; Schmetterer *et al.*, 1997). In many animals (rats, cats, dogs, and rabbits) (Faraci & Brian, 1994; Iadecola *et al.*, 1994; Wang *et al.*, 1995) and human (Schmetterer *et al.*, 1997) studies, inhibiting NO synthase (the rate-limiting enzyme for NO) attenuated the hypercapnia-induced cerebral hemodynamic effects. For example, cerebral vasodilation in response to hypercapnic acidosis was blocked by L-arginine analogs such as N^G-nitro-L-arginine (L-NNA) or N^G-monomethyl-L-arginine (L-NMMA) (Iadecola *et al.*, 1994) which are NO synthase inhibitors. As NO is short lived, diffusible, and highly reactive, it is difficult directly to measure local NO concentration *in vivo* to elucidate this proposed mechanism.

There is also evidence that the cerebroarterial dilational effects of hypercapnia are mediated through adenosine triphosphate (ATP)-sensitive potassium (K_{ATP}) channels (Rosenblum *et al.*, 2001). K_{ATP} channels require L-arginine or L-lysine to maintain an open state (Kontos & Wei, 1996); therefore, L-arginine analogs block the K_{ATP} channels, as well as NO synthase (Kontos & Wei, 1996). Recently, it was shown in an *in vitro* study that K_{ATP} channels in endothelium are pH-sensitive (Xu *et al.*, 2001). As the pH went from 7.4 to 6.6, the K_{ATP} channels shifted from a closed to an opened state. Because the response to CO_2 is a continuum, the responsible mechanism should be affected by increasing or decreasing pH; that is, hypercapnic acidosis triggers K_{ATP} channel opening and hypocapnic alkalosis triggers channel closing. Evidence in support of this hypothesis was recently published by Wei and Kontos (1999).

Respiratory system

Hypocapnia and hypocapnic alkalosis have the potential to worsen lung injury. In an isolated buffer-perfused rabbit lung, Laffey *et al.* (2000) showed that hypocapnic alkalosis damaged the uninjured lung. Prolonged ventilation with hypocapnia – which was maintained with lower inspiratory CO_2 concentrations not by altering ventilation (pH ~7.9, PCO_2 ~12 mmHg) – increased pulmonary artery pressure, airway pressure, and wet-lung weight (Figure 26.2).

High tidal volume ventilatory techniques cause or potentiate a stretch-induced acute lung injury named "ventilator associated lung injury" (VALI). Reducing lung stretch means reducing volumes or pressures applied to the lungs. Unless respiratory rate is altered, smaller tidal volumes often lead to an elevation of P_aCO_2, which eventually leads to permissive hypercapnia. Use of smaller tidal volumes in the presence of elevated P_aCO_2 appears to be beneficial to prevent damage from VALI. Of course, these two phenomena, namely elevated *CO_2* and *smaller tidal volumes*, can be separately controlled by manipulation of respiratory rate. As mentioned by Laffey and Kavanagh (2000), dissecting these factors may be important to intensivists for a couple of reasons. First, permissive hypercapnia is associated with improved outcome (Hickling *et al.*, 1994; Amato *et al.*, 1998). Second, evidence supports that elevated levels of CO_2 might have beneficial effects, independent of lung stretch (Laffey & Kavanagh, 1999). Third, the ARDSNet trial documented that adoption of a low tidal volume ventilatory strategy resulted in a ~25% reduction in mortality in patients suffering from acute respiratory distress syndrome (ARDS) (Network ARDS, 2000). In this latter study, the P_aCO_2 levels were clinically comparable in both groups and not even hypercapnic (35 versus 40 mmHg). In this case, one can hypothesize that reducing lung stretch and permitting hypercapnia could exert additive (or synergistic) benefits (Laffey & Kavanagh, 2000).

Activation of xanthine oxidase, an important enzyme in ischemia–reperfusion injury, has major implications in tissue injury. In one study, Shibata *et al.* (1998), used ischemia–reperfusion, and free-radical injury models in isolated buffer-perfused rabbit lungs to demonstrate that hypercapnic acidosis prevented an increase in capillary permeability after both types

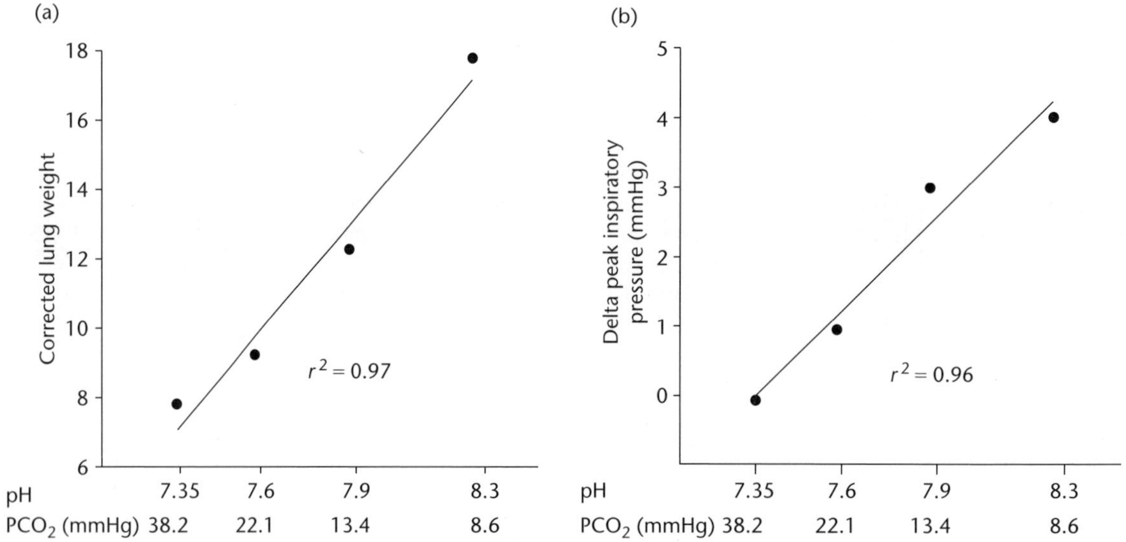

Figure 26.2 (a) Dose–response data for hypocapnic alkalosis versus corrected wet-lung weight ($r^2 = 0.97$; $P < 0.02$). (b) Dose–response data for hypocapnic alkalosis versus elevation in airway pressure ($r^2 = 0.96$; $P < 0.02$). (Reproduced with permission from Laffey, J. & Kavanagh, B. (2000). Biological effects of hypercapnia. *Intensive Care Med.*, **26**: 133–138.)

of lung injury without adverse microvascular effects on the uninjured lung. The mechanism appeared to be the inhibition of xanthine oxidase by hypercapnic acidosis. In a follow-up study from the same research team, investigators studied whether hypercapnia would be protective against ischemia–reperfusion lung injury in an *in vivo* rabbit model. The hypercapnia group ($P_aCO_2 \sim 100$ mmHg, pH ~ 7.10) had attenuated protein leakage, reduced pulmonary edema, improved oxygenation, only minimal increases in tumor necrosis factor alpha (TNF-α) levels, and reduced lung tissue nitrotyrosine (indicating decreased nitration of tissue) (Laffey *et al.*, 2000). All of these findings support the hypothesis that hypercapnic acidosis preserves lung mechanics, attenuates pulmonary inflammation, and reduces free-radical injury. It might also attenuate ischemia–reperfusion injury-induced apoptosis (Figures 26.3 and 26.4).

Circulatory system, heart, and hemodynamics

Hypocapnia alters myocardial oxygenation and cardiac rhythm. Acute hypocapnia decreases myocardial

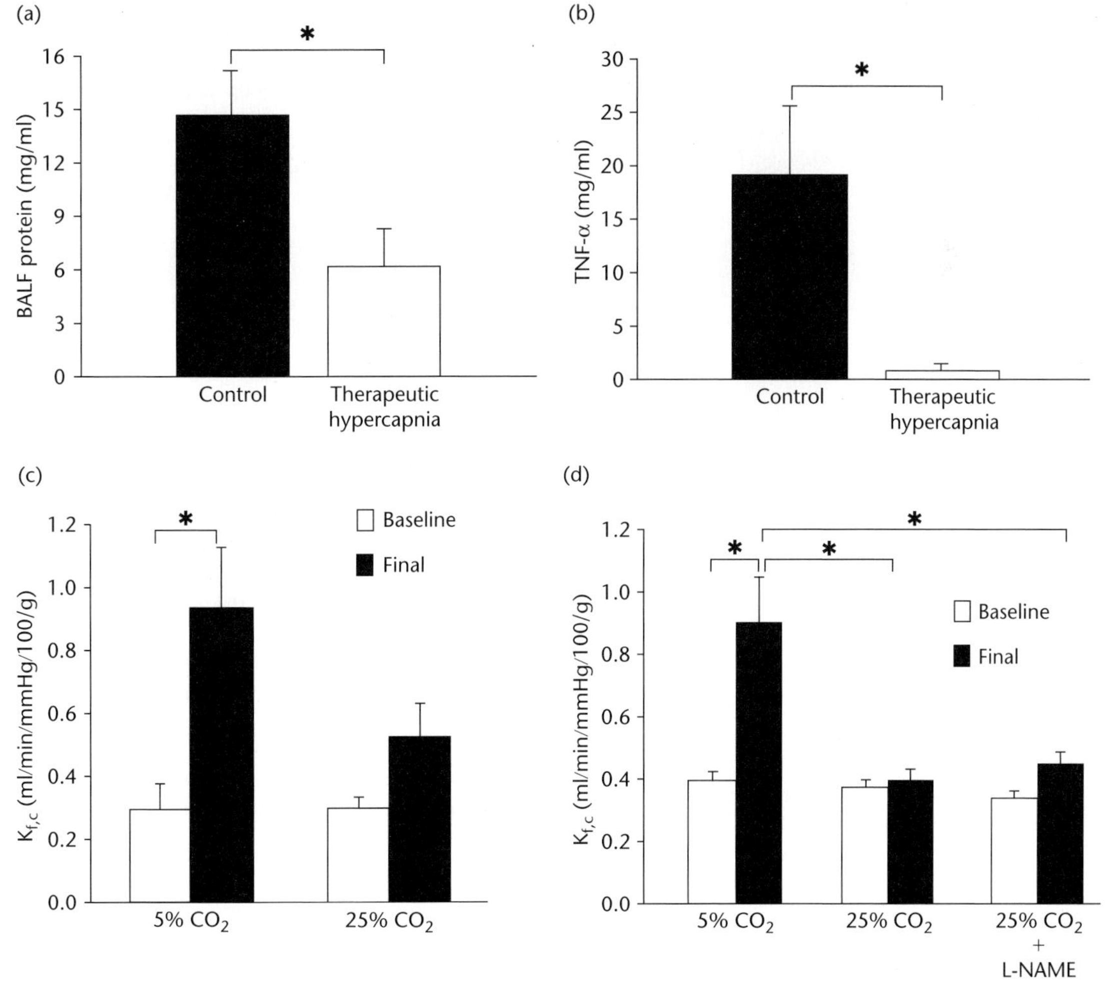

Figure 26.3 Panel (a) *BALF protein.* The protein concentration in the BAL fluid was significantly lower in the hypercapnia than in the control group (*$P < 0.05$). Panel (b) *BALF TNF-α.* BALF TNF-α was significantly lower in the hypercapnia than in control group (*$P < 0.05$). (Reprinted with permission from Laffey *et al.*, 2000.) Panel (c) Pulmonary capillary filtration coefficient ($K_{f,c}$) measured at baseline and after warm ischemia–reperfusion injury. Results are mean ± SEM of the data. Panel (d) $K_{f,c}$ measured at baseline and after injury-induced by addition of purine–xanthine oxidase to perfusate. Results are mean ± SEM of the data (*$P < 0.05$). (Reproduced with permission from Shibata, K., Cregg, N., Engelberts, D., Takeuchi, A., Fedorko, L. & Kavanagh, B. (1998). Hypercapnic acidosis may attenuate acute lung injury by inhibition of endogenous xanthine oxidase. *Am. J. Respir. Crit. Care Med.*, **158**: 1578–1584.)

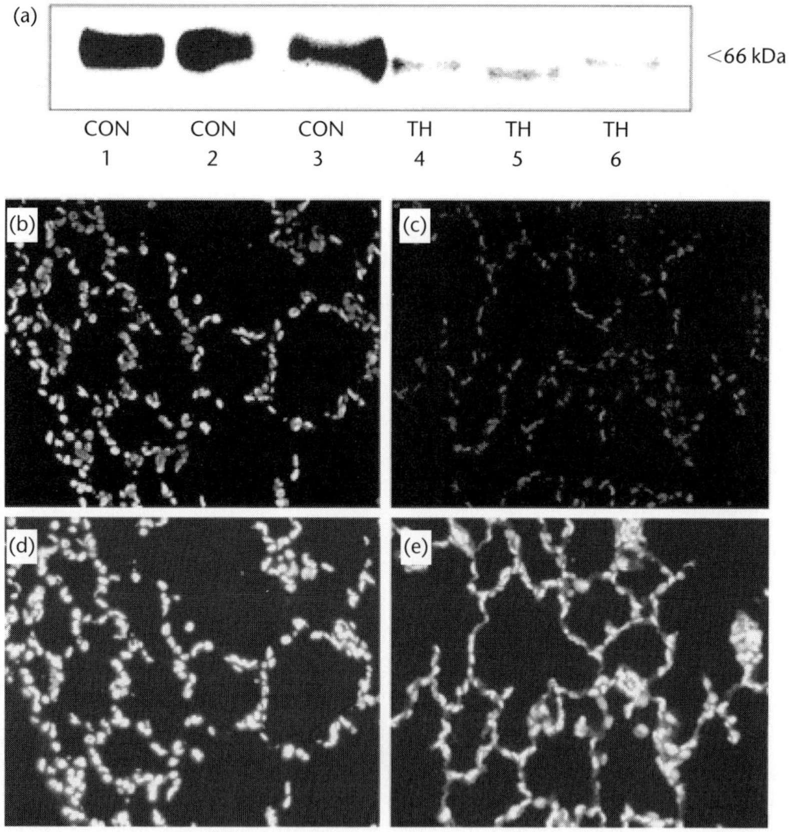

Figure 26.4 Panel (a) Western blot analysis of nitrotyrosine residues from three specimens from each group. A prominent band of nitrotyrosylated protein is demonstrated at approximately 66 kDa. The intensity of the bands is greater in the control (CON) (bands 1–3) than in the hypercapnia (TH) (bands 4–6) group. Panels (b–e) Examples of apoptosis demonstrated by TUNEL assay. Fluorescence is greater in the control than in the hypercapnia group (control group panel (b); hypercapnia group panel (c)), indicating more apoptosis. Comparable tissue DNA profile is demonstrated in the presence of DAPI (control group panel (d); hypercapnia group panel (e)). (Reproduced with permission from Laffey, J. & Kavanagh, B. (2000). Biological effects of hypercapnia. *Intensive Care Med.*, **26**: 133–138.)

oxygen delivery while increasing oxygen demand. Oxygen demand is increased because of the increased myocardial contractility (Boix *et al.*, 1994) and systemic vascular resistance (Richardson *et al.*, 1972). Thus, hypocapnia may contribute to clinically relevant acute coronary syndromes.

Earlier evidence suggested that using fixed acids or buffers to maintain acidotic reperfusion fluids improved recovery of the stunned myocardium (Kitakaze *et al.*, 1988; Matsuda *et al.*, 1991). Therefore, Nomura *et al.* (1994) tested whether hypercapnic acidosis would provide a similar benefit. They used isolated, blood-perfused neonatal lamb hearts to perform the study. After 2 h of cold cardioplegic ischemia at pH 7.4, reperfusion was provided with blood with pH values ranging from 6.8 to 7.8. The pH changes were achieved by altering the fraction of inspired CO_2. In an additional group, hydrochloric acid was used to titrate the pH of the reperfusion blood to 6.8 (metabolic acidotic group). The most hypercapnic acidotic group had the best indices of contractility, coronary blood flow, and myocardial oxygen consumption. Interestingly, the metabolic acidotic group did not get similar protection (Nomura *et al.*, 1994).

Hypercapnia increases tissue perfusion and oxygenation (Akça *et al.*, 2002), mainly through increased cardiac output. For example, increasing the PCO_2 from 20 to 60 mmHg increases the cardiac index about 44%. In a recent study in post-operative cardiac surgery patients, a similar benefit was shown by increasing the PCO_2 from 30 to 50 mmHg. Increasing CO_2 pressure increased the cardiac index, as well as mixed venous oxygen saturation (Ali *et al.*, 2003). This global oxygenation improvement complements the previously mentioned tissue oxygenation effects.

Hypercapnia also causes a complex interaction of altered cardiac output, hypoxic pulmonary vasoconstriction, and intrapulmonary shunt with the result being a net increase in P_aO_2 at a given inspired oxygen concentration (Hickling & Joyce, 1995).

Other known effects

Holmes *et al.* (1994) investigated the effects of hypercapnia, normocapnia, and metabolic acidosis on the retinal vasculature of neonatal rats. Those exposed to hypercapnia had pronounced retardation of normal retinal vascular development. Additionally, hypercapnia exacerbated oxygen-induced retinopathy (Holmes *et al.*, 1997). Similarly, metabolic acidosis-induced neovascularization that appeared similar to retinopathy of prematurity (Holmes *et al.*, 1999). In the light of this evidence, one needs to be concerned about allowing permissive hypercapnia in vulnerable neonates (Laffey & Kavanagh, 2000).

Central sleep apnea causes hypoxemia, increased sympathetic nervous system activity, and in patients with congestive heart failure, increased risk of death (Laffey & Kavanagh, 2002). An enhanced ventilatory response to CO_2 may contribute to the development of central sleep apnea in some patients with congestive heart failure (Javaheri, 1999), and hypocapnia triggers periodic respirations in these patients (Naughton *et al.*, 1994). One of the mechanisms by which application of non-invasive positive airway pressure reduces central sleep apnea is by increasing hemoglobin oxygen saturation and increasing the P_aCO_2 toward or above the apneic threshold (Naughton *et al.*, 1994). In fact, central sleep apnea is predicted by the presence of hypocapnia during waking hours (Sin *et al.*, 1999). Hypocapnia is a common finding in patients with sleep apnea and may be pathogenic.

Sudden exposure to high altitude can result in neurologic impairment. However, the central nervous system impairment seen in previously healthy mountaineers after exposure to extremely high altitudes has been demonstrated to be closely correlated with the degree of hypocapnia – not the level of hypoxia – attained (Hornbein *et al.*, 1989). The cause of acute central nervous system symptoms at high altitudes appears to be due to the alkalosis caused by increased minute ventilation (Laffey & Kavanagh, 2002).

Summary

CO_2 is a significant contributor to the global well being of the organism. It has specific effects on organs and tissues. Oxygenation and perfusion are markedly affected at the tissue–organ- and cellular level by the arterial CO_2 concentration, at least partially because it affects cardiac output. Hypocapnia-induced by hyperventilation is clinically used for treatment of increased intracranial pressure; however, the compromise in tissue perfusion, and thus the resulting secondary ischemia, caused by hypocapnia should be considered when using this treatment. Hypercapnia and hypercapnic acidosis, in contrast, appear to offer protection from ischemia–reperfusion injury. In conclusion, the value of active management of CO_2 to improve tissue-specific outcomes deserves increasing recognition.

References

Adrogue, H. & Madias, N. (1998). Management of life-threatening acid–base disorders. *New Engl. J. Med.*, **338**: 107–111.

Akça, O., Payne, R. & Schurr, A. (2003a) *Hypercapnia Induces Preconditioning against Hypoxic Damage in Rat Hippocampal Slices*. University of Louisville, Louisville, KY.

Akça, O., Doufas, A., Morioka, N., Iscoe, S., Fisher, J. & Sessler, D. (2002). Hypercapnia improves tissue oxygenation. *Anesthesiology*, **97**: 801–806.

Akça, O., Liem, E., Suleman, M.I., Doufas, A., Galandiuk, S. & Sessler, D. (2003). The effect of intraoperative end-tidal carbon dioxide partial pressure on tissue oxygenation. *Anaesthesia*, **58**: 536–542.

Akça, O., Melischek, M., Scheck, T., *et al.* (1999). Postoperative pain and subcutaneous oxygen tension. *Lancet*, **354**: 41–42.

Akça, O., Payne, R., Kehl, F., Sessler, D.I. & Schurr, A. (2003b). Hypercapnic acidosis preconditions brain slices to hypoxia. *American Society of Anesthesiologists Annual Meeting*. Lippincott Williams & Wilkins, San Francisco, CA; p. A-852.

Alberti, E., Hoyer, S., Hamer, J., Stoeckel, H., Paskschiess, P. & Weinhardt, F. (1975). The effect of carbon dioxide on cerebral blood flow and cerebral metabolism in dogs. *Br. J. Anaesth.*, **47**: 941–947.

Ali, S., Hahn, H., Jacobsohn, E., DeWet, C. & Avidan, M. (2003). Therapeutic effects of carbon dioxide administration following cardiac surgery. *American Society of Anesthesiologists (ASA) Annual Meeting*. Lippincott Williams & Wilkins, San Francisco, CA; p. A-431.

Amato, M., Barbas, C., Medeiros, D., *et al.* (1998). Effect of protective-ventilation strategy on mortality in the acute respiratory distress syndrome. *New Engl. J. Med.*, **338**: 347–354.

Arkilic C.F., Taguchi A., Sharma N., *et al.* (2003). Supplemental perioperative fluid administration increases tissue oxygen pressure. *Surgery*, **133**: 49–55.

Boix, J.H., Marin, J., Enrique, E., Monferrer, J., Bataller, A. & Servera, E. (1994). Modifications of tissular oxygenation and systemic hemodynamics after the correction of hypocapnia induced by mechanical ventilation. *Rev. Esp. Fisiol.*, **50**: 19–26.

Bullock, R., Chesnut, R., Clifton, G., *et al.* (2000). Initial management. *J. Neurotrauma*, **17**: 463–469.

Domino, K.B., Lu, Y., Eisenstein, B.L. & Hlastala, M.P. (1993). Hypocapnia worsens arterial blood oxygenation and increases VA/Q heterogeneity in canine pulmonary edema. *Anesthesiology*, **78**: 91–99.

Faraci, F. & Brian, J. (1994). Nitric oxide and the cerebral circulation. *Stroke*, **25**: 692–703.

Faraci, F., Breese, K. & Heistad, D. (1994). Cerebral vasodilation during hypercapnia. Role of glibenclamide-sensitive potassium channels and nitric oxide. *Stroke*, **25**: 1679–83.

Gleason, C., Short, B. & Jones, M.J. (1989). Cerebral blood flow and metabolism during and after prolonged hypocapnia in newborn lambs. *J. Pediatr.*, **115**: 309–314.

Gluck, S. (1998). Acid–base. *Lancet*, **352**: 474–479.

Greif, R., Akça, O., Horn, E., Kurz, A. & Sessler, D.I. (2000). Outcomes Research™ group: supplemental perioperative oxygen to reduce the incidence of surgical wound infection. *New Engl. J. Med.*, **342**: 161–167.

Guzman, J.A. & Kruse, J.A. (1999). Splanchnic hemodynamics and gut mucosal-arterial PCO(2) gradient during systemic hypocapnia. *J. Appl. Physiol.*, **87**: 1102–1106.

Hashimoto, K., Okazaki, K. & Okutsu, Y. (1990). The effect of hypocapnia and hypercapnia on myocardial oxygen tension in hemorrhaged dogs. *Masui*, **39**: 437–441.

Hickling, K. & Joyce, C. (1995). Permissive hypercapnia in ARDS and its effects on tissue oxygenation. *Acta Anaesthesiol. Scand.*, **107**: 201–208.

Hickling, K.G., Walsh, J., Henderson, S. & Jackson, R. (1994). Low mortality rate in adult respiratory distress syndrome using low-volume, pressure-limited ventilation with permissive hypercapnia: a prospective study. *Crit. Care Med.*, **22**: 1568–1578.

Holmes, J., Duffner, L. & Kappil, J. (1994). The effect of raised inspired carbon dioxide on developing rat retinal vasculature exposed to elevated oxygen. *Curr. Eye Res.*, **13**: 779–782.

Holmes, J., Zhang, S., Leske, D. & Lanier, W. (1997). The effect of carbon dioxiode on oxygen-induced retinopathy in the neonatal rat. *Curr. Eye Res.*, **16**: 725–732.

Holmes, J., Zhang, S., Leske, D. & Lanier, W. (1999). Metabolic acidosis-induced retinopathy in the neonatal art. *Invest. Ophthalmol. Vis. Sci.*, **40**: 804–809.

Hornbein, T., Townes, B., Schoene, R., Sutton, J. & Houston, C. (1989). The cost to the central nervous system of climbing to extremely high altitude. *New Engl. J. Med.*, **321**: 1714–1719.

Huizenga, J., Zink, B., Maio, R. & Hill, E. (2000). The penetrance of head injury management guidelines into the practice patterns of Michigan emergency physicians. *Acad. Emerg. Med.*, **7**: 1171.

Huttunen, J., Tolvanen, H., Heinonen, E., *et al.* (1999). Effects of voluntary hyperventilation on cortical sensory responses. Electroencephalographic and magnetoencephalographic studies. *Exp. Brain Res.*, **125**: 248–254.

Iadecola, C., Pellegrino, D., Moskowitz, M. & Lassen, N. (1994). Nitric oxide synthase inhibition and cerebrovascular regulation. *J. Cereb. Blood Flow Metab.*, **14**: 175–192.

Javaheri, S. (1999). A mechanism of central sleep apnea in patients with heart failure. *New Engl. J. Med.*, **341**: 949–954.

Jensen, J.A., Goodson, W.H., Hopf, H.W. & Hunt, T.K. (1991). Cigarette smoking decreases tissue oxygen. *Arch. Surg.*, **126**: 1131–1134.

Kitakaze, M., Weisfeldt, M. & Marban, E. (1988). Acidosis during early reperfusion prevents myocardial stunning in perfused ferret hearts. *J. Clin. Invest.*, **82**: 920–927.

Kontos, H. & Wei, E. (1996). Arginine analogues inhibit responses mediated by ATP-sensitive K channels. *Am. J. Physiol.*, **271**: H1498–H1506.

Kontos, H., Raper, A. & Patterson J. (1977). Analysis of vasoactivity of local pH, PCO_2, and bicarbonate on pial vessels. *Stroke*, **8**: 358–360.

Kurz, A., Sessler, D.I. & Lenhardt, R.A. (1996). Study of wound infections and temperature group: perioperative normothermia to reduce the incidence of surgical-wound infection and shorten hospitalization. *New Engl. J. Med.*, **334**: 1209–1215.

Laffey, J. & Kavanagh, B. (1999). Carbon dioxide and the critically ill- too little of a good thing? *Lancet*, **354**: 1283–1286.

Laffey, J. & Kavanagh, B. (2000). Biological effects of hypercapnia. *Intensive Care Med.*, **26**: 133–138.

Laffey, J. & Kavanagh, B. (2002). Hypocapnia. *New Engl. J. Med.*, **347**: 43–53.

Laffey, J.G., Engelberts, D. & Kavanagh, B.P. (2000a). Injurious effects of hypocapnic alkalosis in the isolated lung. *Am. J. Respir. Crit. Care Med.*, **62**: 399–405.

Laffey, J.G., Tanaka, M., Engelberts, D., *et al.* (2000b). Therapeutic hypercapnia reduces pulmonary and systemic injury following in vivo lung reperfusion. *Am. J. Respir. Crit. Care Med.*, **162**: 2287–2294.

Manley, G., Hemphill, J., Morabito, D., Derugin, N., Erickson, V., Pitts, L. & Knudson, M. (2000). Cerebral oxygenation during hemorrhagic shock: perils of hyperventilation and therapeutic potential of hypoventilation. *J. Trauma*, **48**: 1025–1033.

Marion, D. & Spiegel, T. (2000). Changes in the management of severe traumatic brain injury: 1991–1997. *Crit. Care Med.*, **28**: 16–18.

Mas, A., Saura, P., Joseph, D., Blanch, L., Baigorri, F., Artigas, A. & Fernandez, R. (2000). Effects of acute moderate changes in P_aCO_2 on global hemodynamics and gastric perfusion. *Crit. Care Med.*, **28**: 360–365.

Matsuda, N., Kuroda, H. & Mori, T. (1991). Beneficial actions of acidotic initial reperfusate in stunned myocardium of rat hearts. *Basic Res. Cardiol.*, **86**: 317–326.

Naughton, M., Benard, D., Rutherford, R. & Bradley, T. (1994). Effect of continuous positive airway pressure on central sleep apnea and nocturnal PCO_2 in heart failure. *Am. J. Respir. Crit. Care Med.*, **150**: 1598–1604.

Network ARDS. (2000). Ventilation with lower tidal volumes as compared with traditional tidal volumes for acute lung injury and the acute respiratory distress syndrome. *New Engl. J. Med.*, **342**: 1301–1308.

Nomura, F., Aoki, M., Forbess, J. & Mayer, J. (1994). Effects of hypercarbic acidotic reperfusion on recovery of myocardial function after cardioplegic ischemia in neonatal lambs. *Circulation*, **90**: 321–327.

Okazaki, K., Okutsu, Y. & Fukunaga, A. (1989). Effects of carbon dioxide (hypocapnia and hypercapnia) on tissue blood flow and oxygenation of liver, kidney and skeletal muscle in the dog. *Masui*, **38**: 457–464.

Richardson, D., Kontos, H., Raper, A. & Patterson, J.J. (1972). Systemic circulatory responses to hypocapnia in man. *Am. J. Physiol.*, **223**: 1308–1312.

Rosenblum, W., Kontos, H. & Wei, E. (2001). Evidence for a K_{ATP} ion channel link in the inhibition of hypercapnic dilation of pial artrioles by 7-nitroindazole and tetrodotoxin. *Eur. J. Pharmacol.*, **417**: 203–215.

Ruta, T.S., Drummond, J.C. & Cole, D.J. (1993). The effect of acute hypocapnia on local cerebral blood flow during middle cerebral artery occlusion in isoflurane anesthetized rats. *Anesthesiology*, **78**: 134–140.

Safar, P., Xiao, F., Radovsky, A., *et al.* (1996). Improved cerebral resuscitation from cardiac arrest in dogs with mild hypothermia plus blood flow promotion. *Stroke*, **27**: 105–113.

Schmetterer, L., Findl, O., Strenn, K., *et al.* (1997). Role of NO in the O_2 and CO_2 responsiveness of cerebral and ocular circulation in humans. *Am. J. Physiol.*, **273**: R2005–R2012.

Sheffield, C.W., Sessler, D.I., Hopf, H.W., Schroeder, M., Moayeri, A., Hunt, T.K. & West, J.M. (1997). Centrally and locally mediated thermoregulatory responses alter subcutaneous oxygen tension. *Wound Rep. Reg.*, **4**: 339–345.

Shibata, K., Cregg, N., Engelberts, D., Takeuchi, A., Fedorko, L. & Kavanagh, B. (1998). Hypercapnic acidosis may attenuate acute lung injury by inhibition of endogenous xanthine oxidase. *Am. J. Respir. Crit. Care Med.*, **158**: 1578–1584.

Sin, D., Fitzgerald, F., Parker, J., Newton, G., Floras, J. & Bradley, T. (1999). Risk factors for central and obstructive sleep apnea in 450 men and women with congestive heart failure. *Am. J. Respir. Crit. Care Med.*, **160**: 1101–1106.

Vannucci, R., Brucklacher, R. & Vannucci, S. (1997). Effect of carbon dioxide on cerebral metabolism during hypoxia–ischemia in the immature rat. *Pediatr. Res.*, **42**: 24–29.

Vannucci, R., Towfighi, J., Heitjan, D. & Brucklacher, R. (1995). Carbon dioxide protects the perinatal brain from hypoxic–ischemic damage: an experimental study in the immature rat. *Pediatrics*, **95**: 868–874.

Wang, Q., Pellegrino, D., Baughman, V., Koenig, H. & Albrecht, R. (1995). The role of neuronal nitric oxide synthase in regulation of cerebral blood flow in normocapnia and hypercapnia in rats. *J. Cereb. Blood Flow Metab.*, **15**: 774–778.

Weckesser, M., Posse, S., Olthoff, U., Kemna, L., Dager, S. & Muller-Gartner, H. (1999). Functional imaging of the visual cortex with bold-contrast MRI: hyperventilation decreases signal response. *Magn. Reson. Med.*, **41**: 213–216.

Wei, E. & Kontos, H. (1999). Blockage of ATP-sensitive potassium channels in cerebral arterioles inhibits vasoconstriction from hypocapnoic alkalosis in cats. *Stroke*, **30**: 851–854.

Xu, H., Cui, N., Yang, Z., *et al.* (2001). Direct activation of cloned K_{ATP} channels by intracellular acidosis. *J. Biol. Chem.*, **276**: 12898–12902.

PHYSIOLOGICAL PERSPECTIVES

PART 2

PHYSIOLOGICAL PERSPECTIVES: INTRODUCTION

27

M.B. Jaffe

Rather than repeat basic respiratory physiological concepts, we deemed it important to include several chapters that allowed the reader to delve into the important physiological concepts from a clinical perspective. Therefore, we have included chapters on carbon dioxide (CO_2) pathophysiology, acid–base balance and ventilation/perfusion ($\dot{V}/\dot{Q}$) abnormalities. The chapter titled "Carbon dioxide pathophysiology" (Chapter 28) provides a review of the pathophysiology of CO_2 production and transport. The chapter "acid–base balance" provides a clinically based review of CO_2 and arterial blood gas analysis. A clinical review titled "ventilation/perfusion abnormalities and capnography" is provided so that the reader can better interpret the absolute partial pressure of carbon dioxide at end-tidal ($P_{et}CO_2$), capnogram and arterial–end-tidal differences in view of the presence of $\dot{V}/\dot{Q}$ inequalities resulting from lung disease or hemodynamic factors.

The wealth of information available from the time and volumetric capnogram as described by the varied derived measures are summarized in a chapter titled "capnographic measures". The measures reviewed include the well-known and accepted physiological measures of deadspace and dead-space/tidal volume ratios and slope of phase III as well as more recent concepts such as alveolar ejection fraction. To help the reader better understand the physiological basis of the volumetric capnogram, we have included a chapter that helps the reader using a single-path (Weibel) trumpet-bell anatomical model to appreciate the effects of various anatomic, physical, and physiological parameters on the shape of the volumetric capnogram.

CARBON DIOXIDE PATHOPHYSIOLOGY 28

T.E. Morey

All mammals require transport of carbon dioxide (CO_2) from the intracellular sites of fuel oxidation to the lungs where elimination occurs. This chapter will discuss reduced and increased CO_2 pressures and outline some of the pathophysiology of CO_2 production and transport with special reference to capnography. Conditions that reduce partial pressure of CO_2 (PCO_2) at end-tidal ($P_{et}CO_2$) tension include deviations in CO_2 production in mitochondria and transport by blood that largely depends on functional carbonic anhydrase (CA). In contrast, causes of increased $P_{et}CO_2$ may encompass intravenous sodium bicarbonate administration and CO_2 embolus. In addition, special consideration is made for use of capnography when assessing patients for brain death using the apnea test wherein excessive CO_2 tensions are used to assess the viability of the brain.

Reduced CO_2 pressures

Mitochondrial disorders

Mitochondria serve as the exclusive site for oxidative phosphorylation, an intricate series of biochemical reactions leading to cellular respiration by producing energy laden molecules (i.e. adenosine triphosphate, ATP), water (H_2O), and CO_2 from oxidation of C–C bonds found in various fuel substrates (Nelson & Cox, 2000). Any disruption in normal mitochondrial function manifests as diminished energy reserves and CO_2 production and is most rapidly evident in organs with high-energy requirements such as the brain, heart, kidney, and especially, eye (Nelson & Cox, 2000). Mitochondrial disorders may be classified as inherited or acquired. Inheritance and familial pedigree can be particularly complicated to trace because, unlike other organelles, mitochondria carry a genome independent of nuclear DNA that may result in maternal transmittance of disease that does not fit into classic Mendelian autosomal or sex-linked inheritance patterns (Schon, 1994). Acquired mitochondrial disorders result from exposure of mitochondrial constituents to toxins. Both genetic and acquired mitochondrial disorders are presented herein with an emphasis on CO_2 production and capnography.

Inherited mitochondrial disorders

Inherited mitochondrial defects result from flaws in either mitochondrial (mtDNA) or nuclear DNA (nDNA) encoding for essential proteins needed to enable mitochondrial bioenergetics. This function of mitochondria depends not only on nDNA, but also on mtDNA that originates solely from ova mitochondria because spermatic mtDNA is quickly degraded following union of gametes (Schon, 1994). Each mitochondrion possesses several mtDNA copies that contain 16,569 nucleotide pairs encoding 37 genes. The remaining loci encoding DNA necessary for mitochondrial function are found in the nucleus. Unlike nDNA, mtDNA contains no introns, is rapidly transcribed, and has little ability to self-repair – all of which leads to a 1–2-fold magnitude increase in mutation rate (Poulton, 1997). These mutations cause inherited mitochondrial diseases (e.g. carnitine palmitoyltransferase II deficiency, Leber's optic neuropathy, Kearns–Sayre disease), which can be classified using three systems based on:

1. defects in substrate transport and utilization,
2. types of genetic mutation,
3. chief clinical complaints along with associated symptoms.

Of course, the usefulness of these schemas generally depends on the medical perspective of the respective practitioner (e.g. medical geneticist, neurologist). Overall, the minimum birth prevalence of these respiratory chain diseases is estimated to be approximately 1/7634 (Skladal *et al.*, 2003). In perspective to other myopathies, the annual incidences of Duchenne muscular dystrophy and malignant hyperthermia is approximately 1/3500 live male births and 1/62,000 (with administration of a potent inhalational anesthetic agent and succinylcholine) patients, respectively (Ording, 1985; Skladal *et al.*, 2003).

Although ventilation appears normal in resting patients suffering inherited mitochondrial disorders, provocative exercise stress unmasks differences in ventilatory patterns compared to age- and sex-matched control subjects. That is, although patients with mitochondrial disease appear to have markedly reduced ventilation at peak exercise ($V_{E\,max}$), this ventilatory rate is abnormally high for the actual amount of work being performed on a cycle ergometer as measured by $V_{E\,max}$ divided by the CO_2 output (V_{CO_2}). In one study, $V_{E\,max}$ was 71 ± 31 and 104 ± 23 l/min ($P < 0.001$) for diseased and control subjects, respectively, whereas peak $V_{E\,max}/V_{CO_2}$ was 55 ± 19 and 41 ± 6 ($P = 0.002$), respectively (Flaherty *et al.*, 2001). Notwithstanding this relative overventilation, the $P_{et}CO_2$ appears to be only modestly decreased. That is, the $P_{et}CO_2$ at maximal workloads for diseased and normal subjects was 33 ± 5 and 37 ± 3 mmHg (not significantly different), respectively (Dandurand *et al.*, 1995). Although the cause of this hyperventilatory response is not known, several hypotheses have been proffered for consideration. One suggestion revolves around a tenet that lactic acid is quickly buffered to CO_2 that would potentially increase the central respiratory drive. However, a recent, well-performed study found no differences in lactate clearance between diseased ($t_{1/2}$: 21.27 ± 6.05 min) and control ($t_{1/2}$: 23.50 ± 5.87 min) subjects (Dandurand *et al.*, 1995). An alternative hypothesis speculates that additional mechanoreceptor stimulation due to poor exercise mechanics secondary to mitochondrial myopathy of respiratory muscles may cause this hyperventilation. Indeed, a decrement in respiratory muscle function is evident in patients with mitochondrial disorders. For example, the maximal inspiratory mouth pressure was determined to be $64 \pm 29\%$ and $95 \pm 36\%$ predicted ($P = 0.06$) in diseased and normal patients, respectively, whereas the maximal transdiaphragmatic pressure was 61 ± 23 and 115 ± 31 cm H_2O ($P = 0.01$), respectively (Flaherty *et al.*, 2001). For whatever reason, hyperventilation is present during exercise testing of patients suffering mitochondrial disease and is also associated with a hyperdynamic circulatory state.

These abnormal changes in ventilation in response to exercise stress temptingly allude to the possibility that capnography could potentially contribute to the diagnostic testing of patients suspected to suffer mitochondrial disorders. Although pathological diagnosis of tissue (i.e. muscle biopsy with mitochondrial isolation) still endures as the gold standard, a great fraction of the global population has minimal-to-no access to clinical pathology services, especially in medically underserved, third world nations (Thomason, 1993; Taylor & Turnbull, 1997). As such, capnography may serve as a valuable addition to medical diagnostics either as a stand-alone, point-of-care assay or in combination with other testing such as O_2 consumption. However, some of the aforementioned changes in ventilation and circulation observed in patients with mitochondrial disease probably relate to the associated myopathic changes due to mitochondrial dysfunction. As such, other types of myopathies not due to mitochondrial disorders may cause similar ventilation changes in response to provocative exercise stress testing and will decrease the overall specificity and positive predictive value for this proposed type of testing.

Acquired mitochondrial disorder: cyanide

A number of mitochondrial toxins (e.g. mercury, 1-methyl-4-phenyl-1,2,3,6-tetrahydropyrimidine (MPTP), cyanide) can cause disruption of oxidative phosphorylation and cellular respiration (Sabri *et al.*, 2000). Some of these poisons are particularly useful during the conduct of medical research whereas others have little redeeming scientific value. Cyanide intoxication has inspired public fascination and has been well investigated to uncover its biochemical and physiological effects. In addition, this particular poison may be of interest to clinicians because of a perceived risk of intoxication due to the intravenous administration of sodium nitroprusside. For these reasons, the effects of cyanide on cellular respiration, CO_2 production, and transport will be more extensively presented.

Biochemistry

Cyanide is a small molecule (H—C≡N, molecular weight (MW) 26.02) that was first identified in 1782 and originates from many natural and artificial sources (Kerns *et al.*, 2002). Because of its compact, uncharged nature at physiological pH with consequent rapid egress across membranes, this poison is quickly fatal at relatively small concentrations (200 parts/million) if aerosolized across pulmonary membranes and rapidly lethal (~5 min) if orally ingested (200 mg). Although cyanide interferes with the activity of many enzymes, its inhibitory effect on mitochondrial energetics is most notable for disruption of the activity of cytochrome *c* and resultant abrupt cessation of cellular respiration (Kerns *et al.*, 2002). Cytochrome *c* is a large lipoprotein bound to mitochondrial inner membrane and is composed of 13 subunits that catalyze electron transfer in order to convert lactate and O_2 to water and CO_2 with resultant generation of energy as ATP (i.e. Kreb's cycle). One critical component of cytochrome *c* is the a_3 subunit that is the center wherein electrons and oxygen (O_2) combine. Because cyanide possesses a stronger affinity for the ferric acid (Fe^{3+}) moiety of the a_3 component of cytochrome *c* than does

O_2, this poison does not yield its position to O_2 and, therefore, uncouples oxidative phosphorylation. Consequently, although glycolysis (i.e. anaerobic metabolism) might proceed, aerobic metabolism is halted. Paradoxically, cells suffer asphyxia even in the presence of normal O_2 pressures. As Kreb's cycle slows or stops, minimal or no CO_2 is produced while O_2 consumption is expected to be reduced. As expected, in canine models of sublethal cyanide intoxication, O_2 consumption significantly decreased from 133 ± 19 to 69 ± 21 ml/min, CO_2 production decreased from 128 ± 27 to 103 ± 22 ml/min, and mixed venous lactate concentrations increased from 2.3 ± 0.5 to 7.1 ± 0.7 mM (Breen *et al.*, 1995; 1996).

Sources

Cyanide can be derived from several sources including dietary intake of cyanogens, malicious administration, and iatrogenic production due to administration of sodium nitroprusside.

Cassava

Cyanide intoxication may occur from dietary intake of cassava (*Monihot esculanta*). This tropical root is grown within 30° latitude north or south around the equator and meets the essential carbohydrate demands of approximately a half billion citizens of underdeveloped nations due to its high starch content and hardy nature (Kamalu, 1995; Ravi *et al.*, 1996). For these reasons, the crop is now in global production and is also called manioc, tapioca, mandioca, and yucca. The uncooked plant possesses inherent cyanide glucosides that may be eaten or contaminate subsequent processed foodstuffs such as cassava flour, farofa, used to produce bakery goods (Padmaja, 1995). The cyanide glucosides are converted to active hydrogen cyanide by linamarase that is native to cassava. Two resultant diseases associated with acute and chronic cyanide exposure due to cassava ingestion are *konzo* and tropical ataxic neuropathy, respectively. *Konzo* means "tired legs" in Zairean and is an uncharacterized upper motor neuron disease noted for rapidly developing leg paralysis following large ingestions of cassava (Sreeja *et al.*, 2003). Schoolchildren in Mozambique with *konzo* demonstrate elevated concentrations (225–384 μmol/l) of thiocyanate in urine (Ernesto *et al.*, 2002). Tropical ataxic neuropathy is typified for paresthesias, ataxia, visual changes, and others signs and typically follows a chronic diet of cassava-based foods due to failure of other crops (Oluwole *et al.*, 2000). Other foods potentially laden with cyanogens include almonds, cherry leaves, apricot pits, and other plants (Kerns *et al.*, 2002).

Malicious intent

Cyanide's notoriety as a poison in popular culture stems from its criminal use as an agent of suicide and homicide. For example, 913 members of the People's Temple ministered by James Jones allegedly committed coerced suicide in 1978 at Jonestown, Guyana by ingesting a punch contaminated with cyanide (Lasaga, 1980). Similarly, laboratory scientists and technicians with ready access to chemicals have employed cyanide salts to achieve rapid suicide (Mueller & Borland, 1997). Use of cyanide to achieve homicidal objectives has occurred on both small and large scales. That is, several cases of contaminated pharmaceuticals (e.g. acetaminophen) were reported in recent times (Dershewitz & Levin, 1984). Of greater magnitude, cyanide gas has been repeatedly deployed in military campaigns since the Napoleonic wars to dispatch large formations of enemy soldiers (Kerns *et al.*, 2002). Due to these and other events, cyanide is a chemical well known to the lay public as a potent toxin.

Sodium nitroprusside

Of particular concern to medical professionals, is the potential for iatrogenic cyanide intoxication following the intravenous administration of sodium nitroprusside. This pharmacological agent is administered intravenously, acts to reduce peripheral blood pressure by causing vascular dilation, and structurally is composed of an iron molecule surrounded by a halo of one nitric oxide (NO) and five cyanide moieties. The mechanism whereby blood pressure decreases is due to release of NO from the drug *via* an enzymatic mechanism that also liberates cyanide molecules. Typically, cyanide is rapidly metabolized by rhodanase to an innocuous product, thiocyante. However, several conditions (e.g. large or sustained sodium nitroprusside doses, thiosulfate deficiency, renal failure) may lead to accumulation of cyanide with resultant systemic toxicity.

The few investigators undertaking to determine the effects of sodium nitroprusside on CO_2 production and elimination have published variable findings both between and within human studies (Figure 28.1). One group of 26 patients undergoing major otolaryngological surgery and concurrently induced hypotension caused by sodium nitroprusside experienced no change in arterial PCO_2 (P_aCO_2) (Wildsmith *et al.*, 1975). In this study of anesthetized, ventilated patients, the P_aCO_2 was determined to be 38 ± 4 and 38 ± 3 mmHg before and after infusion of sodium nitroprusside, respectively. In a separate investigation of anesthetized adults undergoing middle-ear surgery with controlled hypotension achieved by sodium nitroprusside infusion, $P_{et}CO_2$ decreased 17%

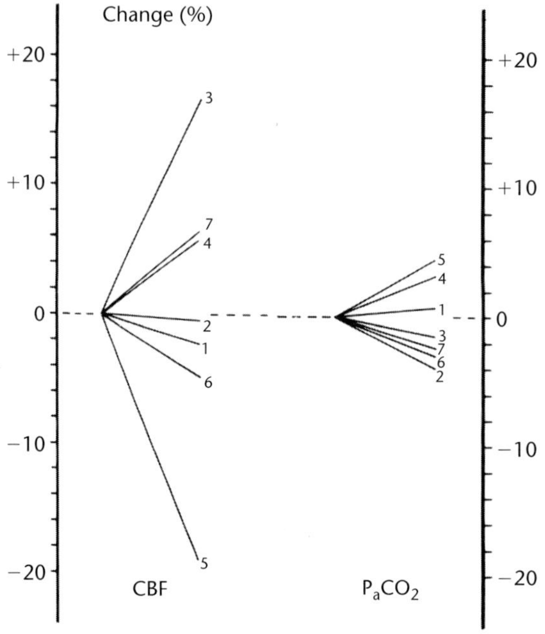

Figure 28.1 The effect of sodium nitroprusside infused intra-arterially in seven awake patients in a dose at the threshold for affecting mean arterial pressure or heart rate. CBF: cerebral blood flow. (Reproduced with permission from Henriksen, L., Paulson, O.B. & Lauritzen, M. (1982). The effects of sodium nitroprusside on cerebral blood flow and cerebral venous blood gases. I. Observations in awake man during and following moderate blood pressure reduction. *Eur. J. Clin. Invest.*, **12**: 383–387.)

whereas P_aCO_2 fell approximately 7% during controlled hypotension to achieve a mean arterial blood pressure of 60 ± 5 mmHg (Ali *et al.*, 2002). The authors noted that decreases in $P_{et}CO_2$ overestimate reductions in P_aCO_2. This significant discrepancy between P_aCO_2 and $P_{et}CO_2$ likely resulted from a large (41.7%) increase in physiological dead space to tidal volume ratio. Different investigators measured changes in P_aCO_2 in awake, spontaneously breathing human subjects subjected to graded reductions in blood pressure caused by intravenous sodium nitroprusside (Henriksen *et al.*, 1982). They determined that P_aCO_2 significantly fell in a dose-dependent manner with mean values of 4.96, 4.81, 4.78, 4.62, and 4.54 kPa during graduated infusions of sodium nitroprusside to achieve 0, 10, 20, 30, and 40% reductions in mean arterial pressure, respectively. (*Note*: The chapter author has not modified the units as originally published by the various journals in order to preserve the integrity of the references. For the readers' benefit, however, the conversion factors for units of pressure are as follows: 1 mmHg = 0.133 kPa or 1 kPa = 7.519 mmHg; 1 cmH_2O = 0.098 kPa or 1 kPa = 10.204 cmH_2O; 1 mmHg = 1.357 cmH_2O or 1 cmH_2O = 0.737 mmHg.) The investigators, however, attributed this change to hyperventilation in subjects, vis-à-vis cyanide toxicity, although no measurement of pulmonary parameters (e.g. respiratory rate, tidal volume) was noted. In the author's view, sodium nitroprusside likely decreases CO_2 production to some extent, but rarely causes notable decrements in cellular respiration at doses of the drug used in clinical medicine.

CA disorders

CA comprises a family name for a group of zinc-dependent enzymes that catalyze the reaction of bicarbonate and a proton to form water and CO_2 (Tripp *et al.*, 2001). The fact that these enzymes originated in deep antiquity (i.e. 3 billion years ago), are ubiquitous, and demonstrate evolutionary convergence between plants and animals attests to their fundamental importance to regulate CO_2 elimination in living organisms (Smith *et al.*, 1999; Tripp *et al.*, 2001; Potter & Harris, 2003). The chemical reaction process occurs in two phases with the first step (Equation (28.1)) occurring instantaneously and the second step (Equation (28.2)) facilitated by CA:

$$CA \cdot Zn - OH^- + H^+ \leftrightarrow CA \cdot Zn - H_2O \quad (28.1)$$

$$HCO_3^- + CA \cdot Zn - H_2O \leftrightarrow H_2O + CO_2 + CA \cdot Zn - OH \quad (28.2)$$

Only diffusion of H^+ away from the active site limits the reaction rate that has an associated Michaelis–Menten k_{cat} value $\sim 8 \times 10^5 s^{-1}$ (Baird *et al.*, 1997; Tripp *et al.*, 2001). Conventionally, the perennial summary equation (28.3) remains more familiar to readers of clinical literature, but does not emphasize the need for CA or the absolute requirement for zinc at this enzyme's active site:

$$HCO_3^- + H^+ \xleftrightarrow{CA} H_2O + CO_2 \quad (28.3)$$

From the CA family found in mammals (i.e., α-class vis-à-vis the vegetative β-class), the cytosolic CA II subtype has inspired and received more study than the others found in cytosol (CA I, III, VII), membranes (CA IV, IX, XII, XIV), mitochondria (CA V), or secreted (CA VI) (Potter & Harris, 2003). Both mutation- and drug-induced inhibition of CA II may lead to changes in CO_2 metabolism and elimination.

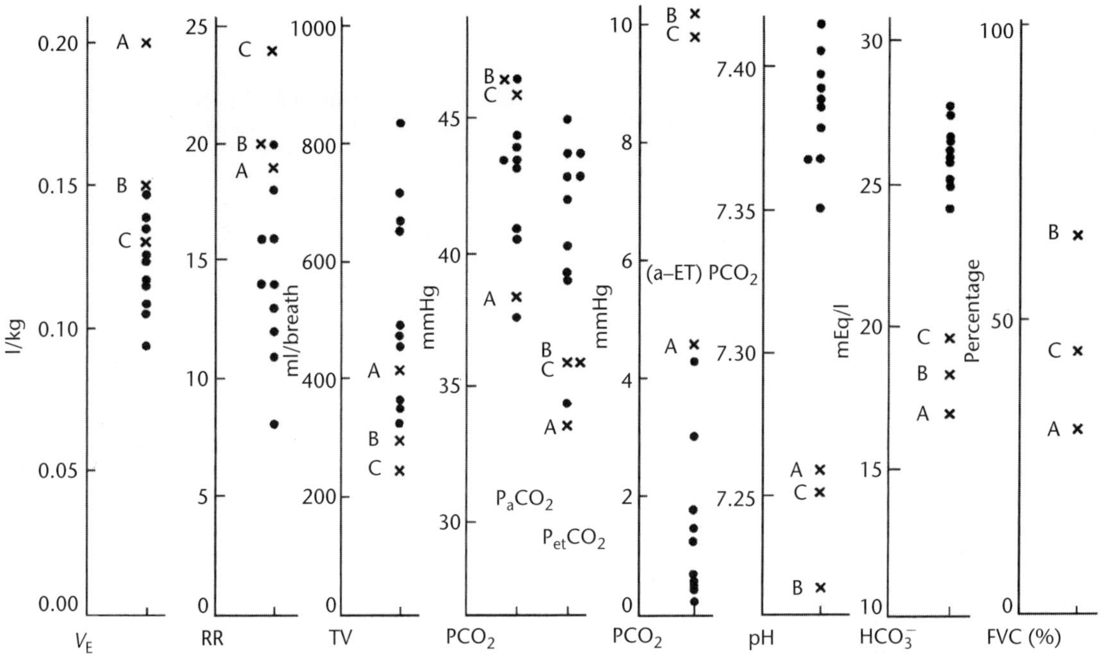

Figure 28.2 Respiratory function parameters in three patients (A, B, and C; noted as ×) with a deficiency of CA II versus 10 healthy volunteers (closed circles). V_E: minute ventilation volume per body weight (l/kg); $P_{et}CO_2$: PCO_2 in end-expiratory gas; pH, P_aCO_2, and HCO_3^- were shown as the values in arterial blood; RR: respiratory rate; TV: tidal volume; FVC: functional vital capacity. (Reproduced with permission from Taki, K., Kato, H. & Yoshida, I. (1999). Elimination of CO_2 in patients with carbonic anhydrase II deficiency, with studies of respiratory function at rest. *Respir. Med.*, **93**: 536–539.)

Inherited CA disorders

CA II disorders encompass a set of autosomal recessive enzymatic diseases caused by point mutations of the DNA sequence (e.g. TAT → TAG) encoding CA or by splice junction mutations (Soda *et al.*, 1995). This rare disease has been reported in several widely dispersed populations of Mediterranean, Arab, and Japanese descent (Sly *et al.*, 1985; Fathallah *et al.*, 1994; Soda *et al.*, 1995). The hallmarks of disease revolve around a clinical triad of renal tubular acidosis, osteoporosis, and cerebral calcification leading to mental retardation (Cumming & Ohlsson, 1985; Whyte, 1993). As expected, this inherited disorder also modifies CO_2 elimination and alveolar CO_2 concentrations. In Japanese patients suffering CA II due to *de nova* mutation or consanguineous parents, $P_{et}CO_2$ was reduced to 35.2 ± 1.3 mmHg compared to a value of 41.2 ± 2.9 mmHg measured in a human cohort (Taki *et al.*, 1999). In addition, P_aCO_2 approached the upper limits of normal values in CA II subjects. Taken together, these two observations yielded increased (a–ET) PCO_2 (difference between P_aCO_2 and $P_{et}CO_2$) of 8.3 ± 3.1 mmHg compared to control values of 1.3 ± 1.3 mmHg (Figure 28.2). Similarly, data from CA II-deficient mice confirmed by western blot analysis also showed elevated P_aCO_2 pressures of 47.4 ± 5.3 mmHg in homozygous recessive animals whereas the wild-type value was 38.1 ± 3.4 mmHg (Lien & Lai, 1998). Furthermore, a sodium bicarbonate challenge (4 mmol/kg) to the mice resulted in an even greater disparity in P_aCO_2 tensions and illustrates the importance of CA II in CO_2 elimination. Unfortunately, $P_{et}CO_2$ was not measured although the animals were anesthetized. Measurement of this parameter is precluded by the fact that currently available capnography technology of either main- or side-stream configuration cannot accommodate extremely rapid respiratory rates (e.g. 160 breaths/min) typical of small rodents, especially when combined with diminutively small tidal volumes (e.g. 0.2 ml/breath). (Similarly, conventional pulse oximetry does not function for small rodents due to extremely high heart rates (e.g. 500 beats/min). Presumably, this problem has little hope of solution in the near future given the relatively small market of animal research when contrasted to that for clinic medicine.) Nevertheless, these studies suggest that P_aCO_2 rises in patients suffering this disease, but cannot be overcome by hyperventilation. The contribution of other types of cytosolic CA (e.g. CA I, III, and VII) to CO_2 transfer in the blood and elimination in the lungs likely mitigates the

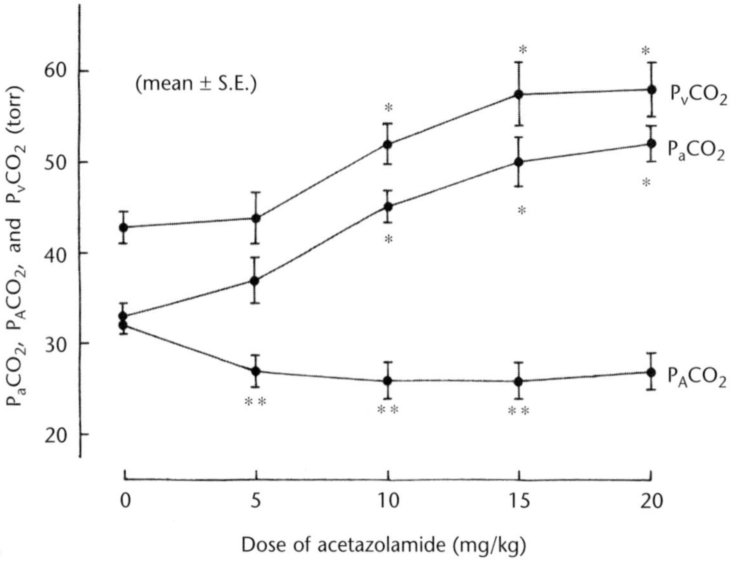

Figure 28.3 The relationship between the dose of acetazolamide and P_aCO_2, P_vCO_2, or P_ACO_2. The P_aCO_2 linearly rises in response to inhibition rate of the red cell CA (RCA) activity and P_vCO_2 rises in parallel with the changes of P_aCO_2. However, P_ACO_2 slightly falls by 16% after administration of 5 mg/kg of acetazolamide and does not change upon further injections of acetazolamide. * shows $P < 0.01$ between control and each value after injection of acetazolamide and ** shows $P < 0.05$. (Reproduced with permission from Taki, K., Mizuno, K., Takahashi, N. & Wakusawa, R. (1986). Disturbance of CO_2 elimination in the lungs by carbonic anhydrase inhibition. *Jpn. J. Physiol.*, **36**: 523–532.)

effects of mutant CA II and allows patients to maintain homeostasis, albeit at abnormal values.

Acquired CA disorders: acetazolamide

A sulfanilamide derivative, acetazolamide remains in widespread clinical use in the treatment of open angle glaucoma recalcitrant to other pharmacological therapies, acute closed angle glaucoma immediately prior to surgical intervention, and chronic obstructive lung disease with hypoventilation. Similar to those changes observed with inherited CA diseases, acetazolamide therapy also increases the difference between P_aCO_2 and alveolar CO_2 as shown in Figure 28.3. This finding has been noted in a number of species including rabbit, cat, and dog. (*Note*: No small rodent species were used, because capnographic investigations are not possible in many small animal models of disease (e.g. Lesh-Nyhan syndrome, muscular dystrophy, phenylketonuria) including transgenic "knock out" mice previously subjected to site directed deletion of DNA sequences (Roemer *et al.*, 1991.) For example, the gap between P_aCO_2 and $P_{et}CO_2$ was less than 0.5 kPa, but rapidly widened to 4.9 kPa following treatment with acetazolamide in rabbits (Lee, 1994). In cats, this difference also increased, but only with intravenous doses of acetazolamide greater than 4 mg/kg of body mass (Wagenaar *et al.*, 1996). Similarly, the P_aCO_2 and $P_{et}CO_2$ measured in anesthetized dog markedly grew from 0.6 ± 1.0 to 21.9 ± 1.0 mmHg after CA inhibition (Taki *et al.*, 1993). This effect was observed to be dose-dependent with additional drug not causing substantial changes in alveolar CO_2 tensions (Taki *et al.*, 1986). The location of this "surplus" CO_2 seems to be in tissue. In the presence of significant CA inhibition caused by acetazolamide, tissue PCO_2 was consistently underestimated by venous PCO_2 (Cardenas *et al.*, 1998). Finally, these changes also occur in spontaneously breathing humans receiving the drug for chronic obstructive pulmonary disease (Krintel *et al.*, 1983). Based on these studies describing acute use of acetazolamide, anesthesiologists should warily consider the actual relationship between $P_{et}CO_2$ and P_aCO_2 in anesthetized, ventilated patients using this drug.

Increased CO_2 pressures

Bicarbonate infusion

Sodium bicarbonate is sometimes intravenously injected to improve acidemia in patients suffering from metabolic acidosis. This buffer rapidly consumes hydrogen ion according to the reaction noted in Equation (28.3) catalyzed very rapidly by CA. If excess H^+ is present, then the quantity of HCO_3^- (i.e. amount of sodium bicarbonate) becomes the limiting factor for CO_2 production. That is, for each HCO_3^- molecule administered, a molecule of CO_2 will be produced. Given that a single adult sized, syringe of factory-packaged sodium bicarbonate contains 50 meq of the drug with only a single negative charge, then the mass of bicarbonate may also be expressed as 50 mmol. Avogadro's law stipulates that the volume (V) of a gas is directly proportional to the moles (n) of the gas (i.e. $V \propto n$) for a fixed temperature and pressure (Silberberg, 1996). Using this law, the volume of CO_2 produced by a single syringe of sodium

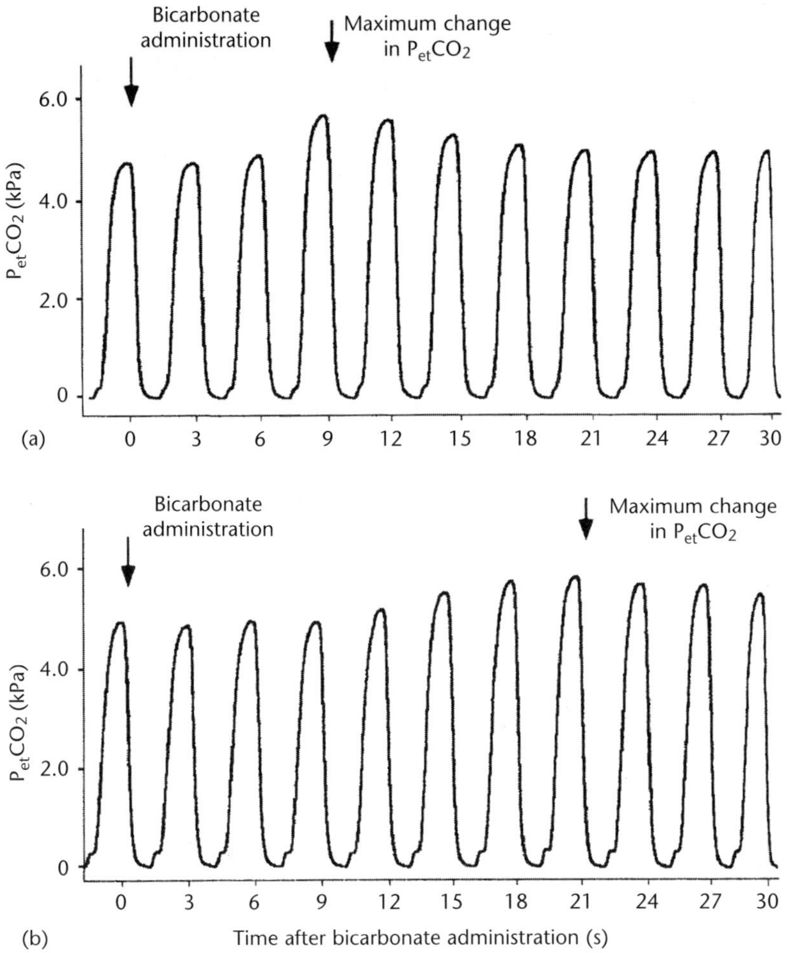

Figure 28.4 Recordings of $P_{et}CO_2$ following an intravenous administration of sodium bicarbonate (0.2 mmol/kg) at a control state ((a) cardiac output = 1.85 l/min) and at a state of decreased cardiac output ((b) cardiac output = 0.83 l/min) in anesthetized, mechanically ventilated dog. When cardiac output decreased, time-max (time for a maximal increase in $P_{et}CO_2$) was prolonged from 3 to 7 breaths-time, with no change in ΔCO_2-max (maximal increases in CO_2) (1 mmHg = 0.133 kPa). (Reproduced with permission from Okamoto, H., Hoka, S., Kawasaki, T., Okuyama, T. & Takahashi, S. (1995). Changes in end-tidal carbon dioxide tension following sodium bicarbonate administration: correlation with cardiac output and haemoglobin concentration. *Acta Anaesthesiol. Scand.*, **39**: 79–84.)

bicarbonate can be calculated as follows:

$$V_{50} = V_{1000} \times \frac{n_{50}}{n_{1000}}, \qquad (28.4)$$

where V_{50} and V_{1000} is the volumes of gas for 50 and 1000 mmol of CO_2, respectively, whereas n_{50} and n_{1000} is the molar masses of 50 and 1000 mmol of CO_2, respectively. Considering gas behavior at standard conditions of temperature (0°C, 273 K) and pressure (760 torr, 1 atmosphere), the standard molar volume of any gas, including CO_2, is always 22.414 l. That is, 1000 mmol (n_{1000}) of CO_2 occupies 22.414 l (V_{1000}) (Silberberg, 1996). Substitution of values yields a calculated volume of 1.121 l of CO_2 for each syringe of bicarbonate injected. However, Spear and colleagues determined that only 80% of expected CO_2 could be recovered from the breath of humans receiving [^{13}C] bicarbonate infusions (Spear *et al.*, 1995). The location of the residual 20% CO_2 remains poorly understood, but may enter metabolic pools or bone of finite capacity as prolonged radiolabeled bicarbonate infusion eventually yields 100% CO_2 recovery. Nevertheless, given this large volume of CO_2 production catalyzed by an extremely rapid, enzyme facilitated reaction, one would expect to observe changes in $P_{et}CO_2$ following injection of sodium bicarbonate.

Although many clinicians have probably noted a $P_{et}CO_2$ increase following sodium bicarbonate injection, Okamoto and colleagues scientifically investigated this phenomenon in a canine model as illustrated in Figure 28.4 (Okamoto *et al.*, 1995). In control dogs, they determined that the time for a maximal increase in $P_{et}CO_2$ was 4 ± 0.3 breaths and that maximal increase in $P_{et}CO_2$ was 6.4 ± 0.5 mmHg (0.85 ± 0.006 kPa). However, the time for maximal increase was inversely dependent on cardiac output (Figure 28.5). That is, the latency to maximal increases in $P_{et}CO_2$ was reduced by increased cardiac output. Furthermore, the maximal increase in $P_{et}CO_2$ was directly correlated to the hemoglobin concentration (Figure 28.6). Probably,

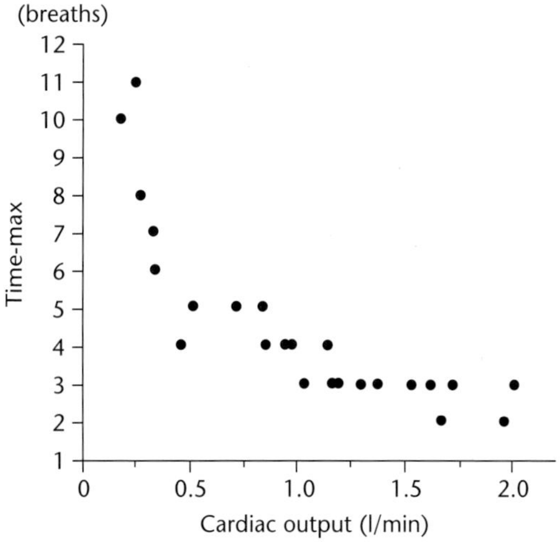

Figure 28.5 Relationship between cardiac output and time-max in anesthetized, mechanically ventilated dog. Cardiac output showed a strong inverse correlation with time-max (time for a maximal increase in $P_{et}CO_2$) ($y = 1.58/x + 1.96$, $r = 0.94$, $P < 0.0001$). (Reproduced with permission from Okamoto, H., Hoka, S., Kawasaki, T., Okuyama, T. & Takahashi, S. (1995). Changes in end-tidal carbon dioxide tension following sodium bicarbonate administration: correlation with cardiac output and haemoglobin concentration. *Acta Anaesthesiol. Scand.*, **39**: 79–84.)

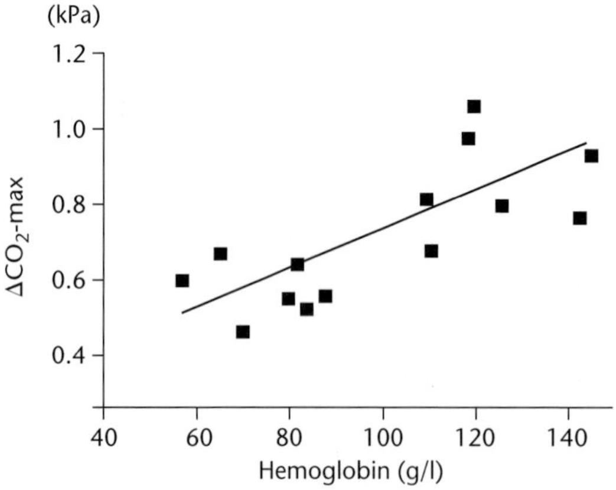

Figure 28.6 Relationship between hemoglobin concentration and ΔCO_2-max (maximal increases in CO_2) in anesthetized, mechanically ventilated dog. A linear correlation was observed. ($y = 0.38x + 1.75$, $r = -0.736$, $P < 0.005$) (1 mmHg = 0.133 kPa). (Reproduced with permission from Okamoto, H., Hoka, S., Kawasaki, T., Okuyama, T. & Takahashi, S. (1995). Changes in end-tidal carbon dioxide tension following sodium bicarbonate administration: correlation with cardiac output and haemoglobin concentration. *Acta Anaesthesiol. Scand.*, **39**: 79–84.)

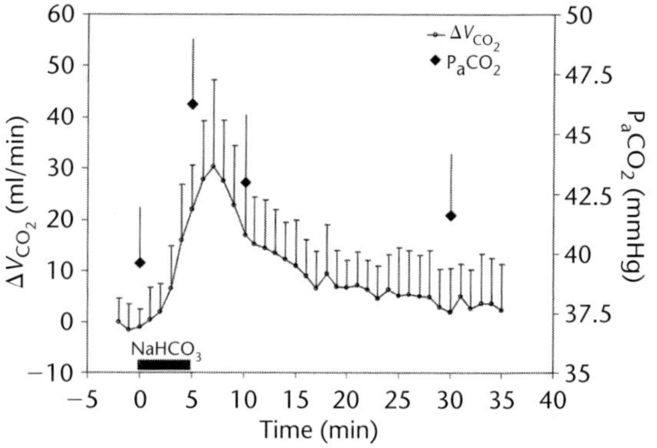

Figure 28.7 Time-course of the changes in V_{CO_2} (ΔV_{CO_2}) and P_aCO_2 in 16 artificially ventilated critically ill patients during and after the infusion of 1.5 mmol/kg sodium bicarbonate over 5 min. (Reproduced with permission from Levraut, J., Garcia, P., Giunti, C., Ichai, C., Bouregba, M., Ciebiera, J.P., Payan, P. & Grimaud, D. (2000). The increase in CO_2 production induced by $NaHCO_3$ depends on blood albumin and hemoglobin concentrations. *Intens. Care Med.*, **26**: 558–564.)

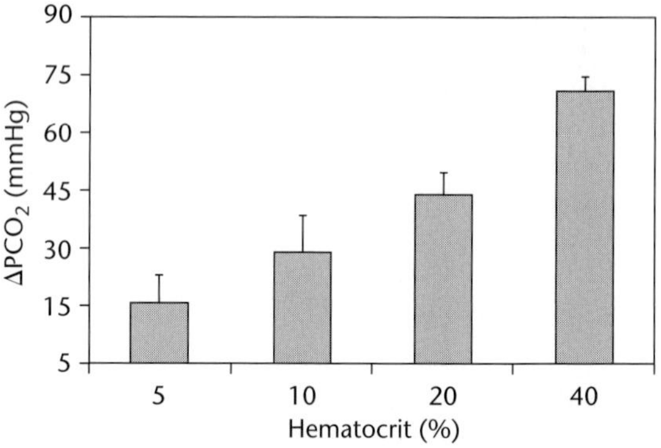

Figure 28.8 Effect of a 25 mM sodium bicarbonate load on the change in PCO_2 (ΔPCO_2) of acidotic regenerated human blood according to the hematocrit level ($n = 5$ for each hematocrit). (Reproduced with permission from Levraut, J., Garcia, P., Giunti, C., Ichai, C., Bouregba, M., Ciebiera, J.P., Payan, P. & Grimaud, D. (2000). The increase in CO_2 production induced by $NaHCO_3$ depends on blood albumin and hemoglobin concentrations. *Intens. Care Med.*, **26**: 558–564.)

this observation may be explained by the absence of CA in plasma, but a rich presence in erythrocytes. Similar data in humans note that CO_2 production is dependent on both hemoglobin and albumin concentrations where the albumin serves as a depot for non-bicarbonate buffers in need of titration as shown in Figures 28.7 and 28.8 (Levraut *et al.*, 2000).

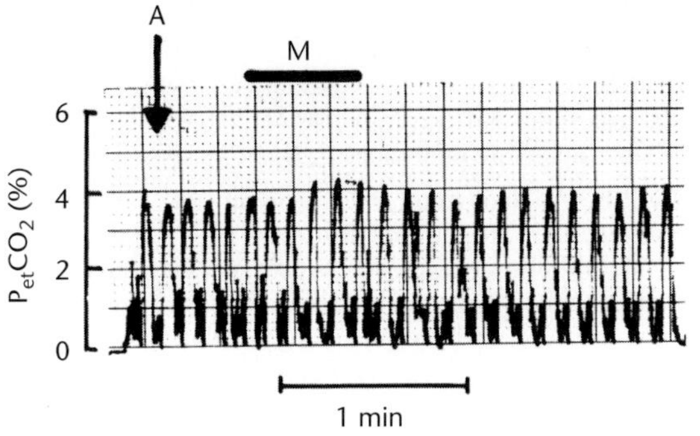

Figure 28.9 Increase in $P_{et}CO_2$ in a woman undergoing laparoscopy and suffering a venous embolism of CO_2. Insufflation of CO_2 started at A. A murmur was heard and insufflation discontinued at M. (Reproduced with permission from Shulman, D. & Aronson, H.B. (1984). Capnography in the early diagnosis of carbon dioxide embolism during laparoscopy. *Can. Anaesth. Soc. J.*, **31**: 455–459.)

CO_2 embolism

CO_2 is commonly used for insufflation of the abdomen during laparoscopy because this gas has a number of favorable characteristics including cost, availability, failure to support combustion, high blood solubility, and others. However, extremely great CO_2 tensions can occur during laparoscopy such that CO_2 is no longer completely solubilized in blood. That is, embolism of CO_2 occurring during laparoscopy can cause cardiovascular collapse and death (Nishiyama & Hanaoka, 1999; Imasogie *et al.*, 2002). It is unclear what changes in $P_{et}CO_2$ to anticipate during a CO_2 embolus. Theoretically, one would expect a rise in $P_{et}CO_2$ until a sufficient volume of CO_2 was embolized to cause right ventricular outflow tract obstruction with subsequent falls in $P_{et}CO_2$ similar to that caused by air embolus. In fact, Shulman and Aronson noted an abrupt rise in $P_{et}CO_2$ from 3.8% to 4.2% in women undergoing laparoscopy as shown in Figure 28.9 (Shulman & Aronson, 1984). Subsequently, the $P_{et}CO_2$ fell to 4.0% over the course of 30 s upon which CO_2 insufflation was terminated after diagnosis of CO_2 embolism. In a second case, Diakun also noted a rise in $P_{et}CO_2$ from 31 to 38 mmHg in a patient undergoing laparoscopy and suffering CO_2 embolism (Diakun, 1991). In most case reports a marked reduction in $P_{et}CO_2$ is first noted and no transient increase in $P_{et}CO_2$ is reported (Beck & McQuillan, 1994; Imasogie *et al.*, 2002). Likely, any increase in $P_{et}CO_2$ is so fleeting and small as to be imperceptible to all but the most fortunate and vigilant anesthesiologist. In addition, one might speculate that an increase or decrease in $P_{et}CO_2$ depends on the rate at which CO_2 is introduced into the venous intravascular space. That is, a rapid injection of CO_2 could cause an abrupt decrease in $P_{et}CO_2$ whereas a small, continuous infusion of CO_2 might lead to transient increases in $P_{et}CO_2$. However, a porcine model in which CO_2 was intravenously injected at rates as low as 0.01 ml/kg/min noted no significant increase in $P_{et}CO_2$ whereas the next higher infusion rate (0.05 ml/kg/min) caused a reduction in $P_{et}CO_2$ from 29 ± 8 to 26 ± 6 mmHg (Couture *et al.*, 1994). In addition, the authors observed that $P_{et}CO_2$ achieved a nadir value at 40 ± 15 s after injection of CO_2 (0.5 ml/kg/min). So, the effects of CO_2 embolus on $P_{et}CO_2$ probably more closely resemble those caused by other embolic material (e.g. air, clot) in clinical practice although a momentary window of time on the order of a few seconds may exist in which increased $P_{et}CO_2$ could be observed by Herculean vigilance.

Apnea testing for brain death

One diagnostic use of increased CO_2 pressures is to establish brain death. The basic principal of this provocative examination is to test the ventilatory response of the respiratory centers of the medulla oblongata to increased pressures of CO_2. If a patient suffering cerebral trauma exerts some respiratory effort with sufficiently increased CO_2 pressures, then the patient is diagnosed with brain injury, but not brain death. Conversely, if no respiratory effort is observed, then brain death is established with subsequent withdrawal of supportive care or consideration of the living remains for organ donation by transplantation professionals in consultation with family members of the patient.

The test is performed a number of ways in various hospitals, but some guidelines stipulate a minimal duration of 10 min of apnea with a P_aCO_2 value in excess of 60 mmHg (Benzel *et al.*, 1992; Dominguez-Roldan *et al.*, 1999). In order to maintain clinically acceptable O_2 tensions in the blood over the duration of 10 min, the patient undergoes preoxygenation so that while experiencing the test apneic oxygenation allows for O_2 delivery to the body. Ventilation is not performed for these patients, as CO_2 elimination is not consistent with performance of the apnea test.

Notwithstanding the years of clinical use for the apnea test, some fundamental problems associated with the examination endure. For example, the rate of rise of CO_2 varies dramatically in patients with various injuries and depends on a number of factors including body temperature, a nonlinear rise in CO_2 pressures dependent on pre-existing P_aCO_2 values, and other factors (Dominguez-Roldan *et al.*, 1999). In addition, this test can be associated with organ damage, such as occurrence of hypoxia, hypotension, and arrhythmias that may damage the patient or potentially life-saving organs for transplantation (al Jumah *et al.*, 1992; Melano *et al.*, 2002). In some patients, a sufficient CO_2 concentration cannot be achieved before complications ensue (Rudolf *et al.*, 1998). For these reasons, several authors have advocated an alternative test to the apnea examination (Melano *et al.*, 2002). In this type of examination, CO_2 is added directly into the inspiratory limb of the airway circuit without any change in ventilatory parameters until the P_aCO_2 exceeds 60 mmHg. The benefits of this type of augmentation are that increases in CO_2 tensions are more easily controlled both in terms of time and overall magnitude and complications due to hypoxia are obviated. Because the patient's lungs remain ventilated, this modified test does not preclude capnography or capnometry. In my opinion, measurement of $P_{et}CO_2$ would be a valuable addition to this test. Capnography allows continuous measurement of CO_2 in contrast to spot tests of arterial blood gas samples. As such, capnography would enable more precise and rapid control of CO_2 flow into the airway circuit and provide mutually independent, corroborative evidence for P_aCO_2 measurement. Given the relative availability of capnography and the gravity of the decision to be considered by physicians and family members, it seems reasonable to add capnometry to the test and thus obtain greater control, flexibility, and quality assurance.

References

al Jumah, M., McLean, D.R., al Rajeh, S. & Crow N. (1992). Bulk diffusion apnea test in the diagnosis of brain death. *Crit. Care Med.*, **20**: 1564–1567.

Ali, S.S., Dubikaitis, A. & al Qattan, A.R. (2002). The relationship between end tidal carbon dioxide and arterial carbon dioxide during controlled hypotensive anaesthesia. *Med. Princ. Pract.*, **11**: 35–37.

Baird, T.T., Waheed, A., Okuyama, T., Sly, W.S. & Fierke, C.A. (1997). Catalysis and inhibition of human carbonic anhydrase IV. *Biochemistry*, **36**: 2669–2678.

Beck, D.H. & McQuillan, P.J. (1994). Fatal carbon dioxide embolism and severe haemorrhage during laparoscopic salpingectomy. *Br. J. Anaesth.*, **72**: 243–245.

Benzel, E.C., Mashburn, J.P., Conrad, S. & Modling, D. (1992). Apnea testing for the determination of brain death: a modified protocol. Technical note. *J. Neurosurg.*, **76**: 1029–1031.

Breen, P.H., Isserles, S.A., Westley, J., Roizen, M.F. & Taitelman, U.Z. (1995). Effect of oxygen and sodium thiosulfate during combined carbon monoxide and cyanide poisoning. *Toxicol. Appl. Pharmacol.*, **134**: 229–234.

Breen, P.H., Isserles, S.A., Tabac, E., Roizen, M.F. & Taitelman, U.Z. (1996). Protective effect of stroma-free methemoglobin during cyanide poisoning in dogs. *Anesthesiology*, **85**: 558–564.

Cardenas, V., Heming, T.A. & Bidani, A. (1998). Kinetics of CO_2 excretion and intravascular pH disequilibria during carbonic anhydrase inhibition. *J. Appl. Physiol.*, **84**: 683–694.

Couture, P., Boudreault, D., Derouin, M., Allard, M., Lepage, Y., Girard, D. & Blaise, G. (1994). Venous carbon dioxide embolism in pigs: an evaluation of end-tidal carbon dioxide, transesophageal echocardiography, pulmonary artery pressure, and precordial auscultation as monitoring modalities. *Anesth. Analg.*, **79**: 867–873.

Cumming, W.A. & Ohlsson, A. (1985). Intracranial calcification in children with osteopetrosis caused by carbonic anhydrase II deficiency. *Radiology*, **157**: 325–327.

Dandurand, R.J., Matthews, P.M., Arnold, D.L. & Eidelman, D.H. (1995). Mitochondrial disease. Pulmonary function, exercise performance, and blood lactate levels. *Chest*, **108**: 182–189.

Dershewitz, R.A. & Levin, G.S. (1984). The effect of the Tylenol scare on parent's use of over-the-counter drugs. *Clin. Pediatr. (Phila.)*, **23**: 445–448.

Diakun, T.A. (1991). Carbon dioxide embolism: successful resuscitation with cardiopulmonary bypass. *Anesthesiology*, **74**: 1151–1153.

Dominguez-Roldan, J.M., Barrera-Chacon, J.M., Murillo-Cabezas, F., Santamaria-Mifsut, J.L. & Rivera-Fernandez, V. (1999). Clinical factors influencing the increment of blood carbon dioxide during the apnea test for the diagnosis of brain death. *Transplant. Proc.*, **31**: 2599–2600.

Ernesto, M., Cardoso, A.P., Nicala, D., Mirione, E., Massaza, F., Cliff, J., Haque, M.R. & Bradbury, J.H. (2002). Persistent konzo and cyanogen toxicity from cassava in northern Mozambique. *Acta Trop.*, **82**: 357–362.

Fathallah, D.M., Bejaoui, M., Sly, W.S., Lakhoua, R. & Dellagi, K. (1994). A unique mutation underlying carbonic anhydrase II deficiency syndrome in patients of Arab descent. *Hum. Genet.*, **94**: 581–582.

Flaherty, K.R., Wald, J., Weisman, I.M., Zeballos, R.J., Schork, M.A., Blaivas, M., Rubenfire, M. & Martinez, F.J. (2001). Unexplained exertional limitation: characterization of patients with a mitochondrial myopathy. *Am. J. Respir. Crit. Care Med.*, **164**: 425–432.

Henriksen, L., Paulson, O.B. & Lauritzen, M. (1982). The effects of sodium nitroprusside on cerebral blood flow and cerebral venous blood gases. I. Observations in awake man during and following moderate blood pressure reduction. *Eur. J. Clin. Invest.*, **12**: 383–387.

Imasogie, N., Crago, R., Leyland, N.A. & Chung, F. (2002). Probable gas embolism during operative hysteroscopy caused by products of combustion. *Can. J. Anaesth.*, **49**: 1044–1047.

Kamalu, B.P. (1995). The adverse effects of long-term cassava (Manihot esculenta, Crantz) consumption. *Int. J. Food Sci. Nutr.*, **46**: 65–93.

Kerns, W., Isom, G. & Kirk, M.A. (2002). Cyanide and hydrogen sulfide. In: Goldfrank, L.R., Flomenbaum, N.E., Lewin, N.A., Howland, M.A., Hoffman, R.S. & Nelson, L.S.

(eds). *Goldfrank's Toxicologic Emergencies*, 7th edition. McGraw-Hill, New York; pp. 1498–1514.

Krintel, J.J., Haxholdt, O.S., Berthelsen, P. & Brockner, J. (1983). Carbon dioxide elimination after acetazolamide in patients with chronic obstructive pulmonary disease and metabolic alkalosis. *Acta Anaesthesiol. Scand.*, **27**: 252–254.

Lasaga, J.I. (1980). Death in Jonestown: techniques of political control by a paranoid leader. *Suicide Life Threat. Behav.*, **10**: 210–213.

Lee, T.S. (1994). End-tidal partial pressure of carbon dioxide does not accurately reflect $PaCO_2$ in rabbits treated with acetazolamide during anaesthesia. *Br. J. Anaesth.*, **73**: 225–226.

Levraut, J., Garcia, P., Giunti, C., Ichai, C., Bouregba, M., Ciebiera, J.P., Payan, P. & Grimaud, D. (2000). The increase in CO_2 production induced by $NaHCO_3$ depends on blood albumin and hemoglobin concentrations. *Intens. Care Med.*, **26**: 558–564.

Lien, Y.H. & Lai, L. W. (1998). Respiratory acidosis in carbonic anhydrase II-deficient mice. *Am. J. Physiol.*, **274**: L301–L304.

Melano, R., Adum, M.E., Scarlatti, A., Bazzano, R. & Araujo, J.L. (2002). Apnea test in diagnosis of brain death: comparison of two methods and analysis of complications. *Transplant. Proc.*, **34**: 11–12.

Mueller, M. & Borland, C. (1997). Delayed cyanide poisoning following acetonitrile ingestion. *Postgrad. Med. J.*, **73**: 299–300.

Nelson, D.L. & Cox, M.M. (2000). Bioenergetics and metabolism. In: *Lehninger Principles of Biochemistry*, 3rd edition. Worth Publishers, New York; pp. 485–904.

Nishiyama, T. & Hanaoka, K. (1999). Gas embolism during hysteroscopy. *Can. J. Anaesth.*, **46**: 379–381.

Okamoto, H., Hoka, S., Kawasaki, T., Okuyama, T. & Takahashi, S. (1995). Changes in end-tidal carbon dioxide tension following sodium bicarbonate administration: correlation with cardiac output and haemoglobin concentration. *Acta Anaesthesiol. Scand.*, **39**: 79–84.

Oluwole, O.S., Onabolu, A.O., Link, H. & Rosling, H. (2000). Persistence of tropical ataxic neuropathy in a Nigerian community. *J. Neurol. Neurosurg. Psychiatry*, **69**: 96–101.

Ording, H. (1985). Incidence of malignant hyperthermia in Denmark. *Anesth. Analg.*, **64**: 700–704.

Padmaja, G. (1995). Cyanide detoxification in cassava for food and feed uses. *Crit. Rev. Food Sci. Nutr.*, **35**: 299–339.

Potter, C.P. & Harris, A.L. (2003). Diagnostic, prognostic and therapeutic implications of carbonic anhydrases in cancer. *Br. J. Cancer*, **89**: 2–7.

Poulton, J. (1997). Pathogenesis of mitochondrial disease. In: Applegarth, D.A., Dimmick, J.E. and Hall, J.G. (eds) *Organelle Diseases*, 1st edition. Chapman & Hall, London; pp. 305–335.

Ravi, V., Aked, J. & Balagopalan, C. (1996). Review on tropical root and tuber crops. I. Storage methods and quality changes. *Crit. Rev. Food Sci. Nutr.*, **36**: 661–709.

Roemer, K., Johnson, P.A. & Friedmann, T. (1991). Knock-in and knock-out. Transgenes, development and disease: a keystone symposium sponsored by Genentech and Immunex, Tamarron, CO, USA, January 12–18, 1991. *New Biol.*, **3**: 331–335.

Rudolf, J., Haupt, W.F., Neveling, M. & Grond, M. (1998). Potential pitfalls in apnea testing. *Acta Neurochir. (Wien.)*, **140**: 659–663.

Sabri, M.I., Spencer, P.S., Baggia, S. & Ludolph, A.C. (2000). Clinical manifestations and mechanisms of action of environmental mitochondrial toxins. In: Sanberg, P.R., Nishino, H.N. & Borlongan, C.V. (eds) *Mitochondrial Inhibitors and Neurodegenerative Disorders*, 1st edition. Humana Press, Totowa; pp. 3–20.

Schon, E.A. (1994). Mitochondrial DNA and the genetics of mitochondrial disease. In: Schapira, A.H. & DiMauro, S. (eds) *Mitochondrial Disorders in Neurology*. Butterworth-Heinemann Ltd, Oxford, pp. 31–48.

Shulman, D. & Aronson, H.B. (1984). Capnography in the early diagnosis of carbon dioxide embolism during laparoscopy. *Can. Anaesth. Soc. J.*, **31**: 455–459.

Silberberg, S. (1996). Gases and the kinetic-molecular theory. In: *Chemistry: The Molecular Nature of Matter and Change*, 3rd edition. Mosby-Year Book, Inc., St. Louis, Missouri; pp. 172–219.

Skladal, D., Halliday, J. & Thorburn, D.R. (2003). Minimum birth prevalence of mitochondrial respiratory chain disorders in children. *Brain*, **126**: 1905–1912.

Sly, W.S., Whyte, M.P., Sundaram, V., Tashian, R.E., Hewett-Emmett, D., Guibaud, P., Vainsel, M., Baluarte, H.J., Gruskin, A. & Al Mosawi, M. (1985). Carbonic anhydrase II deficiency in 12 families with the autosomal recessive syndrome of osteopetrosis with renal tubular acidosis and cerebral calcification. *N. Engl. J. Med.*, **313**: 139–145.

Smith, K.S., Jakubzick, C., Whittam, T.S. & Ferry, J.G. (1999). Carbonic anhydrase is an ancient enzyme widespread in prokaryotes. *Proc. Natl. Acad. Sci. USA*, **96**: 15184–15189.

Soda, H., Yukizane, S., Yoshida, I., Aramaki, S. & Kato, H. (1995). Carbonic anhydrase II deficiency in a Japanese patient produced by a nonsense mutation (TAT → TAG) at Tyr-40 in exon 2 (Y40X). *Hum. Mutat.*, **5**: 348–350.

Spear, M.L., Darmaun, D., Sager, B.K., Parsons, W.R. & Haymond, M.W. (1995). Use of [^{13}C] bicarbonate infusion for measurement of CO_2 production. *Am. J. Physiol.*, **268**, E1123–E1127.

Sreeja, V.G., Nagahara, N., Li, Q. & Minami, M. (2003). New aspects in pathogenesis of konzo: neural cell damage directly caused by linamarin contained in cassava (Manihot esculenta, Crantz). *Br. J. Nutr.*, **90**: 467–472.

Taki, K., Mizuno, K., Takahashi, N. & Wakusawa, R. (1986). Disturbance of CO_2 elimination in the lungs by carbonic anhydrase inhibition. *Jpn. J. Physiol.*, **36**: 523–532.

Taki, K., Hirahara, K., Totoki, T. & Takahashi, N. (1993). Retention of carbon dioxide in tissue following carbonic anhydrase inhibition in dogs. *Clin. Ther.*, **15**: 884–889.

Taki, K., Kato, H. & Yoshida, I. (1999). Elimination of CO_2 in patients with carbonic anhydrase II deficiency, with studies of respiratory function at rest. *Respir. Med.*, **93**: 536–539.

Taylor, R.W. & Turnbull, D.M. (1997). Laboratory diagnosis of mitochondrial disease. In: Applegarth, D.A., Dimmick, J.E. & Hall, J.G. (eds) *Organelle Diseases*, 1st edition. Chapman & Hall, London; pp. 341–349.

Thomason, J.A. (1993). Quality of health services in Papua New Guinea: what do we know? *PNG Med. J.*, **36**: 90–98.

Tripp, B.C., Smith, K. & Ferry, J.G. (2001). Carbonic anhydrase: new insights for an ancient enzyme. *J. Biol. Chem.*, **276**: 48615–48618.

Wagenaar, M., Teppema, L., Berkenbosch, A., Olievier, C. & Folgering, H. (1996). The effect of low-dose acetazolamide on the ventilatory CO_2 response curve in the anaesthetized cat. *J. Physiol.*, **495(Pt 1)**: 227–237.

Whyte, M.P. (1993). Carbonic anhydrase II deficiency. *Clin. Orthop.*, **294**: 52–63.

Wildsmith, J.A., Drummond, G.B. & MacRae, W.R. (1975). Blood-gas changes during induced hypotension with sodium nitroprusside. *Br. J. Anaesth.*, **47**: 1205–1211.

ACID–BASE BALANCE 29

A. Isenberg & P. Boysen

Introduction

Capnography can provide important clues as to the acid–base status of patients. For example, an increase or decrease in the end-tidal carbon dioxide (CO_2) might indicate a primary respiratory acidosis, or a primary respiratory alkalosis, respectively. Alternatively, an increased end-tidal CO_2 tension might be a response to a metabolic alkalosis, and a decreased end-tidal CO_2 tension might be due to compensation for a metabolic acidosis. Certain assumptions, which may not be warranted in some cases, must be made to make appropriate evaluations and diagnoses. Global cardiac output and regional perfusion of the lung must be normal and stable. Similarly, dead space ventilation (Vd/Vt) must be normal and stable. Under these conditions, the end-tidal CO_2 tension and the arterial CO_2 tension are proximate. Beyond these initial clues, arterial blood gas (ABG) analysis is essential to the proper evaluation of acid–base status, and the diagnosis and treatment of underlying disorders.

Normal acid–base homeostasis

Acids and bases are constantly formed in the body as by-products of metabolism and are carefully regulated. The normal pH of the blood ranges from 7.36 to 7.44 (Table 29.1). This narrow range is maintained by a complex system of buffering mechanisms, each designed to regulate the amount of hydrogen ion in the body. These mechanisms include intracellular and extracellular chemical buffers, regulation of CO_2 by the respiratory and central nervous systems (CNS) and control of bicarbonate by the kidney.

Chemical buffering

Acids

The metabolic acids produced are classified as volatile and non-volatile. The primary volatile acid is carbonic acid (H_2CO_3); it is produced during CO_2 reactions and exhaled as CO_2. The non-volatile acids are sulfuric (produced by the breakdown of sulfur containing amino acids), organic acids from the breakdown of carbohydrates and fats, uric acid from nucleic acid metabolism, and inorganic phosphates. The non-volatile acids are buffered by the blood bicarbonate system.

Table 29.1 Normal acid–base composition

	Mean	Range
Arterial blood		
pH	7.40	7.36–7.44
$[H^+]$	40 nM	36–44 neq/l
PCO_2	40 mmHg	36–44 mmHg
$[HCO_3^-]$ actual	24 nM	22–26 meq/l
$[HCO_3^-]$ standard	24 nM	22–26 meq/l
Base excess (BE)	0 mM	−2 to +2 meq/l
Venous blood		
pH	7.38	7.34–7.42
$[H^+]$	42 nM	38–46 neq/l
PCO_2	46 mmHg	42–50 mmHg
Total CO_2	26 mM	23–30 meq/l

Reproduced with permission from Adrogue, H.J. & Madias, N.E. (1998). Arterial blood gas monitoring: acid–base assessment. In: Martin, J. & Tobin, M. (eds) *Principles and Practice of Intensive Care Monitoring*. McGraw Hill, Inc, New York; pp. 217–241.

Bases

Bicarbonate buffers prepare non-volatile acid protons for excretion, a process that consumes the bicarbonate buffer. Bicarbonate diffuses freely between interstitial fluid and plasma along a concentration gradient (Adrogue & Madias, 1998), and carries about 70% of CO_2 (Gravenstein *et al.*, 1989). As bicarbonate is generated, the chloride shift (Hamberger effect) serves to maintain ionic equilibrium in the red blood cells (RBCs) by moving chloride from the RBC into the plasma (Gravenstein *et al.*, 1989). Renal tubular reabsorption serves to preserve bicarbonate. New bicarbonate production (50–100 mmol/day) occurs during renal acidification process whereby protons are secreted to form urinary buffers (phosphate and ammonia) that are then eliminated in the urine.

CO_2 regulation

CO_2 is produced by the metabolism of substrate inside cells. It is then transported in blood to the alveolus where it can be excreted in the gas phase. Some CO_2 travels as gas dissolved in plasma, although the majority of CO_2 is transported in RBCs as bicarbonate. Inside the RBC, CO_2 combines with water to form carbonic acid (or volatile acid), which forms hydrogen ions and bicarbonate as terminal products. The *bicarbonate–carbonic acid equation* is a steady state reaction that is catalyzed by carbonic anhydrase (acetazolamide inhibits this enzyme):

$$CO_2 + H_2O \leftrightharpoons H_2CO_3 \leftrightharpoons H^+ + HCO_3^-$$

Under normal circumstances, CO_2 production and excretion are in equilibrium. The ratio of HCO_3^- to H_2CO_3 is maintained at 20 : 1 (mmol/l) by homeostatic processes (Madias *et al.*, 1979a, b, c; Gennari & Kassirer, 1982). The plasma arterial CO_2 (P_aCO_2) is maintained at 40 mmHg while the venous level is at 46 mmHg, setting up a gradient for the transport of CO_2 from cells into the blood. *Hypercapnia*, or increased CO_2 levels in the blood is produced by the under-excretion of CO_2 and *hypocapnia*, or decreased levels of CO_2 in the blood, evolves from the over-excretion of CO_2.

A buildup of CO_2, such as by hypoventilation will push the bicarbonate–carbonic acid equation to the right, increasing the hydrogen ion concentration thereby decreasing the pH (respiratory acidosis). Conversely, a decrease in the CO_2, as in the case of hyperventilation, pushes this equation to the left, diminishing the hydrogen ion concentration and increasing the pH (respiratory alkalosis).

Changes in the bicarbonate will also affect the equilibrium of the bicarbonate–carbonic acid equation. Loss of bicarbonate (through diarrhea or kidney dysfunction) or addition of acid (diabetic ketoacidosis, DKA) will force the reaction to the right, thereby increasing the H^+ causing metabolic acidosis. Likewise, an increased loss of H^+ through the gastrointestinal (GI) tract (vomiting) or through renal losses, will push the equation to the left and increase the pH (metabolic alkalosis).

CO_2 freely diffuses across cell membranes while HCO_3^- diffuses between the plasma and interstitial fluid in response to concentration gradients. Other buffers, most notably hemoglobin and plasma proteins, are restricted to the vascular compartment.

CO_2 is regulated primarily by the CNS through the medullary chemoreceptors. The P_aCO_2, therefore, is not normally determined by the rate of CO_2 production, but by neural respiratory center output. Increased P_aCO_2 is generally caused by hypoventilation, driven by an aberration in the CNS rather than an augmentation of CO_2 production. Aside from CNS regulation, increases or decreases in P_aCO_2 can be caused by compensation secondary to a primary change in the bicarbonate ion. A volatile acid, CO_2 can be excreted or retained as needed to maintain homeostasis.

Bicarbonate regulation

The kidneys use three mechanisms to regulate plasma bicarbonate. The first method involves reabsorption of filtered bicarbonate, 80%–90% of which is reabsorbed in the proximal tubule of the nephron. The kidney filters approximately 4000 mmol of bicarbonate each day; to reabsorb the filtered bicarbonate ion, the renal tubules must secrete 4000 mmol of hydrogen ions. The distal nephron reabsorbs the remaining 10%–20% of the bicarbonate and secretes 40–60 mmol/day of hydrogen ions to maintain the blood pH. The kidney then uses a second regulatory mechanism to take the remaining 40–60 mmol/day of hydrogen ions and form a titratable acid and NH_4. The excess hydrogen ions are then excreted as NH_4 in the urine as the third process of the kidney for bicarbonate regulation. NH_4 production and excretion will be increased in a metabolic acidosis with normal renal function but will be impaired in chronic renal failure, hyperkalemia, and renal tubular acidosis (RTA) (Schwartz *et al.*, 1959; Goodman *et al.*, 1965; Wall & Knepper, 1990; DuBose, 2003).

Henderson–Hasselbalch equation

The sum of the respiratory and metabolic components that drive the blood pH level can be described by the Henderson–Hasselbalch equation:

$$pH = 6.1\ 1 \log\left[\frac{HCO_3^-}{P_aCO_2 \times 0.0301}\right]$$

This equation is normally used by clinicians to calculate an expected value of bicarbonate that can be compared to the measured bicarbonate as a way to check the accuracy of laboratory values while considering the possibility of a mixed acid–base disorder.

Standard HCO_3^- and base excess

The interdependence of the respiratory and metabolic factors that determine the pH described by the Henderson–Hasselbalch equation have led researchers to derive other parameters, which can be used to describe a metabolic component that is independent from the respiratory component (Adrogue & Madias, 1998). These relationships are only true *in vitro*, because *in vivo*, the presence of buffers other than bicarbonate that are restricted to the vascular compartment confounds the *in vivo* relationship.

The *standard [HCO_3^-]* is a derived parameter corresponding to the plasma bicarbonate concentration in a blood sample fully saturated with oxygen and equilibrated *in vitro* at 38°C having a partial pressure of CO_2 (PCO_2) equal to 40 mmHg (mean is 24 mol/l) (Schwartz & Relman, 1963). This standardized blood oxygen factor is necessary because the level of oxygenation of hemoglobin alters the hemoglobin buffer value, that is, when oxygenated hemoglobin releases oxygen it becomes less acidic, thereby, increasing its buffering capacity (and vice versa when hemoglobin picks up oxygen). The standard HCO_3^-, therefore, can be used to quantify alterations in the buffer systems within a blood sample (Adrogue & Madias, 1998).

The blood BE is another parameter derived from the Henderson–Hasselbalch relationship. It corresponds to the quantity of acid or alkali that must be added to a liter of fully oxygenated blood exposed *in vitro* to PCO_2 of 40 mmHg at 38°C to reach a pH of 7.40 (Adrogue & Madias, 1998). If the initial blood pH is low (acidic), alkali must be added to bring the pH back up to the normal 7.4 value. Thus, the initial blood sample can be said to have a *negative BE* or simply a *base deficit*. With the reverse situation, if a blood sample has a high pH (alkaline), acid must be added to decrease the pH to the normal level, the sample is said to have a *positive BE* or simply a *BE*. The normal value of BE is zero, theoretically but the range of normal values is −2.4 to +2.4 meq/l in women and −3.3 to +1.3 meq/l in men.

Strong ion theory

Traditional acid–base physiology with its basis in the Henderson–Hasselbalch equation has been challenged recently by Peter Stewart's theory, which maintains that hydrogen ion concentration is determined by the dissociation of water ($H_2O \rightarrow H^+ + OH^-$) and not by the addition of hydrogen ions (Stewart, 1981; Kellum, 1998). In short, Stewart found that three independent variables determine the hydrogen ion concentration: the strong ion difference (SID), the total concentration of weak acids, and P_aCO_2. The SID is the net charge balance of all of the "strong ions" in the system; that is, the ions that are essentially inert and completely dissociated (not water and not bicarbonate because it readily combines with CO_2 or OH^-). The SID discounts the other ions present in low concentrations; one must remember that they are present (Figge *et al.*, 1992).

$$\text{SID} = \text{Na} + \text{K} + \text{Ca} + \text{Mg} + \text{PO}_4 - (\text{Cl} - \text{lactate})$$

Thus, when strong ions are added to a system, neutrality is maintained by altering weak electrolyte dissociation. For example, when sodium bicarbonate is given to a patient, the serum bicarbonate does not increase because of simply giving bicarbonate in the fluid but because the solution contained the strong cation, sodium, which causes the water dissociation reaction to shift left resulting in fewer hydrogen ions and thus a higher pH (Gauthier & Szerlip, 2002). This Stewart approach is of aid particularly when considering the acidosis, especially those of "dilutional" origin that have been found to be correctable via treatment with the administration of a strong ion, such as chloride (Waters *et al.*, 1999; Constable, 2003), and with mortality prediction in the pediatric intensive care unit (ICU) (Balasubramanyan *et al.*, 1999).

Diagnosis of acid–base disorders

ABG

A critical step in diagnosing an acid–base disorder, after a thorough history and physical, is to collect and analyze an ABG (Gennari *et al.*, 1982a, b; Harrington *et al.*, 1982; Valtin, 1987a, b; Adrogue & Wesson, 1994; Adrogue & Tobin, 1997). The ABG should be drawn using a low-friction syringe that uses blood pressure as the driving force; negative pressure syringes can cause gas bubble formation that can induce errors as the bubbles equilibrate with the blood gases. Excessive heparin (>0.2 ml) should not be used in the collection tube as it can lead to a low P_aCO_2 and low HCO_3^- (dilutional effect) and a high partial pressure of oxygen in arterial blood (P_aO_2) (Bloom *et al.*, 1985); lyophilized heparin syringes may be used. At least 3 ml of blood should be collected using a small needle. The ABG should be analyzed immediately because RBC anaerobic metabolism will quickly acidify a sample. Samples that cannot be analyzed quickly should be placed on ice and cooled to 4°C (Adrogue & Madias, 1998). Remember also that a respiratory alkalosis may be temporarily induced by a painful blood draw in an anxious patient.

ABGs are thought to provide the best assessment of pulmonary exchange and tissue oxygenation. However, central venous and mixed venous blood gases are evolving as an important means to assess perfusion (Weil *et al.*, 1986; Benjamin *et al.*, 1987; Bakker *et al.*, 1992; Zhang & Vincent, 1993). With circulatory insufficiency, venous pH and P_aCO_2 have been shown to change earlier and with greater magnitude than arterial values (Oropello *et al.*, 1996). Further, it has been documented that in patients with circulatory failure, it may be misleading to use only arterial blood samples to monitor acid–base status (Adrogue *et al.*, 1989a, b). Severity of the discrepancy between arterial and venous draws becomes greater with declining circulatory function and extreme during cardiac arrest.

It is important to remember that venous blood HCO_3^- is approximately 2 meq/l higher than the arterial value because the majority of the metabolically produced CO_2 that is added to venous blood is carried as bicarbonate. Venous blood also has a greater quantity of carbamino compounds and dissolved CO_2 than arterial blood (Adrogue & Madias, 1998).

Capillary blood samples can be used, particularly in children, to measure ABG. Care must be taken to warm the area prior to the procedure (about 5 min) to secure a dilated vascular bed (Harrison *et al.*, 1997). Acid–base status can also be measured using a peripheral vein in the dorsum of the hand that has been warmed (to 45°C for 10 min); the resulting values are very close to those from an arterial draw (Adrogue & Madias, 1998). Lastly umbilical cord gases should use arterial rather than venous blood as arterial acidemia may be present with a normal venous pH; the lower range of normal for the arterial pH is 7.10 (Thorp & Rushing, 1999).

The ABG measures the arterial pH and the PCO_2 in the arterial blood. Electrolytes should be drawn simultaneously to obtain a *measured* HCO_3^-, which should be used to compare the *calculated* HCO_3^- from the Henderson–Hasselbalch equation. The two values should agree within 2 mmol/l. Otherwise, errors have been introduced in the laboratory, math, or the blood draw itself (commonly a non-simultaneous draw of electrolytes and ABG). As the blood sampling is intermittent, transient changes in the acid–base composition can exist and not be detected (Adrogue & Madias, 1998). Serum albumin should also be measured with a suspected acidosis to aid in consideration of anion gap (AG) issues. A serum creatinine (CR) may be helpful in many cases when considering dysfunction or compensation by the kidneys. Urine pH and osmolar gap are also useful values to consider in the face of their respective acid–base scenarios.

Other important issues to explore when diagnosing an acid–base disorder are patient history and drug use. Chronic renal failure predisposes a patient to metabolic acidosis, as do diarrheal diseases. Vomiting can cause a metabolic alkalosis while those with pneumonia, sepsis, or cardiac failure frequently have respiratory alkalosis. Air trapping diseases or sedative overdoses can cause a respiratory acidosis (DuBose, 2003). Drug history is an important factor. Loop and thiazide diuretics can cause metabolic alkalosis and carbonic anhydrase inhibitors can cause a metabolic acidosis. Overdoses of drugs can also cause mixed acid–base disorders such as the combined metabolic acidosis and respiratory alkalosis caused by salicylate overdose.

Approach to simple acid–base disorders

Acid–base disorders are shown in Figure 29.1 and Table 29.2.

1 Thorough history and physical.
2 Draw the arterial blood for ABG. Examine the *pH* first. If the $pH < 7.38$, there is an acidemia. If the pH is >7.44, there is an alkalemia.
3 Decide whether the primary disorder is *metabolic or respiratory*:
   – If acidemia: Respiratory acidosis if $P_aCO_2 > 45$
   Metabolic acidosis if $HCO_3^- < 22$
   – If alkalemia: Respiratory alkalosis if $P_aCO_2 < 35$
   Metabolic alkalosis if $HCO_3^- > 26$
4 If the primary disorder is metabolic, is there appropriate *compensation* (use the compensation equations (see pages 274–275)). If the primary disorder is respiratory, decide if it is acute or chronic (use the compensation equations).
5 Consider accuracy of laboratory values (true versus spurious results) and entertain possibility of *mixed AB disorder*.
6 Calculate *AG*:

   $$AG = Na - [Cl + HCO_3^-]$$

   The normalAG value is 10–12 meq/l.

   If there is a metabolic acidosis and the AG is >12, there is a high AG acidosis. If the AG is 12 or less, there is a normal AG (hypochloremic) acidosis. If the AG is >20, there is an underlying AG acidosis in the face of any other acid–base disturbances present.
7 If there is an elevated AG, calculate the *corrected serum bicarbonate*:

   Corrected bicarbonate
   $= \text{excess AG} + \text{measured } HCO_3^-$
   If the corrected bicarbonate is *low* (<24 meq/l), there is an underlying non-AG acidosis; if *high* (>24 meq/l) there is an underlying metabolic alkalosis.
8 Calculate *ancillary laboratory values* with respect to suspected diagnosis (albumin, serum/urine osmolar gap, electrolytes (potassium, blood urea nitrogen (BUN), CR, glucose, etc.), blood/urine screens for toxins).

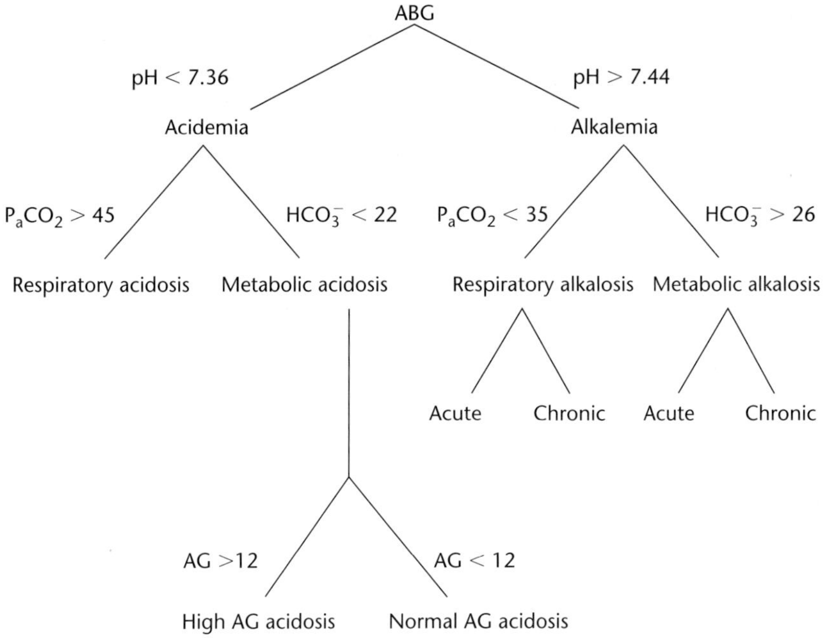

Figure 29.1 Acid–base diagnostic algorithm. (Reproduced with permission from Feibusch, K.C., Breaden, R.S., Bader, C.D. & Gomperts, S.N. (1998). *Prescription for the Boards: USMLE Step 2*, 2nd edition. Lippincott-Raven, Philadelphia.)

Table 29.2 Secondary response to simple acid–base disorders

Condition	Expected response	Maximal response
Metabolic acidosis	$\Delta P_aCO_2 \approx 1.2\ \Delta[HCO_3^-]$	10 mmHg
Metabolic alkalosis	$\Delta P_aCO_2 \approx 0.7\ \Delta[HCO_3^-]$	65 mmHg
Respiratory acidosis		
Acute	$\Delta[HCO_3^-] \approx 0.1\ \Delta P_aCO_2$	30 meq/l
Chronic	$\Delta[HCO_3^-] \approx 0.3\ \Delta P_aCO_2$	45 meq/l
Respiratory alkalosis		
Acute	$\Delta[HCO_3^-] \approx 0.2\ \Delta P_aCO_2$	16–18 meq/l
Chronic	$\Delta[HCO_3^-] \approx 0.4\ \Delta P_aCO_2$	12–15 meq/l

Reproduced with permission from Adrogue, H.J. & Madias, N.E. (1998). Arterial blood gas monitoring: acid–base assessment. In: Martin, J. & Tobin, M. (eds) *Principles and Practice of Intensive Care Monitoring*. McGraw Hill, Inc, New York; pp. 217–241.

Simple acid–base disorders

Acid–base disorders can be described as *simple*, wherein one acid–base disturbance exists, or *mixed*, where there are two or more acid–base disorders present simultaneously (Harrington *et al.*, 1982; Valtin, 1987a, b). Simple acid–base disorders involve a primary abnormality in either metabolism (change in the bicarbonate) or respiration (change in arterial CO_2) that causes a secondary change, or compensatory response, in the other component. The compensation response serves to ameliorate the primary disturbance in an effort to bring the pH back to baseline (Giebisch *et al.*, 1955; Brackett *et al.*, 1965). Secondary compensation for a primary acid–base disorder, however, does not constitute a mixed acid–base disorder because compensation in itself is not a separate acid–base disturbance.

Compensation

Primary respiratory disturbances will cause secondary changes in the metabolism (renal acid production/secretion alterations) and primary metabolic disturbances will invoke compensatory changes in the

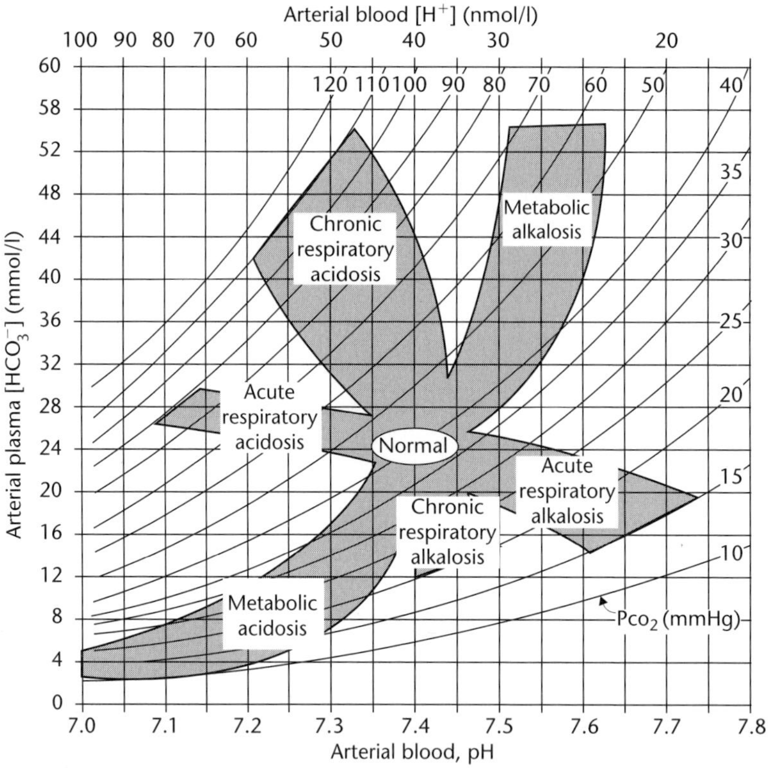

Figure 29.2 Acid–base nomogram. Figure showing the 90% confidence limits of normal respiratory and metabolic compensations for primary acid–base disturbances. Values for mixed disturbances will fall outside of the shaded areas. (Reproduced with permission from DuBose Jr, T.D. *Acid–base disorders*. In: Brenner and Rector's The Kidney, 6th edition, Brenner, B.M. (ed.). Philadelphia, Saunders; 2000, pp. 925–997.)

respiration (increased or decreased ventilation). The amount of compensation can be predicted from the *compensation equations* listed below. If the compensation values differ from predicted values, a mixed acid–base disorder should be considered.

For example, a primary respiratory acidosis will invoke a secondary metabolic alkalosis to compensate for the effects of the excess acid in the system. To illustrate, a comatose victim may develop a respiratory acidosis because an injured ventilation stimulation pathway (e.g. due to cerebral edema secondary to a head injury) leads to hypoventilation and CO_2 trapping. The pH will decrease because of the increased P_aCO_2 and a shift in the carbonic acid equation. The kidneys recognize the acidosis and effect changes in the acid titration process to secrete less HCO_3^- to compensate for the respiratory acidosis.

The four cardinal simple acid–base disorders are as follows: metabolic acidosis, metabolic alkalosis, respiratory acidosis, and respiratory alkalosis. Secondary responses to each of these four disorders follow a predictable pattern (Flenley, 1971). Classically, the acid–base nomogram (sometimes referred to as the Davenport diagram) can be used to graph a patient's HCO_3^- and pH to determine which type of disorder the patient has. The modified acid–base nomogram (Figure 29.2) has shaded intervals that mark the appropriateness of compensation. Values that fall outside of the shaded areas indicate a mixed disturbance. Further, compensation equations can be used to assess responses to acid–base disorders and to decide whether a mixed acid–base disturbance may be present.

Compensation equations

Disorder	Rule of compensation
Metabolic acidosis	$P_aCO_2 = (1.5 \times HCO_3^-) + 8$ or P_aCO_2 will ↓ 1.25 mmHg per mmol/l ↑ in HCO_3^- or $P_aCO_2 = HCO_3^- + 15$

Metabolic alkalosis	P_aCO_2 will ↑ 0.75 mmHg per mmol/l ↑ in HCO_3^- or P_aCO_2 will ↑ 6 mmHg per 10 mmol/l ↑ in HCO_3^- or $P_aCO_2 = HCO_3^- + 15$
Respiratory alkalosis	
Acute	HCO_3^- will ↓ 2 mmol/l per 10 mmHg ↓ in P_aCO_2
Chronic	HCO_3^- will ↓ 4 mmol/l per 10 mmHg ↓ in P_aCO_2
Respiratory acidosis	
Acute	HCO_3^- will ↑ 1 mmol/l per 10 mmHg ↑ in P_aCO_2
Chronic	HCO_3^- will ↑ 4 mmol/l per 10 mmHg ↑ in P_aCO_2

Mixed acid–base disorders

Mixed acid–base disorders occur when a person has more than one independent acid–base disorder (Narins & Emmett, 1980; Adrogue & Madias, 1998); mixed acid–base disorders are very common in hepatic failure (Tyor & Sieker, 1959; Prytz *et al.*, 1976) and in ICU (Cohen & Schwartz, 1966; Aberman & Fulop, 1972; Roncoroni *et al.*, 1976; Gauthier & Szerlip, 2002). Many combinations of acid–base disorders are possible; there may be two acidotic disorders paired together (respiratory acidosis with metabolic acidosis), two alkalotic disorders together (respiratory alkalosis with metabolic alkalosis), two disorders working towards opposite pH poles that can normalize pH (respiratory acidosis and metabolic alkalosis and vice versa), or even three or more disorders simultaneously.

For example, a person with DKA (a metabolic acidosis), may begin to decrease his respirations as he becomes more acidemic and less conscious (as a result of the DKA) and develop a separate respiratory acidosis. Or a person can overdose on sedatives and salicylates and have a mixed acid–base disorder in response to the individual drugs taken (metabolic and respiratory acidosis with sedatives and respiratory alkalosis with salicylates). In the case, where a metabolic acidosis and a metabolic alkalosis exist in the same patient, the pH may be normal and checking the *AG* is the next step in the evaluation (an increased AG in this case indicates a metabolic acidosis is present) (Tables 29.3 and 29.4).

Table 29.3 Classification of mixed acid–base disorders

Co-existence of different simple disorders
Additive combination of two disorders
Metabolic acidosis and respiratory acidosis
Metabolic alkalosis and respiratory alkalosis
Counterbalancing combination of two disorders
Metabolic alkalosis and respiratory acidosis
Metabolic acidosis and respiratory alkalosis
Metabolic acidosis and metabolic alkalosis
Respiratory acidosis and respiratory alkalosis
Combination of two or more disorders
Respiratory and metabolic acidosis and metabolic alkalosis
Respiratory and metabolic alkalosis and metabolic acidosis
Respiratory and metabolic alkalosis and respiratory alkalosis
Respiratory and metabolic alkalosis and respiratory acidosis
Co-existence of two or more entities of a simple disturbance
Metabolic simple disorder
Mixed high AG metabolic acidosis
Mixed hyperchloremic metabolic acidosis
Hyperchloremic and high AG metabolic acidosis
Mixed chloride sensitive metabolic alkalosis
Mixed chloride resistant metabolic alkalosis
Chloride sensitive and chloride resistant metabolic alkalosis
Respiratory simple disorder
Acute on chronic respiratory acidosis
Acute on chronic respiratory alkalosis
Co-existence of different simple disorders and simple disorder entities
Subgroups
Acute on chronic respiratory acidosis and metabolic acidosis or alkalosis
Acute on chronic respiratory alkalosis and metabolic acidosis or alkalosis
Mixed high AG metabolic acidosis and respiratory acidosis or alkalosis
Mixed high AG metabolic acidosis and metabolic alkalosis

Reproduced with permission from Adrogue, H.J. & Madias, N.E. (1998). Arterial blood gas monitoring: acid–base assessment. In: Martin, J. & Tobin, M. (eds) *Principles and Practice of Intensive Care Monitoring*. McGraw Hill, Inc, New York; pp. 217–241.

Metabolic acidosis

Metabolic acidosis can be caused by either an increase in endogenous acid production (lactic or ketoacids in DKA), a decrease in bicarbonate (diarrhea), or by an accumulation of endogenous acids (renal failure). There will be a decrease in the pH and in the HCO_3^-. The secondary response to metabolic acidosis is

Table 29.4 Characterization of the mixed acid–base disorders

Disorder type	pH	P_aCO_2 (mmHg)	HCO_3^- (meq/l)	Na (meq/l)	K (meq/l)	Cl^- (meq/l)	AG (meq/l)	Clinical notes
Metabolic and respiratory acidosis	7.10	50	15	140	5.0	102	23	Renal failure and hypercapnic respiratory failure
	6.99	34	8	141	6.0	105	28	Cardiopulmonary arrest
Metabolic and respiratory alkalosis	7.69	30	35	134	4.0	84	15	Hepatic failure and nasogastric suction
	7.60	40	38	131	3.6	77	16	Congestive heart failure (CHF) and diuretics chronic obstructive pulmonary disease (COPD) and diuretics
Metabolic acidosis and respiratory alkalosis	7.44	55	36	135	3.8	84	15	
	7.45	48	32	133	4.2	85	16	Acute respiratory distress syndrome (ARDS) and acetate-rich TPN
Metabolic acidosis and respiratory alkalosis	7.44	12	8	136	5.5	106	22	Renal failure and Gram-negative septicemia
	7.40	15	9	138	4.1	110	19	Salicylate intoxication
Metabolic acidosis and alkalosis	7.43	39	25	132	3.7	84	23	Alcoholic liver disease and diuretics
	7.37	35	20	138	4.0	93	25	DKA after $NaHCO_3$ therapy
Respiratory acidosis and alkalosis	7.54	41	34	140	3.8	93	13	COPD with mechanical ventilation
	7.68	28	32	137	3.5	91	14	COPD with mechanical hyperventilation
Respiratory and metabolic acidosis, metabolic alkalosis	7.38	57	33	134	4.7	77	24	COPD, diuretics, and shock
Respiratory and metabolic alkalosis, metabolic acidosis	7.43	25	16	135	3.2	97	22	CHF, diuretics, and shock
Hyperchloremic and high AG acidosis	7.12	16	5	137	3.6	114	18	DKA with adequate salt and water balance
Acute on chronic respiratory acidosis	7.22	80	32	141	4.3	99	10	COPD and high oxygen
Acute on chronic respiratory alkalosis	7.54	12	10	132	3.2	107	15	Alcoholic liver disease and cerebral bleeding
Acute on chronic respiratory acidosis and metabolic acidosis	7.09	65	19	136	3.3	105	12	COPD and diarrhea
Mixed high AG, metabolic acidosis and respiratory acidosis	7.18	44	16	133	5.7	100	17	Hepatic, renal, and pulmonary failure
Mixed high AG	7.36	31	17	132	4.0	89	26	Alcoholic liver disease, vomiting, and lactic acidosis
Metabolic acidosis and metabolic alkalosis	7.40	40	24	143	5.5	95	24	DKA, lactic acidosis, HCO_3 therapy

Reproduced with permission from Adrogue, H.J. & Madias, N.E. (1998). Arterial blood gas monitoring: acid–base assessment. In: Martin, J. & Tobin, M. (eds) *Principles and Practice of Intensive Care Monitoring*. McGraw Hill, Inc, New York; pp. 217–241.

hyperventilation, which in an attempt to increase the pH back to baseline, releases the volatile acid CO_2 from the lungs and results in hypocapnia (Asch *et al.*, 1969; Bone *et al.*, 1974; Fulop, 1997).

The reduction in pH can cause several effects on the respiratory, cardiac, and nervous systems. Tidal volume increases with increased ventilation, which can lead to Kussmaul respirations. The decreased pH sensitizes the peripheral chemoreceptors, increasing minute ventilation, which within hours can bring about an almost complete respiratory compensation (Asch *et al.*, 1969; Gauthier & Szerlip, 2002).

Metabolic acidosis decreases cardiac contractility but inotropic activity is maintained because of the sympathetic catecholamine release; cardiac output and heart rate will increase with mild academia ($pH > 7.2$) (Wildenthal *et al.*, 1968; Mehta & Kloner, 1987). With a rapidly developing acidosis, left ventricular performance has been found to decrease, with decreases in stroke work and mean rate of ejection (Wildenthal *et al.*, 1968). Peripheral arterial vasodilation is common with central venoconstriction (Carrier *et al.*, 1964), a scenario that predisposes the patient to pulmonary edema due to the decrease in vascular compliance. Additionally, acidemia shifts the oxyhemoglobin dissociation curve to the right, unloading oxygen more effectively while an acidemia-induced decrease in 2–3 DPG moves the curve to the left (Mines, 1992).

Additionally, metabolic acidosis leads to hyperkalemia as hydrogen ions are exchanged for K^+ or Na^+ on a cellular level. Every pH decrease of 0.10 leads to an increase in plasma potassium of 0.6 mmol/l. Hypokalemia can be caused in some metabolic acidosis by urinary wasting of K^+ (RTA, DKA, lactic acidosis, and diarrhea) (DuBose, 2003).

Signs and symptoms

Metabolic acidosis causes CNS depression causing headaches, lethargy, stupor, or coma. Glucose intolerance can occur. Metabolic acidosis is a particularly common finding in the ICU (Gaulthier & Szerlip, 2002).

Two types of metabolic acidosis

There are two types of metabolic acidosis: high AG metabolic acidosis and non-AG (normal AG or hyperchloremic) metabolic acidosis. Both types of metabolic acidosis will have similar capnographic findings, however. Assuming normal cardiac output and pulmonary perfusion, both the end-tidal CO_2 and the P_aCO_2 will be low.

AG metabolic acidosis

The AG, represents the unmeasured anions in plasma, such as anionic proteins, phosphate, sulfate, and other organic anions. Determination of the AG is invaluable in assessing a metabolic acidosis (DeTroyer *et al.*, 1977; Emmett & Narins, 1977; Oh *et al.*, 1985; Madias *et al.*, 1979b; Adrogue *et al.*, 1982; Gabow, 1985). The normal value is 8–12 mmol/l (Winter *et al.*, 1992) and can be calculated from the following formula:

$$AG = Na - (Cl + HCO_3^-)$$

A high AG is usually due to an increase in unmeasured anions, such as acetoacetate or lactate, that is the addition of acid (usually non-volatile), endogenous or exogenous, to the system. It is less commonly due to a decrease in the unmeasured cations (calcium, magnesium, potassium). An increased AG cannot be caused by loss of alkali or by decreased acid excretion by the kidney.

In the case of the high AG, typically the loss of bicarbonate is not paralleled by an increase in chloride ions, thus a wide gap is created. With a normal albumin level, a high AG is usually due to non-chloride containing acids that contain inorganic (phosphate, sulfate), organic (ketoacids, lactate, uremic organic anions), exogenous (salicylate or other ingested toxins which cause organic acid production), or other unidentified anions. A high AG may occur with an increased albumin concentration or alkalosis (alkalosis alters the charge on albumin). Even in the presence of a normal or alkalotic pH, the high AG points to the presence of the addition of excess acid in the body system (Gauthier & Szerlip, 2002).

A normal AG can be caused by an increase in unmeasured cations or by the addition of atypical cations like lithium (overdose) or cationic immunoglobulins (plasma cell dyscrasia) (De Troyer *et al.*, 1977). In non-AG acidosis, the loss of base is offset by a rise in chloride that maintains the normal level of anionic charge in the system. A decrease in the albumin concentration can cause a low AG, such as with nephrotic syndrome. Hypoalbuminemia can also lead to a spuriously low AG and mask an acidosis (Gauthier & Szerlip, 2002). With acidosis, the anionic charge on albumin can be reduced and cause a low AG. Therefore, it is necessary to correct the serum AG by 2.5–3.0 meq/l for every decrease in serum albumin below 4 g/dl (Gabow, 1985). Also, hyperviscosity and severe hyperlipidemia can cause a spuriously low AG and lead to the underestimation of sodium and chloride concentrations (Figure 29.3 and Table 29.5).

High AG metabolic acidosis

There are two mechanisms behind a high AG metabolic acidosis (Kreisberg, 1984). The first mechanism involves an excessive load of a non-HCl acid (lactate, ketoacid, ingested toxins) that overwhelms the breakdown or excretory processes of the body.

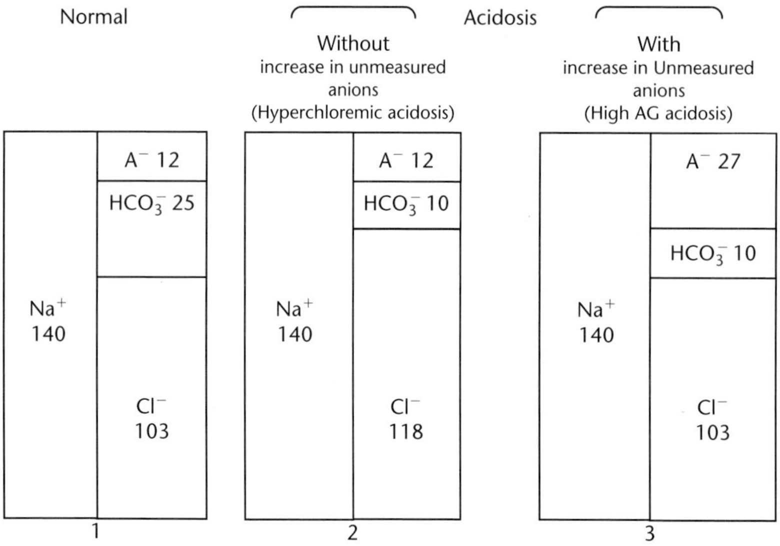

Figure 29.3 Schematic representation of the AG. *Hyperchloremic acidosis* is marked by a decreased serum bicarbonate without an increase in unmeasured anions above normal value; chloride ions are increased to make up the remainder of the negative charge (column 2). In *high AG acidosis* (column 3), increased amounts of fixed acids or other anions (A^-) are present, bicarbonate is decreased, and the level of chloride ions is at its normal value. (Reproduced with permission from Brackett Jr, N.C. (1974). An approach to clinical disorders of acid–base balance. *South. Med. J.*, **67**: 1084–1101.)

Table 29.5 Causes of metabolic acidosis

High AG	Normal AG
Endogenous acid load	*Renal diseases*
Ketoacidosis	Proximal RTA
Diabetes	Classic distal tubular acidosis
Alcoholism	Hyperkalemic distal tubular acidosis
Starvation	Interstitial nephritis
Uremia	Urinary tract obstruction
Lactic acidosis	Early renal failure
Exogenous toxins	*GI loss of bicarbonate*
Osmolar gap present	Diarrhea
Methanol	Small bowel losses
Ethylene glycol	Anion exchange resins
Osmolar gap absent	*Drugs*
Salicylates	Acetaxolamide
Paraldehyde	Mafenide
	Amphotericin B
	Amiloride
	Spironolactone
	Toluene ingestion
	Acid infusion
	HCl
	Arginine HCl
	Lysine HCl

Reproduced with permission from Adrogue, H.J. & Madias, N.E. (1998). Arterial blood gas monitoring: acid–base assessment. In: Martin, J. & Tobin, M. (eds) *Principles and Practice of Intensive Care Monitoring*. McGraw Hill, Inc, New York; pp. 217–241.

The second mechanism involves a diminished capacity of the kidneys to excrete the normal load of endogenous acids typically produced by the body (acute and chronic renal failure).

To diagnose a high AG acidosis, take a thorough history, with particular attention to drug or toxin ingestion, and keep in mind the typical diseases associated with high AG metabolic acidosis, such as diabetes or alcoholism. An ABG should then be performed to check for a concomitant acid–base disorder (such as respiratory alkalosis with salicylate overdose). Check β-hydroxybutyrate in alcoholics (alcoholic ketoacidosis) and analyze urine for oxalate crystals in suspected ethylene glycol ingestions. Look for clinical signs of uremia (uremic acidosis) and examine the BUN. Recognize the clinical settings in which lactate levels may be increased (lactic acidosis), such as with cardiac failure, shock, cancer, hypotension, thiamine deficiency, or drug/toxin ingestion (DuBose, 2003; Sterns, 2003), and that hyperventilation and respiratory alkalosis may also accompany some of these states, especially hemorrhagic shock (Benjamin *et al.*, 1987).

Remember to calculate a corrected bicarbonate (excess AG + measured bicarbonate) as this value represents the baseline bicarbonate that existed before the development of the high AG metabolic acidosis (Madias *et al.*, 1979; Adrogue *et al.*, 1982; Adrogue & Madias, 1998), and will be important in calculating alkali replacement (Garella *et al.*, 1973).

Excessive acid load causes of high AG metabolic acidosis

The three main causes of high AG acidosis that result from an excessive load of non-HCl acid are: (1) lactic acidosis, (2) ketoacidosis, and (3) ingested toxins.

Lactic acidosis

Lactic acidosis (lactate > 5 mmol/l, pH < 7.25) is most commonly caused by an increase in the plasma L-lactate isomer. L-lactate is produced as a result of decreased tissue perfusion in conditions, such as shock, circulatory failure, severe anemia, mitochondrial enzyme defects, and metabolic inhibitors (carbon monoxide, cyanide) and is commonly followed on surgical units to monitor postoperative progress. L-lactate acidosis appears with malignancies, diabetes mellitus, renal or hepatic failure, severe infections (cholera, malaria), seizures, acquired immune deficiency syndrome, or drugs/toxins (biguanides, ethanol, methanol, isoniazid, AZT analogs, and fructose) (DuBose, 2003). Bowel ischemia or infarction (especially while receiving vasopressors) is also a common cause of increased L-lactate. A D-lactate acidosis can be caused by formation of this isomer by gut bacteria and is seen in patients with jejunoileal bypass or by intestinal obstruction (Uribarri *et al.*, 1998) or in patients in which D-lactate metabolism is impaired (Oh *et al.*, 1985); hyperchloremia may also be seen with the D-lactate acidosis.

Lactic acidosis can also be categorized as type A, where tissue mitochondria function normally but oxygen delivery cannot meet metabolic requirements and type B where there is adequate oxygen yet acidosis occurs due to abnormal carbohydrate breakdown (phenformin intoxication, hepatic failure, diabetes mellitus, fructose ingestion) (Hindman, 1990). Patients with one type may develop the other type as their acidosis progresses.

It is important to remember that patients with lactic acidosis may have a normal AG (Iberti *et al.*, 1990; Aduen *et al.*, 1995), even in with high levels of blood lactate. Blood lactate concentrations higher than 5 mmol/l in an ICU patient are associated with a mortality rate of 59% at 3 days and 83% at 10 days (Stacpoole *et al.*, 1994). General treatment strategies for lactic acidosis involve correcting the underlying disruption of lactate metabolism with a restoration of tissue perfusion. Avoid vasoconstrictors as they may worsen tissue perfusion. Alkali therapy is encouraged in acute, severe academia (pH < 7.1) and usually avoided in the mild to moderate cases. $NaHCO_3^-$ therapy is generally discouraged as $NaHCO_3^-$ may depress cardiac performance and increase lactate production ($NaHCO_3^-$ stimulates phosphofructokinase) (Fraley *et al.*, 1980; Arieff *et al.*, 1982; Graf *et al.*, 1985; Cooper *et al.*, 1990; Mathieu *et al.*, 1991). It may also cause fluid overload, hypertension, and an overshoot alkalosis in those for whom the acidosis is remedied. If $NaHCO_3^-$ is used, titrate to raise the pH to no >7.2 over 30–40 min (DuBose, 2003).

Ketoacidosis

DKA DKA is caused by an increase in fatty acid metabolism with the accumulation of ketoacids, acetoacetate, and β-hydroxybutyrate. Lactic acidosis and hyperchloremic acidosis may also occur as well with uncontrolled diabetes mellitus (Atchley *et al.*, 1933). Although DKA usually occurs when a patient with type 1 diabetes does not take the required insulin dosage or has an illness or infection that acutely disrupts insulin requirements, a recent study has shown that 27% of patients in a series with DKA were type 2 diabetics (Westphal, 1996). Hyperglycemia (glucose > 300 mg) occurs as well. In recent studies, end-tidal CO_2 has been used to predict the severity of acidosis in the pediatric population with DKA (Fearon & Steele, 2002). The treatment strategy for DKA is to start fluids, restart or adjust the insulin (inhibits ketone production), and correct potassium deficits. Bicarbonate therapy is needed only for pH < 7.1 and has been shown to be of particular use in DKA patients admitted with a pure hyperchloremic acidosis as opposed to a pure high AG acidosis (Adrogue *et al.*, 1982).

Alcoholic ketoacidosis Alcoholic ketoacidosis occurs in alcoholics who acutely stop drinking, develop nausea and vomiting, and then cease to eat. Glucose is typically low to normal (from starvation) and the acidosis is caused by elevated ketones, particularly β-hydroxybutyrate. Mild lactic acidosis and low insulin levels may be present with increased levels of triglyceride, cortisol, glucagon, and growth hormone (DuBose, 2003). Electrolyte abnormalities are also common. Patients with alcoholic ketoacidosis can also present with a metabolic alkalosis from vomiting or respiratory alkalosis from liver disease (Wrenn *et al.*, 1991) and may have hypoalbuminenia from liver disease that may further confound the acid–base evaluation. Treatment for alcoholic ketoacidosis is intravenous (i.v.) fluids with glucose (and concurrent thiamine to avoid precipitating Wernicke's encephalopathy) and the correction of deficits of potassium, magnesium, and phosphate. Watch for rhabdomyolysis that can occur secondary to the phosphate deficiency (and is exacerbated by glucose infusion).

High AG acidosis from ingested toxins

Salicylates Salicylate overdose in adults usually causes respiratory alkalosis (panting); a mixed metabolic acidosis–respiratory alkalosis, or less commonly, a pure high AG metabolic acidosis also can result (Farber *et al.*, 1949; Winters *et al.*, 1959). In the latter case, only part of the acidosis is due to the salicylates, most is due to increased lactic acid production. Treatment is by gastric lavage with isotonic saline (not

$NaHCO_3^-$), followed by activated charcoal. In a purely acidotic patient, consider i.v. $NaHCO_3^-$ to alkalinize the urine. Acetazolamide can be used if an alkaline diuresis cannot be achieved but HCO_3^- must be replaced adequately or a metabolic acidosis will ensue. Potassium and glucose must be replaced during treatment. Consider hemodialysis, if the patient has renal failure.

Alcohols

The two main alcohols that are causes of a high AG metabolic acidosis are ethylene glycol and methanol, both of which can cause respiratory depression and coma. If such intoxication is suspected by history, the osmolar gap can be used to identify the presence of extraneous osmolytes.

Osmolar gap: Plasma osmolality is normally determined by sodium, urea, and glucose and is calculated by:

$$P_{osm} = 2Na + \frac{Glu}{18} + \frac{BUN}{2.8}$$

[Glu and BUN in mg/dl]

The measured and calculated osmolality should agree within 10–15 mmol/kg H_2O.

If there is a discrepancy, serum sodium is spuriously low (hyperlipidemia or hyperproteinemia) or osmolytes other than sodium, urea, and glucose have accumulated in the plasma. Mannitol, radiocontrast media, isopropyl alcohol, ethylene glycol, ethanol, methanol, and acetone can all raise the osmolality.

Ethylene glycol, one of the principal ingredients in antifreeze, causes a high AG metabolic acidosis and severe CNS, heart, lung, and kidney damage when ingested. The increased osmolar gap results from ethylene glycol and its metabolites (oxalic, glycolic, and lactic acid) (Gabow *et al.*, 1986). Oxalate crystals will be found in the urine. Bicarbonate may be <5 meq/l (Burkhart & Kulig, 1990). Treatment should be instituted immediately (half-life of ethylene glycol is 3 h (Peterson *et al.*, 1981)) with saline or osmotic diuresis, thiamine and pyridoxine supplements, ethanol or fomepizole (both compete with ethylene glycol for metabolism by alcohol dehydrogenase), and hemodialysis.

Methanol (wood alcohol) ingestion can cause severe optic nerve ("snowfield" vision) and CNS damage in addition to the metabolic acidosis (Burkhart & Kulig, 1990). The increased osmolar gap is a result of its low molecular weight. Lactic acid and ketoacids are thought to contribute to the acidosis. Treatment is similar to that of ethylene glycol.

Decreased kidney function as a cause of high AG metabolic acidosis

Uremic acidosis is a disorder of advanced renal failure (moderate renal insufficiency leads to normal (hyperchloremic) metabolic acidosis). As renal disease progresses, diseased nephrons have a diminished capacity for filtration and reabsorption of organic anions. As nephrons die and the net number decreases, organic acids build up. Uremic acidosis is therefore characterized by a reduced rate of NH_4 production and excretion (Litzow *et al.*, 1967; Widmer *et al.*, 1979); the excess acid (up to 20 mmol/day), is buffered by alkaline salts from bone (Pellegrino & Biltz, 1965). As a result of the calcium carbonate buffering, the HCO_3^- rarely falls below 15 mmol/l and the AG rarely rises above 20 mmol/l. Treatment involves hemodialysis or oral alkali replacement to maintain the HCO_3^- between 20 and 24 mmol/l to prevent bone breakdown and to inhibit muscle catabolism. If patients are hypokalemic, add furosemide.

Non-AG (hyperchloremic) metabolic acidosis

Non-AG (normal or hyperchloremic) metabolic acidosis results from a loss of base (HCO_3^-), as opposed to the addition of acid as in the case of high AG metabolic acidosis. A non-AG metabolic acidosis occurs primarily through disturbances of the HCO_3^-, either through a primary loss of bicarbonate or a failure to replace bicarbonate stores (Reynolds, 1958; Schwartz *et al.*, 1959; Watten *et al.*, 1959; Goodman *et al.*, 1965; Halperin *et al.*, 1974; Widmer *et al.*, 1979; Arruda & Kurtzman, 1980; Batlle *et al.*, 1981; DuBose & Caflisch, 1985; Adrogue & Madias, 1998). Excess HCl is another mechanism that produces this condition. A loss of alkali in the system causes reciprocal changes in the HCO_3^- and Cl^- that result in a normal, non-elevated AG. The increased level of chloride (hyperchloremia) that results will approximate the value of the decrease in bicarbonate; the SID theory helps to explain this relationship and to explain the effectiveness of treating hyperchloremic acidosis with sodium bicarbonate (Constable, 2003). If this relationship is absent, a mixed disorder must be considered.

There are four main groups of causes of a non-AG metabolic acidosis: (1) GI, (2) renal diseases, (3) drugs, and (4) acid infusions.

GI

The primary GI cause of non-AG metabolic acidosis is diarrhea. Diarrheal stools contain a higher level of HCO_3^- than normal stools and are relatively chloride poor, so along with volume depletion, a metabolic acidosis develops (Watten *et al.*, 1959). The urine pH, however, is not acidic as expected with a systemic acidosis. The urine pH will be around 6 because the hypokalemia that develops with the metabolic acidosis as a result of intestinal losses increases the renal production and excretion of NH_4 that buffers the normally acidic urine.

To differentiate a non-AG metabolic acidosis due to GI losses from RTA, one must consider the urine NH_4 levels; urine NH_4 is high with diarrhea and low with RTA. Urinary NH_4 levels can be estimated by calculating the urine AG (UAG) (Batlle *et al.*, 1988).

UAG:

$$UAG = [Na^+ + K^+]urine - [Cl^-]urine$$

When $Cl > Na + K$, the urine ammonium level is appropriately increased which points to an extrarenal cause of the metabolic acidosis (DuBose, 2003).

Other causes of GI loss mediated non-AG metabolic acidosis include: surgical drainage of the intestinal tract, GI fistulas (secrete bicarbonate-rich fluid), or ureters that have been appended to the intestines.

Renal disease

Progressive renal disease leads to non-AG metabolic acidosis when the glomerular filtration rate (GFR) is 20–50 ml/min and then to AG metabolic acidosis (uremic acidosis) as the GFR falls below 20 ml/min. The renal tubular acidoses are a common cause of the non-AG metabolic acidosis (Reynolds, 1958; Schwartz *et al.*, 1959; Watten *et al.*, 1959; Goodman *et al.*, 1965; Halperin *et al.*, 1974; Widmer *et al.*, 1979; Arruda & Kurtzman, 1980; Batlle *et al.*, 1981; DuBose & Caflisch, 1985; Adrogue & Madias, 1998).

RTA (type 2) is caused by an excessive loss of HCO_3^- because of dysfunction of the proximal tubules; this produces glycosuria, animoaciduria, and phosphaturia (Fanconi syndrome). The urine pH is acidic ($pH > 5.5$). Do not treat with $NaHCO_3^-$ because it is not reabsorbed in the dysfunctional proximal tubule. Treatment is therefore very difficult.

RTA (types 1 and 4) affect the distal tubules and result in a metabolic acidosis as the kidney is unable to replace the HCO_3^- stores that are lost during fixed acid production. In type 1 ("classic distal") RTA, urine pH is high ($pH > 5.5$) because patients are unable to acidify their urine. In addition to a non-AG metabolic acidosis, findings include hypokalemia, positive UAG (low urine NH_4), hypocitraturia, and hypercalciuria. Type 4 includes hyperkalemia that is disproportionate to the GFR reduction and thought to be the mechanism supporting the ammonium excretion (Wall & Knepper, 1990), and a urine pH that is low because distal acidification is normal. Treatment for both includes bicarbonate and correction of potassium, if needed (Table 29.6). Hyporeninemic hypoaldosteronism will also cause non-AG metabolic acidosis in patients with renal dysfunction and will cause a hyperkalemic distal RTA by a mechanism of aldosterone resistance (Adrogue & Madias, 1998). Hyperkalemia and the acidosis will be out of proportion to the decrease in the GFR.

Table 29.6 Comparison of the renal tubular acidoses

Test	Proximal RTA	Classic distal RTA	Hyperkalemic distal RTA
Plasma [HCO_3^-]	14–18 meq/l	Variable	15–20 meq/l
Plasma [Cl^-]	Increased	Increased	Increased
Plasma [K^+]	Mild decrease	Mild to severe decrease	Mild to severe increase
Plasma AG	Normal	Normal	Normal
GFR	Normal or decreased	Normal or decreased	Normal or decreased
Urine pH during acidosis	≤ 5.5	>6.0	≤ 5.5
Urine pH after acid loading	≤ 5.5	>6.0	≤ 5.5
U–B PCO_2 in alkaline	Normal	Decreased	Decreased
Urine fractional excretion	>15%	<5%	<5%
Of HCO_3^- at normal P[HCO_3^-] and Tm HCO_3^-	Decreased	Normal	Normal
Nephrolithiasis	Absent	Present	Absent
Nephrocalcinosis	Absent	Present	Absent
Osteomalacia	Present	Present	Absent
Phosphaturia	Present	Absent	Absent
Aminoaciduria	Present	Absent	Absent
Alkali therapy	High dose	Low dose	Low dose

U–B PCO_2: difference between PCO_2 values in urine and arterial blood. (Reproduced with permission from Adrogue, H.J. & Madias, N.E. (1998). Arterial blood gas monitoring: acid–base assessment. In: Martin, J. & Tobin, M. (eds) *Principles and Practice of Intensive Care Monitoring*. McGraw Hill, Inc, New York; pp. 217–241.)
Tm HCO_3^-: maximum absorption of bicarbonate.

Drugs

Several drug types can incite a non-AG metabolic acidosis in patients with renal dysfunction: non-steroidal anti-inflammatory drugs (NSAIDs), trimethoprim, pentamidine, and angiotensin-converting enzyme (ACE) inhibitors. A hyperkalemic state will also be present. Inhalation of paint and glue, which contain toluene, can cause metabolic acidosis (Taher *et al.*, 1974; Carlisle *et al.*, 1991).

Acid infusion

Acid infusions, especially HCl, are occasionally given as treatment for patients with metabolic alkalosis (Wilson *et al.*, 1972; Harken *et al.*, 1975), particularly when prompt correction of the disturbance is imperative. Other agents that may be used are NH_4Cl and arginine monohydrochloride.

Parenteral nutrition with excess of cationic amino acids (usually the L-amino acid preparations) can lead to a metabolic acidosis (Heird *et al.*, 1972). The newer formulas that use protein solutions rather than the older protein hydrosylate formulations, are thought to be more beneficial (Gauthier & Szerlip, 2002). To minimize the possibility of metabolic acidosis, total parenteral nutrition (TPN) solutions should be buffered with acetate or other organic anions.

Metabolic alkalosis

Metabolic alkalosis is characterized by an elevated blood pH, an increase in HCO_3^-, and later, an augmentation of the P_aCO_2 secondary to hypoventilation. Rarely, it can be caused by a net gain in HCO_3^-, an unusual scenario because it would require a large continuous infusion of alkali to the body (milk-alkali syndrome or an alkali infusion in the face of renal insufficiency). More commonly, metabolic alkalosis is caused by a loss of non-volatile acid from the extracellular fluid (usually HCl via vomiting); it is usually accompanied by hypochloremia and hypokalemia. It can also be caused by hypermineralocorticoid states and severe potassium deficiency (Bleich *et al.*, 1966; Kassirer *et al.*, 1970) (Table 29.7).

Table 29.7 Causes of metabolic alkalosis

Chloride responsive	Chloride resistant
GI Cl^- losses	*Mineralocorticoid excess*
Vomiting	Primary aldosteronism
Nasogastric suction	Cushing syndrome
Villous adenoma of the colon	Adrenocorticotropic hormone (ACTH)-secreting tumor
Congenital choridorrhea	Adrenogenital syndromes
Renal Cl^- losses	Renovascular disease
Loop diuretics	Accelerated hypertension
Furosemide	Renin-secreting tumors
Bumetanide	*Drugs*
Ethacrynic acid	Fludrocortisone
Organomercurials	Corticosterone
Early distal diuretics	Prednisone
Thiazides	Prednisolone
Metolazone	Cortisone, hydorcortisone
Methylprednisolone	Licorice
Indapamide	
Post-hypercapnic state	*Miscellaneous conditions*
Poorly reabsorbed anions	Bartter syndrome
Bartter syndrome	Gitelman syndrome
Gitelman syndrome	Liddle syndrome
Alkali administration	Severe K^+ depletion
$NaHCO_3$	Milk-alkali syndrome
Organic anions	
Citrate, lactate, acetate	

Reproduced with permission from Adrogue, H.J. & Madias, N.E. (1998). Arterial blood gas monitoring: acid–base assessment. In: Martin, J. & Tobin, M. (eds) *Principles and Practice of Intensive Care Monitoring*. McGraw Hill, Inc, New York; pp. 217–241.

The development of a metabolic alkalosis involves two stages. In the first stage, a loss of acid invokes the alkalosis. In the second stage, the alkalosis can continue if the kidneys are unable to compensate by excreting the excess HCO_3^- due to volume contraction, a low GFR, or because of hypochloremia or hypokalemia (Madias *et al.*, 1980; DuBose, 2003).

The above tetrad increases distal tubule H^+ secretion and can be treated with NaCl or KCl. However, if the hypokalemia is due to autonomous hypoaldosteronism, the alkalosis must be repaired surgically or pharmacologically (Melby, 1984).

The secondary compensation response to metabolic alkalosis is hypoventilation that serves to retain CO_2 (hypercapnia) and decrease the pH back to baseline (Bone *et al.*, 1974).

Alkali administration

An increased alkali load in a patient with normal kidney function will not typically cause a metabolic alkalosis. Bicarbonate given in the operating room will generally increase the end-tidal CO_2 to balance the infusion. If there are hemodynamic disturbances, however, alkali excretion may be slowed. Watch patients with oral or parenteral citrate loads (transfusions), parenteral hyperalimentation, or exchange resins (polystyrene sulfonate and aluminum hydroxide).

Diagnosis

Capnographic findings, with normal cardiac output and perfusion, will show an increased CO_2 in the non-mechanically ventilated patient and increased P_aCO_2. It is useful to assess the patient's extracellular fluid volume (ECFV) and blood pressure to establish the cause for the metabolic alkalosis. Urine electrolytes are also helpful. Additionally, it may be useful to categorize metabolic alkalosis into those that are chloride sensitive (responsive to NaCl) and those that are chloride resistant (not responsive to NaCl) (Table 29.7).

Chloride sensitive alkalosis

In this type of metabolic alkalosis, chloride depletion is the key factor in the pathogenesis (Schwartz *et al.*, 1961; DeGraeff *et al.*, 1964; Cannon *et al.*, 1965; Kassirer *et al.*, 1965; Wallace *et al.*, 1968; Kassirer *et al.*, 1970; Luke & Galla, 1983; Rosen *et al.*, 1988). Urine chloride excretion is decreased with a urine chloride concentration of <10 meq/l (normal is 10–20 meq/l); disorders that are chloride sensitive are typically characterized by low fluid volume. The paucity of chloride causes a reabsorption of sodium that results in excretion of hydrogen ions and increased production of bicarbonate, which worsens the alkalosis. By treating this disorder with NaCl, the alkalotic cycle can be broken because bicarbonate excretion will be increased.

GI disorders

The chloride sensitive alkaloses include several GI disorders (vomiting, gastric drainage, villous adenoma of the colon, and chloride-rich diarrhea). Basically, as hydrogen ions are lost through inappropriate GI motion, bicarbonate is retained. The loss of fluid and NaCl in vomitus or nasogastric suction will cause volume contraction that will invoke the renin/aldosterone system. The GFR will be reduced and HCO_3^- will be reabsorbed. Chloride is depleted in this process when the HCO_3^- is continually added to plasma in exchange for chloride. The kidney will then conserve chloride. Treat these disorders with fluids for volume expansion, give NaCl, and repair any potassium depletions.

Drugs

Certain diuretics, specifically the thiazides and loops, can cause a chloride sensitive alkalosis; ethacrynic acid in particular causes a contraction alkalosis (Cannon *et al.*, 1965). These two classes induce a chloruresis while causing an acute reduction in ECFV. Chronic use of these drugs will cause a metabolic alkalosis by increasing distal tubule salt recovery thereby forcing an increased secretion of hydrogen ions and potassium (DuBose, 2003). Secondary hypoaldosterism also results. Isotonic saline will correct the deficit.

Large doses of penicillin or carbenicillin contain non-reabsorbable anions that can increase distal tubule acidification and potassium loss through a trans-epithelial potential difference.

Other causes

Chloride sensitive alkalosis has several other causes. Magnesium deficiency results in hypokalemic alkalosis by renal distal tubule acidification with increased action of the rennin/aldosterone system. Hypokalemia causes alkalosis by increasing potassium reabsorption at the expense of hydrogen ions – give potassium to correct. After lactic or ketoacidosis, the acids that caused the original acidosis are metabolized to bicarbonate. Subsequent to a hypercapnic episode, a surplus of HCO_3^- exists in much the same manner as with other post-acidotic episodes. Correct chloride and the alkalosis should subside. Cystic fibrosis, milk-alkali syndrome (McMillan & Freeman, 1965), and excessive skin loss of NaCl can cause a metabolic alkalosis. Treatment with acid is not useful; treat the underlying disorder and use sodium or potassium salts.

Chloride resistant alkalosis

A normal level of chloride excretion characterizes this type of metabolic alkalosis (McMillan & Freeman, 1965; Kassirer & Schwartz, 1966; Gill & Bartter, 1978; Dunn, 1981; Melby, 1984; Rosen *et al.*, 1988). Urine chloride concentration is >20 meq/l. This type of alkalosis includes several mineralocorticoid disorders (hyperaldosteronism, Cushing syndrome, licorice intake, Bartter syndrome) and profound hyperkalemia. The increased aldosterone will increase acid excretion leading to alkalosis, particularly with hypokalemia (Kassirer *et al.*, 1970). Excess salts will cause the ECVF to expand causing hypertension. The effects of aldosterone resulting in polydipsia, polyuria, and hypo-osmolar urine will continue to increase potassium excretion. The underlying disorder must be treated to relieve these metabolic alkaloses, as they are chloride independent, sodium or potassium salts will not be useful.

Useful hints

A patient with a high HCO_3^- and a low chloride has either metabolic alkalosis or a chronic respiratory acidosis. Remember that the pH will establish the difference between these two options: high pH with metabolic alkalosis and low pH with the chronic respiratory acidosis.

A patient with alkalosis and chronic hypokalemia suggests mineralocorticoid excess or diuretic use in a hypertensive patient. Low plasma rennin activity and normal chloride in a patient who is not taking diuretic medication indicates a primary mineralocorticoid disturbance. Alkalosis and hypokalemia in a normotensive, non-edematous patient suggests Bartter's syndrome, Gitelman's syndrome, magnesium deficiency, or vomiting. Determine urine electrolytes. Alkaline urine with increased sodium suggests vomiting or alkali ingestion. Acidic urine with low sodium, potassium, and chloride can suggest vomiting, a post-hypercapnic state, or prior diuretic ingestion. If urine sodium, potassium, or chloride are not decreased, magnesium level, Bartter's or Gitelman's syndrome, or current diuretic ingestion should be considered (DuBose, 2003).

Respiratory acidosis

Respiratory acidosis is an acid–base disorder where the primary disturbance is invoked by an increase in the blood CO_2 tension. It is diagnosed by an increase in the P_aCO_2 and a decrease in the blood pH. The secondary compensation response is an increase in HCO_3^- (McFadden & Lyons, 1968; Avery *et al.*, 1970; Madias & Adrogue, 1983; Madias *et al.*, 1985). Acutely, the small increase in HCO_3^- is due to the body's non-HCO_3^- buffers, which promotes movement of bicarbonate to the interstitial fluid from the intravascular compartment. This will cause a small decrease in the standard bicarbonate and a somewhat larger decrease in the blood BE (Adrogue & Madias, 1998). Chronically, renal adaptations lead to much larger increases in HCO_3^- with a parallel increase in standard bicarbonate and blood BE (Adrogue & Madias, 1998). Renal acidification processes responding to hypercapnia require 3–5 days to perform maximally (Adrogue & Madias, 1998). Additionally, hypochloremia is a common finding with respiratory acidosis due to the chloride shift into RBCs as well as renal losses from the secondary response (Schwartz *et al.*, 1961; Adrogue and Madias, 1998).

Using the compensation equations, it can be determined that in the case of an acute respiratory acidosis, the HCO_3^- will increase 1 mmol/l for every 10 mmHg increase in the P_aCO_2. With a chronic (>24 h duration) respiratory acidosis, renal compensation increases the HCO_3^- at 4 mmol/l for every 10 mmHg increase in P_aCO_2. Serum HCO_3^- typically will not increase above 38 mmol/l.

Diagnosis

To diagnose a respiratory acidosis, perform ABG and electrolyte analysis. History and physical examination should suggest the cause. Non-pulmonary parameters to be assessed include a detailed drug history, hematocrit, upper airway assessment, chest wall rigidity/trauma, and neuromuscular function. Capnographic findings should demonstrate a high end-tidal CO_2 and a high P_aCO_2.

Clinically respiratory acidosis manifests with symptoms that vary according to the severity and duration of the acidosis, the underlying disease, and whether there is an accompanying hypoxemia. Acute increases in P_aCO_2 can cause anxiety, dyspnea, confusion, psychosis, hallucinations, and coma (Table 29.8). Chronic increases in P_aCO_2 cause sleep disturbances, memory loss, daytime somnolence, personality changes, coordination impairment, and motor dysfunctions such as tremor, myoclonic jerks, and asterixis (Table 29.9). Increased P_aCO_2 may mimic the signs and symptoms of increased intracranial pressure with headaches, papilledema, abnormal reflexes, focal muscle weakness; each of these symptoms is due to vasoconstriction secondary to loss of the vasodilatory effects of CO_2 (DuBose, 2003).

Causes

There are several causes of primary respiratory acidosis: (1) central, (2) airway, (3) parenchyma, (4) neuromuscular, and (5) miscellaneous (See Tables 29.8 and 29.9).

Central causes

Central causes of respiratory acidosis include drugs, such as anesthetics, alcohol, morphine, and sedatives. The main mechanism is through the depression of the neural respiratory center (medullary chemoreceptors) that lead to shallow breathing and CO_2 trapping. Strokes and infections, such as encephalitis, can also lead to respiratory acidosis through this mechanism.

Airway causes

Several types of airway disturbances can lead to respiratory acidosis. Acute obstruction by foreign body or secretions (pulmonary edema (Avery *et al.*, 1970)), and asthma can compromise normal breathing and lead to a respiratory acidosis; status asthmaticus may cause metabolic acidosis or respiratory alkalosis (Roncoroni *et al.*, 1976). Generalized bronchospasm due to anaphylaxsis, inhalational burn, or toxin ingestion will also lead to respiratory acidosis.

Parenchymal causes

Emphysema, pneumoconiosis, and bronchitis will cause a chronic respiratory acidosis as a result of air trapping. Restrictive disorders will lead to a respiratory acidosis because of the high metabolic cost of breathing against stiff lungs and/or chest wall.

Table 29.8 Causes of acute respiratory acidosis

Normal airways and lungs	Abnormal airways and lungs
CNS depression	*Upper airways obstruction*
General anesthesia	Coma induced
Sedative overdose	Aspiration/foreign body
Head trauma	Laryngospasm
Cerebrovascular accident	Angioedema
Central sleep apnea	Obstructive sleep apnea
Cerebral edema	Inadequate intubation
Brain tumor	*Lower airways obstruction*
Encephalitis	Generalized bronchospasm
Neuromuscular impairment	Severe asthma/status asthmaticus
High spinal cord injury	Bronchiolitis
Guillain–Barre syndrome	*Alveolar obstruction*
Status epilepticus	Severe pneumonia or ARDS
Botulism	Severe pulmonary edema
Myasthenic crisis	*Pulmonary perfusion defect*
Hypokalemic myopathy	Cardiac arrest
Familial periodic paralysis	Severe circulatory failure
Drugs/toxins (curare, succinylcholine, organophosphates, aminoglycosides)	Massive pulmonary embolus
Ventilatory restriction	Fat/air embolism
Rib fractures with flail chest	
Pneumothorax	
Hemothorax	
Impaired diaphragmatic function (ascites, etc.)	
Iatrogenic events	
Misplaced/displaced airway	
Inappropriate mechanical ventilation	

Reproduced with permission from Adrogue, H.J. & Madias, N.E. (1998). Arterial blood gas monitoring: acid–base assessment. In: Martin, J. & Tobin, M. (eds) *Principles and Practice of Intensive Care Monitoring*. McGraw Hill, Inc, New York; pp. 217–241.

Neuromuscular causes

Abnormalities or disease in the motor neurons, neuromuscular junction, and skeletal muscle can cause hypoventilation via respiratory muscle fatigue. Mechanical ventilation may cause respiratory acidosis if it is incorrectly supervised/monitored, if sudden CO_2 production arises (because of fever, agitation, sepsis, or overfeeding) or if pulmonary function suddenly worsens and alveolar ventilation declines.

Miscellaneous causes

High levels of positive end-expiratory pressure (PEEP) in the presence of reduced cardiac output can cause hypercapnia as a result of increases in alveolar dead space. Permissive hypercapnia is being used with increasing frequency because of studies suggesting lower mortality than with conventional mechanical ventilation, especially with severe CNS or heart disease. Although the potential benefits of permissive hypercapnia may be mitigated by correction of the academia, it is prudent to keep the pH in the range of 7.2–7.3 by administering $NaHCO_3^-$ (DuBose, 2003).

Treatment

Acute respiratory acidosis

Acute respiratory acidosis can be life threatening in many cases and measures to reverse the underlying cause should be taken simultaneously with steps to ensure proper ventilation. Tracheal intubation and mechanical ventilation may be required. Care should be taken with oxygen administration in patients with underlying COPD and chronic CO_2 retention, as the respiratory drive for these patients is based on a higher level of CO_2 than the average, healthy patient. Additionally, rapid correction of hypercapnia can cause cardiac arrhythmias, reduced cerebral perfusion, and seizures.

Table 29.9 Causes of chronic respiratory acidosis

Normal airways and lungs
CNS depression
Sedative overdose
Methadone/heroin addiction
Primary alveolar hypoventilation
Obesity–hypoventilation syndrome (Pickwickian syndrome)
Brain tumor
Bulbar poliomyelitis
Neuromuscular impairment
Poliomyelitis
Multiple sclerosis
Muscular dystrophy
Amyotrophic lateral sclerosis
Diaphragmatic paralysis
Myxedema
Myopathic disease (polymyositis)
Ventilatory restriction
Kyphoscoliosis, spinal arthritis
Obesity
Fibrothorax
Hydrothorax
Abnormal airways and lungs
Upper airways obstruction
Tonsillar and peritonsillar hypertrophy
Paralysis of vocal cords
Tumor of the vocal cords or pharynx
Airways stenosis after prolonged intubation
Thymoma, aortic aneurysm
Lower airways obstruction
COPD (bronchitis, bronchiolitis, emphysema, bronchiectasis)
Disorders involving alveoli
Severe chronic pneumonitis
Diffuse infiltrative disease (alveolar proteinosis)
Interstitial fibrosis

Reproduced with permission from Adrogue, H.J. & Madias, N.E. (1998). Arterial blood gas monitoring: acid–base assessment. In: Martin, J. & Tobin, M. (eds) *Principles and Practice of Intensive Care Monitoring*. McGraw Hill, Inc, New York; pp. 217–241.

Chronic respiratory acidosis

This condition can be difficult to correct, but measures can be taken to improve the underlying lung function. The P_aCO_2 should be lowered gradually in these patients, with a goal of restoring P_aCO_2 to baseline levels and to provide sufficient potassium and chloride to enhance the renal excretion of HCO_3^-.

Respiratory alkalosis

Respiratory alkalosis is an acid–base disorder marked by an elevated pH and a decreased P_aCO_2. It evolves from hyperventilation, which lowers the P_aCO_2 and increases the ratio of HCO_3^- to P_aCO_2, thereby increasing the pH; the hydrogen ion concentration falls because of the reduction of H_2CO_3 in the body (Gennari & Kassirer, 1982; Valtin, 1987b; Adrogue & Tobin, 1997). Acutely, non-bicarbonate cellular buffers, through non-renal mechanisms, respond by consuming HCO_3^- (Kety & Schmidt, 1946; Kazemi *et al.*, 1967; Arbus *et al.*, 1969; Gledhill *et al.*, 1975); this adaptation takes 5–10 min.

Hypocapnia sustained longer than 2–6 h is further compensated by a decrease in renal ammonium and titratable acid excretion and a reduction in filtered HCO_3^- reabsorption. Renal adaptation to respiratory alkalosis takes several days (2–3) with normal volume status and normal kidney function (Manfredi, 1967; Gennari *et al.*, 1972; Gougoux *et al.*, 1975; Cohen *et al.*,1976; Madias *et al.*, 1990; Krapf *et al.*, 1991). The reduction in bicarbonate with chronic respiratory alkalosis is accompanied by a parallel decrease in the standard bicarbonate and in blood BE; these changes are not observed in acute respiratory alkalosis (Adrogue & Madias, 1998).

In chronic respiratory alkalosis, each 1 mmHg fall in P_aCO_2 causes a .4–5 mmol/l decrease in the HCO_3^- and a .3 mmol/l decrease in the hydrogen ion concentration (.003 rise in the pH). Additionally, plasma chloride will be increased in chronic respiratory alkalosis to offset the decrease in HCO_3^- (Adrogue & Madias, 1998).

Signs and symptoms

Symptoms of respiratory alkalosis relate primarily to the underlying disease. Typically with a rapid decrease in the P_aCO_2, decreased cerebral blood flow can result in dizziness, confusion, and seizures, even without hypoxemia. The cardiovascular effects of respiratory alkalosis in a conscious patient are minimal. In the anesthetized or mechanically ventilated patient, however, cardiac output and blood pressure may fall as a result of the effects of anesthesia and PEEP on heart rate, systemic resistance, and venous return. Arrhythmias may occur in patients with heart disease as a result of changes in oxygen unloading by blood from a left shift in the hemoglobin–oxygen dissociation curve (Bohr effect). Acute respiratory alkalosis causes intracellular shifts of sodium, potassium, and phosphate and reduces free calcium ion 2+ concentration by increasing the protein-bound fraction. Hypocapnia-induced hypokalemia is minor (DuBose, 2003). Capnographic findings will show a reduced end-tidal CO_2 and a reduced P_aCO_2 (Table 29.10).

Causes

Respiratory alkalosis is the most common acid–base disturbance in critically ill patients. If the alkalosis is

Table 29.10 Comparison of acute and chronic respiratory acidosis and alkalosis

Condition	P_aCO_2 (mmHg)	$[HCO_3]$ (meq/l)	$[H^+]$ (neq/l)	pH	$[Na^+]$ (meq/l)	$[Cl^-]$ (meq/l)	AG (meq/l)
Normal	40	24	40	7.40	140	104	12
Respiratory acidosis							
Acute	60	26	55	7.26	141	104	11
Chronic	60	29	50	7.30	140	99	12
Respiratory alkalosis							
Acute	20	20	24	7.62	138	104	14
Chronic	20	16	30	7.52	140	111	14

Reproduced with permission from Adrogue, H.J. & Madias, N.E. (1998). Arterial blood gas monitoring: acid–base assessment. In: Martin, J. & Tobin, M. (eds) *Principles and Practice of Intensive Care Monitoring*. McGraw Hill, Inc, New York; pp. 217–241.

severe, prognosis tends to be poor. Respiratory alkalosis is common in mechanically ventilated patients, as well as being a frequent finding in early to moderate heart failure and in the early stages of respiratory failure. Common causes of respiratory alkalosis include CNS stimulation, hypoxemia, drugs/hormones, stimulation of chest receptors, and miscellaneous origins (Table 29.11).

Hyperventilation syndrome

Hyperventilation syndrome occurs as a result of many underlying causes, including episodes of acute anxiety. It includes many neurologic symptoms: paresthesias, circumoral numbness, chest wall tightness or pain, dizziness, inability to take adequate breaths, and tetany. These symptoms themselves may be sufficiently stressful to perpetuate the disorder. ABG demonstrates an acute or chronic respiratory alkalosis with P_aCO_2 in the range of 15–30 mmHg and no hypoxemia.

CNS stimulation

Hyperventilation can be invoked by such stimuli as pain, fear, anxiety, or psychosis and can lead to respiratory alkalosis if the stimulus is prolonged. Cerebrovascular insult or infection, tumor, or trauma can initiate similar responses. Different patterns of hyperventilation may be produced with P_aCO_2 at 20–30 mmHg.

Hypoxemia or tissue hypoxia

Hypoxic states can arise from a variety of causes from high altitudes (Lenfant & Sullivan, 1971). Lifelong residents of high altitude have almost complete pH compensation (Gledhill *et al.*, 1975). Pneumonia, anemia, and asthma (McFadden & Lyons, 1968; Roncoroni *et al.*, 1976) are also causes of respiratory alkalosis.

Drugs or hormones

Salicylates are the most common cause of drug-induced respiratory alkalosis (Farber *et al.*, 1949;

Table 29.11 Causes of respiratory alkalosis

Hypoxemia or tissue hypoxia
Decreased inspired oxygen tension
High altitude
Pneumonia
Aspiration/foreign body
Laryngospasm
Drowning
Cyanotic heart disease
Severe anemia
Left shift of HbO_2 curve
Hypotension
Severe circulatory failure
Pulmonary edema

Stimulation of chest receptors
Pneumonia
Asthma
Pneumothorax
Hemothorax
Flail chest
ARDS
Cardiac failure
Non-cardiogenic pulmonary edema
Pulmonary embolism
Pulmonary fibrosis

CNS stimulation
Voluntary
Pain/anxiety/psychosis
Fever
Subarachnoid hemorrhage
Cerebrovascular accident
Meningoencephalitis
Tumor
Trauma

Drugs or hormones
Nikethamide, ethamivan
Doxapram
Xanthines
Salicylates
Catecholamines
Angiotensin II
Vasopressors
Progesterone
Medroxyprogesterone
Dinitrophenol
Nicotine

Miscellaneous
Pregnancy
Gram-positive septicemia
Gram-negative septicemia
Hepatic failure
Mechanical hyperventilation
Heat exposure

Reproduced with permission from Adrogue, H.J. & Madias, N.E. (1998). Arterial blood gas monitoring: acid–base assessment. In: Martin, J. & Tobin, M. (eds) *Principles and Practice of Intensive Care Monitoring*. McGraw Hill, Inc, New York; pp. 217–241.

Winters *et al.*, 1959) because they directly stimulate the medullary chemoreceptors. Methylxanthines, theophylline, and aminophylline stimulate ventilation and increase the ventilatory response to CO_2. Increased progesterone levels in pregnancy lead to a respiratory alkalosis through the hormonal induction of increased ventilation (arterial P_aCO_2 is lowered by as much as 5–10 mmHg).

Stimulation of chest receptors

Hemothorax, flail chest, cardiac failure, pulmonary embolism can incite a respiratory alkalosis.

Miscellaneous

Respiratory alkalosis is a common finding of hepatic failure with the severity of failure correlating with the severity of the alkalosis (Tyor & Sieker, 1959; Prytz *et al.*, 1976; DuBose, 2003). It is also an early finding in Gram-negative septicemia (prior to the development of fever, hypoxemia, or hypotension) (Simmons *et al.*, 1960), and in the pure form associated with a good prognosis (Blair, 1971).

Treatment

Management of respiratory alkalosis involves efforts to treat the underlying disorder. Beta-blockers may ameliorate the peripheral manifestations of a hyperadrenergic state.

References

Aberman, A. & Fulop, M. (1972). The metabolic and respiratory acidosis of acute pulmonary edema. *Ann. Intern. Med.*, **76**: 173–184.

Adrogue, H.J. & Madias, N.E. (1998). Arterial blood gas monitoring: acid–base assessment. In: Martin, J. & Tobin, M. (eds) *Principles and Practice of Intensive Care Monitoring*. McGraw Hill, Inc, New York; pp. 217–241.

Adrogue, H.J. & Tobin, M.J. (1997). Clinical picture of respiratory failure. In: Adrogue, H.J. & Tobin, M.J. (eds) *Blackwell's Basics of Medicine.* Blackwell Scientific, Boston; pp. 213–308.

Adrogue, H.J. & Wesson, D.E. (1994). Introductory concepts. In: Adrogue, H.J. & Wesson, D.E. (eds) *Blackwell's Basics of Medicine, Vol. 1: Acid–base*. Blackwell, Boston; pp. 1–47.

Adrogue, H.J., Rashad, M.N., Gorin, A.B., Yacoub, J. & Madias, NE. (1989a). Arteriovenous acid–base disparity in circulatory failure: studies on mechanism. *Am. J. Physiol.*, **257**: F1087–F1093.

Adrogue, H.J., Rashad, M.N., Gorin, A.B., Yacoub, J. & Madias, N.E. (1989b). Assessing acid–base status in circulatory failure. Differences between arterial and central venous blood. *New Engl. J. Med.*, **320**: 1312–1316.

Adrogue, H.J., Wilson, H., Boyd III, A.E., Suki, W.N. & Eknoyan, G. (1982). Plasma acid–base patterns in diabetic ketoacidosis. *New Engl. J. Med.*, **307**: 1603–1610.

Aduen, J., Bernstein, W.K. & Miller, J., *et al.* (1995). Relationship between blood lactate concentrations and ionized calcium, glucose, and acid–base status in critically ill and noncritically ill patients. *Crit. Care Med.*, **23**: 246–252.

Arbus, G.S., Herbert, L.A., Levesque, P.R., Etsten, B.E. & Schwartz, W.B. (1969). Characterization and clinical application of the "significance band" for acute respiratory alkalosis. *New Engl. J. Med.*, **280**: 117–123.

Arieff, A.I., Leach, W., Park, R. & Lazarowitz, V.C. (1982). Systemic effects of $NaHCO_3$ in experimental lactic acidosis in dogs. *Am. J. Physiol.*, **242**: F586–F591.

Arruda, J.A. & Kurtzman, N.A. (1980). Mechanisms and classification of deranged distal urinary acidification. *Am. J. Physiol.*, **239**: F515–F523.

Asch, M.J., Dell, R.B., Williams, G.S., Cohen, M. & Winters, RW. (1969). Time course for development of respiratory compensation in metabolic acidosis. *J. Lab. Clin. Med.*, **73**: 610–615.

Atchley, D., Loeb, R.F., Richards, D.W., Benedict, E.M. & Driscoll, M.E. (1933). On diabetic acidosis: a detailed study of electrolyte balances following the withdrawal and reestablishment of insulin therapy. *J. Clin. Invest.*, **12**: 297–326.

Avery, W.G., Samet, P. & Sackner, M.A. (1970). The acidosis of pulmonary edema. *Am. J. Med.*, **48**: 320–324.

Bakker, J., Vincent, J.L., Gris, P., Leon, M., Coffernils, M. & Kahn, R.J. (1992). Veno-arterial carbon dioxide gradient in human septic shock. *Chest*, **101**: 509–515.

Balasubramanyan, N., Havens, P.L. & Hoffman, G.M. (1999). Unmeasured anions identified by the Fencl–Stewart method predict mortality better than base excess, anion gap, and lactate in patients in the pediatric intensive care unit. *Crit. Care Med.*, **27**: 1577–1581.

Batlle, D.C., Arruda, J.A. & Kurtzman, N.A. (1981). Hyperkalemic distal renal tubular acidosis associated with obstructive uropathy. *New Engl. J. Med.*, **304**: 373–380.

Batlle, D.C., Hizon, M., Cohen, E., Gutterman, C. & Gupta, R. (1988). The use of the urinary anion gap in the diagnosis of hyperchloremic metabolic acidosis. *New Engl. J. Med.*, **318**: 594–599.

Benjamin, E., Paluch, T.A., Berger, S.R., Premus, G., Wu, C. & Iberti, T.J. (1987). Venous hypercarbia in canine hemorrhagic shock. *Crit. Care Med.*, **15**: 516–518.

Blair, E. (1971). Acid–base balance in bacteremic shock. *Arch. Intern. Med.*, **127**: 731–739.

Bleich, H.L., Tannen, R.L. & Schwartz, W.B. (1966). The induction of metabolic alkalosis by correction of potassium deficiency. *J. Clin. Invest.*, **45**: 573–579.

Bloom, S.A., Canzanello, V.J., Strom, J.A. & Madias, N.E. (1985). Spurious assessment of acid–base status due to dilutional effect of heparin. *Am. J. Med.*, **79**: 528–530.

Bone, J.M., Cowie, J., Lambie, A.T. & Robson, J.S. (1974). The relationship between arterial pCO_2 and hydrogen ion concentration in chronic metabolic acidosis and alkalosis. *Clin. Sci. Mol. Med.*, **46**: 113–123.

Brackett Jr, N.C. (1974). An approach to clinical disorders of acid–base balance. *South. Med. J.*, **67**: 1084–1101.

Brackett, N., Cohen, J.J. & Schwartz, W.B. (1965). Carbon dioxide titration curve of normal man. *New Engl. J. Med.*, **272**: 6–12.

Burkhart, K.K. & Kulig, K.W. (1990). The other alcohols. Methanol, ethylene glycol, and isopropanol. *Emerg. Med. Clin. North Am.*, **8**: 913–928.

Cannon, P., Heinemann, H.O., Albert, M.S., Laragh, J.H. & Winters, R.W. (1965). "Contraction" alkalosis after diuresis of edematous patients with ethacrynic acid. *Ann. Intern. Med.*, **62**: 979–990.

Carlisle, E.J., Donnelly, S.M., Vasuvattakul, S., Kamel, K.S., Tobe, S. & Halperin, M.L. (1991). Glue-sniffing and distal renal tubular acidosis: sticking to the facts. *J. Am. Soc. Nephrol.*, **1**: 1019–1027.

Carrier, O., Cowsert, M., Hancock, J. & Guyton, A.C. (1964). Effect of hydrogen ion on vascular resistance in isolated artery segments. *Am. J. Physiol.*, **207**: 168–172.

Cohen, J.J. & Schwartz, W.B. (1966). Evaluation of acid–base equilibrium in pulmonary insufficiency. An approach to a diagnostic dilemma. *Am. J. Med.*, **41**: 163–167.

Cohen, J.J., Madias, N.E., Wolf, C.J. & Schwartz, W.B. (1976). Regulation of acid–base equilibrium in chronic hypocapnia. Evidence that the response of the kidney is not geared to the defense of extracellular (H^+). *J. Clin. Invest.*, **57**: 1483–1489.

Constable, P.D. (2003). Hyperchloremic acidosis: the classic example of strong ion acidosis. *Anesth. Analg.*, **96**: 919–922.

Cooper, D.J., Walley, K.R., Wiggs, B.R. & Russell, J.A. (1990). Bicarbonate does not improve hemodynamics in critically ill patients who have lactic acidosis. A prospective, controlled clinical study. *Ann. Intern. Med.*, **112**: 492–498.

De Troyer, A., Stolarczyk, A., De Beyl, D.Z. & Stryckmans, P. (1977). Value of anion-gap determination in multiple myeloma. *New Engl. J. Med.*, **296**: 858–860.

DeGraeff, J., Struyvenberg, A. & Lameijer, L.D.F. (1964). The role of chloride in hypokalemic alkalosis. *Am. J. Med.*, **37**: 778–788.

DuBose Jr, T.D. (2003). *Acidosis and Alkalosis*. Harrisons Online: McGraw Hill, Inc.

DuBose Jr, T.D. & Caflisch, C.R. (1985). Validation of the difference in urine and blood carbon dioxide tension during bicarbonate loading as an index of distal nephron acidification in experimental models of distal renal tubular acidosis. *J. Clin. Invest.*, **75**: 1116–1123.

Dunn, M.J. (1981). Prostaglandins and Bartter's syndrome. *Kidney Int.*, **19**: 86–102.

Emmett, M. & Narins, R.G. (1977). Clinical use of the anion gap. *Medicine (Baltimore)*, **56**: 38–54.

Farber, H., Yiengst, M.J. & Shock, N.W. (1949). The effect of therapeutic doses of aspirin on the acid–base balance of the blood in normal adults. *Am. J. Sci.*, **217**: 256–262.

Fearon, D.M. & Steele, D.W. (2002). End-tidal carbon dioxide predicts the presence and severity of acidosis in children with diabetes. *Acad. Emerg. Med.*, **9**: 1373–1378.

Feibusch, K.C., Breaden, R.S., Bader, C.D. & Gomperts, S.N. (1998). *Prescription for the Boards: USMLE Step 2*, 2nd edition. Lippincott-Raven, Philadelphia.

Figge, J., Mydosh, T. & Fencl, V. (1992). Serum proteins and acid–base equilibria: a follow-up. *J. Lab. Clin. Med.*, **120**: 713–719.

Flenley, D.C. (1971). Another non-logarithmic acid–base diagram? *Lancet*, **1**: 961–965.

Fraley, D.S., Adler, S., Bruns, F.J. & Zett, B. (1980). Stimulation of lactate production by administration of bicarbonate in a patient with a solid neoplasm and lactic acidosis. *New Engl. J. Med.*, **303**: 1100–1102.

Fulop, M. (1997). A guide for predicting arterial CO_2 tension in metabolic acidosis. *Am. J. Nephrol.*, **17**: 421–424.

Gabow, P.A. (1985). Disorders associated with an altered anion gap. *Kidney Int.*, **27**: 472–483.

Gabow, P.A., Clay, K., Sullivan, J.B. & Lepoff, R. (1986). Organic acids in ethylene glycol intoxication. *Ann. Intern. Med.*, **105**: 16–20.

Garella, S., Dana, C.L. & Chazan, J.A. (1973). Severity of metabolic acidosis as a determinant of bicarbonate requirements. *New Engl. J. Med.*, **289**: 121–126.

Gauthier, P.M. & Szerlip, H.M. (2002). Metabolic acidosis in the intensive care unit. *Crit. Care Clin.*, **18**: 289–308, vi.

Gennari, F. & Kassirer, J.P. (1982). Respiratory alkalosis. In: Cohen, J.J. (ed.) *Acid–Base*. Little, Brown, Boston; pp. 349–376.

Gennari, J., Cohen, J.J. & Kassirer, J.P. (1982a). Normal acid–base values. In: Cohen, J.J. (ed.) *Acid–Base*. Little, Brown, Boston; pp. 107–110.

Gennari, J.F., Cohen, J.J. & Kassirer, J.P. (1982b). Measurement of acid–base status. In: Cohen, J.J. (ed.) *Acid–Base*. Little, Brown, Boston; pp. 97–106.

Gennari, F.J., Goldstein, M.B. & Schwartz, W.B. (1972). The nature of the renal adaptation to chronic hypocapnia. *J. Clin. Invest.*, **51**: 1722–1730.

Giebisch, G., Berger, L. & Pitts, R.F. (1955). The extrarenal response to acute acid–base disturbances of respiratory origin. *J. Clin. Invest.*, **34**: 231–245.

Gill Jr, J.R. & Bartter, F.C. (1978). Evidence for a prostaglandin-independent defect in chloride reabsorption in the loop of Henle as a proximal cause of Bartter's syndrome. *Am. J. Med.*, **65**: 766–772.

Gledhill, N., Beirne, G.J. & Dempsey, J.A. (1975). Renal response to short-term hypocapnia in man. *Kidney Int.*, **8**: 376–384.

Goodman, D., Lemann, J., Lennon, E.J. & Relman, A.S. (1965). Production, excretion, and net balance of fixed acid in patients with renal acidosis. *J. Clin. Invest.*, **44**: 495–506.

Gougoux, A., Kaehny, W.D. & Cohen, J.J. (1975). Renal adaptation to chronic hypocapnia: dietary constraints in achieving H^+ retention. *Am. J. Physiol.*, **229**: 1330–1337.

Graf, H., Leach, W. & Arieff, A.I. (1989). Metabolic effects of sodium bicarbonate in hypoxic lactic acidosis in dogs. *Am. J. Physiol.*, **249**: F630–F635.

Gravenstein, J.S., Paulus, D.A. & Hayes, T.J. (1989). *Capnography in Clinical Practice*. In: Gravenstein, Paulus, Hayes (eds) Butterworths, Boston, MA.

Halperin, M.L., Goldstein, M.B., Haig, A., Johnson, M.D. & Stinebaugh, B.J. (1974). Studies on the pathogenesis of type I (distal) renal tubular acidosis as revealed by the urinary PCO_2 tensions. *J. Clin. Invest.*, **53**: 669–677.

Harken, A.H., Gabel, R.A., Fencl, V. & Moore, F.D. (1975). Hydrochloric acid in the correction of metabolic alkalosis. *Arch. Surg.*, **110**: 819–821.

Harrington, J., Cohen, J.J. & Kassirer, J.P. (1982). Mixed acid–base disturbances. In: Cohen, J.J. (ed.) *Acid–Base*. Little, Brown, Boston, MA; pp. 377–390.

Harrison, A.M., Lynch, J.M., Dean, J.M. & Witte, M.K. (1997). Comparison of simultaneously obtained arterial and capillary blood gases in pediatric intensive care unit patients. *Crit. Care Med.*, **25**: 1904–1908.

Heird, W.C., Dell, R.B., Driscoll Jr, J.M., Grebin, B. & Winters, R.W. (1972). Metabolic acidosis resulting from intravenous alimentation mixtures containing synthetic amino acids. *New Engl. J. Med.*, **287**: 943–948.

Hindman, B.J. (1990). Sodium bicarbonate in the treatment of subtypes of acute lactic acidosis: physiologic considerations. *Anesthesiology*, **72**: 1064–1076.

Iberti, T.J., Leibowitz, A.B., Papadakos, P.J. & Fischer, E.P. (1990). Low sensitivity of the anion gap as a screen to detect hyperlactatemia in critically ill patients. *Crit. Care Med.*, **18**: 275–277.

Kassirer, J.P. & Schwartz, W.B. (1966). The response of normal man to selective depletion of hydrochloric acid. Factors in the genesis of persistent gastric alkalosis. *Am. J. Med.*, **40**: 10–18.

Kassirer, J.P., Berkman, P.M., Lawrenz, D.R. & Schwartz, W.B. (1965). The critical role of chloride in the correction of hypokalemic alkalosis in man. *Am. J. Med.*, **38**: 172–189.

Kassirer, J.P., London, A.M., Goldman, D.M. & Schwartz, W.B. (1970). On the pathogenesis of metabolic alkalosis in hyperaldosteronism. *Am. J. Med.*, **49**: 306–315.

Kazemi, H., Shannon, D.C. & Carvallo-Gil, E. (1967). Brain CO_2 buffering capacity in respiratory acidosis and alkalosis. *J. Appl. Physiol.*, **22**: 241–246.

Kellum, J.A. (1998). Lactate and pHi: our continued search for markers of tissue distress. *Crit. Care Med.*, **26**: 1783–1784.

Kety, S. & Schmidt, C.F. (1946). The effects of active and passive hyperventilation on cerebral blood flow, cerebral oxygen consumption, cardiac output, and blood pressure of normal young men. *J. Clin. Invest.*, **25**: 107–119.

Krapf, R., Beeler, I., Hertner, D. & Hulter, H.N. (1991). Chronic respiratory alkalosis. The effect of sustained hyperventilation on renal regulation of acid–base equilibrium. *New Engl. J. Med.*, **324**: 1394–1401.

Kreisberg, R.A. (1984). Pathogenesis and management of lactic acidosis. *Ann. Rev. Med.*, **35**: 181–193.

Lenfant, C. & Sullivan, K. (1971). Adaptation to high altitude. *New Engl. J. Med.*, **284**: 1298–1309.

Litzow, J.R., Lemann Jr, J. & Lennon, E.J. (1967). The effect of treatment of acidosis on calcium balance in patients with chronic azotemic renal disease. *J. Clin. Invest.*, **46**: 280–286.

Luke, R.G. & Galla, J.H. (1983). Chloride-depletion alkalosis with a normal extracellular fluid volume. *Am. J. Physiol.*, **245**: F419–F424.

Madias, N.E. & Adrogue, H.J. (1983). Influence of chronic metabolic acid–base disorders on the acute CO_2 titration curve. *J. Appl. Physiol.*, **55**: 1187–1195.

Madias, N.E., Adrogue, H.J. & Cohen, J.J. (1980). Maladaptive renal response to secondary hypercapnia in chronic metabolic alkalosis. *Am. J. Physiol.*, **238**: F283–F289.

Madias, N.E., Adrogue, H.J., Cohen, J.J. & Schwartz, W.B. (1979a). Effect of natural variations in P_aCO_2 on plasma $[HCO_3^-]$ in dogs: a redefinition of normal. *Am. J. Physiol.*, **236**: F30–F35.

Madias, N.E., Adrogue, H.J., Horowitz, G.L., Cohen, J.J. & Schwartz, W.B. (1979b). A redefinition of normal acid–base equilibrium in man: carbon dioxide tension as a key determinant of normal plasma bicarbonate concentration. *Kidney Int.*, **16**: 612–618.

Madias, N.E., Ayus, J.C. & Adrogue, H.J. (1979c). Increased anion gap in metabolic alkalosis: the role of plasma-protein equivalency. *New Engl. J. Med.*, **300**: 1421–1423.

Madias, N.E., Cohen, J.J. & Adrogue, H.J. (1990). Influence of acute and chronic respiratory alkalosis on preexisting chronic metabolic alkalosis. *Am. J. Physiol.*, **258**: F479–F485.

Madias, N.E., Wolf, C.J. & Cohen, J.J. (1985). Regulation of acid–base equilibrium in chronic hypercapnia. *Kidney Int.*, **27**: 538–543.

Manfredi, F. (1967). Effects of hypocapnia and hypercapnia on intracellular acid–base equilibrium in man. *J. Lab. Clin. Med.*, **69**: 304–312.

Mathieu, D., Neviere, R., Billard, V., Fleyfel, M. & Wattel, F. (1991). Effects of bicarbonate therapy on hemodynamics and tissue oxygenation in patients with lactic acidosis: a prospective, controlled clinical study. *Crit. Care Med.*, **19**: 1352–1356.

McFadden Jr, E.R. & Lyons, H.A. (1968). Arterial-blood gas tension in asthma. *New Engl. J. Med.*, **278**: 1027–1032.

McMillan, D.E. & Freeman, R.B. (1965). The milk alkali syndrome: a study of the acute disorder with comments on the development of the chronic condition. *Medicine (Baltimore)*, **44**: 485–501.

Mehta, P.M. & Kloner, R.A. (1987). Effects of acid base disturbance, septic shock, and calcium and phosphorous abnormalities on cardiovascular function. *Crit. Care Clin.*, **3**: 747–758.

Melby, J.C. (1984). Primary aldosteronism. *Kidney Int.*, **26**: 769–778.

Mines, A. (1992). Oxygen carriage by blood. In: Johnson, L. (ed.) *Essential Medical Physiology*. Raven Press, New York.

Narins, R.G. & Emmett, M. (1980). Simple and mixed acid–base disorders: a practical approach. *Medicine (Baltimore)*, **59**: 161–187.

Oh, M.S., Uribarri, J., Alveranga, D., Lazar, I., Bazilinski, N. & Carroll, H.J. (1985). Metabolic utilization and renal handling of D-lactate in men. *Metabolism*, **34**: 621–625.

Oropello, J.M., Manasia, A., Hannon, E., Leibowitz, A. & Benjamin, E. (1996). Continuous fiberoptic arterial and venous blood gas monitoring in hemorrhagic shock. *Chest*, **109**: 1049–1055.

Pellegrino, E.D. & Biltz, R.M. (1965). The composition of human bone in uremia. Observations on the reservoir functions of bone and demonstration of a labile fraction of bone carbonate. *Medicine (Baltimore)*, **44**: 397–418.

Peterson, C.D., Collins, A.J., Himes, J.M., Bullock, M.L. & Keane, W.F. (1981). Ethylene glycol poisoning: pharmacokinetics during therapy with ethanol and hemodialysis. *New Engl. J. Med.*, **304**: 21–23.

Prytz, H., Holst-Christensen, J., Korner, B. & Liehr, H. (1976). Portal venous and systemic endotoxaemia in patients without liver disease and systemic endotoxaemia in patients with cirrhosis. *Scand. J. Gastroenterol.*, **11**: 857–863.

Reynolds, T. (1958). Observations on the pathogenesis of renal tubular acidosis. *Am. J. Med.*, **25**: 503–515.

Roncoroni, A.J., Adrougue, H.J., De Obrutsky, C.W., Marchisio, M.L. & Herrera, M.R. (1976). Metabolic acidosis in status asthmaticus. *Respiration*, **33**: 85–94.

Rosen, R.A., Julian, B.A., Dubovsky, E.V., Galla, J.H. & Luke, R.G. (1988). On the mechanism by which chloride corrects metabolic alkalosis in man. *Am. J. Med.*, **84**: 449–458.

Schwartz, W.B. & Relman, A.S. (1963). A critique of the parameters used in the evaluation of acid–base disorders. *New Engl. J. Med.*, **268**: 1382–1388.

Schwartz, W., Hall, P.W., Hays, R.M. & Relman, A.S. (1959). On the mechanism of acidosis in chronic renal disease. *J. Clin. Invest.*, **38**: 39–52.

Schwartz, W., Hays, R.M., Polak, A. & Haynie, G.D. (1961). Effects of chronic hypercapnia on electrolyte and acid–base equilibrium. II. Recovery, with special reference to the influence of chloride intake. *J. Clin. Invest.*, **40**: 1238–1249.

Simmons, D., Nicoloff, J. & Guze, L.B. (1960). Hyperventilation and respiratory alkalosis as signs of Gram-negative bacteremia. *J. Am. Med. Assoc.*, **174**: 2196–2199.

Stacpoole, P.W., Wright, E.C., Baumgartner, T.G., Bersin, R.M., Buchalter, S., Curry, S.H., Duncan, C., Harman, E.M., Henderson, G.N., Jenkinson, S., *et al.* (1994). Natural history and course of acquired lactic acidosis in adults. DCA-Lactic Acidosis Study Group. *Am. J. Med.*, **97**: 47–54.

Sterns, R. (2003). Fluid, electrolyte, and acid–base disturbances. *J. Am. Soc. Nephrol.*, **2**: 1–42.

Stewart, P. (1981). How to understand acid–base. Elsevier North Holland, Inc., New York.

Taher, S.M., Anderson, R.J., McCartney, R., Popovtzer, M.M. & Schrier, R.W. (1974). Renal tubular acidosis associated with toluene "sniffing". *New Engl. J. Med.*, **290**: 765–768.

Thorp, J.A. & Rushing, R.S. (1999). Umbilical cord blood gas analysis. *Obstet. Gynecol. Clin. North. Am.*, **26**: 695–709.

Tyor, M. & Sieker, H.O. (1959). Biochemical, blood gas and peripheral circulatory alterations in hepatic coma. *Am. J. Med.*, **27**: 50–59.

Uribarri, J., Oh, M.S. & Carroll, H.J. (1998). D-lactic acidosis. A review of clinical presentation, biochemical features, and pathophysiologic mechanisms. *Medicine (Baltimore)*, **77**: 73–82.

Valtin, H.G.F. (1987a). Approach to the patient: useful tools. In: Valtin, H.G.F. (ed.) *Acid–Base Disorders*. Little, Brown, Boston; pp. 61–86.

Valtin, H.G.F. (1987b). Respiratory alkalosis: clinical examples. In: Valtin, H.G.F. (ed.) *Acid–Base Disorders*. Little, Brown, Boston; pp. 143–157.

Wall, S.M. & Knepper, M.A. (1990). Acid–base transport in the inner medullary collecting duct. *Semin. Nephrol.*, **10**: 148–158.

Wallace, M., Richards, P., Chesser, E. & Wrong, O. (1968). Persistent alkalosis and hypokalaemia caused by surreptitious vomiting. *Quart. J. Med.*, **37**: 577–588.

Waters, J.H., Miller, L.R., Clack, S. & Kim, J.V. (1999). Cause of metabolic acidosis in prolonged surgery. *Crit. Care Med.*, **27**: 2142–2146.

Watten, R., Morgen, F.M., Songkhla, Y.N., Vanikiati, B. & Phillips, R.A. (1959). Water and electrolyte studies in cholera. *J. Clin. Invest.*, **38**: 1879–1889.

Weil, M.H., Rackow, E.C., Trevino, R., Grundler, W., Falk, J.L. & Griffel, M.I. (1986). Difference in acid–base state between venous and arterial blood during cardiopulmonary resuscitation. *New Engl. J. Med.*, **315**: 153–156.

Westphal, S.A. (1996). The occurrence of diabetic ketoacidosis in non-insulin-dependent diabetes and newly diagnosed diabetic adults. *Am. J. Med.*, **101**: 19–24.

Widmer, B., Gerhardt, R.E., Harrington, J.T. & Cohen, J.J. (1979). Serum electrolyte and acid base composition. The influence of graded degrees of chronic renal failure. *Arch. Intern. Med.*, **139**: 1099–1102.

Wildenthal, K., Mierzwiak, D.S., Myers, R.W. & Mitchell, J.H. (1968). Effects of acute lactic acidosis on left ventricular performance. *Am. J. Physiol.*, **214**: 1352–1359.

Wilson, RF, Gibson, D, Percinel, AK, Ali, M.A., Baker, G., LeBlanc, L.P. & Lucas, C. (1972). Severe alkalosis in critically ill surgical patients. *Arch. Surg.*, **105**: 197–203.

Winter, S.D., Pearson, J.R., Gabow, P.A., Schultz, A.L. & Lepoff, R.B. (1990). The fall of the serum anion gap. *Arch. Intern. Med.*, **150**: 311–313.

Winters, R.W., White, J.S., Hughes, M.C. & Ordway, N.K. (1959). Disturbances of acid–base equilibrium in salicylate intoxication. *Pediatrics*, **23**: 260–285.

Wrenn, K.D., Slovis, C.M., Minion, G.E. & Rutkowski, R. (1991). The syndrome of alcoholic ketoacidosis. *Am. J. Med.*, **91**: 119–128.

Zhang H. & Vincent J.L. (1993). Arteriovenous differences in PCO_2 and pH are good indicators of critical hypoperfusion. *Am. Rev. Respir. Dis.*, **148**: 867–871.

VENTILATION/PERFUSION ABNORMALITIES AND CAPNOGRAPHY 30

A. Gabrielli & A.J. Layon

Introduction

The lung may be considered a simple oxygen (O_2) and carbon dioxide (CO_2) exchanger with both gas and blood flow in and out (Figure 30.1). When there is equilibrium between these two components gas exchange will be optimal, assuming that ventilation/perfusion ($\dot{V}/\dot{Q}$) are distributed in the same proportion.

Mismatching of ventilation and blood flow (perfusion) within the diseased lung is the most common cause of hypoxemia and hypercapnia, and this process may result in both hypoxic and hypercapnic respiratory failure. Despite the great practical importance of this subject, many aspects remain obscure. Indeed, only a few advances in understanding this concept have been made in the past century.

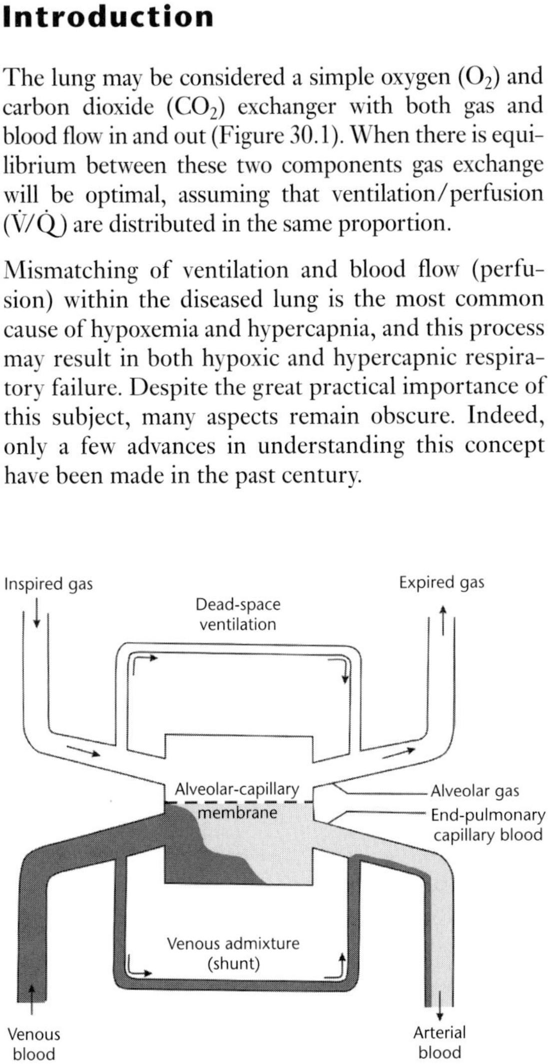

Figure 30.1 Functional representation of gas exchange in the lung. At equilibrium of alveolar gas and end-pulmonary capillary flow the end expiratory gas is the result of venous admixture and dead-space ventilation. (Reproduced with permission from Andrew, B.L. & Nunn, J.F. (2000). *Nunn's Applied Respiratory Physiology*, 5th edition. Butterworth-Heinemann, Boston; p. 46, 164, 243–245.)

The first was the recognition that the gas exchange taking place in any lung unit is determined by the ratio of ventilation to blood flow. Haldane first recognized that this mechanism was a potential cause of hypoxemia, although he concluded that this mismatching of ventilation and blood flow would not cause CO_2 retention but only hypoxemia, a misconception that still surfaces from time to time (Haldane & Priestley, 1905). In the mid-portion of the 20th century, Riley & Cournard (1949) clarified the quantitative relationship among ventilation, blood flow, and gas exchange. This important advance in knowledge led to the introduction of the O_2–CO_2 diagram, which allowed a graphic analysis of relationships between these two gases that were not amenable to algebraic manipulation (Figure 30.2).

Finally in the mid 1960s the introduction of computers allowed to describe the O_2 and CO_2 dissociation curves (Figure 30.3).

Ventilation in relation to perfusion

In the last few years there has been increased interest in considering the properties of $\dot{V}/\dot{Q}$ distributions to be composed of three alveolar compartments: ventilated underperfused, perfused and underventilated, and ideally matched. The breakthrough in the analysis of $\dot{V}/\dot{Q}$ ratio was the application of the computer methods for analyzing the behavior of distributions originally described by Riley & Cournard (1949). One way of approaching $\dot{V}/\dot{Q}$ ratio is to construct it from the distribution of ventilation and blood flow. While at rest, an average sized individual would have about 4 l of ventilating alveolar area for a cardiac output of approximately 5 l, resulting in an "ideal" $\dot{V}/\dot{Q}$ matching of 0.8. In reality, all possible ranges of $\dot{V}/\dot{Q}$ ratios are described in Figure 30.2, where expired gas results in a mixture of "ideal" alveolar with inspired gas (dead-space) and arterial blood results in a mixture of fully oxygenated with mixed venous blood.

Posture and rate of alveolar filling both effect the distribution of inspired gas. For example, normal tidal

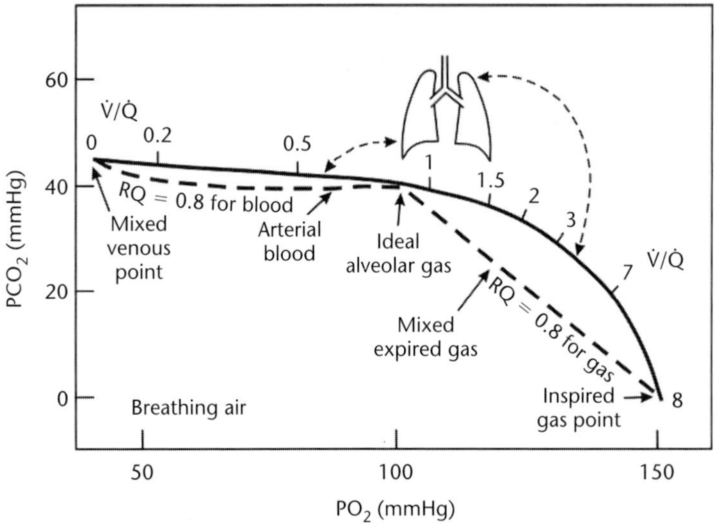

Figure 30.2 O_2–CO_2 diagram showing a $\dot{V}/\dot{Q}$ ratio line. PO_2 and PCO_2 is predicted along the line from the inspired gas point ($\dot{V}/\dot{Q}$ = infinite) to the mixed venous point ($\dot{V}/\dot{Q}$ = 0). (Reproduced with permission from West, J.B. (2000). *Respiratory Physiology, The Essentials*, 6th edition. Lippincot, Philadelphia, p. 53.)

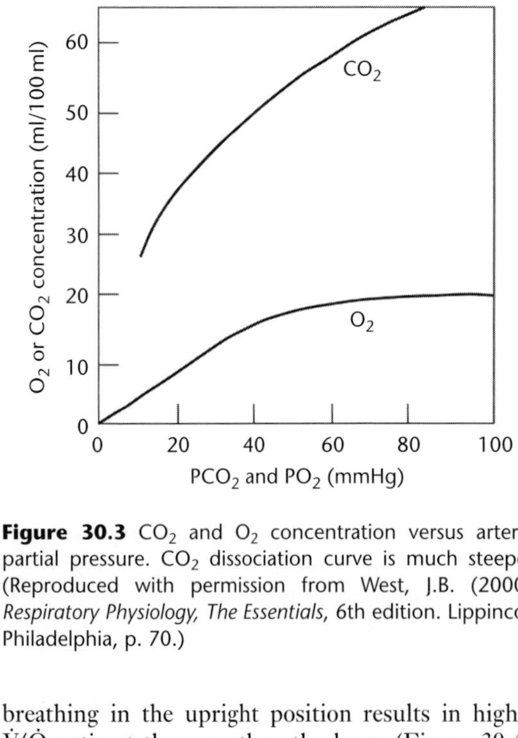

Figure 30.3 CO_2 and O_2 concentration versus arterial partial pressure. CO_2 dissociation curve is much steeper. (Reproduced with permission from West, J.B. (2000). *Respiratory Physiology, The Essentials*, 6th edition. Lippincot, Philadelphia, p. 70.)

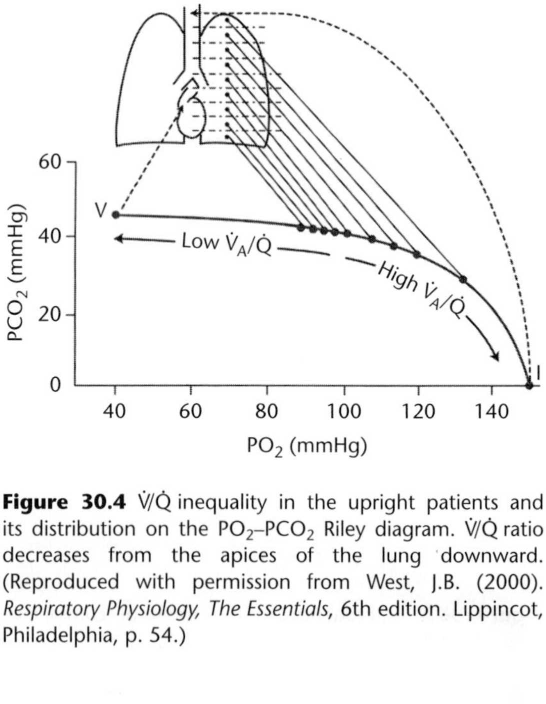

Figure 30.4 $\dot{V}/\dot{Q}$ inequality in the upright patients and its distribution on the PO_2–PCO_2 Riley diagram. $\dot{V}/\dot{Q}$ ratio decreases from the apices of the lung downward. (Reproduced with permission from West, J.B. (2000). *Respiratory Physiology, The Essentials*, 6th edition. Lippincot, Philadelphia, p. 54.)

breathing in the upright position results in higher $\dot{V}/\dot{Q}$ ratio at the apex than the bases (Figure 30.4). However, this relationship changes in the supine position, as it results in preferential perfusion of the posterior portion of the lung as compared with the anterior portion. In general, the effect of gravity on ventilation seems to be of a minor importance as compared to its effect on perfusion.

The rate of inflation of the lungs is the function of inflation pressure, compliance, and airway resistance. This concept is summarized in the term of time constant which is the product of the compliance and resistance and is:

1. The time required for inflation to 63% of the final volume attained if inflation is prolonged indefinitely.
2. The time that would be required for inflation of the lungs if the initial gas flow rate were maintained throughout inflation.

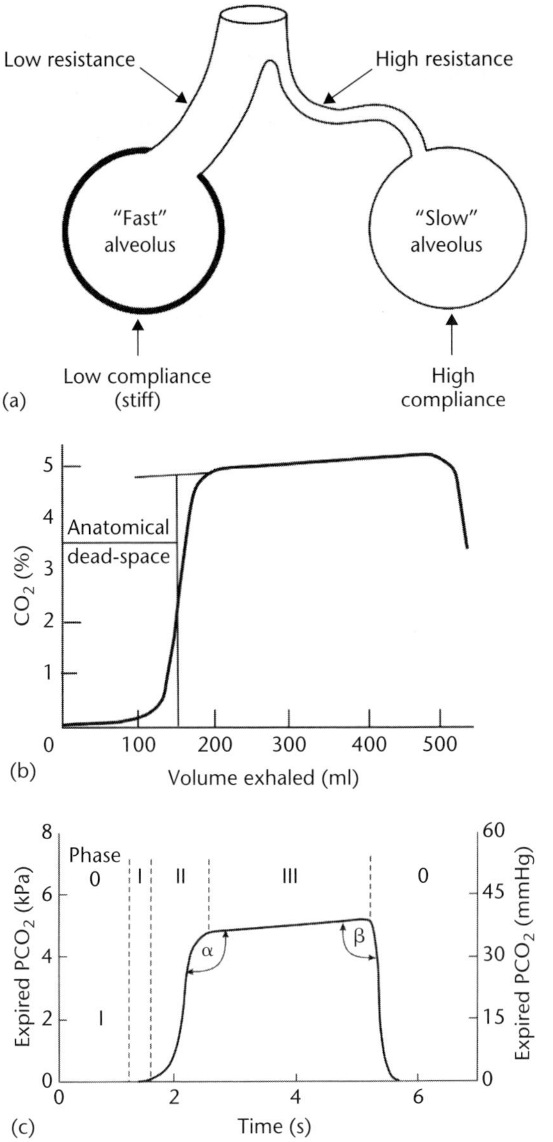

Figure 30.5 Heterogeneous distribution of compliance and resistance resulting in sequential emptying of exhaled gas from different alveola. (a): Volumetric capnography: CO_2 rise on exhalation is plotted against the volume exhaled. (b): Time capnography: exhalation and inhalation are plotted against time.

If the time constants were equal in all alveoli, the buildup of pressure in the different units would be identical at all times during inflation and therefore:

1. Distribution of inspired gas would be independent of the rate, duration, and frequency of inspiration.
2. Compliance would not be effected by changes in frequency.
3. There would be no redistribution of gas in the lungs.

This "ideal" condition is never encountered in critically ill patients on mechanical ventilation where time constants vary and are associated with sequential alveolar emptying during exhalation.

In this setting, the alveoli with a higher ventilation in relation to perfusion (high $\dot{V}/\dot{Q}$ alveoli) have a resultant lower CO_2 compared to alveoli with low $\dot{V}/\dot{Q}$ ratio, which would, conversely, have a higher CO_2. The actual overall concentration of CO_2 in the alveoli is determined by the extent of $\dot{V}/\dot{Q}$ of the alveoli ($\dot{V}/\dot{Q}$ ratio) (Figure 30.5).

Dead-space ventilation

In general, dead-space is defined as areas of ventilation without perfusion. Anatomical dead-space is the volume of the conducting airways and is rarely changed by pathophysiology. Alveolar dead-space can be defined as part of the inspired volume that passes through the anatomical dead-space to mix with gas at the alveoli level, but which does not take part in gas exchange. The physiologic dead-space is defined as the sum of the anatomical and alveolar dead-spaces that represent all parts of the tidal volume (V_T) that do not participate in gas exchange. The calculation of dead-space became possible with the presentation of an important mathematical equation by Bohr (1891). For a single breath, the equation consists of four terms including the:

1. V_T,
2. mixed expired CO_2 concentration,
3. alveolar CO_2 concentration,
4. dead-space (V_D/V_T).

Knowing three of these components, one can always calculate the dead-space. Modern interpretation of the Bohr equation defines V_D/V_T:

$$\frac{V_D}{V_T} = \frac{P_aCO_2 - P_{et}CO_2}{P_aCO_2},$$

where P_aCO_2 is partial pressure of carbon dioxide in arterial blood and $P_{et}CO_2$ is partial pressure of carbon dioxide at end-tidal.

Several factors can affect the interpretation of this measurement, including:

1. age;
2. posture;
3. size of individual;
4. position of neck and jaw;
5. lung volume at end inspiration;

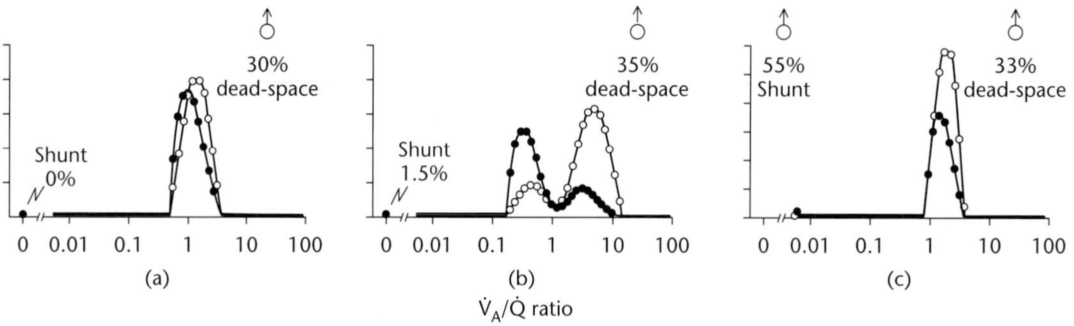

Figure 30.6 Distribution of $\dot{V}/\dot{Q}$ with the multiple gas elimination technique (MIGET). (a): Narrow distribution of $\dot{V}$ and $\dot{Q}$ in a healthy subject. Note that there is considerable blood flow going to the compartments with $\dot{V}_A/\dot{Q}$ ratio between .03 and .3. There is also an excess of ventilations in lung units with $\dot{V}_A/\dot{Q}$ ratio up to 6, however, all ventilation blood flow goes to the compartment closest to normal ventilation ratio, at about 1, and in particular, there is no blood flow to the unventilated compartment. (b): Bimodal both $\dot{V}$ and $\dot{Q}$ distribution in a patient with chronic obstructive pulmonary disease and V_D/V_T of 35%). Considerable blood flow is going to the compartment with $\dot{V}/\dot{Q}$ ratio between 0.1 and 1, while relatively low perfusion is noticed above the $\dot{V}/\dot{Q}$ of 1. (c): Increased shunt in a patient with ARDS. Late perfusion surge (approximately 0.9–1 $\dot{V}/\dot{Q}$ ratio) followed by exaggerated ventilations at above 5 $\dot{V}/\dot{Q}$ ratio. (Reproduced with permission from Roca, J. & Wagner, P.D. (1994). Contribution of multiple inert gas elimination technique to pulmonary medicine. 1. Principles and information content of the multiple inert gas elimination technique. *Thorax*, **49**: 815–824.)

6 tracheal intubation or tracheostomy;
7 V_T and respiratory rate;
8 drugs;
9 gender;
10 different clinical conditions including pulmonary embolism, smoking, anesthesia, and artificial ventilation.

Volumetric capnography as a plot of CO_2 concentration and expired volume has been utilized as a method of real-time calculation of anatomical and physiological dead-space ventilation in patients with $\dot{V}/\dot{Q}$ mismatch (Figure 30.6(a)). As anatomical dead-space generally does not change over time, alterations of physiological dead-space measured in real time can be used to indicate changes in the alveolar dead-space component. While the information obtained from volumetric capnography could be theoretically useful to titrate ventilator parameter, its use is not widespread. Time capnography, a plot of CO_2 concentration against time contains information on both inhalation and exhalation and is of widespread clinical use (Figure 30.6(b)).

Although very similar in shape to volume capnograms, time capnograms provide information in real time which is useful to the clinician, including:

1 expiratory and *inspiratory* CO_2 measurement;
2 respiratory rate;
3 slope of the exhalation curve;
4 a value for end-expiratory partial pressure of CO_2 (PCO_2), which may be correlated with the arterial PCO_2 to reveal an arterial–end-expiratory CO_2 difference. This value is useful in the titration of positive end-expiratory pressure (PEEP)/continuous positive airway pressure (CPAP), for example, in acute respiratory failure.

Perfusion in relation to ventilation

Shunt or venous admixture can be seen as the opposite of dead-space, and is defined as perfusion without ventilation, by far the most important cause of hypoxemia in critically ill patients. This is a useful index of $\dot{V}/\dot{Q}$ inequality and is related to an alteration in the ideal alveolar $-P_aO_2$ difference caused by blood flow to the lung units with abnormally low $\dot{V}/\dot{Q}$ ratio. In healthy subjects a 5% physiologic shunt is present, mostly from the thebesian and bronchial veins emptying directly in the central circulation. A certain degree of $\dot{V}/\dot{Q}$ scatter is also present in healthy individuals. In fact, as the pulmonary circulation operates at low pressure, it is rarely distributed evenly to all parts of the lungs and the degree of non-uniformity of perfusion is usually greater than that for ventilation. In the supine position, the difference is in blood flow between apices and bases are replaced by differences between anterior and posterior aspects of the lung.

While absolute distinctions between true shunt and $\dot{V}/\dot{Q}$ scatter are impossible due to the heterogeneous nature of pulmonary diseases, a few methods have been suggested to better define their pathophysiology. In the mid-1970s, the multiple inert gas elimination technique (MIGET) was established as the gold standard

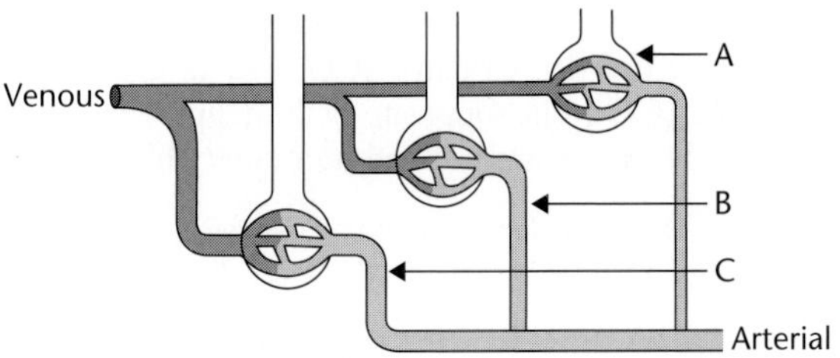

Figure 30.7 Arterial blood O_2 and CO_2 concentration is the average of "ideal alveolar gas tension (B) and scatter of $\dot{V}/\dot{Q}$ ratios (A and C). (Reproduced with permission from Andrew, B.L. & Nunn, J.F. (2000). *Nunn's Applied Respiratory Physiology*, 5th edition. Butterworth-Heinemann, Boston; p. 46, 164, 243–245.)

to provide qualitative and quantitative information on $\dot{V}/\dot{Q}$ mismatch and pulmonary gas exchange in patients with lung disease (Wagner *et al.*, 1974a, b; Evans & Wagner, 1977). The MIGET uses simultaneous venous infusion of six inert gases in trace concentrations, covering a broad spectrum of partition coefficients, to characterize the distribution of the $\dot{V}/\dot{Q}$ within the entire lung.

In summary, mixed expired gas always represents a mixture of ideal alveolar gas, dead-space, and under-ventilated alveoli. As a result, arterial blood O_2 and CO_2 concentrations represent a mixture of blood with gas tensions of "ideal" alveolar gas and scattered $\dot{V}/\dot{Q}$ ratio blood (Figure 30.7).

Capnography in patients with $\dot{V}/\dot{Q}$ abnormalities

The use of capnography as a means to monitor "the presence" of exhaled breath has been set as a monitoring standard of care by the American Society of Anesthesiology for approximately the past 15 years. Closed claim analysis studies conducted by anesthesiologists (Caplan *et al.*, 1990) and intraoperative events reviews (Tinker *et al.*, 1989; Cote *et al.*, 1991) concluded that intraoperative measurement of the end-tidal CO_2 partial pressure ($P_{et}CO_2$) provides an early warning of potentially catastrophic anesthetic mishaps. In a world of increasingly complex clinical monitoring, capnography has also been only recently used as a tool to provide information on pulmonary perfusion, alveolar ventilation, and respiratory patterns. Therefore, its value as a monitor/diagnostic tool in patients with $\dot{V}/\dot{Q}$ mismatch is not yet well defined.

Extensive clinical reviews of the time capnograph are available in other chapter of this book, review articles (Bhavani-Shankar *et al.*, 1992), and websites (www.capnography.com). In this section we will briefly review the appropriate terminology used to describe different phases of the inspiratory and expiratory capnographic tracing and the physiologic meaning of these wave-forms in the setting of a patient with $\dot{V}/\dot{Q}$ abnormalities (Bhavani-Shankar *et al.*, 1992; Nunn, 2000). A time capnograph is a plot of CO_2 and time that can be divided into inspiratory and expiratory segments, each one grouped in phases (Figure 30.5(b)).

Inspiratory segment: The inspiratory phase, phase 0, is usually a flat line overlapping the zero (baseline) CO_2 concentration line, unless rebreathing is present. The later part of the horizontal base line is the phase I of expiratory segment. Phase 0 represents the dynamics of inspiration.

Expiratory segment: The expiratory segment, similar to a single breath CO_2 curve, is divided into phases I, II, and III, and occasionally, phase IV, which represents the terminal rise in CO_2 concentration.

Phase I: Phase I represents CO_2-free gas from the apparatus and anatomical dead-space.

Phase II: Phase II consists of a rapid S-shaped upswing on the tracing, due to mixing of dead-space gas with alveolar gas.

α-angle: The angle between phases II and III, has been referred to as the α-angle, and increases as the slope of phase III increases. Changes of the α-angle correlate with sequential emptying of alveoli. In general, the more heterogeneous are functional units of the lung, the wider is the α-angle.

Phase III: Phase III is the link between the α-angle and the $P_{et}CO_2$. Its slope is the core of $\dot{V}/\dot{Q}$ mismatch abnormalities (Nunn & Hill, 1960; Bhavani-Shankar *et al.*, 1995). $\dot{V}/\dot{Q}$ mismatch within the unit may be due either to incomplete gas mixing (alveolar mixing defect) or as a result of late gas distribution to alveoli with low $\dot{V}/\dot{Q}$ ratio (higher PCO_2). Regional variation between respiratory units produce a large spectrum of $\dot{V}/\dot{Q}$ ratios. Under these circumstances, the slope of phase III is determined by the gas emptying sequence of the alveolar units. If the units empty synchronously, the CO_2 expired results in a smooth flat or slightly upsloping phase III. In patients with severe $\dot{V}/\dot{Q}$ scatter and longer time constants, CO_2 emptying is sequential resulting in a steeper rising slope of phase III (Figure 30.8(a)). In general the more severe the mismatch, the steeper the slope. This attribute makes capnography a useful diagnostic tool to detect abnormalities in $\dot{V}/\dot{Q}$ mismatch of the lung. Factors, such as changes in cardiac output, CO_2 production, airway resistance, and functional residual capacity (FRC) may further affect the $\dot{V}/\dot{Q}$ status of the

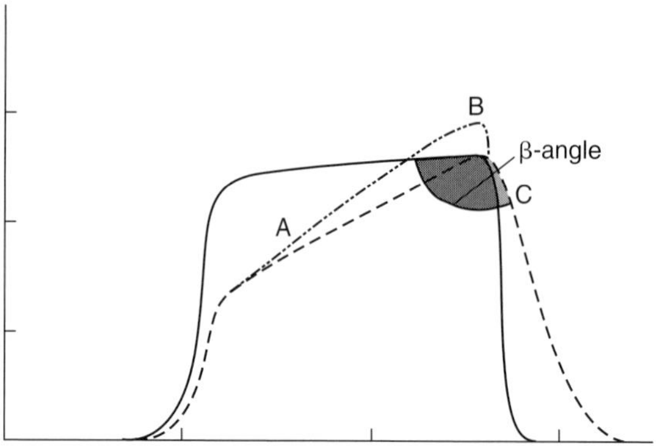

Figure 30.8 (a): Upsloping of phase III as an index of $\dot{V}/\dot{Q}$ mismatch, variable with inspiratory time and time constant of the lung. (b): Sequential emptying in patients with low lung compliance (decreased FRC), short inspiratory time (low respiratory rate, large V_T) and severe $\dot{V}/\dot{Q}$ mismatch can result in "reverse" P_aCO_2–$P_{et}CO_2$ gradient. The distance between the apex of the phase III B tracing and baseline is phase IV. (c): Increased β-angle as an index of rebreathing. The capnograph may or may not go back to baseline.

various units in the lung, and thus influence the height or the slope of phase III.

Other mechanisms affecting CO_2 mixing that can contribute to the phase III slope are the breathing pattern (breathing frequency (f_R), V_T, and incompetent expiratory valves (Strömberg & Gustafsson, 2000).

In hyperventilating subjects, the time for diffusive gas mixing is reduced and localized more peripherally, resulting in a steeper phase III slope of the capnograph which is not representative of $\dot{V}/\dot{Q}$ mismatch in the lung. An incompetent expiratory valve resulting in rebreathing may affect the α-angle and upslope the phase III of the capnograph. A simultaneous recording of flow rate waveforms is potentially used to differentiate this technical problem from an abnormal plateau of phase III of the capnograph.

$P_{et}CO_2$ and P_aCo_2–$P_{et}CO_2$ gradient

In healthy adults, the $P_{et}CO_2$ is lower than P_aCO_2 (average of all alveoli) by approximately 5 mmHg. The P_aCO_2–$P_{et}CO_2$ difference [(a–ET)PCO_2] is due to the $\dot{V}/\dot{Q}$ mismatch in the lungs (alveolar dead-space) as a result of temporal, spatial, and alveolar mixing defects. Healthy infants and children have the best $\dot{V}/\dot{Q}$ matching and lowest alveolar dead-space resulting in a smaller difference than in adults (Fletcher, 1988; Rich & Sconzo, 1991).

Reduction in cardiac output and pulmonary blood flow result in a decrease in $P_{et}CO_2$ and an increase in P_aCO_2–$P_{et}CO_2$; the opposite will happen with an increase in cardiac output and pulmonary blood.

The (a–ET)PCO_2 fraction is a measure of, and correlates well with, alveolar dead-space. In general, an increase in (a–ET)PCO_2 suggests an increase in dead-space ventilation as an indirect estimate of $\dot{V}/\dot{Q}$ mismatching of the lung (Nunn & Hill, 1960).

Despite the widespread use of end-tidal CO_2, the appropriate use of this non-invasive method of assessing blood gases is unclear. In patients with lung disease, $P_{et}CO_2$ can differ from P_aCO_2 because of $\dot{V}/\dot{Q}$ mismatching. As a result, changes in $P_{et}CO_2$ may be seen with a corresponding increase, decrease, or no change in P_aCO_2 depending on what happens to $\dot{V}/\dot{Q}$ mismatch. However, the $P_{(a-ET)}CO_2$ may be the most appropriate use for $P_{et}CO_2$ monitoring.

Under conditions of constant lung ventilation, $P_{et}CO_2$ monitoring can be used as a monitor of pulmonary blood flow. Increases in cardiac output and pulmonary blood flow result in better perfusion of the alveoli and a rise in $P_{et}CO_2$. Consequently, alveolar dead-space is reduced as is (a–ET)CO_2. The relationship between $P_{et}CO_2$ and pulmonary artery blood flow was studied during separation from cardiopulmonary bypass (Maslow *et al.*, 2001). The decrease in $P_{(a-ET)}CO_2$ is due to an increase in the alveolar CO_2 with a relatively unchanged arterial CO_2 concentration, suggesting better pulmonary excretion of CO_2. The improved CO_2 excretion is due to better perfusion of upper parts of the lung (Askrog, 1966).

Although, $P_{et}CO_2$ is related to the P_aCO_2, the difference between the two values may be of clinical value in cases such as acute respiratory distress syndrome (ARDS), in patients receiving PEEP, and those being considered for weaning from mechanic ventilation. In general, the difference between P_aCO_2 and $P_{et}CO_2$ will increase if there is a contribution of ventilation from high $\dot{V}_A/\dot{Q}$ ratios. This concept will be more extensively reviewed in the clinical application section.

A phase III variation consisting of an exaggerated increase of $P_{et}CO_2$ with an up-sloping trend at the very end of the phase III waveform is occasionally referred to as a terminal rise or phase IV (Figure 30.8b). The upslope is primarily linked to an increase in time constants within the lung and is an indirect indication of $\dot{V}/\dot{Q}$ status of the lung. A "two lung compartments" theory has been proposed to explain this variant, where two different lung regions with mechanical and $\dot{V}/\dot{Q}$ properties empty in time sequence (Fletcher *et al.*, 1981).

A fast alveolar compartment, with high initial expiratory flow rate and rapid emptying of gases, has a rather constant CO_2 output and is responsible for the near-horizontal initial part of phase III trace. A slow alveolar component, when expiratory flow decreases towards the end of expiration, causes a steep rise of exhaled CO_2 and, therefore, a terminal upslope in the tracing. Normally, the alveolar gases contained in the slow alveolar component remain within the airways and participate in the anatomical dead-space; these are not usually analyzed by the CO_2 sensor at the mouth. However, exaggerated alveolar PCO_2 fluctuations during the respiratory cycle due decreased FRC, combined with the use of large V_T, and low-frequency ventilation increase the chances of higher CO_2-containing exhaled gas reaching the mouth. This has been observed frequently during general anesthesia. Under these circumstances, as the expiratory flow rate decreases towards the end of expiration, low $\dot{V}/\dot{Q}$ areas (alveoli with higher PCO_2) make a more substantial contribution to the gas exchange (Fletcher & Jonson, 1984).

In rare circumstances, the slope of phase III increases steadily to a level that reverses the "normal" (a–ET)PCO_2 difference, resulting in a negative (a–ET)PCO_2 value. It should go without saying, but often does not, that more obvious reasons for measurement errors, such as device malfunctioning, rebreathing or inadvertent addition of CO_2 to the inspired gases, should be ruled out before making a more complicated interpretation of the finding.

The presence of an $P_{et}CO_2$ exceeding P_aCO_2, has been observed in obese and pregnant subjects. Therefore, (a–ET)PCO_2 may not reflect alveolar dead-space when phase III has a steeper slope or when a terminal "step up knee" of the waveform is appreciated.

The (a–ET)PCO_2 could be zero or negative even in the presence of alveolar dead-space ventilation. For example, it has been observed during cardiac surgery that alveolar dead-space was increased at the end of cardiopulmonary bypass but as the slope of phase III was also increased, there was no change in (a–ET)PCO_2 (Fletcher *et al.*, 1986).

In conclusion, changes in alveolar dead-space correlate with (a–ET)PCO_2 only when phase III is flat or has a minimal slope.

β-angle

Phase III terminates in the β-angle. The descending limb that follows phase III is normally of 90° and represents the inspiratory phase during which the fresh gases (CO_2-free gases) are inhaled and CO_2 concentration falls rapidly to zero. An increase of the β-angle and the delay or lack of return of the capnograph to a zero baseline has been observed during rebreathing (Figure 30.8(c).) (Berman & Pyles, 1988; Podraza *et al.*, 1991; Kumar *et al.*, 1992) or as an artifact (Badgwell *et al.*, 1993) and with defective inspiratory valves.

Clinical correlation of $\dot{V}/\dot{Q}$ ratio mismatch and capnography abnormalities

The attention of physiologists and physicians for many years has been focused on how best to assess the quality and quantity of $\dot{V}/\dot{Q}$ inequality. While, ideally, we would like to know the actual distribution of $\dot{V}/\dot{Q}$ ratios for each patient, in most instances we must rely on indirect information from the arterial blood gas interpretations.

The difference in and the ratio of PO_2 between alveolar gas and arterial blood are often useful in assessing the degree of $\dot{V}/\dot{Q}$ inequality. These indexes have the advantage of being less sensitive to the patient's level of ventilation than is the arterial PO_2 alone.

In the ideal lung, when atmospheric O_2 (21%) has reached the alveoli (i.e. A), the P_AO_2 will approximate 100 mmHg, losing about one-third of initial concentration due to the presence of water vapor and alveolar CO_2. Alveolar O_2 is determined by measurement of O_2 from pulmonary capillary blood, a process in which there is minimal variability at rest with continuous alveolar ventilation. If venous blood enters the arterial system without being ventilated at all the admixture is calculated as the shunt fraction:

$$\frac{Q_S}{Q_T} = \frac{C_cO_2 - C_aO_2}{C_cO_2 - C_vO_2},$$

where Q_S is the shunted blood, Q_T the total blood flow, and C_aO_2, C_vO_2 and C_cO_2 are the content of the arterial, mixed venous and capillary blood, respectively.

The most important feature of an absolute shunt is the lack of an increase in the P_aO_2 in response to breathing 100% O_2. The P_aO_2 is often a useful measure of the degree of $\dot{V}/\dot{Q}$ inequality in a diseased lung. For example, a patient with chronic obstructive pulmonary disease (COPD), whose P_aO_2 is 50 mmHg, is likely to have more $\dot{V}/\dot{Q}$ inequality than one whose arterial P_aO_2 is 70 mmHg, all other things (such as fraction of inspired O_2 (F_IO_2)) being equal. The main disadvantage of P_aO_2 as a measure of $\dot{V}/\dot{Q}$ inequality is that its value is affected by the level of ventilation and by other causes of hypoxemia.

$\dot{V}_A/\dot{Q}$ mismatch, absolute shunt, dead-space, and diffusion limitations are the most important intrapulmonary factors regulating the P_aO_2. Extrapulmonary factors of importance are:

1 F_IO_2;
2 total ventilation;
3 cardiac output;
4 O_2 consumption;
5 CO_2 production.

In a single alveolar unit, it is easy to conceptualize the predicted exhaled CO_2 changes during $\dot{V}/\dot{Q}$ mismatch. If blood flow is obstructed, alveolar CO_2 will fall, eventually reaching the composition of inspired gas when blood flow is totally abolished. If ventilation is decreased or abolished, the CO_2 of alveolar gas will be similar to that of mixed venous blood. It is not so easy, however, to predict the composition of mixed venous blood CO_2 composed of a very large number of lung units. In general, the blood PCO_2 is unlikely to be raised. In fact, an increase of CO_2 in the pulmonary venous circuit will trigger the chemoreceptors and increase spontaneous ventilation, thereby reducing the PCO_2 of the unshunted blood to normal. If hypoxia greatly increases respiratory drive, the resultant hyperventilation may even result in decreased P_aCO_2 (hypocapnia), as is typically observed in the arterial blood gas analysis of spontaneously breathing patients affected by pulmonary emboli. The importance of $\dot{V}/\dot{Q}$ inequality in producing hypercapnia in patients with lung disease has only recently been pointed out (West, 1971; *et al.*, 1994). However, in general, P_aCO_2 is often of no value in assessing the amount of $\dot{V}/\dot{Q}$ inequality because the gas is highly diffusible and very sensitive to the level of ventilation. As volumetric and time capnography find more clinical and research applications in critically ill patients our understanding of $\dot{V}/\dot{Q}$ abnormalities will improve.

Capnography in anesthesia

Capnography is considered a standard of care during anesthesia (American Society of Anesthesiologists: Standards for basic anesthetic monitoring (1998). Available at: http//www.asahq.hq) and is strongly recommended by the American College of Emergency Physicians as an adjunctive method to ensure endotracheal tube position.[1] However, how well end-tidal CO_2 reflects changes in P_aCO_2 is still debated. For example, a recent Medline literature search of the leading anesthesia journals seems to indicate that the (a–ET)PCO_2 difference may change widely and unpredictably during surgical procedures (Wahba & Tessler, 1996).

Capnography as an index of $\dot{V}/\dot{Q}$ mismatch in obstructive lung disease

Alteration of the slopes of phases II and III of the volumetric capnograph have been extensively studied in patients with obstructive airway diseases as an index of $\dot{V}/\dot{Q}$ alteration, where phase II is due to progressive recruitment of alveoli during gas transit. Furthermore, normal lung models have demonstrated that during the phase III slope of the time capnograph, CO_2 is continuously excreted into the alveoli, which become progressively smaller as expiration continues. Sequential emptying of the lung occurs with better-ventilated compartments contributing relatively more to the early portion of exhalation, and the more slowly ventilated compartments contributing to the latter part of exhalation (van Meerten, 1970). This steady increase in alveolar PCO_2 towards the end of expiration explains the mild rising positive slope of phase III as expiration proceeds in normal lung.

Intuitively, phase III in a time capnograph in patients with severe $\dot{V}/\dot{Q}$ mismatch will represent sequential CO_2 release from high $\dot{V}/\dot{Q}$ alveolar unit first (low CO_2) and low $\dot{V}/\dot{Q}$ alveolar unit last (high CO_2) (Strömberg & Gustafsson, 2000).

Interestingly, the relationship between spirometrically measured exhaled volume and $\dot{V}/\dot{Q}$ ratio in patients with obstructive lung diseases has been poor (Ballester *et al.*, 1990; Wagner *et al.*, 1996), as has been the relationship between forced expiratory volume at 1 s (FEV_1) and gas trapping (Gustafsson *et al.*, 1994). When the multiple inert gas washout technique has been used to assess ventilation maldistribution in patients with chronic obstruction, it has been demonstrated that the $\dot{V}/\dot{Q}$ ratio remains essentially normal until FEV_1 is below 40% of predicted. In these chronically obstructed patients, capnograph may appear normal.

Conversely, a significantly higher degree of $\dot{V}/\dot{Q}$ mismatch has been found in patients with acute, severe obstruction where compensation to $\dot{V}/\dot{Q}$ inequality (increase cardiac output, hyperventilation, increased hemoglobin, and hypoxic pulmonary vasoconstriction) cannot be readily achieved (Ballester *et al.*, 1990). This probably explains why treatment with β_2

[1] American College of Emergency Physicians. Clinical Policies Committee. Verification of endotracheal tube placement. (2002). *Ann. Emerg. Med.*, **40(5)**: 551–552. Guidelines 2000 for Cardiopulmonary resuscitation and emergency cardiovascular care: international consensus on science. *Circulation* 2000; **102(8)**: I1-I370.

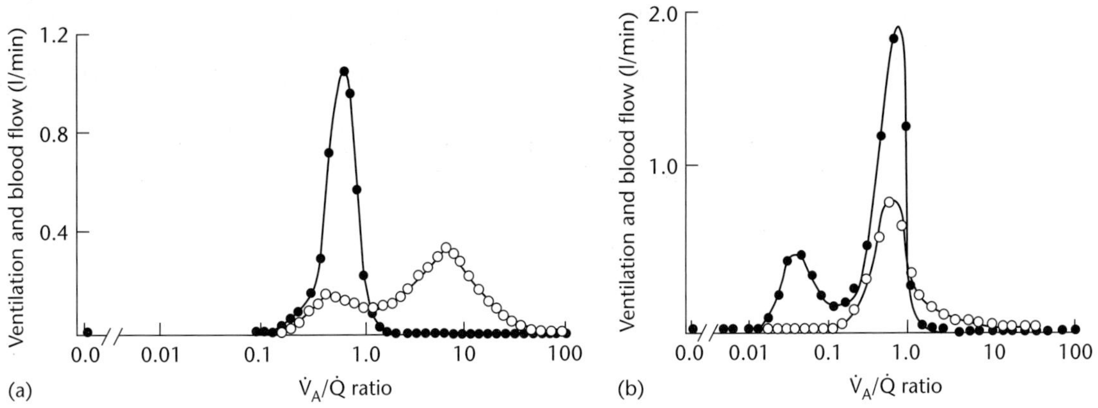

Figure 30.9 $\dot{V}/\dot{Q}$ distribution in a patient with an emphysema-type COPD and two bronchitis-type COPD. Note the different bimodal distribution. (Reproduced with permission from Wagner, P.D., Dantzker, D.R., Dueck, R., Clausen, J.L. & West, J.B. (1997). Ventilation–perfusion in chronic obstructive pulmonary disease. *J. Clin. Invest.*, **59**: 203–216.)

agonists in acute or chronic severe asthma has been shown to improve FEV_1, but not $\dot{V}/\dot{Q}$ mismatch (Ballester *et al.*, 1989).

In summary, a volumetric capnographic phase II and III positive slope, and a time capnographic phase III positive slope are both seen more often in the more severe chronic patients and in most patients with acute pulmonary disease. In patients with lung disease, the $P_{et}CO_2$ can differ from P_aCO_2 because of $\dot{V}/\dot{Q}$ mismatching, and changes in the $P_{et}CO_2$ may be seen with a corresponding increase, decrease, or no change in P_aCO_2 depending on what happens to $\dot{V}_A/\dot{Q}$ mismatch.

Single values of $ETCO_2$ have proven unreliable as differential diagnosis indexes in patients with COPD versus asthma, as well as in patients with increased extravascular lung water (Brown *et al.*, 1998).

However, $ETCO_2$ during weaning from mechanical ventilation has been used with success to prevent dangerous, and frequently unrecognized, hypercapnia in patients with increased dead-space ventilation (Suara *et al.*, 1996). Unfortunately, clinically relevant hypercapnic episodes (change of $ETCO_2$ of greater than 3 mmHg) can only be detected with a sensitivity of 82% and a specificity of 76%, making arterial sampling during the weaning a frequent necessity. Despite these limitations, capnography may substantially reduce the number of arterial blood gas analyses necessary during weaning from mechanical ventilations (Niehoff *et al.*, 1988).

Two different patterns of $\dot{V}_A/\dot{Q}$ mismatch have been observed with COPD when MIGET was applied (Wagner *et al.*, 1977). Both depict a bimodal distribution of perfusion or ventilation. Irrespective of the type of COPD (emphysema (type A) or bronchitis (type B)), the severity of anatomical emphysema seems to correlate with the dispersion of ventilation and blood flow distribution (Figure 30.9(a) and (b)). The relative influence of these two MIGET patterns on dead-space ventilation capnography waveforms and (a–ET)PCO_2 difference is not known.

Capnography as an index of $\dot{V}/\dot{Q}$ mismatch in ARDS

ARDS is an example of severe $\dot{V}/\dot{Q}$ scatter. Low lung compliance and an increase in resistance imply longer time constants and sequential CO_2 emptying, resulting in a steeper rising slope of phase III of time capnograph (Figure 30.8(a)). Therefore ventilatory disturbance in ARDS can be monitored with a real-time capnograph.

Ventilatory disturbances in ARDS have been also studied to establish a relationship between volumetric capnography and respiratory system mechanics (Romero *et al.*, 1997). Interestingly, change in V_T does not alter capnographic indexes in ARDS patients. After adjusting for breathing pattern, the ratio between alveolar ejection volume to tidal volume (VA_E/V_T) exhibited the best correlation with mechanical parameters, suggesting that ventilatory disturbances could be monitored in a patient with ARDS by volumetric capnography.

The (ET-a)PCO_2 difference has been used as a tool for real-time bedside monitor in ventilated neonates. It has been suggested that this difference can be used to assess improved $\dot{V}/\dot{Q}$ matching when surfactant therapy is used in ARDS (Wenzel *et al.*, 1999). Unfortunately, the (a–ET)PCO_2 difference is not always predictable and constant because conditions both of increased and decreased $\dot{V}/\dot{Q}$ ratio are present. Nevertheless, when low $\dot{V}/\dot{Q}$ units are predominant (physiologic shunt) the change of PCO_2 is minimal and the (a–ET)PCO_2 difference is predicted to be reliable, although occasionally widened.

On the contrary, dead-space ventilation can significantly increase the (a–ET)PCO_2 difference, resulting in the measurement becoming progressively less reliable. Direct measurement of dead-space ventilation with volumetric capnography is therefore useful to predict the relationship between P_aCO_2 and $P_{et}CO_2$.

Measurement of dead-space ventilation has also been used to assess efficacy of therapeutic interventions in patients with acute lung injury and severe $\dot{V}/\dot{Q}$ mismatch. For example, capnography has been used to assess alveolar and physiologic dead-space changes in models of ARDS in animals both pre- and post-bronchial alveolar lavage and with the use of surfactant (Wenzel *et al.*, 1999).

Recent reports in pediatric and adult populations suggest that a V_D/V_T ratio of 60% is a critical ratio for lack of reliability of $P_{et}CO_2$ in patients with increased extravascular lung water (Hubble *et al.*, 2000).

This observation mirrors our personal experience in adult ARDS patients (see Chapter 23). Furthermore, a V_D/V_T of less than 50% has seemed to acquire statistical importance in reliably predicting successful extubations, while a V_D/V_T more than 65% identifies patients at risk for respiratory failure following extubation in the pediatric population (Hubble *et al.*, 2000); a similar value, V_D/V_T of 63%, identifies patients at risk of death in adult ARDS (Nuckton *et al.*, 2002).

The studies of Hubble *et al.* (2000) and Nuckton *et al.* (2002) suggest that the direct calculation of dead-space ventilation should be an important parameter to assist with decision-making, and that an increased (a–ET) PCO_2 difference – generally more than 10 mmHg – might be the trigger to measure this important clinical parameter. Other important causes of a widening gap and decrease in $P_{et}CO_2$ also need to be ruled out. Of particular significance is the low cardiac output state and pulmonary embolism.

In patients with severe $\dot{V}_A/\dot{Q}$ mismatch, capnography may still be helpful in the selection of ventilator settings to achieve a desired P_aCO_2 or to insure that the P_aCO_2 is not lowered too rapidly. Sudden change of $P_{et}CO_2$ may indicate a ventilator circuit disconnection, a leak or an obstruction in the circuit, or a malfunctioning ventilator (Napolitano, 1999). The (a–ET)PCO_2 difference in ARDS patients has recently found another interesting application. It has been theorized that the narrowing of this difference, while positive end-inspiratory pressure is applied in patients with ARDS, indicates the best possible recruitment of unstable alveoli without overdistension (Murray *et al.*, 1984). In other words, calculating V_D/V_T in patients with a large (a–ET)PCO_2 difference could be strategically useful to optimize PEEP, thereby limiting promotion of excessive "West zone 1" in the lung (Figure 30.10). Our experience at the University of Florida confirms the utility of using V_D/V_T in titrating PEEP in ARDS patients (Rose & Banner, 2000). Furthermore, we have noted that exhaled CO_2/min (LCO_2), calculated in real time

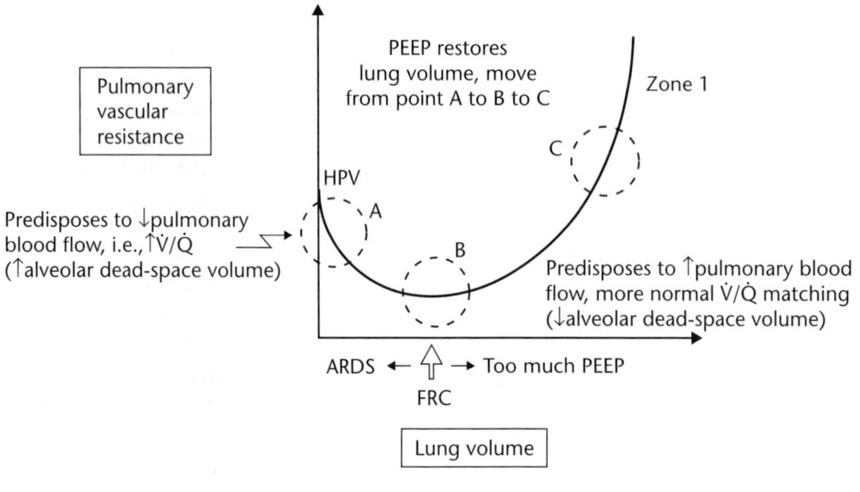

Figure 30.10 Titration of PEEP in patients with low FRC (point A to point B) restores lung volume, decreases pulmonary vascular resistance, *decreases* V_D/V_T and improves $\dot{V}/\dot{Q}$ matching. Excess of PEEP (point B to point C) overdistend the lung, *increases* V_D/V_T without improving and potentially deteriorating $\dot{V}/\dot{Q}$ matching. (Courtesy of M.J. Banner, University of Florida, Gainesville, modified.)

with volumetric capnography closely correlates with V_D/V_T (yielding a $r^2 = 0.71$) and is another potential means to titrate PEEP to its "best physiologic value" (Rose & Banner, 2000). Nonetheless, this enhanced, if as yet theoretical, utility of capnometry in clinical practice has been neither fully validated (Jardin *et al.*, 1985) nor generally accepted.

Capnography as an index of $\dot{V}/\dot{Q}$ mismatch in pulmonary fibrosis

Hypoxemia at rest that worsens during exercise is the hallmark of the respiratory pathophysiology known as pulmonary fibrosis (Barbera *et al.*, 1990; Crystal *et al.*, 1976). In general, the measurement of the diffusing capacity of CO_2 in these patients provides an indication of degree of gas exchange impairment and correlates with both $\dot{V}/\dot{Q}$ mismatch and the degree of vascular reactivity to a high concentration of O_2 and exercise. The effect of $\dot{V}/\dot{Q}$ mismatch is unequal for PCO_2 and O_2. The reason for the different behavior of the two gases is the different shaped dissociation curves of CO_2 and O_2 (Figure 30.3). With an increase in $\dot{V}/\dot{Q}$ mismatch, the increase of PCO_2 augments ventilatory drive. As the CO_2 dissociation curve is nearly linear in the physiologic range, increased ventilation will increase CO_2 output in both high and low $\dot{V}/\dot{Q}$ ratio units. This is not true for O_2, whose relatively flat dissociation curve does not allow an increase of O_2 concentration in the unit with high $\dot{V}/\dot{Q}$ ratio. The net result is that the mixed PaO_2 rises only modestly with increased ventilation, and some hypoxemia remains.

In conclusion, the pattern of $\dot{V}_A/\dot{Q}$ mismatch in patients with pulmonary fibrosis is highly predictable. There is little clinical experience with the use of capnography in these patients (Augusti & Barbera, 1994).

Capnography as an index of $\dot{V}/\dot{Q}$ mismatch in one lung ventilation, lung resection and lung transplantation

Simplified lung models of one lung ventilation have demonstrated an upslope in phase III of the capnograph. This appears to be due to sequential emptying of the lung, with better-ventilated compartments contributing relatively more to the early part of the exhalation while slowly ventilated compartments contribute more to the latter part of exhalation (van Meerten, 1970). Delayed alveolar emptying in the phase III capnogram as also been demonstrated by separate bronchospirometry and capnography of the two lungs in a patient with occlusion of the right pulmonary artery (van Meerten, 1971).

More recently, capnography has been used to evaluate $\dot{V}/\dot{Q}$ mismatch of a single lung after regional lung surgery, utilizing sequential endobronchial intubation with a fiberoptic bronchoscope (Yoshimasu *et al.*, 1996). During surgery, gas flow is expected to decrease from the surgical site and increase from opposite, non-operative site. Post-operatively, perfusion to the operative site is more severely reduced than is ventilation. In these cases, increased $\dot{V}/\dot{Q}$ mismatch is consistent with widened (a–ET)PCO_2 gradient and seems to correlate with hyperinflation of the remaining lobe after resection. A possible vagal nerve denervation-related reduction of blood flow and alveolar wall stretching of the remaining lung seems to correlate with the decreased capillary circulation (Schmitz & Shapiro, 1995).

Capnography has not been reliable during rapid change of alveolar dead-space ventilation, and/or ischemia–reperfusion lung injury, as may occur immediately after lung transplantation. However, the narrowing of the (a–ET)PCO_2 difference shortly after transplantation may be temporally related to successful readjustment of the recipient pulmonary circulation to the transplanted lung (Jellinek *et al.*, 1993).

Capnography as an index of $\dot{V}/\dot{Q}$ mismatch in pulmonary embolism

The recent introduction of commercially available volumetric capnography has contributed to the widespread knowledge of the change in dead-space ventilation during pulmonary embolism. However, the scientific basis for the use of time capnography for pulmonary embolism has been recognized for more than 30 years (Robin *et al.*, 1964; Burki, 1986). Pulmonary embolism causes several characteristic clinical symptoms. Among others, the most statistically significant seem to be dyspnea, chest pain, increased minute ventilation, tachycardia, and hypoxemia. However, the most common physiologic alteration is the development of increased alveolar dead-space. As discussed in the introductory portion of this chapter, pulmonary embolism results in a decrease in blood flow to well-ventilated alveoli (Dantzker *et al.*, 1978). As a result of decreased transport of CO_2 via the pulmonary artery to functional lung units, the expiratory breath content of CO_2 decreases and the plateau of the CO_2 volume capnogram flattens (Schreiner *et al.*, 1993). Alveolar hypoxia and increased alveolar dead-space results in increased minute ventilation with resultant hypocarbia. A minimal *decrease* of large airway dead-space ventilation is noticed, mostly secondary to hypocarbic bronchoconstriction (Elliott, 1992). With ablation of this compensation, as in a patient who is chemically paralyzed, heavily sedated, or anesthetized, the P_aCO_2 always increases from baseline and the (a–ET)PCO_2 gap widens (Nikodymova *et al.*, 1968). While the pulmonary artery angiogram, spiral chest computerized tomography, and scintillation $\dot{V}/\dot{Q}$ lung scan remain the gold standards for the diagnosis of pulmonary embolism, capnography has the advantage of not requiring arterial puncture, and using equipment that is essentially portable, lightweight, and commercially available (Eriksson *et al.*, 1989; Fletcher & Jonson, 1994). Decreased $P_{et}CO_2$ by time capnography has also been noticed to correlate quantitatively with lung perfusion defect and pulmonary artery pressure when low perfusion was due to pulmonary embolism (Kline *et al.*, 2000).

A sophisticated neural network has been used recently to interpret data collected from the capnogram of patients who have an established diagnosis of pulmonary embolism. Despite the fact that capnometer and flowmeter measurements were integrated into the network, as were vital signs typically seen in pulmonary embolism, sensitivity of nearly 100% was achieved, however with a low specificity of about 27% (Patel *et al.*, 1999).

In conclusion, pulmonary embolism can significantly affect both volumetric and time capnography. However, in spite of its potential, capnography cannot be considered a replacement for the above gold standard diagnostic techniques.

Capnography as an index of $\dot{V}/\dot{Q}$ mismatch in low cardiac output state

Decreased cardiac output decreases $P_{et}CO_2$ due to a relative change in the volume of perfused lung. The percent decrease in $P_{et}CO_2$ directly correlated with the percent decrease in cardiac output ($r^2 = 0.82$) in 24 patients undergoing aortic aneurysm surgery with constant ventilation (Leigh *et al.*, 1961). Additionally, a $P_{et}CO_2$ greater than 30 and 34 mmHg were, respectively, invariably associated with cardiac index greater than 2 l/min/m^2 (Askrog, 1966) and 2.5 l/min/m^2, respectively (Maslow *et al.*, 2001). When cardiac output is severely decreased, reduced alveolar blood flow will prevent CO_2 elimination from matching with systemic CO_2 production. As a result, $P_{et}CO_2$ will decrease while the mixed venous PCO_2 will continue to increase (Weil *et al.*, 1985). More sophisticated work in animals showed that the end-tidal CO_2 correlates well with left ventricular stroke volume index when transesophageal echocardiographic measurements were used to calculate stroke volume index in a pig model of ventricular fibrillation and resuscitation by chest compression (Pernat *et al.*, 2003). While the correlation between capnography and cardiac output in subjects with healthy lungs has been encouraging, results in patients with lung disease are still controversial (Pianosi & Hochman, 1996).

Capnography as an index of $\dot{V}/\dot{Q}$ mismatch in trauma

Major advantages of capnography are that it does not require collections of arterial blood, is essentially portable and lightweight, and easily commercially available. It is therefore of no surprise that the use of capnography in monitoring critically ill patients in transport, such as trauma victims, has been extensively described. The following is a short review of the clinical experience of time capnography "in trauma action".

$\dot{V}/\dot{Q}$ mismatch is predictably increased in trauma patients. However, the mechanism is thought to be largely secondary to an increase in alveolar dead-space related to blood loss and low cardiac output and, therefore, somewhat predictable. The most important clinical use of capnography has been found in the "targeting" of ventilation during prehospital care of major trauma victims before it is possible to obtain arterial blood gas analysis (Helm *et al.*, 2003). The implications of this use ought be obvious, as a considerable number of these patients, including those with associated head injuries, can be inadvertently hyperventilated with potentially worsened outcomes from decreased cerebral perfusion. In fact, it is relatively well known that profound and persistent hyperventilation can significantly increase the risk of cerebral ischemia and a subsequent poor long-term outcome (Muizelaar *et al.*, 1991; Prough & Lang, 1997).

Contrasting studies have also been seen in the trauma literature. For example, the incidence of normocapneic ventilation has been increased by following $P_{et}CO_2$ in trauma victims (Helm *et al.*, 2003) during transport (Ratnasabapathy *et al.*, 2002), as long as the patient is maintained in the same position (i.e. supine). Unfortunately, as frequent changes in position alter $\dot{V}/\dot{Q}$ matching, the correlation coefficient of P_aCO_2 versus $P_{et}CO_2$ has been disappointingly low ($r = 0.46$–0.62; $P < 0.001$) (Grenier *et al.*, 1999), thus possibly limiting the clinical usefulness of this technique when positioning is not "fixed".

In general, the application of CPAP in these patients decreases shunt and improves $\dot{V}/\dot{Q}$ matching, as long as the patient has been adequately resuscitated and there is no further "West zone I" produced. The application of CPAP has been shown to decrease functional dead-space in a swine model of acute lung injury from chest wall disruption when $\dot{V}/\dot{Q}$ ratio was measured by the MIGET technique (Schweiger *et al.*, 2003).

Artifacts affecting the interpretation of capnography in patients with $\dot{V}/\dot{Q}$ mismatch

The American Association of Respiratory Care (AARC) strongly recommends use of capnography in patients mechanically ventilated in the intensive care unit (ICU).

However, when capnography is used as an indirect monitor of the critically ill patient's P_aCO_2, one has to consider several limitations that can affect the accuracy of this technology:

1 The composition of the respiratory gas mixture may affect the capnogram, such as the use of high O_2 concentrations in critically ill patients (Ammann & Galvin, 1968) or the use of helium.[2]
2 The f_R may alter the slope of phase III and the $P_{et}CO_2$ measured value (Graybeal & Russell, 1994).
3 The presence of Freon®, used as a propellant in metered dose inhalers, can cause an artificial increase of the $P_{et}CO_2$ reading (Elliott *et al.*, 1991).
4 Contamination of the monitor or sampling system by secretions or condensate, a sample tube of excessive length, a sampling rate that is too high, or obstruction of the sampling chamber can lead to unreliable results.
5 Use of filters can lead to falsely low $P_{et}CO_2$ readings (Hardman *et al.*, 1997).
6 Small V_T delivery, especially in neonates and pediatric patients, with low continuous flow rates leaks into the ventilator circuit, around the tracheal tube cuffs, or in the presence of uncuffed tubes can result in a factitiously low $P_{et}CO_2$ value (Branson, 1990).
7 A low cardiac output state may result in an artificially low $P_{et}CO_2$ value.
8 In the presence of a carbonated beverage in the stomach, one may see several breaths with a factitiously elevated $P_{et}CO_2$ value (Li, 2001).

[2] Perkin-Elmer, M.G.A. (1982). *1100 Operation and maintenance manual*, p. 6–26.

Conclusion

Mismatching of ventilation and blood flow is common, and may become very severe in diseased lungs. The attention of physiologists and physicians has been recently focused on time and volume capnography to monitor dynamics of CO_2 in critically ill patients. It has been proven that both alveolar dead-space and venous admixture can contribute to abnormalities of the capnogram as a single entity or can coexist (Riley & Cournard, 1949). Therefore, capnographic features such as absolute $P_{et}CO_2$ value, capnographic waveform interpretation, as well as the (a–ET)PCO_2 differences need to be interpreted in view of the presence of $\dot{V}/\dot{Q}$ inequality from lung disease or hemodynamic factors. Despite its limitations, capnography can provide significant and clinically useful information, data of a type that may enable diagnostic and therapeutic data. As capnographic technology improves and clinical experience accumulates, we anticipate a greater use of this monitoring modality.

References

AARC Clinical Practice Guideline (2003). Capnography/capnometry during mechanical ventilation 2003, revision and update. *Respir. Care*, **48**: 534–539.

Agusti, A.G.N. & Barbera, J.A. (1994). Contribution of multiple inert gas elimination technique to pulmonary medicine. 2. Chronic pulmonary diseases: Chronic obstructive pulmonary disease and idiopathic pulmonary fibrosis. *Thorax*, **48**: 924–932.

Ammann, E.C. & Galvin, R.D. (1968). Problems associated with the determination of carbon dioxide by infrared absorption. *J. Appl. Physiol.*, **25**: 333–335.

Andrew, B.L. & Nunn, J.F. (2000). *Nunn's Applied Respiratory Physiology*, 5th edition. Butterworth-Heinemann, Boston; p. 46, 164, 243–245.

Askrog, V. (1966). Changes in (a–A)CO_2 difference and pulmonary artery pressure in anesthetized man. *J. Appl. Physiol.*, **21**: 1299–1305.

Badgwell, J.M., Kleinman, S.E. & Heavner, J.E. (1993). Respiratory frequency and artifact affect capnographic baseline in infants. *Anesth. Analg.*, **77**: 708–712.

Ballester, E., Reyes, A., Roca, J., Guitart, R., Wagner, P.D. & Rodriguez-Roisin, R. (1989). Ventilation–perfusion mismatching in acute severe asthma: effects of salbutamol and 100% oxygen. *Thorax*, **44**: 258–267.

Ballester, E., Roca, J., Ramis, L., Wagner, P.D. & Rodriguez-Roisin, R. (1990). Pulmonary gas exchange in chronic asthma response to 100% oxygen and salbutamol. *Am. Rev. Respir. Dis.*, **141**: 558–562.

Barbera, J.A., Ramirez, J., Roca, J., Wagner, P.D., Sanchez-Lloret, J. & Rodriguez-Roisin, R. (1990). Lung structure and gas exchange in mild chronic obstructive pulmonary disease. *Am. Rev. Respir. Dis.*, **141**: 895–901.

Berman, L.S., Pyles, S.T. (1988). Capnographic detection of anesthesia circle valve malfunctions. *Can. J. Anaesth.*, **35**: 473–475.

Bhavani-Shankar, K., Kumar, A.Y., Moseley, H.S. & Ahyee-Hallsworth, R. (1995). Terminology and the current limitations of time capnography: a brief review. *J. Clin. Monit.*, **11**: 175–182.

Bhavani-Shankar, K., Moseley, H., Kumar, A.Y. & Delph, Y. (1992). Capnometry and anaesthesia. *Can. J. Anaesth.*, **39**: 617–632.

Bohr, C. (1891). Uber die Lungenathmund. *Skand. Arch. Physiol.*, **2**: 236.

Branson, R.D. (1990). The measurement of energy expenditure: instrumentation, practical considerations, and clinical application. *Respir. Care*, **35**: 640–656.

Brown, L.H., Gough, J.E. & Seim, R.H. (1998). Can quantitative capnometry differentiate between cardiac and obstructive causes of respiratory distress? *Chest*, **113**: 323–326.

Burki, N.K. (1986). The dead space to tidal volume ratio in the diagnosis of pulmonary embolism. *Am. Rev. Respir. Dis.*, **133**: 679–685.

Caplan, R.A., Posner, K.L., Ward, R.J. & Cheney, F.W. (1990). Adverse respiratory events in anesthesia: a closed claims analysis. *Anesthesiology*, **72**: 828–833.

Cote, C.J., Rolf, N. & Liu, L.M., *et al.* (1991). A single-blind study of combined pulse oximetry and capnography in children. *Anesthesiology*, **74**: 980–987.

Crystal, R.G., Fulmer, J.D., Roberts, W.C., Moss, M.L., Line, B.R. & Reynolds, H.Y. (1976). Idiopathic pulmonary fibrosis. Clinical, histological, radiographic, physiologic, scintigraphic, cytologic and biochemical aspects. *Ann. Intern. Med.*, **85**: 769–788.

Dantzker, D.R., Wagner, P.D., Tornabene, V.W., Alazraki, N.P. & West, J.B. (1978). Gas exchange after pulmonary thromboembolization in dogs. *Circ. Res.*, **42**: 92–103.

Elliott, C.G. (1992). Pulmonary physiology during pulmonary embolism. *Chest*, **101**: 163S–171S.

Elliott, W.R., Raemer, D.B., Goldman, D.B. & Philip, J.H. (1991). The effects of bronchodilator-inhaler aerosol propellants on respiratory gas monitors. *J. Clin. Monit.*, **7**: 175–180.

Eriksson, L., Wollmer, P., Olsson, C., Albrechtsson, U., Larusdottir, H., Nilsson, R., Sjogren, A., Jonson, B. (1989).Diagnosis of pulmonary embolism based upon alveolar dead space analysis. *Chest*, **96**: 357–362.

Evans, J.W. & Wagner, P.D. (1977). Limits on VA/Q distributions from analysis of experimental inert gas elimination. *J. Appl. Physiol.*, **42**: 889–898.

Fletcher, R. (1988). Invasive and noninvasive measurement of the respiratory deadspace in anesthetized children with cardiac disease. *Anesth. Analg.*, **67**: 442–447.

Fletcher, R. & Jonson, B. (1984). Deadspace and the single breath test for carbon dioxide during anaesthesia and artificial ventilation. Effects of tidal volume and frequency of respiration. *Br. J. Anaesth.*, **56**: 109–119.

Fletcher, R., Jonson, B., Cumming, G. & Brew, J. (1981). The concept of dead space with special reference to the single breath test for carbon dioxide. *Br. J. Anaesth.*, **53**: 77–88.

Fletcher, R., Malmkvist, G., Niklason, L. & Jonson, B. (1986). On-line measurement of gas-exchange during cardiac surgery. *Acta Anaesthesiol. Scand.*, **30**: 295–299.

Graybeal, J.M. & Russell, G.B. (1994). Relative agreement between Raman and mass spectrometry for measuring end-tidal carbon dioxide. *Respir. Care*, **39**: 190–194.

Grenier, B., Verchère, E. & Mesli, A. *et al.* (1999). Capnography monitoring during neurosurgery: reliability in relation to various intraoperative positions. *Anesth. Analg.*, **88:** 43–48.

Gustafsson, P.M., Johansson, H.J. & Dahlbäck, G.O. (1994). Pneumotachographic nitrogen washout method for measurement of the volume of trapped gas in the lungs. *Pediatr. Pulmonol.*, **17**: 258–268.

Haldane, J.S. & Priestley, J.G. (1905). The regulation of the lung ventilation. *J. Physiol.* **32**: 225–266.

Hardman, J.G., Curran, J. & Mahajan, R.P. (1997). End-tidal carbon dioxide measurement and breathing system filters. *Anaesthesia*, **52**: 646–648.

Helm, M., Schuster, R., Hauke, J. & Lampl, L. (2003). Tight control of prehospital ventilation by capnography in major trauma victims. *Brit. J. Anaesth.* **90**: 327–332.

Hubble, C.L., Gentile, M.A., Tripp, D.S., Craig, D.M., Meliones, J.N. & Cheifetz, I.M. (2000). Deadspace to tidal volume ratio predicts successful extubation in infants and children. *Crit. Care Med.*, **28**: 2034–2040.

Jardin, F., Genevray, B., Pazin, M. & Margairaz, A. (1985). Inability to titrate PEEP in patients with acute respiratory failure using end-tidal carbon dioxide measurements. *Anesthesiology*, **62**: 530–533.

Jellinek, H., Hiesmayr, M., Simon, P., Klepetko, W. & Haider, W.A. (1993). Arterial to end-tidal CO_2 tension difference after bilateral lung transplantation. *Crit. Care Med.*, **21**: 1035–1040.

Kline, J.A., Kubin, A.K., Patel, M.M., Easton, E.J. & Seupal, R.A. (2000). Alveolar dead space as a predictor of severity of pulmonary embolism. *Acad. Emerg. Med.*, **7**: 611–617.

Kumar, A.Y., Bhavani-Shankar, K., Moseley, H.S. & Delph, Y. (1992). Inspiratory valve malfunction in a circle system: pitfalls in capnography. *Can. J. Anaesth.*, **39**: 997–999.

Leigh, M.D., Jones, J.C. & Motley, H.L. (1961). The expired carbon dioxide as a continuous guide of the pulmonary and circulatory systems during anesthesia and surgery. *J. Thoracic Cardiovasc. Surg.*, **41**: 597–610.

Li, J. (2001). Capnography alone is imperfect for endotracheal tube placement confirmation during emergency intubation. *J. Emerg. Med.*, **20**: 223–229.

Maslow, A., Stearns, G. & Bert, A. *et al.* (2001). Monitoring end-tidal carbon dioxide during weaning from cardiopulmonary bypass in patients without significant lung disease. *Anesth. Analg.*, **92**: 306–313.

Muizelaar, J.P., Marmarou, A. & Ward, J.D. *et al.* (1991). Adverse effects of prolonged hyperventilation in patients with severe head injury: A randomized clinical trial. *J. Neurosurg.*, **75**: 731–739.

Murray, I.P., Modell, J.H., Gallagher, T.J. & Banner, M.J. (1984). Titration of PEEP by the arterial minus end-tidal carbon dioxide gradient. *Chest*, **85**: 100–104.

Napolitano, L.M. (1999). Capnography in critical care. Accurate assessment of ARDS therapy? *Crit. Care Med.*, **27**: 862–863.

Niehoff, J., DelGuercio, C., LaMorte, W., Hughes-Grasberger, S.L., Heard, S., Dennis, R. & Yeston, N. (1988). Efficacy of pulse oximetry and capnometry in postoperative ventilatory weaning. *Crit. Care Med.*, **16**: 701–705.

Nikodymova, L., Daum, S., Stiksa, J. & Widimsky, J. (1968). Respiratory changes in thromboembolic disease. *Respiration*, **25**: 51–66.

Nuckton, T.J., Alonso, J.A., Kallet, R.H., Daniel, B.M., Pittet, J.F., Eisner, M.D. & Matthay, M.A. (2002). Pulmonary dead-space fraction as a risk factor for death in the acute respiratory distress syndrome. *New. Eng. J. Med.*, **346**: 1281–1286.

Nunn, J.F., Hill, D.W. (1960). Respiratory dead space and arterial to end-tidal carbon dioxide tension difference in anesthetized man. *J. Appl. Physiol.*, **15**: 383–389.

Patel, M.M., Rayburn, D.B., Browning, J.A. & Kline, J.A. (1999). Neural network analysis of the volumetric capnogram to detect pulmonary embolism. *Chest*, **116**: 1325–1332.

Pernat, A., Weil, M.H., Sun, S. & Tang, W. (2003). Stroke volumes and end-tidal carbon dioxide generated by precordial compression during ventricular fibrillation. *Crit. Care Med.*, **31**: 1819–1823.

Pianosi, P. & Hochman, J. (1996). End-tidal estimates of arterial PCO_2 for cardiac output measurements by CO_2 rebreathing: a study in patients with cystic fibrosis and healthy controls. *Pediatr. Pulmonol.*, **22**: 154–160.

Podraza, A.G., Salem, M.R., Joseph, N.J. & Brencley, J.L. (1991). Rebreathing due to incompetent unidirectional valves in the circle absorber system. *Anesthesiology*, **75**: A422.

Prough, D.S. & Lang, J. (1997). Therapy of patients with head injuries: key parameters for management. *J. Trauma*, **42**: S10–S18.

Ratnasabapathy, U., Allam, S. & Souter, M.J. (2002). Apparatus: evaluation of an expired fraction carbon dioxide monitor. *Anaesthesia*, **57**: 900–904.

Rich, G.F. & Sconzo, J.M. (1991). Continuous end-tidal CO_2 difference sampling within the proximal endotracheal tube estimates arterial CO_2 tension in infants. *Can. J. Anaesth.*, **38**: 201–203.

Riley, R.L. & Cournard, A. (1949). "Ideal" alveolar air and the analysis of ventilation–perfusion relationships in the lung. *J. Appl. Physiol.*, **1**: 825–847.

Robin, E.D., Julian, D.G., Travis, D.M. & Crump, C.H. (1964). A physiologic approach to the diagnosis of acute pulmonary embolism. *New. Engl. J. Med.*, **260**: 586–591.

Roca, J. & Wagner, P.D. (1994). Contribution of multiple inert gas elimination technique to pulmonary medicine. 1. Principles and information content of the multiple inert gas elimination technique. *Thorax*, **49**: 815–824.

Romero, P.V., Lucangelo, U., Lopez-Aguilar, J., Fernandez, R. & Blanch, L. (1997). Physiologically based indices of volumetric capnography in patients receiving mechanical ventilation. *Eur. Respir. J.*, **10**: 1309–1315.

Rose, J.T. & Banner, M.J. (2000). Effects of positive end expiratory pressure (PEEP) on physiologic deadspace volume to tidal volume ratio (V_D/V_T), abstracted. *Crit. Care Med.*, **28**: A86.

Saura, P., Blanch, L., Lucangelo, U., Fernandez, R., Mestre, J. & Artigas, A. (1996). Use of capnography to detect hypercapnic episodes during weaning from mechanical ventilation. *Intensive Care Med.*, **22**: 374–381.

Schmitz, B.D. & Shapiro, B.A. (1995). Capnography. *Respir. Care Clin. N. Am.*, **1**: 107–117.

Schreiner, M.S., Leksell, L.G., Gobran, S.R., Hoffman, E.A., Scherer, P.W. & Neufeld, G.R. (1993). Microemboli reduce phase III slopes of CO_2 and invert phase II slopes of infused SF6. *Respir. Physiol.*, **91**: 137–154.

Schweiger, J.W., Downs, J.B. & Smith, R.A. (2003). Chest wall disruption with and without acute lung injury: effects of continuous positive airway pressure therapy on ventilation and perfusion relationships. *Crit. Care Med.*, **31**: 2364–2370.

Strömberg, N.O.T. & Gustafsson, P.M. (2000). Ventilation inhomogeneity assessed by nitrogen washout and ventilation–perfusion mismatch by capnography in stable and induced airway obstruction. *Ped. Pulm.*, **29**: 94–102.

Tinker, J.H., Dull, D.L., Caplan, R.A., Ward, R.J. & Cheney, F.W. (1989). Role of monitoring devices in prevention of anesthetic mishaps: a closed claims analysis. *Anesthesiology*, **71**: 541–546.

van Meerten, R.J. (1970). Expiratory gas concentration curves for examination of uneven distribution of ventilation and perfusion in the lung. First communication: theory. *Respiration*, **27**: 552–564.

van Meerten, R.J. (1971). Expiratory gas concentration curves for examination of uneven distribution of ventilation and perfusion in the lung. Second communication: experiments. *Respiration*, **28**: 167–185.

Wagner, P.D., Naumann, P.F. & Laravuso, R.B. (1974a). Simultaneous measurement of eight foreign gases in blood by gas chromatography. *J. Appl. Physiol.*, **36**: 600–605.

Wagner, P.D., Saltzman, H.A. & West, J.B. (1974b). Measurement of continuous distributions of ventilation–perfusion ratios: theory. *J. Appl. Physiol.*, **36**: 588–599.

Wagner, P.D., Dantzker, D.R., Dueck, R., Clausen, J.L. & West, J.B. (1977). Ventilation–perfusion in chronic obstructive pulmonary disease. *J. Clin. Invest.*, **59**: 203–216.

Wagner, P.D., Hedenstierna, G. & Rodriguez-Roisin, R. (1996). Gas exchange, expiratory flow obstruction and the clinical spectrum of asthma. *Eur. Respir. J.*, **9**: 1278–1282.

Wahba, R.W. & Tessler, M.J. (1996). Misleading end-tidal CO_2 tensions. *Can. J. Anaesth.*, **43**: 862–866.

Weil, M.H., Bisera, J., Trevino, R.P. & Rackow, E.C. (1985). Cardiac output and end-tidal carbon dioxide. *Crit. Care Med.*, **13**: 907–909.

Wenzel, U., Rudiger, M., Wagner, M.H. & Wauer, R.R. (1999). Utility of deadspace and capnometry measurements in determination of surfactant efficacy in surfactant-depleted lungs. *Crit. Care Med.*, **27**: 946–952.

West, J.B. (1971). Causes of carbon dioxide retention in lung disease. *New. Engl. J. Med.*, **284**: 1232–1236.

Yoshimasu, T., Miyoshi, S., Maebeya, S., Hirai, I. & Naito, Y. (1996). Evaluation of effect of lung resection on lobar ventilation and perfusion using intrabronchial capnography. *Chest*, **109**: 25–30.

CAPNOGRAPHIC MEASURES 31

U. Lucangelo, A. Gullo, F. Bernabè & L. Blanch

Introduction

Capnography is a graphic display of carbon dioxide (CO_2) during the breathing cycle. CO_2 levels may be represented as a trace versus time (time capnography) or expiratory volume (volumetric capnography) with the single-breath test for CO_2 (SBT-CO_2). In this chapter, the clinical data obtained by the morphologic analysis of a capnogram and by the derived measurements are studied.

Initially, the morphology of a theoretical capnogram will be examined, with a single alveolus with compliance (C), in series with an airway with resistance (R). The understanding of the physiologic processes that make up this ideal model, allows a correct interpretation of normal and pathologic capnographic waveforms. Time and volumetric capnographic measures will then be compared in a theoretical model, in a healthy subject, and in pathologic conditions.

Time capnography

In time capnography, the whole breathing cycle is analyzed. Figure 31.1 shows a comparison between the capnogram derived by the ideal lung model and that of a healthy subject. In the ideal capnogram, the inspiratory phase (I) may be singled out, where PCO_2 is zero (as external air virtually contains no CO_2) and an expiratory phase (E), which is divided into four segments. At the beginning, PCO_2 is still zero (a–b segment), coming from airways that are not involved in gas exchange. The b–c segment corresponds to the sharp increase in PCO_2 concentration from the alveoli that produce the gas exchange; the attained value remains constant in time (c–d segment), and then sharply drops again to zero, corresponding with the beginning of the next breath. The square waveform of the theoretical capnogram is due to a situation of perfect homogeneity in the model, as the whole system is regulated by alveolar compliance and by airway resistance to the expiratory flow. Hence, CO_2 elimination depends on a single time constant ($\tau = R \times C$), and on a single ventilation/perfusion ($\dot{V}/\dot{Q}$) ratio (Mangalaboyi *et al.*, 1992).

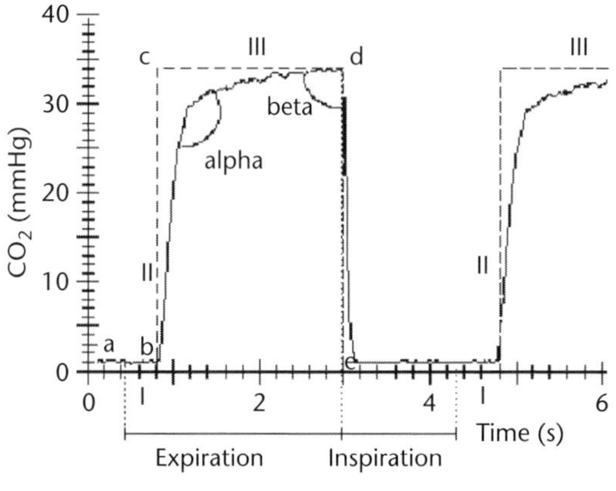

Figure 31.1 Normal time capnogram.

This is why the b–c and d–e segments are perfectly orthogonal, and the c–d segment is parallel to the time axis, thus forming a 90° angle between them. Basically, the lung is made of approximately 300–400 million alveoli, each having its own τ, and a gravitational variation in the $\dot{V}/\dot{Q}$ ratio (Hess, 1990; Bhavani-Shankar *et al.*, 1995). Therefore, in the capnogram of a healthy subject, variations in angle width and in inclination of its segments may be observed (Swedlow, 1986; Bhavani-Shankar *et al.*, 1995). As in the theoretical model, an inspiratory phase (I) and an expiratory phase (E) made of three segments may be singled out. The first phase (a–b) represents the beginning of expiration. The analyzed gas fills in the anatomic dead-space (V_d) made of those structures that are not suitable for gas exchange, such as pharynx, larynx, trachea, and bronchi. In mechanically ventilated subjects, the endotracheal tube or the tracheostomy probe are included in the V_d. Therefore, the concentration of CO_2 from these regions is close to zero up to point b.

From this point on, a second phase starts (wall of the capnogram), which is a mixed air zone. It is a segment with an S-shaped trend and with a sharp upswing due to mixing of air coming from the V_d with air coming

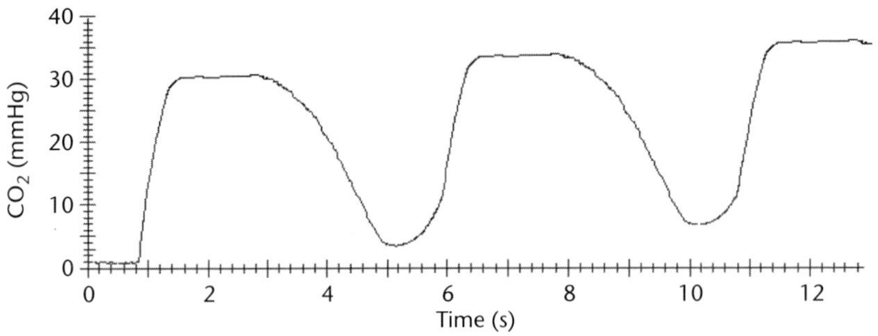

Figure 31.2 Malfunctioning in the inspiratory valve, characterized by a rise in the baseline, by an extension of phase III, and by a widening of the beta angle.

from alveoli with rapid depletion. The third phase (c–d), otherwise called "alveolar plateau" represents exhalation of pure alveolar gas, and it rises slightly due to the mild inhomogeneity of the $\dot{V}/\dot{Q}$ ratio and of alveolar CO_2 concentration. Hoffbrand (1966) has demonstrated a mean capnograph slope of 1.84 mmHg/l in normal subjects.

The highest value of CO_2 during the alveolar plateau (point d), which is normally present at end expiration, is called end-expiratory partial pressure or end-tidal CO_2 ($P_{et}CO_2$).

Once phase III is completed, the capnographic wave sharply descends towards zero (d–e), due to the irrelevant amount of CO_2 usually present in inspiratory gas, thus forming an approximately right angle (beta angle). The descending limb of the capnogram represents the inspiratory phase in which CO_2-free gas from the airways is inhaled, thus determining the rapid fall of PCO_2 to zero. In conclusion, the portion of the capnographic wave from beginning of inspiration to beginning of expiration is termed as phase 0; it consists of the descending limb of the capnogram, and the initial portion of the baseline. The final part of the baseline represents phase I of the expiratory segment. Phase 0 represents the inspiratory portion of the breathing cycle (Bhavani-Shankar *et al.*, 1992; 1995).

At the end of phase III, a terminal upswing may occasionally be seen, called phase IV. In the absence of lung disease, this finding is caused by alveolar characteristics under circumstances such as pregnancy and obesity. In both populations, due to a decrease in lung compliance and in functional residual capacity (FRC), two lung compartments are determined, each having different mechanical properties and different $\dot{V}/\dot{Q}$ ratio (fast- and slow-depletion compartments). The action of slower alveoli, richer in CO_2, is more evident in anesthesia and in artificial ventilation with high tidal volumes and low breathing frequency.

Finally, in the capnogram of a normal subject it is possible to separate the alpha angle between phases II and III (100–110°), and the beta angle (≅90°) between phase III and inspiratory phase (Figure 31.1) (Bhavani-Shankar *et al.*, 1995).

Pathologic time capnogram

The main variations in the morphology of the capnographic wave are now discussed.

Phase I (a–b segment)

The length of the a–b segment may be artificially increased, thus modifying the breathing circuit by addition of airway adapters, and antibacterial filters that increase the instrument dead-space (V_d). The main factors that may cause a progressive rise in the baseline are connected with the presence of CO_2 in inspiratory gas. This may occur with modern ventilators because of a malfunctioning of the inspiratory valve that, apart from raising the baseline, makes the beta angle more obtuse. When low-flow or closed-circuit anesthesia ventilators are used, the rise in the baseline may be caused by depletion of the CO_2 absorbent system, which occurs in the absence of changes in the beta angle (Figure 31.2) (Pyles *et al.*, 1984; Berman & Pyles, 1988; Podraza *et al.*, 1991; Yasodananda *et al.*, 1992). A sharp rise in the baseline is a typical sign of contamination of the device that analyzes gas exhaled in combination with water, mucus or impurities (Figure 31.3).

Alterations in phases II and III

Bronchial obstruction makes regional alveolar ventilation inhomogeneous, thus altering the normal $\dot{V}/\dot{Q}$ ratio. This determines different readings of CO_2 alveolar pressure that are asynchronously exhaled, flattening the verticality of phase II. As a consequence, phase III increases its slope and the alpha angle becomes more obtuse. The main clinical causes of obstruction of the expiratory flow are asthma, bronchospasm, and chronic obstructive pulmonary disease (COPD). Even emphysema produces a slanted upstroke of phase II. Furthermore, obstruction of exhaled gas may be caused by external factors such as

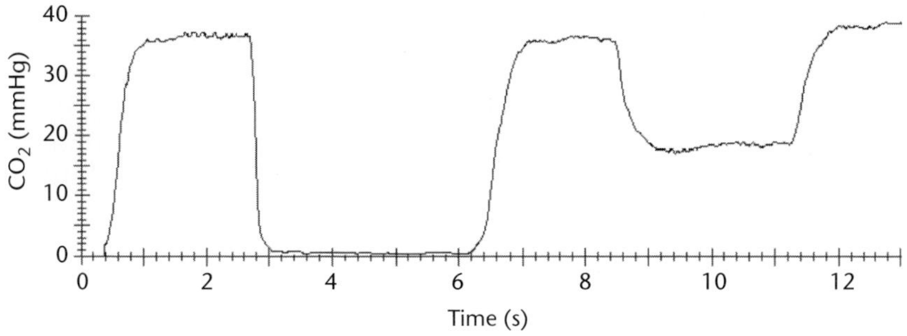

Figure 31.3 Malfunctioning in the cell that analyzes exhaled gas.

a kinked tracheal tube (Leigh *et al.*, 1961; Cote *et al.*, 1986; Weingarten, 1986; van Ganderingen *et al.*, 1987; Weingarten, 1990).

The variations in phase III slope can be ascribed to the following physiologic phenomena (Bhavani-Shankar *et al.*, 1992).

1 Cyclic variation in alveolar CO_2 during ventilation (greater during expiration than during inspiration). CO_2 is constantly poured into the alveoli, which progressively reduce their volume as expiration proceeds. The produced effect is a constant increase in alveolar PCO_2 until end expiration, followed by an increase in the slope in phase III.
2 Late emptying of the alveoli with the lowest $\dot{V}/\dot{Q}$ ratio and, thus, with relatively higher PCO_2. If all the alveoli had the same PCO_2, phase III would be almost horizontal. In effect, this "ideal" situation does not occur even in normal lungs, which have a wide range of $\dot{V}/\dot{Q}$. Some alveoli have a higher $\dot{V}/\dot{Q}$ ratio (overventilated) than that of "ideal" alveoli and, therefore, have a relatively lower PCO_2. Others have a lower $\dot{V}/\dot{Q}$ ratio (underventilated) than that of ideal alveoli, resulting in a relatively higher PCO_2. Delayed emptying of the alveoli with a low $\dot{V}/\dot{Q}$ ratio (high PCO_2) contributes to the increase in the slope of phase III. The mechanisms by which this effect can be produced are the following:
   - *Within the terminal respiratory units:* The difference in $\dot{V}/\dot{Q}$ between units can be caused by both incomplete mixing of the gases (alveolar mixing defect), and by the fact that the maximum ventilation and the maximum perfusion of that unit are out of phase (temporal mismatching – the perfusion is greater during the last part of expiration when ventilation is less).
   - *Between the terminal respiratory units:* This can be the consequence of regional variations in the ventilation per unit of perfusion, which produces a range of $\dot{V}/\dot{Q}$ ratios (spatial mismatching). In this case the phase III slope is determined by the nature of the alveolar emptying: synchronous or asynchronous. If the alveolar units empty synchronously, the gas from well-perfused and poorly perfused alveoli is exhaled simultaneously, resulting in a horizontal or slightly inclined phase III slope. If the units empty in an asynchronous manner, the units with a higher time constant, and thus a higher PCO_2, empty later (sequential emptying), resulting in a steeper phase III slope.

Other factors such as changes in cardiac output (CO), CO_2 production, airway resistance, and FRC can further influence the $\dot{V}/\dot{Q}$ ratio of the various lung units affecting the height or slope of the phase III curve. This pattern is evidenced as a normal physiologic variation even during pregnancy (Bhavani-Shankar *et al.*, 1995).

Deformation of phases II and III: capnographic measures

As the the geometric form of the whole capnographic wave is the result of a continuing process of elimination of alveolar gas, pathologies affecting phase II also affect the alveolar plateau and, for this reason, will be dealt with in the same section. Lung pathologies globally interact with CO_2 washout, thus altering both convective processes (flow rate, breathing frequency, tidal volume, and conducting airway volume) and diffusive processes, time, available cross section, and intra airway concentration gradient (Neufeld *et al.*, 1991). The shape of the capnogram is modified by airway obstruction (Hoffbrand, 1966), and the evaluation of this deformation, using measurable indexes, has been previously analyzed as a measurement of bronchial patency. Worth (1986) reported on the most important indexes applied in the literature for quantitative description of time capnography in patients with chronic airflow limitation; these indexes include phases II and III. These indexes have been calculated as the change in partial pressure per second, as percentage of the initial end-tidal amplitude or as time interval between 25% and 75% of the inspiratory/end-tidal partial pressure difference. Another index has been proposed, which calculates the minimum radius of curvature of the alpha angle as a direct measurement of the time constant.

Recently, several studies confirmed that the slope of phase III is connected with asthma, COPD, and respiratory system resistance (R_{rs}) in intubated and in spontaneously breathing patients (Blanch *et al.*, 1994; Yaron, 1996).

The slope of expired CO_2 (mmHg/s) can be calculated in several ways: by linear regression during phase III of the expired capnogram. The initial 25% of the expired capnogram is rejected for calculation, as it consists of gas exhaled in phases I and II (Blanch *et al.*, 1994) or as in the study of You *et al.* (1992), during the half-second preceding the end-expiratory CO_2 peak, or else calculated at 0.36 s before the end of expirogram (Kumar *et al.*, 1992). Yaron (1996) calculated the derivative (dCO_2/dt) of the alveolar plateau versus time. Both studies proved that there is an increase in the slope in phase III in subjects affected by COPD and/or asthma, rather than in a control group without lung disease. In particular, in the population studied by Blanch *et al.* (1994), which included intubated and mechanically ventilated subjects affected by COPD, ischemic heart disease, septic shock, acute respiratory distress syndrome (ARDS), asthma, and coma, the slope in phase III ranged from 0.69 to 12.3 mmHg, with an average of 3.61 ± 0.40 mmHg. Furthermore, average expired CO_2 slope was 1.62 ± 0.13 mmHg in patients without auto-positive end-expiratory pressure (autoPEEP) and 4.88 ± 0.51 mmHg in patients with autoPEEP ($P < 0.01$). These findings suggest that a steeper average slope in phase III is associated with a higher degree of alveolar inhomogeneity, confirmed by the presence of high autoPEEP readings. Although the population analyzed (41 patients) was heterogeneous concerning the lung pathologies presented, this study demonstrates a fair overall correlation between autoPEEP and R_{rs} ($r = 0.75$; $P < 0.001$), and between autoPEEP and expired CO_2 slope ($r = 0.74$; $P < 0.001$). Furthermore, as evidence of the importance of total resistances (including the action of the airways, and of flow resistance properties of the endotracheal tube and of the equipment), in the process of CO_2 elimination a linear correlation was evidenced between R_{rs} and the slope in phase III ($r = 0.86$; $P < 0.001$). However, due to the inhomogeneity of the patients analyzed, and to the high prediction interval limits (±7.89 cmH_2O/l/s), R_{rs} readings cannot be accurately determined.

Furthermore, the slope of the alveolar plateau was considered in relation with spirometric readings in asthma patients, expecting to use the capnogram during bronchospasm, and considering its response to bronchodilators that are known to influence spirometric indexes.

You *et al.* (1992) studied a group of 24 asthma patients, with an average slope in phase III of 0.3 ± 0.23%/s, with a statistically significant difference from a control group (0.08 ± 0.06%/s). In asthma patients, a very significant correlation was evidenced between the slope of phase III and forced expired volume in 1 s (FEV1) ($r = 0.83$; $P < 0.001$). Furthermore, in 13 asthma patients the effect of the bronchodilating therapy was assessed, which produced an increase in FEV1, and a decrease in the slope of phase III ($r = 0.96$; $P < 0.001$).

Similar results were obtained by Yaron (1996), who found an important correlation between expiratory slope of phase III (dCO_2/dt) and peak expiratory flow rate (PEFR) in spontaneously breathing asthmatic patients and in normal healthy volunteers. The average dCO_2/dt readings in asthma patients (0.26 ± 0.06), and PEFR readings (274 ± 96 l/min) were significantly different ($P < 0.001$) from readings in normal healthy subjects ($dCO_2/dt = 0.13 \pm 0.06$; PEFR = 527 ± 96 l/min).

After bronchodilating therapy in 18 of the asthma patients, percentage PEFR readings increased from 58 ± 17% to 74 ± 17% of predicted value ($P < 0.001$), in association with a decrease in dCO_2/dt from 0.27 ± 0.05 to 0.19 ± 0.07 ($P < 0.005$).

This study suggests that the capnogram is useful in determining the greater effectiveness of inhaled bronchodilating therapy rather than spirometry, as an effort-independent, non-invasive method, easily performed at the patient's bedside (Figure 31.4).

The great disadvantage of these indexes is that they are based on a partial pressure–time plot. When expiratory partial pressure is plotted versus time, even in healthy subjects, curve-deforming influences, like expiratory flow, have to be taken into account (Smidt, 1976).

Alterations of the inspiratory phase

In instances when the CO_2 exhaled by external air or by fresh gas flow is diluted, $P_{et}CO_2$ and beta angle readings may present artifacts (Figure 31.5).

If the inspiratory valve in a closed-circuit respiratory system is malfunctioning or in a sidestream capnograph with a high response time (Figure 31.6), there may be an extension and/or a decrease in the slope of the descending limb (van Ganderingen *et al.*, 1987; Berman & Pyles, 1988; Pascucci *et al.*, 1989; Kumar *et al.*, 1992).

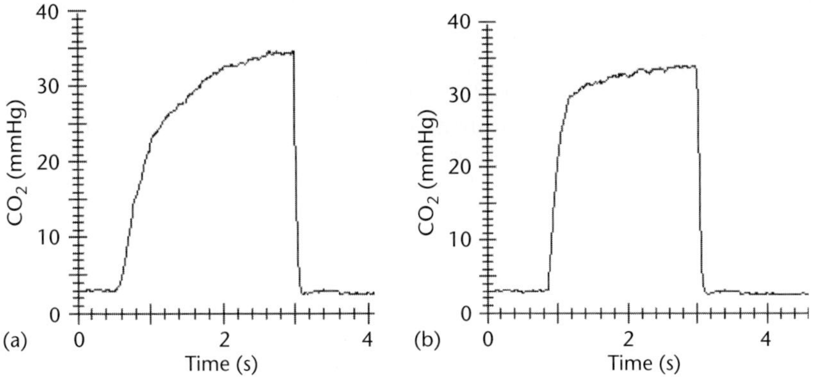

Figure 31.4 Capnogram before (a) and after (b) bronchodilating therapy. Note that in figure (a) phases II and III are extended, and the alpha angle is wider.

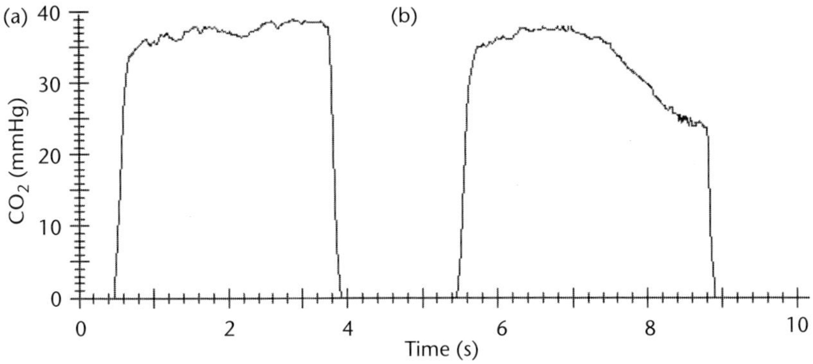

Figure 31.5 In (a) a normal wave is seen. On the other hand in (b), the wave presents artifacts due to inadequate sample rate and/or dilution of exhaled gas by the continuing gas flow.

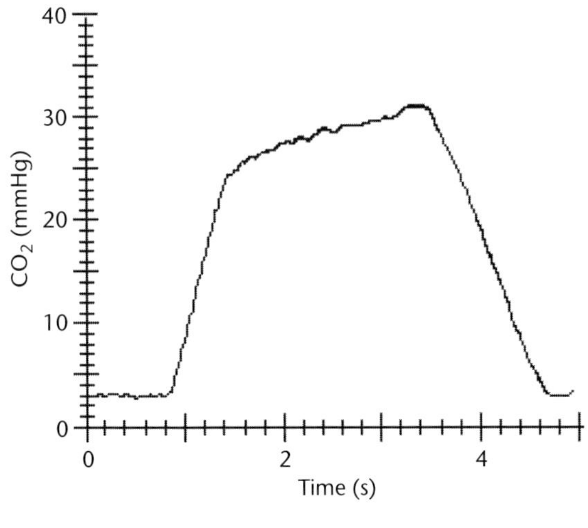

Figure 31.6 Extension of the inspiratory descending limb due to vaporization of gas on the sample line or to the high response time of the analyzer. It occurs in children, who have a shorter breathing cycle.

Volumetric capnography

In the previous chapter, the usefulness of the capnogram was explained, when CO_2 is measured versus time. It was also hinted that CO_2 may be measured versus volume, resembling a single-breath test of nitrogen (SBT-N_2) washout, which is normally used in pulmonary pathophysiology studies to determine closure volume and anatomic dead-space (Fowler, 1948; Comroe & Fowler, 1951). The physiologic mechanism responsible for phases I, II, and III in a time capnogram is similar to the one responsible for the phases seen in a SBT-CO_2 curve or an SBT-N_2 curve (Bhavani-Shankar *et al.*, 1995).

A typical SBT-CO_2 is shown in Figure 31.7, where the three phases that characterize it can be clearly distinguished (Bhavani-Shankar *et al.*, 1992). Phase I represents the gas without CO_2 arriving from the airways (anatomic and instrument dead-space). The following phase II consists of a rapid S-shaped rise (the result of mixing of dead-space gas and alveolar gas). Finally, phase III (alveolar plateau) represents the CO_2-rich gas coming from the alveoli. Even in this case, phase II forms with phase III an alpha angle.

The study of the phase III slope of the volumetric capnogram gives a more accurate picture of the state of pulmonary $\dot{V}/\dot{Q}$ ratio than the corresponding CO_2 versus time trace (Hoffbrand, 1966).

This may occur because a smaller volume of expired gas (approximately the final 15%) occupies half the

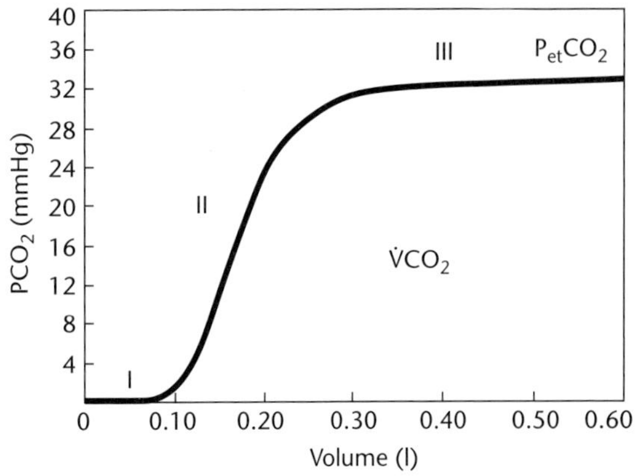

Figure 31.7 Normal volumetric capnogram.

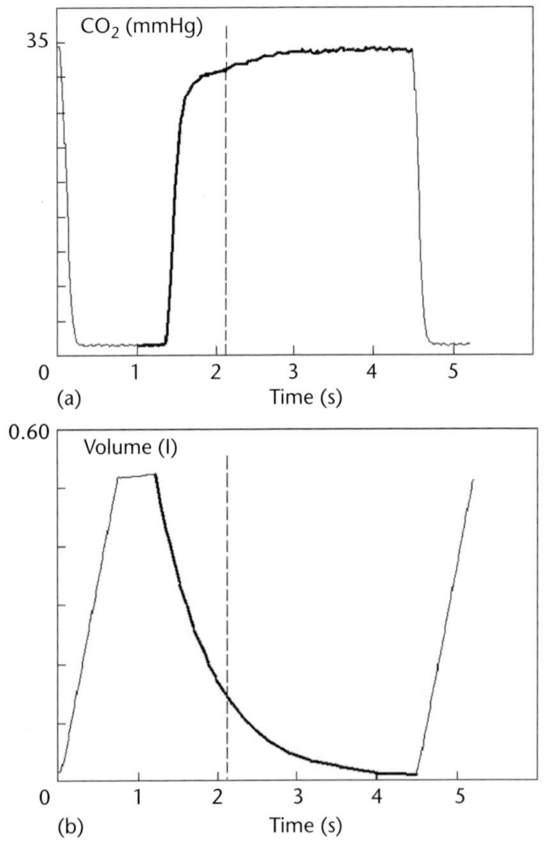

Figure 31.8 CO_2 elimination (a) and expiratory volume (b) are plotted versus time. Alveolar plateau corresponds to the lowest part of expired volume as depicted by the dotted line.

time available for expiration (Figure 31.8). In this case, CO_2 alterations are distributed in a relative long period of time, which results in a decrease in the slope of the alveolar plateau (Bhavani-Shankar *et al.*, 1995).

The advanced technology combination of airway flow monitoring and mainstream capnography allows the pulmonary V_d and CO_2 production ($\dot{V}CO_2$) to be calculated. The SBT-CO_2 system allows breath-by-breath calculation of this and other important parameters of ventilatory monitoring.

For these reasons, the use of volumetric capnography is clinically more profitable than time capnography.

Deformation of phase II: volume capnographic measures

Worth (1986) proved that the analysis of phase II versus exhaled volume (ranging from 25–50% to 50–75% of the expiratory CO_2 tension) separates healthy subjects from asthma and emphysema patients. These findings prove that serial inhomogeneity due to different airway morphology may be expressed by the variations in the slope of phase II versus volume. However, the discrimination degree of this index is lower when healthy subjects are compared with emphysema patients, characterized by mild airway obstruction (Kars *et al.*, 1995).

Deformation of phase III: volume capnographic measures

Ream *et al.* (1995), analyzed the pattern of the capnographic wave in healthy children, with age ranging from 5 months to 17 years, which evidenced a progressive normalization of the slope of phase III with increasing age. In fact, lung growth involves an increase in the number of acinar cells, which in turn leads to an increase in alveolar surface and to a decrease in resistance to gas diffusion. Morphologic lung growth determines a decrease in the arterial–alveolar CO_2 gradient, with a flattening and normalization of the slope of phase III.

This study proves that any interpretation of the capnographic wave must be considered in relation with the patient's age, and the delay in stabilization of the slope of phase III could be a sign of silent pulmonary disease.

Further studies evidenced the role of the slope of phase III, which turns out to be correlated with FRC in a surfactant-depleted animal mode (McRae & Neufeld, 1993) and it separates, in another model, healthy from ARDS animals.

Recently, from a global analysis of SBT-CO_2, it was evidenced that the slope of phase III was one of the most robust predictors of lung volume variations in healthy animals during control ventilation (Stenz *et al.*, 1998) and in a model with acute lung injury (Arnold *et al.*, 2000).

Volume capnography in dead-space evaluation (V_d)

From the analysis of SBT-CO_2, it is possible to determine the airway, physiologic, and alveolar V_d (Fletcher *et al.*, 1981) (Figure 31.9).

The measurement of Fowler V_d (airway V_d) is based on the geometric method of equivalent areas (p = q), obtained by crossing the back extrapolation of phase III with a vertical line traced so as to have equal p and q areas. Airway V_d is then measured from the beginning of expiration to the point where the vertical line crosses the volume axis (Fowler, 1948).

Figure 31.10 differs from Figure 31.9 with a line parallel to the volume axis, equal to the CO_2 arterial pressure value (P_aCO_2).

In this case, it is possible to determine the readings from areas Y and Z, which represent the values of alveolar and airway V_d, respectively. Table 31.1 summarizes SBT-CO_2 parameters and those derived from the added P_aCO_2 readings.

Last, if these values are referred to the tidal volume (V_t), it is possible to single out several dead-space components (Fletcher *et al.*, 1981):

$$\frac{V_{d\ phys}}{V_t} = \frac{Y + Z}{X + Y + Z}$$

$$\frac{V_{d\ alv}}{V_t} = \frac{Y}{X + Y + Z}$$

$$\frac{V_{d\ alv}}{V_{t\ alv}} = \frac{Y}{X + Y}$$

$$\frac{V_{d\ aw}}{V_t} = \frac{Z}{X + Y + Z}.$$

An alternative method to measure airway dead-space is the one introduced by Langley *et al.* (1976), which is based on determination of the $\dot{V}CO_2$ value, which corresponds to the area inscribed within the CO_2 versus volume curve (indicated in the figure as X area). Further on, $\dot{V}CO_2$ is plotted versus expired volume (Figure 31.11). Airway V_d can be calculated from the value obtained on the volume axis by back extrapolation of the first linear part of the $\dot{V}CO_2$ versus volume curve (Fletcher *et al.*, 1981).

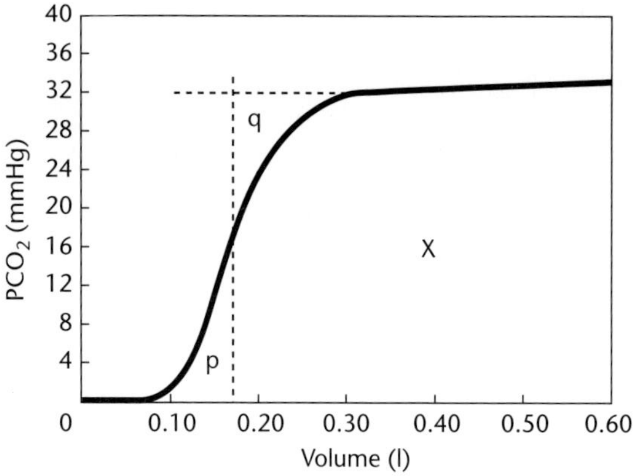

Figure 31.9 Analysis of SBT-CO_2 to determine the airway, physiologic, and alveolar V_d.

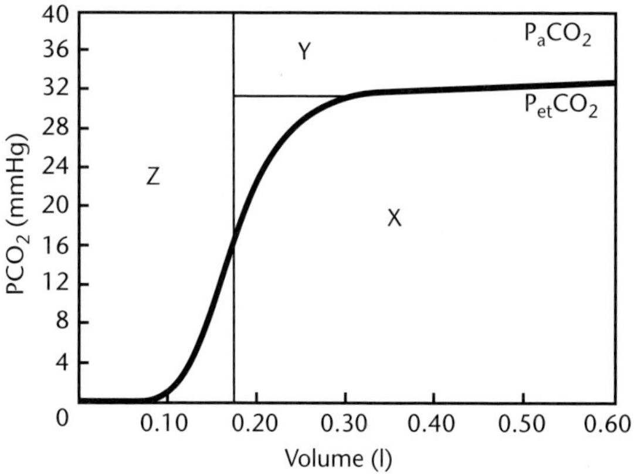

Figure 31.10 This figure differs from Figure 31.9 with a line parallel to the volume axis, equal to the P_aCO_2.

Table 31.1 SBT-CO_2 parameters and those derived from the added P_aCO_2 readings

SBT-CO_2 measures the following:	
Airway dead-space	Anatomic dead-space
Tidal alveolar volume	Actual air volume in gas exchange
Alveolar ventilation per minute	Actual air volume in gas exchange per minute
V_d/V_t	Airway dead-space/tidal volume ratio
CO_2 production	Amount of CO_2 produced by the metabolism
Arterial CO_2 allows to measure the following parameters:	
Physiologic dead-space	Volume of inspired gas, not active in gas exchange (combination of airway alveolar dead-space)
Alveolar dead-space	Ventilated area not involved in gas exchange
Physiologic V_d/V_t	Physiologic dead-space/tidal volume ratio

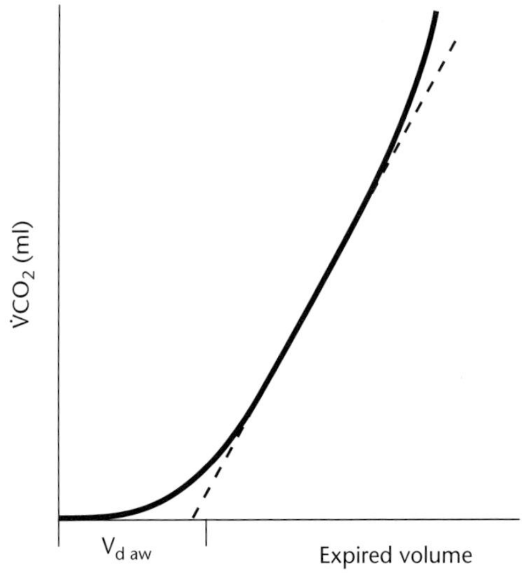

Figure 31.11 The method of Langley and others for estimation of airway dead-space.

Although these indexes are clinically useful, they are always bound to visual criteria for the definition of phase III. Often, the geometric analysis establishing the separation between the second and third phases of the capnogram is hardly seen even in healthy subjects. Another drawback is the morphologic need to represent the third phase as a straight line, ignoring the possibility that a rise in expiration PCO_2 may not be linear (You *et al.*, 1994).

Volumetric capnography as non-invasive determination of cardiac output

It is generally known that all situations producing a decrease in lung flow (pulmonary embolism, severe hemorrhage, cardiac arrest, etc.) affect the capnographic wave, which exponentially decreases in width. This phenomenon is due to the so-called CO_2 "dilution" effect, caused by a decrease in pulmonary blood flow, alveolar ventilation being equal. In this situation, the phases of the capnogram versus time do not vary (except in height) and, in particular, phase III preserves its initial slope. Similarly, SBT-CO_2 undergoes morphologic changes during the alterations of the hemodynamic conditions that, as proposed by Arnold *et al.* (1996), may be used for a non-invasive determination of CO. The authors analyzed in a sheep 21 indexes derived from SBT-CO_2 during cardiac output (CO) alterations. After an initial bivariate linear regression analysis, 20 of the 21 analyzed indexes turned out to be connected with CO, thus proving a close association between volumetric capnography and CO measured by ultrasonic flow probe. A following stepwise linear regression analysis was used to create a multivariate predictive equation of CO. From the statistical analysis, only two variables were singled out; when these variables were associated, they conveyed a higher predictive value to the experimental model ($r^2 = 0.94$, $P < 0.0001$): the angle between the slope line for phases II and III, divided by the volume of CO_2 per breath (angle/mlCO_2), and the slope of phase II. The equation of predicted CO is as follows:

$$CO = b + (-0.408)X_1 + 0.044\,X_2,$$

where b represents the baseline CO measure, X_1 = angle/mlCO_2 and X_2 = slope phase II.

It must be underlined that the only variable not related to CO is the slope of phase III, which, as evidenced by Arnold *et al.* (1996), is an accurate predictor of lung volume change.

The encouraging results of this study suggest a clinical use of SBT-CO_2 in the field of non-invasive hemodynamic and ventilatory monitoring. Recently, Murias *et al.* (2002) have shown that using a partial rebreathing method to measure CO compared to thermodilution yielded a bias and precision calculation of -0.07 ± 0.91 l/min for lower or intermediate CO values in critical care patients. Therefore, the non-invasive partial CO_2 rebreathing technique may be an alternative method for CO determination in mechanically ventilated critically ill patients.

Alveolar ejection volume/tidal volume

Finally, a different approach to volumetric capnography is that of using the CO_2 elimination curve versus volume ($\dot{V}CO_2/V_t$) curve. Furthermore, using the $\dot{V}CO_2/V_t$ curve, the fraction of volume flow corresponding to alveolar gas exhalation can be calculated.

Alveolar ejection volume (V_{ae}) can be defined as the fraction of V_t with minimal V_d contamination. This may be inferred from the asymptotic pattern of the $\dot{V}CO_2/V_t$ curve at end expiration, where by definition V_d is equal to zero. We defined Vae as the volume that characterizes this relationship up to a 5% variation (Romero *et al.*, 1997).

The method of Vae determination is presented in a normal subject and in an ARDS patient (Figure 31.11) where $\dot{V}CO_2/V_t$ curves in a representative breath are recorded. After a given volume has been exhaled, $\dot{V}CO_2$ progressively increases to reach a total amount of CO_2 elimination in a single expiration ($\dot{V}CO_{2\,tot}$). The increase in $\dot{V}CO_2$ is slightly non-linear because of alveolar inhomogeneity, that is the presence of a certain amount of alveolar gas contaminated by

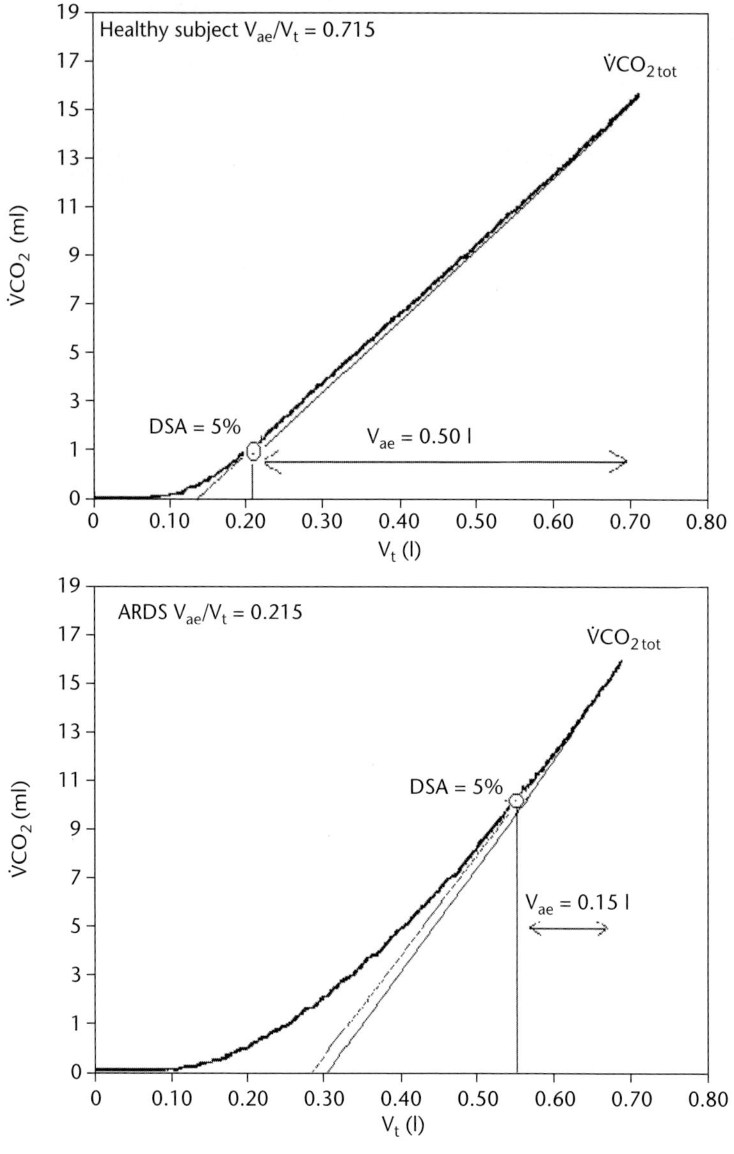

Figure 31.12 Determination of V_{ae}/V_t in a healthy and an ARDS patient.

parallel V_d. At the very end of expiration, exhaled gas comes only from alveoli, thus being pure alveolar gas. Assuming a fixed amount of V_d contamination (V_d allowance, DSA), we can obtain a point on the $\dot{V}CO_2/V_t$ curve representing the beginning of the V_{ae}. The Vae was then measured from the $\dot{V}CO_2/V_t$ curve as follows.

First, the slope of the last 50 points of every cycle was obtained by linear fitting, using the least squares method. Then Vae was obtained as the value of the volume at the intersection between the $\dot{V}CO_2/V_t$ curve and a straight line, having a maximal value at end expiration and a slope equal to 0.95 (1 − DSA) times the calculated slope (Figure 31.12). Vae is expressed as a fraction of V_t (V_{ae}/V_t) (Romero *et al.*, 1997).

V_{ae}/V_t has been shown to be a good index in that, it demonstrates different behaviors between healthy subjects undergoing general anesthesia and patients with ARDS, it retains this discriminative capacity independent of the tidal volume and PEEP applied. Finally, apart from the phase III slope, which bears no relation to any index of respiratory mechanics, V_{ae}/V_t is inversely correlated with resistances and directly correlated with compliance of the respiratory system. It follows that V_{ae}/V_t can have clinical applications in all those lung disorders characterized by marked alveolar inhomogeneity (Lucangelo *et al.*, 1995; Romero *et al.*, 1995; 1997; Blanch *et al.*, 1999).

Recently (Bernabé *et al.*, 2003) Vae/Vt prognostic value for outcome has been tested in 25 mechanically ventilated patients with acute lung injury. The change in V_{ae}/V_t between admission and after 48 hours (dV_{ae}/V_t) was greater in patients who died (0.07 ± 0.09), compared to patients who survived (-0.03 ± 0.06, $P < 0.01$), concluding that dV_{ae}/V_t can predict mortality in patients with acute lung injury.

Conclusions

Time capnography is universally acknowledged as a safety tool during anesthesia. As an easy-to-use, non-invasive method, capnography is also used in intensive care settings, both in intubated and in non-intubated patients. However, with new contributions to the literature, it is evident that volumetric capnography represents a logical evolution from time capnography. Technologic improvements enabled the use of combined sensors for simultaneous measurement and recording of expiratory flow and CO_2 elimination at the patient's bedside. These recordings establish several parameters for hemodynamic and ventilatory monitoring. Although a standard for these indexes is not yet available, and further clinical studies are required, the practical and theoretical advantage of volume on time capnography is unquestionable.

References

Arnold, J.H., Stenz, R.I., Thompson, J.E. & Arnold, L.W. (1996). Noninvasive determination of cardiac output using single breath CO_2 analysis. *Crit. Care Med.*, **24**: 1701–1705.

Arnold, J.H., Stenz, R.I., Grenier, B. & Thompson J.E. (2000). Single-breath CO_2 analysis as a predictor of lung volume change in a model of acute lung injury. *Crit. Care Med.*, **28**: 760–764.

Berman, L.S. & Pyles, S.T. (1988). Capnographic detection of anesthesia circle valve malfunctions. *Can. J. Anaesth.*, **35**: 473–475.

Bernabé, F., Vatua, S., Lucangelo, U., Villagrá, A., Saura, P., Romero, P. & Blanch, L. (2003). Alveolar ejection volume predicts death in patients with acute lung injury. *Am. J. Resp. Crit. Care Med.*, **167**, A934.

Bhavani-Shankar, K., Moseley, H., Kumar, A.Y. & Delph, Y. (1992). Capnometry and anaesthesia. Review article. *Can. J. Anaesth.*, **39**: 617–632.

Bhavani-Shankar, K., Kumar, A.Y., Moseley, H. & Hallsworth, R.A. (1995). Terminology and the current limitations of time capnography: a brief review. *J. Clin. Monit.*, **11**: 175–182.

Blanch, L., Fernandez, R., Saura, P., Baigorri, F. & Artigas, A. (1994). Relationship between expired capnogram and respiratory system resistance in critically ill patients during total ventilatory support. *Chest*, **105**: 219–223.

Blanch, L., Lucangelo, U., Lopez, J., Fernandez, R. & Romero, P. (1999). Volumetric capnography and respiratory system mechanics in patients with acute lung injury: effects of positive end expiratory pressure. *Eur. Respir. J.*, **13**: 1048–1054.

Comroe, J.H.J. & Fowler, W.S. (1951). Lung function studies: IV. Detection of uneven alveolar ventilation during a breath of oxygen. *Am. J. Med.*, **10**: 408–413.

Cote, C.J., Liu, L.M.P., Szyfelbein, S.K., *et al.* (1986). Intraoperative events diagnosed by expired carbon dioxide monitoring in children. *Can. Aaesth. Soc. J.*, **33**: 315–320.

Fletcher, R., Jonson, B., Cumming, G. & Brew, J. (1981). The concept of deadspace with special reference to the single breath test for carbon dioxide. *Br. J. Anaesth.*, **53**: 77–88.

Fowler, W.S. (1948). Lung function studies: II. The respiratory dead space. *Am. J. Physiol.*, **154**: 405–416.

Hess, D. (1990). Capnometry and capnography: technical aspects, physiologic aspects, and clinical applications. *Resp. Care*, **35**: 557–576.

Hoffbrand, B.I. (1966). The expiratory capnogram: a measure of ventilation–perfusion inequalities. *Thorax*, **21**: 518–523.

Kars, A.H., Goorden, G., Stijnen, T., Bogaard, J.M., Verbraak, A.F.M. & Hilvering, C. (1995). Does phase 2 of the expiratory PCO_2 versus volume curve have diagnostic value in emphysema patients? *Eur. Respir. J.*, **8**: 86–92.

Kumar, A.Y., Bhavani-Shankar, K., Moseley, H.S.L. & Delph, Y. (1992). Inspiratory valve malfunction in a circle system: pitfalls in capnography. *Can. J. Anaesth.*, **39**: 997–999.

Langley, F., Even, P. & Duroux, P. (1976). Ventilatory consequences of unilateral pulmonary artery occlusion. In: *Distribution des Echanges Gaseaux Pulmonaires*. INSERM, France, Paris; pp. 209–212.

Leigh, M.D., Jones, J.C. & Mottley, H.L. (1961). The expired carbon dioxide as continuous guide of the pulmonary and circulatory systems during anaesthesia and surgery. *J. Thoracic Cardiovasc. Surg.*, **41**: 597–610.

Lucangelo, U., Lopez, J., Fernandez, R., Blanch, L. & Romero, P. (1995). Capnographic indexes and lung mechanics in patients with acute lung injury receiving mechanical ventilation. Effect of PEEP. *Int. Care Med.*, **21**: S45.

Mangalaboyi, J., Chopin, C. & Chambrin, M.C. (1992). Utilisation de la capnographie en réanimation. In: *Monitorage Non Invasive en Réanimation*. Masson, Paris; pp. 31–51.

McRae, K.M. & Neufeld, G.R. (1993). Capnogram reflects the severity of acute lung injury in a surfactant depletion model. *Anesthesiology*, **79**: A301.

Murias, G.E., Villagrá, A., Vatua, S., *et al.* (2002). Evaluation of a noninvasive method for cardiac output measurement in critical care patients. *Intens. Care Med.*, **28**: 1470–1474.

Neufeld, G.R., Gobran, S., Baumgardner, J.E., Aukburg, S.J., Schreiner, M. & Scherer, P.W. (1991). Diffusivity, respiratory rate and tidal volume influence inert gas expirograms. *Respir. Physiol.*, **84**: 31–47.

Pascucci, R.C., Schena, J.A. & Thompson, J.E. (1989). Comparison of sidestream and mainstream capnometers in infants. *Crit. Care Med.*, **17**: 560–562.

Podraza, A.G., Salem, M.R., Joseph, N.J. & Brencley, J.L. (1991). Rebreathing due to incompetent unidirectional valves in the circle absorber system. *Anesthesiology*, **75**: A422.

Pyles, S.T., Berman, L.S. & Modell, J.H. (1984). Expiratory valve dysfunction in a semiclosed circle anesthesia circuit – verification by analysis of carbon dioxide waveform. *Anesth. Analg.*, **63**: 536–537.

Ream, R.S., Schreiner, M.S., Neff, J.D., *et al.* (1995). Volumetric capnography in children: influence of growth on the alveolar plateau slope. *Anesthesiology*, **82**: 64–73.

Romero, P., Lucangelo, U., Lopez, J. & Blanch, L. (1995). Alveolar ejection ratio elucidated from VCO_2 versus Vt curves. *Crit. Care Med.*, **21**: S45.

Romero, P., Lucangelo, U., Lopez, J. & Blanch, L. (1997). Physiologically based indices of volumetric capnography in patients receiving mechanical ventilation. *Eur. Respir. J.* **10**: 1309–1315.

Smidt, U. (1976). Emphysema as possible explanation for the alteration of expiratory PO_2 and PCO_2 curves. *Bull. Eur. Physiopathol. Respir.*, **12**: 605–624.

Stenz, R.I., Grenier, B.T., Arnold, J.H. (1998). Single breath CO_2 analysis as a predictor of lung volume in a healthy animal model during controlled ventilation. *Crit. Care Med.*, **26**: 1409–1413.

Swedlow, D.B. (1986). Capnometry and capnography: the anesthesia disaster early warning system. *Semin. Anesth.* **5**: 194–205.

van Ganderingen, H.R., Gravenstein, N., Van der Aa, J.J. & Gravenstein, J.S. (1987). Computer-assisted capnogram analysis. *J. Clin. Monit.*, **3**: 194–200.

Weingarten, M. (1986). Anesthetic and ventilator mishaps: prevention and detection. *Crit. Care Med.*, **14**: 1084–1086.

Weingarten, M. (1990). Respiratory monitoring of carbon dioxide and oxygen a ten-year perspective. *J. Clin. Monit.*, **6**: 217–225.

Worth, H. (1986). Expiratory partial pressure curves in the diagnosis of emphysema. *Bull. Eur. Physiopathol. Respir.*, **22**: 191–199.

Yaron, M. (1996). Utility of the expiratory capnogram in the assessment of bronchospasm. *Ann. Emerg. Med.*, **28**: 403–407.

Yasodananda Kumar, A., Bhavani-Shankar, K., Moseley, H.S.L. & Delph, Y. (1992). Inspiratory valve malfunction in a circle system: pitfalls in capnography. *Can. J. Anaesth.*, **39**: 997–999.

You, B., Mayeux, D., Rkiek, B., Autran, N., Dang, V. & Grilliat, J.P. (1992). La capnographie expiratoire dans l'asthme. Perspectives d'utilisation chez l'enfant et comme méthode de monitorage. *Rev. Mal. Resp.*, **9**: 547–552.

You, B., Duvivier, C., Dang, V.V. & Grilliat, J.P. (1994). Expiratory capnography in asthma: evaluation of various shape indices. *Eur. Respir. J.*, **7**: 318–323.

ANATOMICAL AND PHYSIOLOGICAL BASIS OF VOLUME CAPNOGRAPHY STUDIED BY THE SINGLE PATH MODEL

32

P.W. Scherer & K. Zhao

Introduction

Volume-based capnography as opposed to time-based capnography is useful since it is possible to immediately relate the concentration of carbon dioxide (CO_2) exiting the mouth to the region in the airways from which the gas originated at the beginning of expiration. This can be done by the use of well-known anatomical airway models such as those proposed by Weibel (see Weibel, 1963; 1991; Haefeli-Bleuer & Weibel, 1988). This leads naturally to the use of the capnogram to measure airway dead-space and alveolar gas concentration from phases I, II, and III (alveolar plateau) of the curve. The sigmoid shape of the capnogram is due to the interplay of bronchial airway structure, the physics of gas convection and diffusion, and the physiology of CO_2 evolution from alveolar capillary blood. The single path model (SPM) is the simplest possible reasonably accurate mathematical model of these processes. Since its introduction by Scherer *et al.* in 1972, the SPM has been very useful in understanding the effect of various anatomical, physical, and physiological parameters on the shape of the capnogram and in suggesting further possible clinical uses of the capnogram. We review some of these findings in what follows.

Relation of SPM to real asymmetric airway anatomy

The human respiratory airways are a system of asymmetric dichotomously branching tubes that are divided into conducting and respiratory airways depending on the presence of alveoli in the tube walls. There are on average about 23 generations of branching between the trachea and the terminal alveolar sacs. In Weibel's (1991) symmetric model of the bronchial tree, alveolation begins at generation 14 and the subsequent generations of alveolated tubes are called acini with 2^{15} or 32,768 total acini in both the lungs.

Figure 32.1 shows how the real three-dimensional (3-D) asymmetric dichotomously branching airways are mapped into a single path "one-dimensional, trumpet bell" surface of revolution enclosing the volume of the original asymmetric system.

In doing this mapping it is very important to note that the shape of the single path trumpet bell, or the variation of its cross-sectional area with distance or generation, $A(x)$ or $A(z)$, depends on both the branching structure of the original airways and the manner in which these airways fill or empty in time. For example, Figure 34.1 shows a moment during inspiration in which gas volume V_2 lies between volumes V_1 and V_3 and has flowed into this location due to the way in which the alveolated functional residual capacity (FRC) airways have expanded and pulled gas into the conducting airways. If the FRC airways had expanded differently, V_2 would not lie as it does in Figure 32.1. Figure 32.1 also shows that the particular cross-sectional area of the trumpet bell $A_2(z)$ is the sum of a_{21}, a_{22}, and a_{23} which form the forward front of the volume V_2. Similarly, the gas concentration in the 1-D trumpet bell located at $A_2(z)$ is the average of the concentration c_{21}, c_{22}, and c_{23}.

It is obvious from Figure 32.1 that any 3-D asymmetric airway structure filling or emptying in any way can be mapped into an equivalent $A(z)$ trumpet bell which is the anatomical basis of the SPM. Differences in the original asymmetric airways or in the ways they fill will translate into different rates of "flaring" of the $A(z)$ function. In this way both healthy and diseased, for example chronic obstructive pulmonary disease (COPD) airways can be modeled by the SPM.

In addition to the airways modeled as rigid, the SPM also contains an expandable alveolar volume surrounding the airways and an alveolar capillary blood distribution along the acinus. It is the expansion and contraction of the alveolar volume that moves air into and out of the lung during inspiration and expiration. These are shown schematically in Figure 32.2 as the gray and black areas surrounding the acinar airway generations. It is from the pulmonary arterial mixed venous blood with $PCO_2 = C_B$ that CO_2 gas evolves into the alveolated airways.

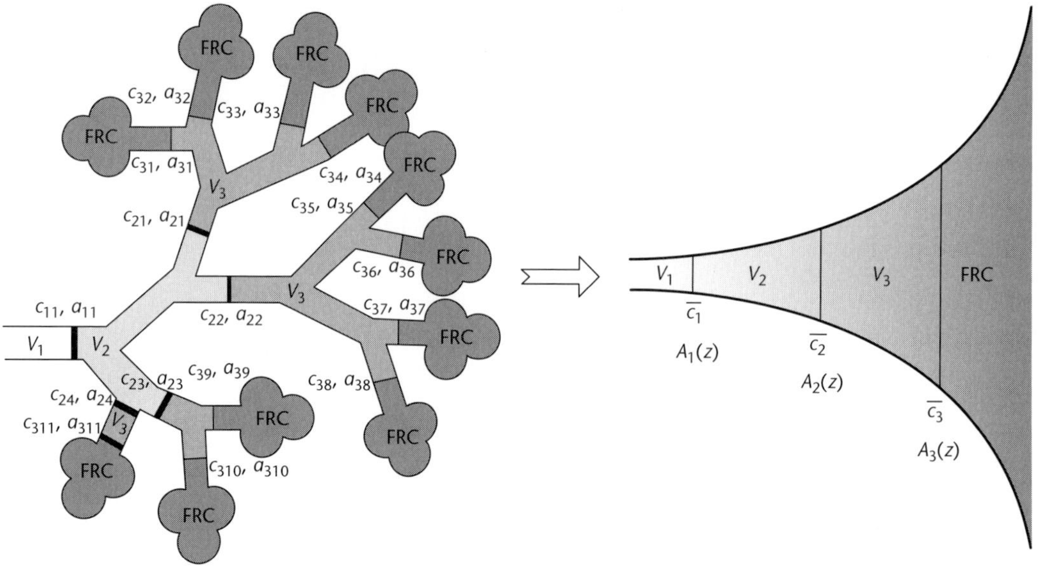

Figure 32.1 Schematic diagram of gas flow through a 3-D airway system mapped into the flow through a single path surface of revolution (SPM) airway model. The SPM depends on both the anatomy of the 3-D model and the way in which the air flows through it. (Reproduced with permission from Huang, J.W. (2000). Non-invasive estimation of cardiac output and mixed venous PCO_2 using the single path model of gas exchange. Ph.D. Dissertation, University of Pennsylvania, Philadelphia.)

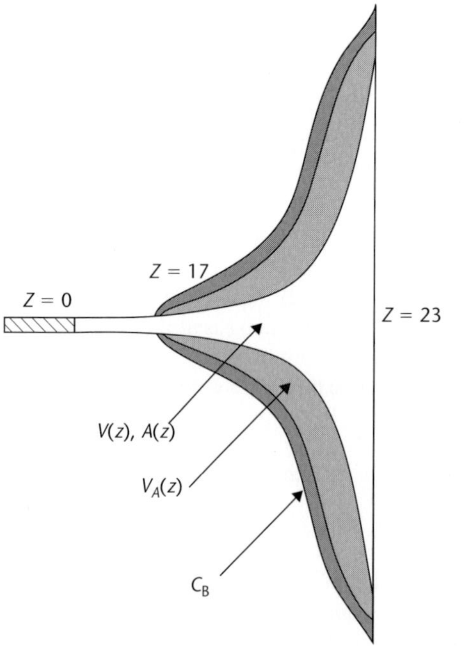

Figure 32.2 Schematic diagram of the SPM showing the rigid airways, surrounding expandable alveolar volume, and alveolar capillary mixed venous blood flow distribution. (Reproduced with permission from Schwardt, J.D., Gobran, S.R., Neufeld, G.R., Aukburg, S.J. & Scherer, P.W. (1991). Sensitivity of CO_2 washout to changes in acinar structure in a single-path model of lung airways. *Ann. Biomed. Eng.*, **19**: 679–697.)

In order to specify the $A(z)$ function of the SPM trumpet bell shown in Figures 32.1 and 32.2, it is necessary to have an anatomical model of the airways and the manner in which they fill and empty. For this purpose, most authors have used Weibel's symmetric dichotomy airway model (Weibel, 1963; 1988; 1991). It should be noted however that this is strictly a matter of convenience and does not indicate that the SPM is limited to a symmetric model airway system of regular dichotomous branching that fills and empties uniformly. At this time there is not enough experimental data in the literature on airway filling and emptying to make any other choice more attractive. In fact, it is found in practice that for use in the SPM and for best agreement with CO_2 washout data in both healthy and diseased lungs, the Weibel airway model must be narrowed and lengthened somewhat by introducing an airway reduction parameter, β, which puts in the effects on $A(z)$ of real airway asymmetry and non-uniform filling and emptying. More on the use of β will be discussed below.

Equations of the SPM

We present here only the basic governing equations of the SPM and not the details of their derivation. Those interested in these details should see the references (Scherer *et al.*, 1972; 1988; Gobran, 1991; Neff, 1996). The fundamental equation of the SPM is the "one (spatial) dimensional" partial differential convective diffusion equation:

$$\left(1+\frac{V_A}{V}\right)\frac{\partial c}{\partial t}+\left(\frac{\dot{Q}}{V}\right)\frac{\partial c}{\partial z} = \frac{1}{V}\frac{\partial}{\partial z}\left[\frac{D_{\text{mol}}A}{l}\frac{\partial c}{\partial z}\right]+\frac{N_{\text{A}}(z)\dot{Q}_B\lambda(\sqrt{c_B}-\sqrt{c})}{VN_{\text{T}}}. \tag{32.1}$$

See list of symbols in the Appendix. Equation (32.1) describes the time, t, and spatial z, changes, in CO_2 gas concentration $c(z, t)$ during inhalation and exhalation in the trumpet bell single path airway model shown in Figure 32.2 and is derived by doing a CO_2 mass balance on a "slice" of the trumpet bell.

The last term on the right in Equation (32.1) is a source term $S(z, t)$ which describes the evolution of CO_2 from the mixed venous alveolar capillary blood into the respiratory airways. By changing the form of this source term, Equation (32.1) can be used to model any type of gas being emitted or taken up by the alveolar blood. In writing the source term as shown in Equation (32.1) we are assuming that: (a) cardiac output is distributed equally to all alveoli and that blood flow to a specific generation is given by $(\dot{Q}_{\text{B}})(N_{\text{A}}(z)/N_T)$ (b) the inlet pulmonary arterial side of each generation has the constant mixed venous pCO_2 concentration given by C_{B}, and (c) the exit pulmonary venous side of each generation has blood pCO_2 concentration in equilibrium with local alveolar airway gas. In addition, the auxiliary equation giving airway gas flow rate,

$$\dot{Q}(z, t) = \dot{V}_{\text{T}}(t)\left[1-\int_0^z \frac{N_{\text{A}}}{N_{\text{T}}}\text{d}s\right], \tag{32.2}$$

must be solved simultaneously with Equation (32.1). A constant molecular diffusivity, D, for CO_2 (D_{mol}) ($0.17\,\text{cm}^2/\text{s}$) is used in Equation (32.1) since other more complex diffusivities such as the Taylor diffusivity are only applicable in the upper airways and have very little effect on the shape (especially on phase III) of the capnogram. Equations (32.1) and (32.2) are solved numerically on a computer with appropriate boundary and initial conditions specified (Scherer *et al.*, 1988; Neff, 1996). The model is started from some initial condition such as CO_2 airway gas concentration constant at the typical end-tidal value and run for several breath cycles until steady-state periodicity is established – usually about three breath cycles. One can then plot the numerical calculation of CO_2 concentration seen at the mouth as a function of volume expired to obtain a numerical prediction of the capnogram as shown in Figure 32.3.

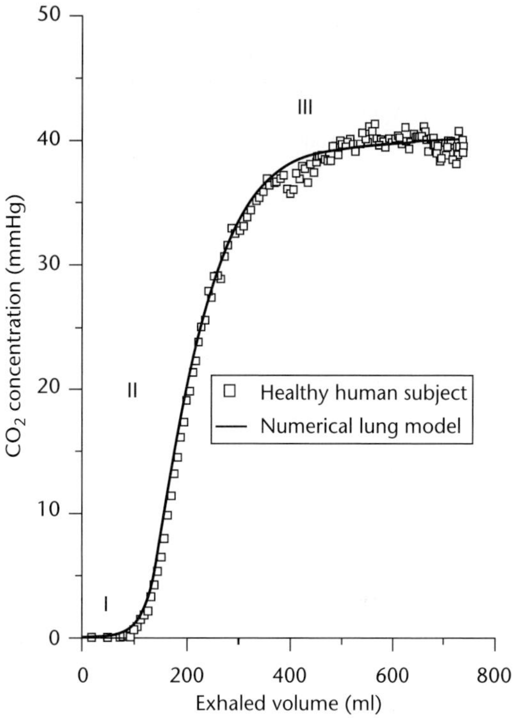

Figure 32.3 Experimentally measured capnogram from a healthy human subject (FRC = 3307 ml, V_{T} = 742 ml, and f = 10.3 bpm) compared to a computed washout curve obtained from the SPM using the same parameter values. Distinct phases I, II, and III are shown. (Reproduced with permission from Schwardt, J.D., Gobran, S.R., Neufeld, G.R., Aukburg, S.J. & Scherer, P.W. (1991). Sensitivity of CO_2 washout to changes in acinar structure in a single-path model of lung airways. *Ann. Biomed. Eng.*, **19**: 679–697.)

If Equation (32.1) is integrated from a given generation z to the end of the model at $z = 23$, and the resulting equation rearranged to solve for $\partial c/\partial V = (1/Al)(\partial c/\partial z)$ one obtains:

$$\left.\frac{\partial c}{\partial V}\right|_z = \left.\frac{1}{D_{\text{mol}}A^2}\right|_z\left[\left.\dot{Q}c\right|_z - \int_z^{23}\left\{(V+V_{\text{A}})\frac{\partial c}{\partial t}\right\}\text{d}z + \int_z^{23} S(z, t)\,\text{d}z\right], \tag{32.3}$$

which shows that at any instant, the volume slope $\partial c/\partial V$ of the CO_2 concentration profile at any point in the airways is caused by a combination of gas diffusion, convection, evolution, and accumulation, and is also very sensitive to airway total cross-sectional area, $A(z)$. Equation (32.3) is useful in answering the long-standing question of what causes the slope $\partial c/\partial V$ of the alveolar plateau seen in the capnogram and in other respiratory gas washout curves; that is, it is seen to have many causes.

Equation (32.1) without the source term and Equation (32.2) were originally derived for the single path trumpet bell airway model shown in Figure 32.2 by Shendalman in the late 1960s in the Department of Chemical Engineering at Yale University. The model was initially applied to N_2 washout and first published by Scherer *et al.* in 1972. Simultaneously and independently, Paiva (1972) in Belgium published a model containing an equation similar to Equation (32.1) without the source term and without an expanding alveolar volume and applied it also to N_2 washout. The source term was added to Equation (32.1) by Scherer *et al.* in 1988 and the SPM has since been applied to CO_2 and other gas washout by the author and many other workers.

Figure 32.3 shows an example of a capnogram computed using the SPM and an experimental curve obtained from a healthy human subject. The agreement for all three phases of the curve is seen to be quite good. The parameters used in both the curves are listed in the figure caption.

An example of the SPM prediction of CO_2 concentration variation within the airways is shown in Figure 32.4.

Intra-airway CO_2 gas concentration profiles predicted by an SPM simulation of a tidal breath of 750 cc with a breathing rate of 12 bmp are shown. It is seen that most of the CO_2 enters the incoming tidal volume (V_T) during the last half of inspiration as shown by the large Gaussian-shaped hump on the time axis. While CO_2 gas is entering the incoming V_T during inspiration, its concentration is seen to drop in the peripheral alveolated airways and then to rise again there during expiration as the alveolar plateau is washed out. Thus the SPM can provide insight into intra-airway CO_2 concentration events that have never been and cannot be easily measured.

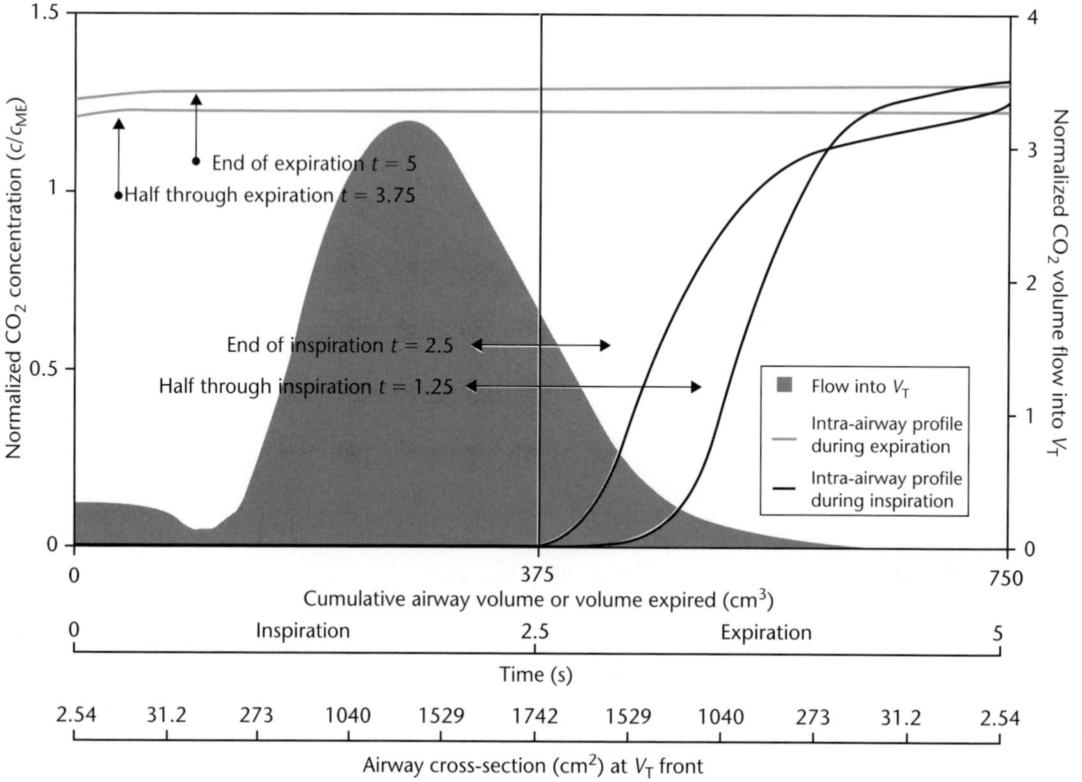

Figure 32.4 Normalized intra-airway CO_2 gas concentration (c/c_{ME}) and CO_2 volume flow rate into the V_T (750 ml) as computed by the SPM for sinusoidal breathing (f = 12 bpm) in a healthy adult lung. CO_2 volume flow into the V_T is normalized by dividing by the average $\dot{V}CO_2$ per breath. The computation shows that most CO_2 is transferred into the V_T during the second half of inspiration and that CO_2 concentration rises in the acinar airways during expiration due to evolution from the pulmonary capillary blood. (Reproduced with permission from Huang, J.W., Yang, G.C., Scherer, P.W. & Neufeld, G.R. (2000). Airway cross section strongly influences alveolar plateau slope of capnograms for smaller tidal volumes. *Respir. Physiol.*, **119**: 51–55.)

SPM parameter sensitivity study for CO_2 washout

It is evident that the SPM contains a large number of parameters. Schwardt *et al.* (1991) systematically investigated the effect of many of these parameters on the shape of the capnogram. He summarized these in the three "spidergrams" shown in Figures 32.5–32.7. Horizontal axes correspond to order of symbols in boxes. Figure 32.5 shows the computed results for a group of parameters that affect the Fowler dead-space, V_{Daw}. Similar to the case in Figures 32.6 and 32.7, the curves all cross at the point representing the "standard" SPM lung model. This model is defined to represent the case of resting tidal breathing in a healthy adult lung. Parameters for this lung include V_T of 750 ml, sinusoidal breathing frequency of 12 bpm, cardiac output, $\dot{Q}_B$, of 6.6 l/min, mixed venous PCO_2, C_B, of 48 mmHg, and FRC of 2500 ml. In addition, in the standard lung, the alveolar capillary blood flow is distributed to the acinar generations in proportion to the (Haefeli-Bleuer & Weibel, 1988) number of alveoli per generation.

The horizontal axes show the variation of the various parameters and in each case, all other parameters were held constant at standard values while the one indicated on a given axis was varied. The first two axes labeled R (later called β) refer to the effect of narrowing and lengthening or narrowing without lengthening, each of the Weibel's acinar generations. As discussed below, this change in acinar anatomy is especially relevant to the airway destruction that occurs in emphysema. The last parameter varied in Figure 32.5 is the acinar blood flow distribution which is shown to vary from all blood flow directed to the proximal generation, $z = 17$, to all blood flow directed to the last acinar generation, $z = 23$. This type of parameter variation occurs during micro-embolic obstruction of alveolar blood flow and is discussed more below. It can be seen that most parameters have a significant effect on V_{Daw} with the exception of cardiac output and mixed venous PCO_2.

Figures 32.6 and 32.7 show similar sensitivity plots for computed phase III slope (%/l) and for computed $\dot{V}CO_2$ of the capnogram. Of particular note is the numerical prediction that phase III slope will become negative when blood is distributed only to the 17th acinar generation.

Figure 32.8 shows some of the computed washout curves corresponding to cases in Figure 32.6 where the slope of phase III of the capnogram is decreased below normal including the case of all acinar blood flow distributed only to the 17 generation.

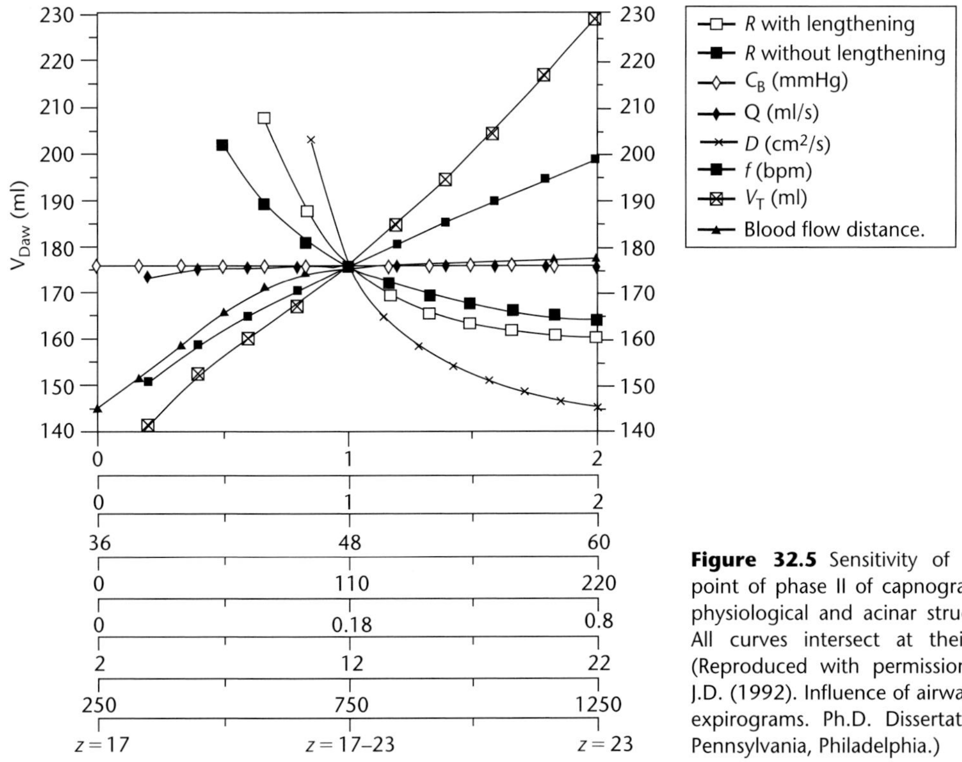

Figure 32.5 Sensitivity of V_{Daw} (~inflection point of phase II of capnogram) to changes in physiological and acinar structural parameters. All curves intersect at their normal values. (Reproduced with permission from Schwardt, J.D. (1992). Influence of airway structure on gas expirograms. Ph.D. Dissertation, University of Pennsylvania, Philadelphia.)

Figures 32.5–32.8 imply that the SPM can be a powerful tool for investigating the effect of various anatomical and physiological parameters on the shape of the capnogram. It is also clear that much of this investigation could not easily be performed experimentally in animals or humans. Some of these parameter effects however have been experimentally investigated, and we now report on some of these cases.

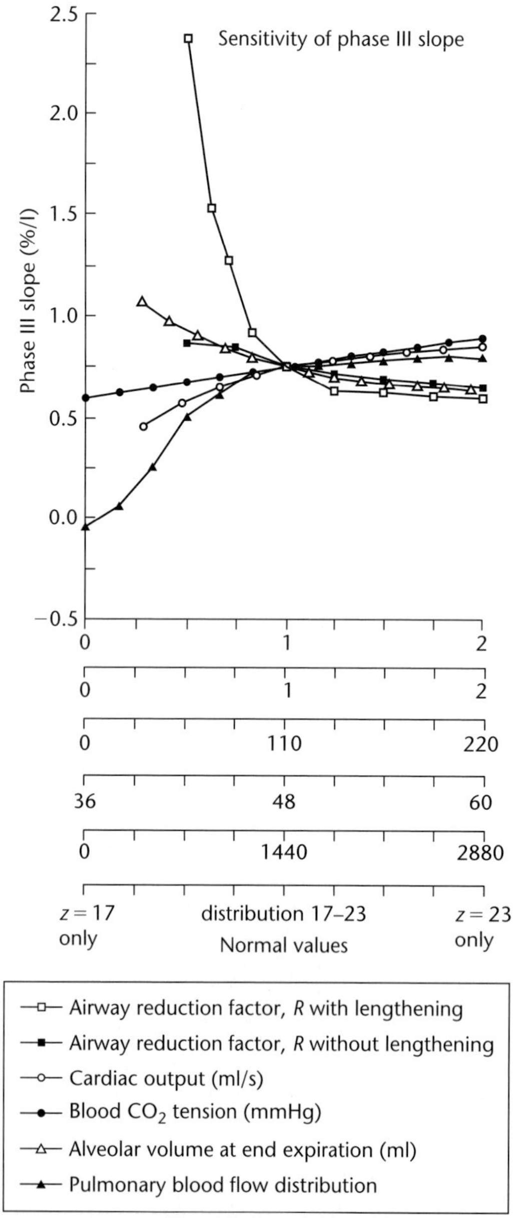

Figure 32.6 Sensitivity of phase III slope of capnogram to changes in physiological and acinar structural parameters. All curves intersect at their normal values. (Reproduced with permission from Schwardt, J.D., Gobran, S.R., Neufeld, G.R., Aukburg, S.J. & Scherer, P.W. (1991). Sensitivity of CO_2 washout to changes in acinar structure in a single-path model of lung airways. *Ann. Biomed. Eng.*, **19**: 679–697.)

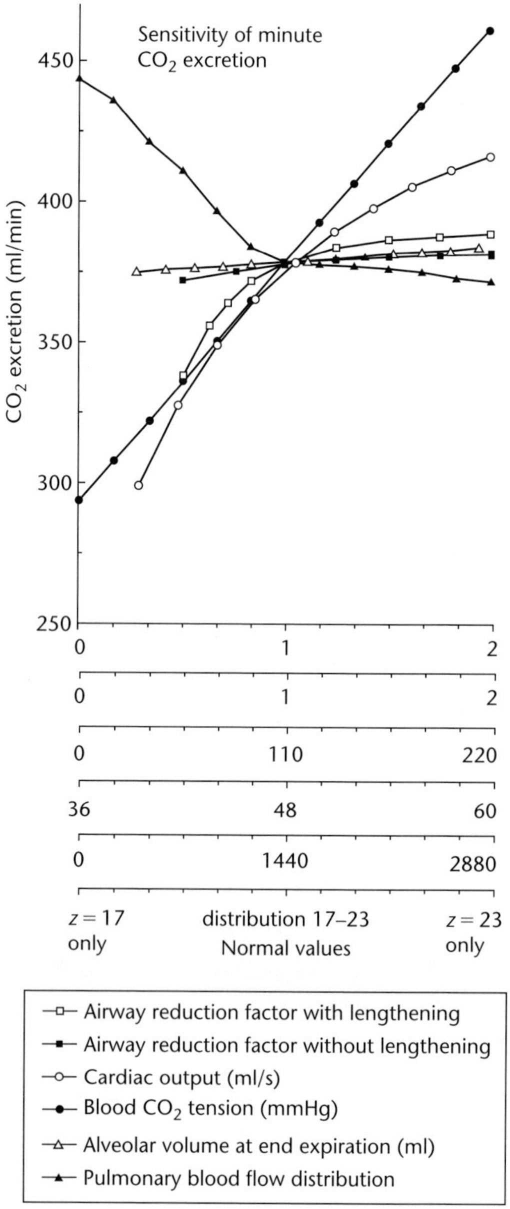

Figure 32.7 Sensitivity of $\dot{V}CO_2$ to changes in physiological and acinar structural parameters. Parameter ranges are identical to those in Figure 32.6. (Reproduced with permission from Schwardt, J.D., Gobran, S.R., Neufeld, G.R., Aukburg, S.J. & Scherer, P.W. (1991). Sensitivity of CO_2 washout to changes in acinar structure in a single-path model of lung airways. *Ann. Biomed. Eng.*, **19**: 679–697.)

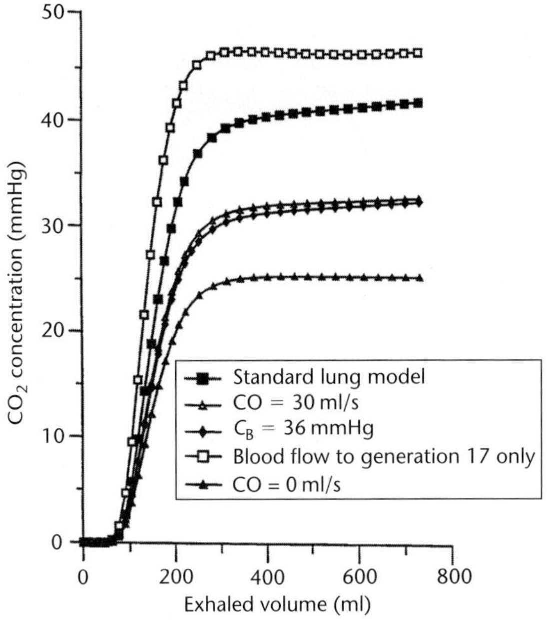

Figure 32.8 Specific examples from Figure 32.6 of computed capnograms that exhibit phase III flattening. (Reproduced with permission from Schwardt, J.D., Gobran, S.R., Neufeld, G.R., Aukburg, S.J. & Scherer, P.W. (1991). Sensitivity of CO_2 washout to changes in acinar structure in a single-path model of lung airways. *Ann. Biomed. Eng.*, **19**: 679–697.) CO: cardiac output.

Experimental studies correlated with SPM results

Neufeld *et al.* (1991; 1992) studied the periodic steady-state simultaneous pulmonary elimination of He, SF_2, and CO_2 in spontaneously breathing human subjects. They compared their experimental results with SPM simulations and found that:

a V_{Daw} increased with V_T at a rate that was inverse to the diffusivity of the evolving gas;

b normalized slope, NS, of phase III $((\partial c/\partial V)/c_{ME})$ decreased with increasing V_T for all gases; and

c as shown in Figure 32.9, for given breathing conditions, the NS was inversely proportional to gas diffusivity.

They concluded that gas diffusivity and cross-sectional area of the acinus strongly affect V_{Daw} and NS and that the SPM was accurate in simulating these physiological variables.

Schwardt *et al.* (1994) studied the effects of COPD on the shape of the capnogram in a group of six patients at the Veterans Affairs Medical Center in Philadelphia. They found that the NS of phase III of the capnogram (slope divided by mixed expired CO_2 concentration, $((\partial c/\partial V)/c_{ME})$ were much higher in the COPD patients than in healthy subjects for a given V_T inhaled. They also found that this effect could be simulated

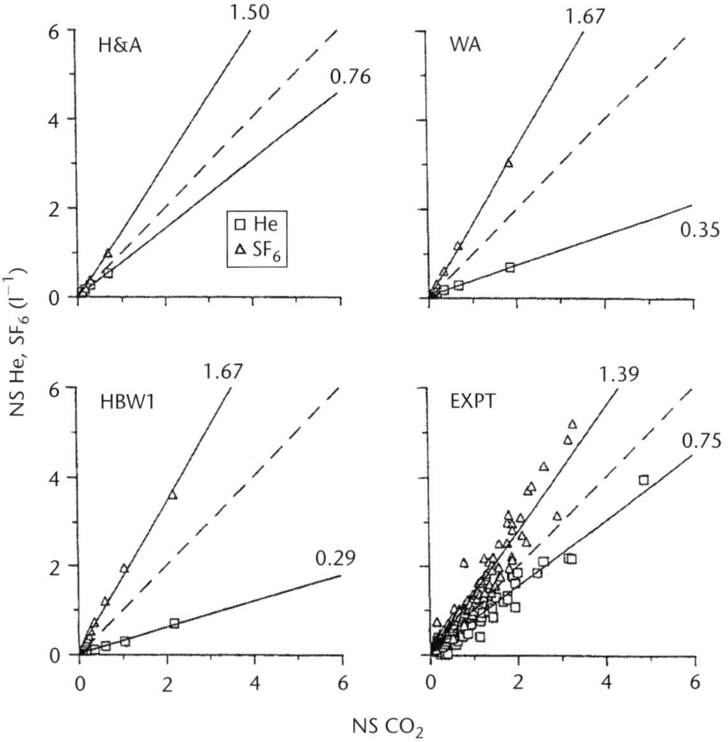

Figure 32.9 Phase III NS of He and SF_6 versus CO_2. The figure includes experimentally measured, computed, and normalized phase III washout slopes (EXPT) $(d(c/c_{ME})/dV)$ over a range of V_T (5–22 ml/kg) in several airway models including Weibel A (WA), Haefeli-Bleuer–Weibel (HBW1), and Hansen and Ampaya (H&A). In each model, the identity line (dashed line) and the regression lines determined from the simulation are shown. The diffusivity dependence of phase III slope is inversely proportional to the rate of cross-sectional area expansion between generations 16 and 19 in of the morphometric model chosen. (Reproduced with premission from Neufeld, G.R., Schwardt, J.D., Gobran, S.R., Baumgardner, J.E., Schreiner, M.S., Aukburg, S.J. & Scherer, P.W. (1992). Modelling steady state pulmonary elimination of He, SF_6 and CO_2: effect of morphometry. *Respir. Physiol.*, **88**: 257–275.)

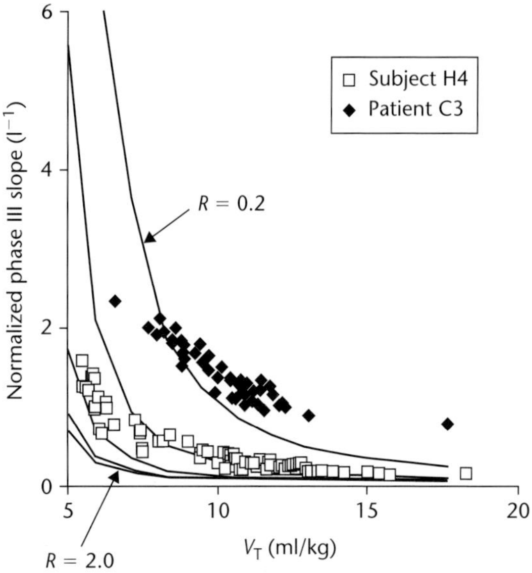

Figure 32.10 Experimental normalized phase III capnogram slope versus V_T data from one healthy (open squares) and one COPD (solid diamonds) human subject are plotted over SPM computed curves of area reduction with lengthening factors from $R(\beta) = 0.2$–2.0. The optimization algorithm chooses the curve (R value) that best fits each data set. Note that the COPD patients have much steeper phase III slopes than the healthy subjects at all V_T. (Reproduced with permission from Schwardt, J.D., Neufeld, G.R., Baumgardner, J.E. & Scherer, P.W. (1994). Noninvasive recovery of acinar anatomic information from CO_2 expirograms. *Ann. Biomed. Eng.*, **22**: 293–306.)

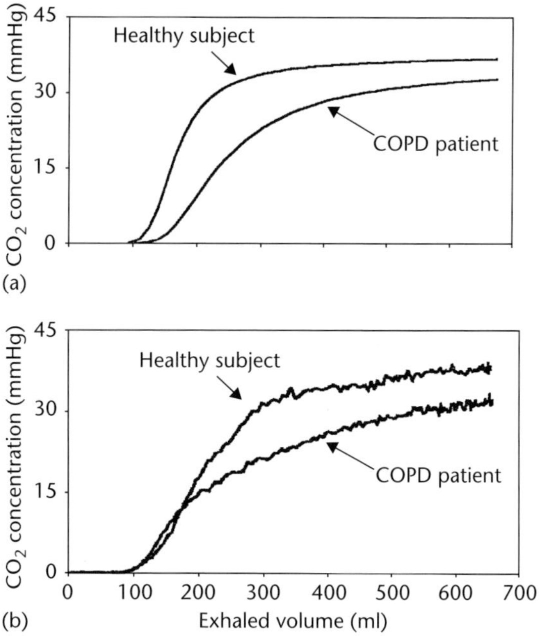

Figure 32.11 SPM simulation capnograms from a healthy subject and a COPD patient (a) compared with experimentally measured capnograms form the same two subjects (b). It is evident that the lengthening and reduction in acinar airway cross-section used in the COPD SPM computation obtained from data as shown in Figure 32.10 well simulates the clinical washout curve. (Reproduced with permission from Schwardt, J.D. (1992). Influence of airway structure on gas expirograms. Ph.D. Dissertation, University of Pennsylvania, Philadelphia.)

in the SPM by reducing the cross-sectional area of the acinar generations by a constant factor R (or β) while simultaneously lengthening the generations by the factor of $1/\beta$ to preserve the volume of each generation and of the FRC. These effects are shown in Figures 32.10 and 32.11.

They then modeled the acinar anatomical changes characteristic of severe emphysema as the replacement of a large number of small spherical airspaces (diameter d_H) in each generation in the healthy lung by a smaller number of much larger airspaces (diameter d_D) in a COPD diseased lung. Using this model, they showed that the area reduction factor, β, which was obtained by matching the SPM predictions to the patient data, could be related to the average diameters of the acinar airspaces, d, and the average acinar diffusive conductance, $\overline{G}$, by the equation:

$$\beta = \frac{A_D(z)}{A_H(z)} = \frac{\mathrm{FRC_D}/\mathrm{FRC_H}}{d_D/d_H} = \sqrt{\frac{\mathrm{FRC_D}}{\mathrm{FRC_H}} \cdot \frac{\overline{G}_D}{\overline{G}_H}}. \tag{32.4}$$

In Equation (32.4), the H and D subscripts refer to healthy and diseased lungs, respectively. They thus showed that the SPM could be used to non-invasively recover acinar anatomical information from the capnogram.

Motivated by SPM predictions, Schreiner *et al.* (1993) studied the effect on the capnogram and on infused SF_6 (using SF_6 saturated saline) washout curves of microsphere infusion into the venous circulation of an anesthetized and mechanically ventilated goat. After establishing steady-state baseline conditions, they produced pulmonary micro-embolization by infusing 125 μm diameter glass microspheres. The results of the experiment are shown in Figures 32.12–32.14. Figure 32.12(a) shows the baseline capnogram and SF_6 washout curves while Figure 32.12(b) shows the same curves after embolization.

Negative phase III slopes following embolization are evident for both the gases with the slope of SF_6 being steeper than that of CO_2 because of the lower air phase diffusivity of SF_6.

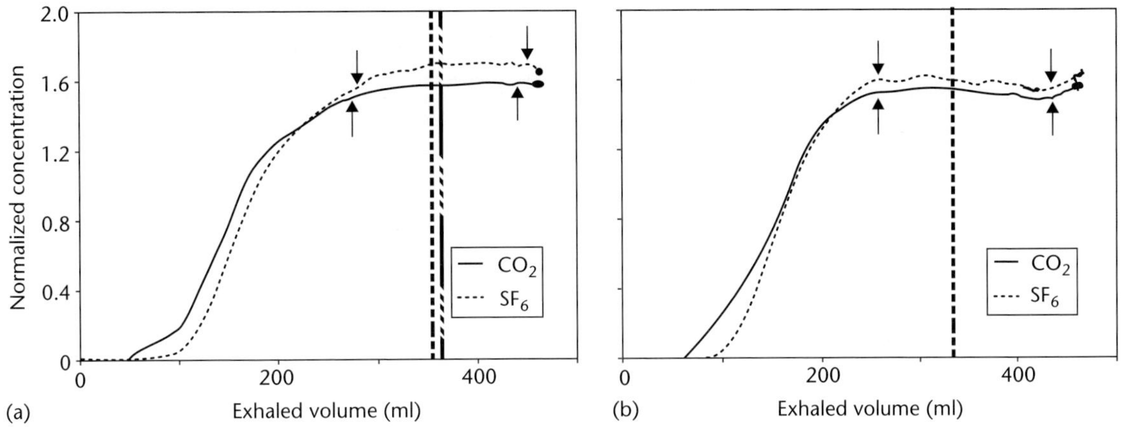

Figure 32.12 Simultaneous washout curves for CO_2 and SF_6 before and after micro-embolization with 15 g of 125 μm glass beads. The vertical dashed lines mark the exhaled volume at which 60% of the CO_2 and SF_6 have been exhaled. Phase III slope is computed by linear regression between the two arrows. Prior to embolization (a) the SF_6 curve shows a steeper phase III slope and larger V_{Daw} than the capnogram, due to the smaller gas phase molecular diffusivity of SF_6. After embolization (b) both the alveolar plateaus show a negative slope with the SF_6 curve more negative than the capnogram again due to the smaller SF_6 gas phase diffusivity. For both the curves post-embolization, V_{Daw} is similar and in comparison to the pre-embolization curves, there is a rise in gas concentration at the beginning of phase III due to more gas being evolved in the earlier generations of the acinar airways. (Reproduced with permission from Schreiner, M.S., Leksell, L.G., Gobran, S.R., Hoffman, E.A., Scherer, P.W. & Neufeld, G.R. (1993). Microemboli reduce phase III slopes of CO_2 and invert phase III slopes of infused SF_6. *Respir. Physiol.*, **91**: 137–154.)

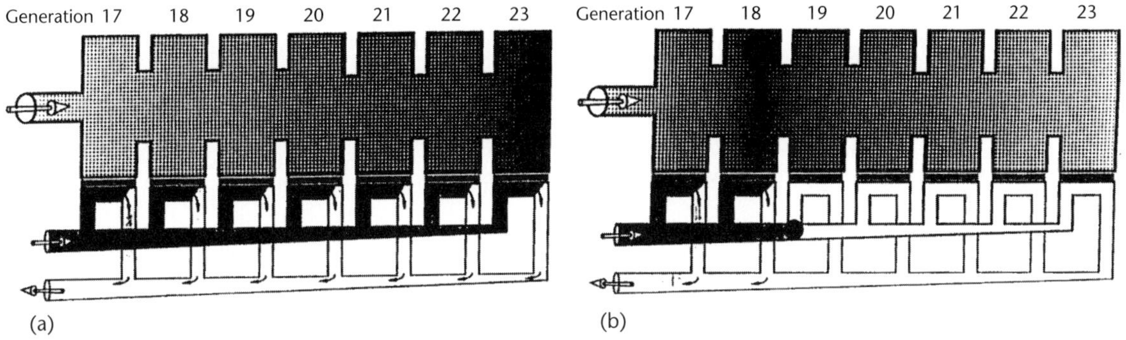

Figure 32.13 A schematic representation of the alveolar blood and gas flow in an acinar structure (modified from Weibel, 1981). In the healthy, normal condition (a), blood flow is distributed to each generation in proportion to the number of alveoli in that generation, while ventilation is greatest in the proximal generations and less in the distal generations. This results in a diffusive ventilation/perfusion ($\dot{V}/\dot{Q}$) gradient within the acinus with the highest concentration of evolving gas (denser shading) at the 23rd generation and the lowest concentration at the 17th. After embolization (b), blood flow is limited to the upper generations while the inhaled V_T moves into distal non-perfused regions of the lung. This results in a bi-directional airway gas concentration gradient decreasing in both the directions away from generation 18 where the alveolar capillary blood flow obstruction has occurred, and a reversal in the ($\dot{V}/\dot{Q}$) gradient depicted in A. The gas washout profile seen at the mouth on exhalation (see Figure 32.12) reflects these changes in airway gas concentration. (Reproduced with permission from Schreiner, M.S., Leksell, L.G., Gobran, S.R., Hoffman, E.A., Scherer, P.W. & Neufeld, G.R. (1993). Microemboli reduce phase III slopes of CO_2 and invert phase III slopes of infused SF_6. *Respir. Physiol.*, **91**: 137–154.)

Figure 32.13(a, b) show in schematic form using Weibel's airway model, the most likely effect of the embolization on acinar gas and blood flow.

In Figure 32.13(b), acinar blood flow is confined to the proximal generations 17 and 18 only while tidal gas flow ventilates the whole acinus. This produces CO_2 and SF_6 concentration gradients in both directions within the acinus leading to the negative phase III slopes of the washout curves seen in Figure 32.12(b) above.

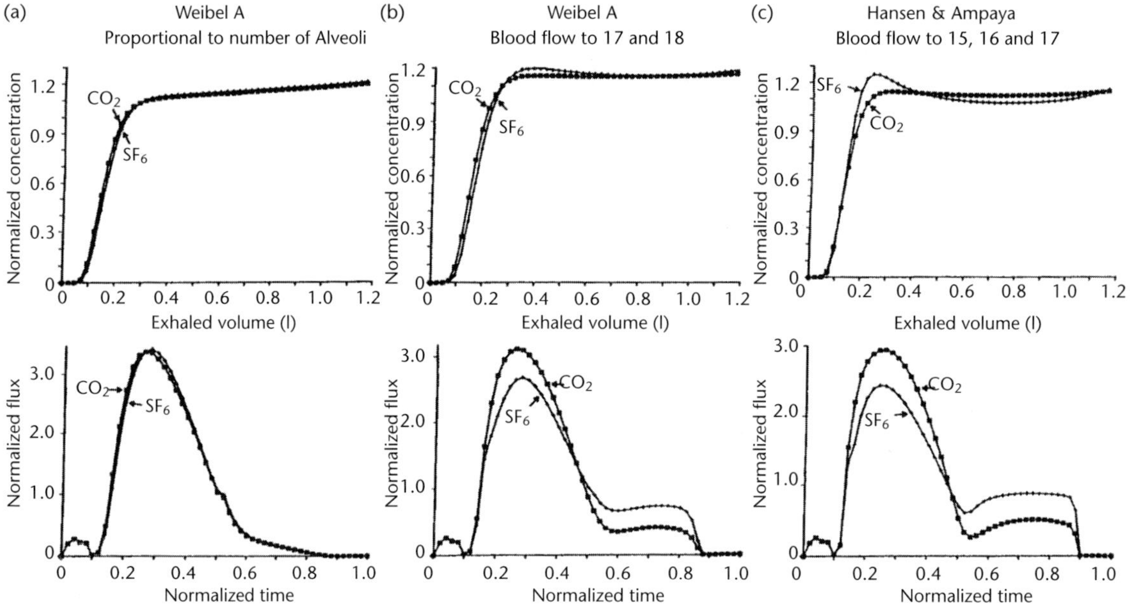

Figure 32.14 SPM simulations in a 70 kg man of the microsphere embolization experiment in a goat described in Figures 32.12 and 32.13 showing the CO_2 and SF_6 washout curves (upper panels) and the computed gas flux into the moving V_T (lower panels). The healthy pre-embolization expirogram is shown in (a), while (b) and (c) show simulations of post-embolization expirograms using the Weibel, and Hansen and Ampaya airway models, respectively. In agreement with the experimental data shown in Figure 32.12, both the post-embolic simulations show negative sloping phase IIIs with upward concavity, and higher gas concentrations at the beginning of phase III in comparison with the pre-embolic simulation. The bottom panels show that both of these post-embolic effects on the washout curve are due to continuing gas evolution into the V_T on exhalation as it passes beneath the obstructed capillary gas source in the proximal acinar generations. In agreement with experiment, both the effects are more pronounced for SF_6 due to its lower gas phase diffusivity. (Reproduced with permission from Schreiner, M.S., Leksell, L.G., Gobran, S.R., Hoffman, E.A., Scherer, P.W. & Neufeld, G.R. (1993). Microemboli reduce phase III slopes of CO_2 and invert phase III slopes of infused SF_6. *Respir. Physiol.*, **91**: 137–154.)

Figure 32.14(b) and also Figure 32.8 above show an SPM simulation of the experiment where all alveolar capillary blood flow is distributed only to generations 17 and 18.

Similar to the experimental results, phase III slopes are predicted to be negative after embolization as evolved gas diffuses in both the directions along the acinus. The figures also show the higher rising phase II and the greater amount of CO_2 expired (also seen in the experimental results shown in Figure 32.12) due to the continuing flow of CO_2 into the V_T from the proximal alveolar wall blood source during exhalation following embolization.

The results shown in Figures 32.12–32.14 are similar to clinical observations in humans following pulmonary embolization and show that the SPM is effective in modeling this phenomenon.

In a study of the effect of age on the shape of the capnogram, Ream *et al.* (1995) also compared their experimental results to predictions of the SPM. They studied the change in normalized phase III slope ($(\partial c/\partial V)/c_{ME}$) for CO_2) and Fowler dead-space, V_{Daw}, with age in children aged 5 months–18 years who were mechanically ventilated during minor elective surgery. They collected data for V_T of 8.5 and 12.5 ml/kg and compared their data with the predictions of SPM calculations in Weibel's lung models altered to represent pediatric lungs at various stages of growth (Neff, 1996). Figures 32.15 and 32.16 show the results.

The NS of phase III is seen to decrease with age in a curvilinear fashion while the dead-space increases with age in a more linear trend. Noting Fick's first law of diffusion, they attributed the decrease in NS to an increase in total acinar airway cross-sectional area with lung growth. Farmery (1995) objected to this interpretation and showed that the predictions of a single well-mixed alveolar volume model fit the NS data just as well as the SPM simulations. He suggested that the decrease in NS with growth could simply be due to increase in FRC.

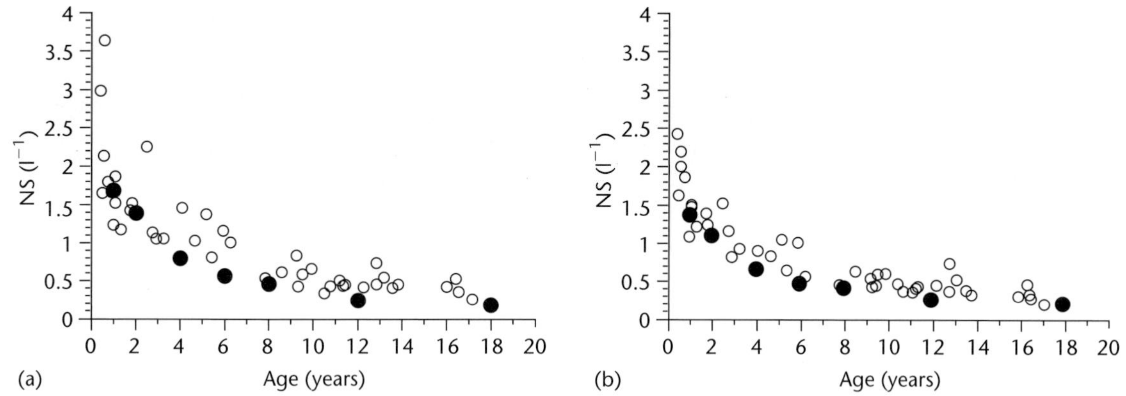

Figure 32.15 Comparison of normalized phase III capnogram slope determined by patient measurements (open circles) with SPM simulated CO_2 washout using a "growing" pediatric airway model (closed circles) as a function of age for V_T of 8.5 ml/kg (a) and 12.5 ml/kg (b). (Reproduced with permission from Ream, R.S., Schreiner, M.S., Neff, J.D., McRae, K.M., Jawad, A.F., Scherer, P.W. & Neufeld, G.R. (1995). Volumetric capnography in children. Influence of growth on the alveolar plateau slope. *Anesthesiology*, **82**: 64–73.)

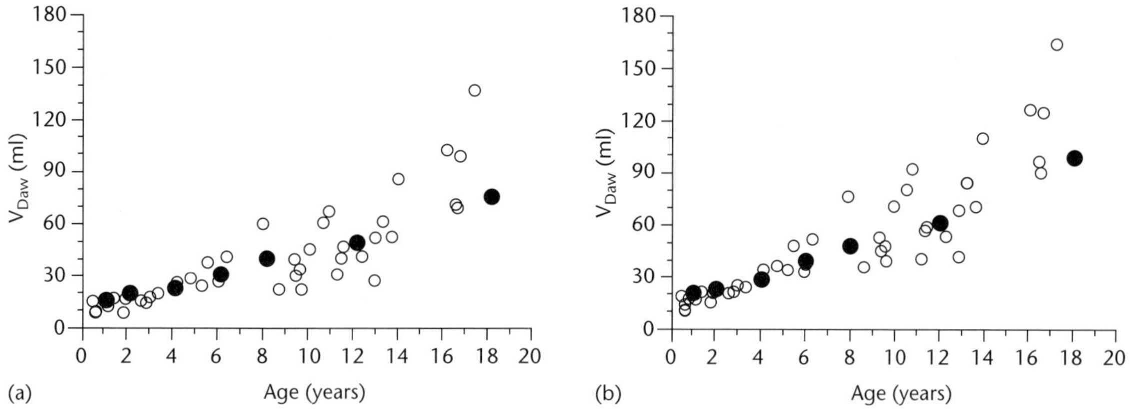

Figure 32.16 Comparison of airway dead-space (V_{Daw}) determined by patient measurements (open circles) with SPM capnogram simulations on a "growing" pediatric lung model (closed circles) as a function of age for V_T of 8.5 ml/kg (a) and 12.5 ml/kg (b). (Reproduced with permission from Ream, R.S., Schreiner, M.S., Neff, J.D., McRae, K.M., Jawad, A.F., Scherer, P.W. & Neufeld, G.R. (1995). Volumetric capnography in children. Influence of growth on the alveolar plateau slope. *Anesthesiology*, **82**: 64–73.)

To investigate the question further, Huang (2000) studied the variation of NS with V_T during resting spontaneous breathing in three adult males and compared their results with the predictions of SPM simulations and the predictions of Farmery's well-mixed alveolar volume (SAM) model. The results, which lead to deeper physical insight, are shown in Figure 32.17.

It is seen that for high V_T, greater than about 15 ml/kg, the NS predictions of both SPM and the SAM agree but that for lower V_T, typical of those used in the Ream *et al.* (1995) experiments, the SPM gives better agreement with the experimental data. The physical reason for this is that at high V_T, most of the inhaled gas penetrates deep into the acinus where mixing by molecular diffusion is rapid and the acinus indeed behaves as a single large well-mixed alveolar volume. At low V_T however, most of the inhaled gas does not penetrate deeply into the acinus. Mixing by diffusion is less rapid since total airway cross-sectional area is not as large, and steeper alveolar concentration gradients persist throughout exhalation leading to steeper values of the NS.

Recently, Whiteley *et al.* (2002) have used an extremely accurate finite element form of the SPM to investigate the effect of ventilation pattern on the arterial PCO_2–end-tidal PCO_2 difference. They found that the difference depends strongly on ventilation pattern and, among other things, that when V_T are

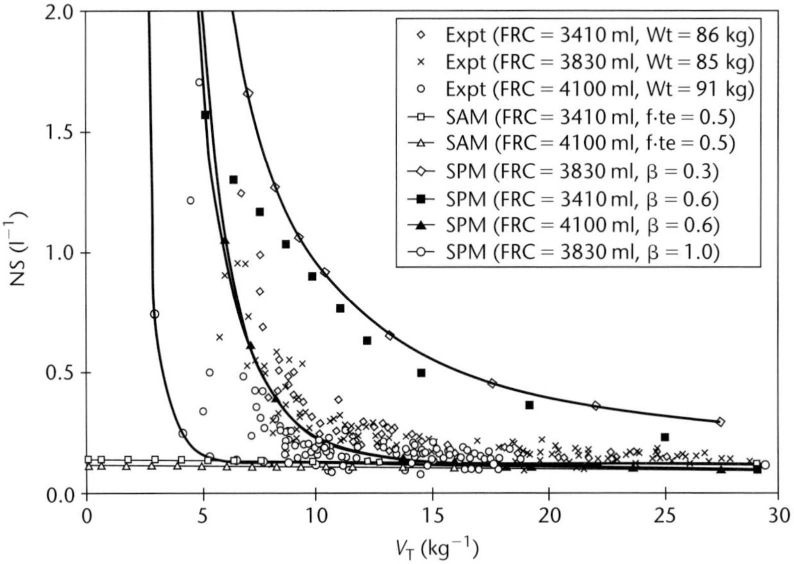

Figure 32.17 Comparison of the NS generated by the SPM and the SAM with experimental (Expt.) data collected from three healthy human subjects. The V_T is varied from 450–2500 ml. FRCs of 3410 and 4100 ml are used for both the models to reflect the lowest and highest FRC of the subjects. The β (=R) values used in the SPM represent the fractional reduction (e.g. $\beta = 0.6 =$ 40% reduction) in the acinar generational total cross-sectional areas used in a given SPM calculation. The SAM agrees with the SPM for the larger V_T. (Reproduced with permission from Huang, J.W., Yang, G.C., Scherer, P.W. & Neufeld, G.R. (2000). Airway cross section strongly influences alveolar plateau slope of capnograms for smaller tidal volumes. *Respir. Physiol.*, **119**: 51–55.)

decreased while breathing rate is increased to maintain constant alveolar ventilation, the SPM predicts an increase in the $P_aCO_2 - P_{et}CO_2$ difference.

Future possible uses of the SPM and capnogram

I Huang (2000) developed a technique to non-invasively recover cardiac output ($\dot{Q}_B$) and mixed venous PCO_2 (C_B) from the capnogram of spontaneously breathing or mechanically ventilated human subjects. The method consists of finding those values of $\dot{Q}_B$ and C_B that minimize the difference between the predictions of the SPM for $\dot{V}CO_2$ and NS and the recorded capnogram values for a given subject V_T and breathing rate. An example of the minimization applied to data from a mechanically ventilated goat is shown in Figure 32.18. The white dot represents the minimum difference between the SPM predictions and the recorded goat capnogram measurements found by a numerical searching technique.

Figures 32.19 and 32.20 show comparisons of the cardiac output ($\dot{Q}_B$) and the mixed venous PCO_2 (C_B), recovered using the SPM recovery method with values obtained by direct measurement in a mechanically ventilated goat.

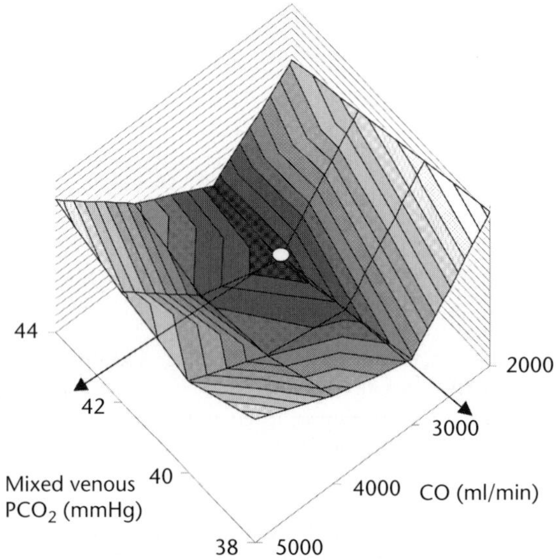

Figure 32.18 Combined $\dot{V}CO_2$ and NS topology. The minimum point on this surface (white dot) is found by high-definition cubic spline interpolation. (Reproduced with permission from Huang, J.W. (2000). Non-invasive estimation of cardiac output and mixed venous PCO_2 using the single path model of gas exchange. Ph.D. Dissertation, University of Pennsylvania, Philadelphia.)

The C_B was measured in blood withdrawn from pulmonary artery catheterization and the $\dot{Q}_B$ was measured by a mass balance on PO_2 between the pulmonary artery and the left atrium. As shown, most of the SPM C_B data lie within 5% and most of the $\dot{Q}_B$ data lie within 15% of the direct measurements. The SPM method of recovery also has the advantage that it can be applied to spontaneously breathing exercising subjects and is not restricted to use only during mechanical ventilation.

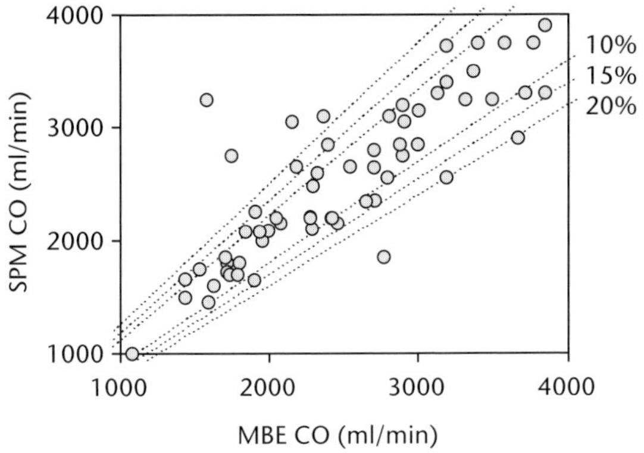

Figure 32.19 Goat cardiac output ($\dot{Q}_B$) recovery results. Comparison of the CO recovered using the SPM with the goat experimental data calculated by direct O_2 mass balance (MBE) on blood entering and leaving the lung. The three diagonal lines are the error rates of ±10%, 15%, and 20%, respectively. Most recovered CO values are within the 15% error lines. (Reproduced with permission from Huang, J.W. (2000). Non-invasive estimation of cardiac output and mixed venous PCO_2 using the single path model of gas exchange. Ph.D. Dissertation, University of Pennsylvania, Philadelphia.)

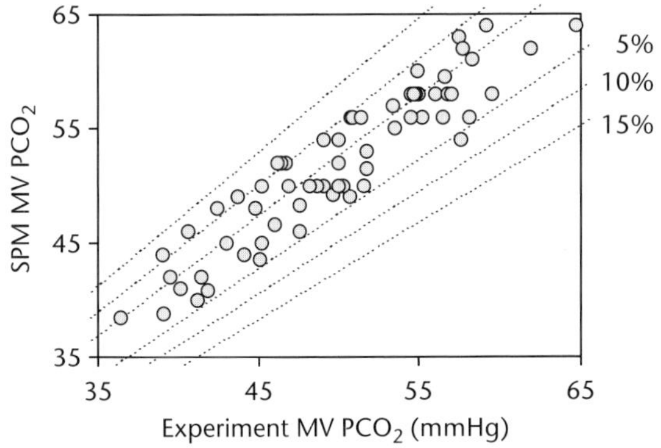

Figure 32.20 Goat mixed venous (MV) PCO_2 (C_B) recovery results. Comparison of the C_B recovered using the SPM with the goat PCO_2 data obtained by catheterization and blood withdrawal from the pulmonary artery. The three diagonal lines are the error rates of ±5%, 10%, and 15%, respectively. Most recovered C_B values are within the 5% error lines. (Reproduced with permission from Huang, J.W. (2000). Non-invasive estimation of cardiac output and mixed venous PCO_2 using the single path model of gas exchange. Ph.D. Dissertation, University of Pennsylvania, Philadelphia.)

II Equation (32.3) above suggests that it might be possible to use the slope of phase III of the capnogram $\partial c/\partial V$ to obtain an estimate of total acinar airway cross-sectional area by inverting the equation to solve for $A(V)$ as:

$$A(V) = \sqrt{\frac{1}{D_{\mathrm{mol}}\dfrac{\partial c}{\partial V}}\left[\dot{Q}c - \int_z^{23}(V+V_A)\frac{\partial c}{\partial t}\mathrm{d}z + \int_z^{23}S(z,t)\mathrm{d}z\right]}. \tag{32.5}$$

Numerical computation using the SPM shows that the $c(V)$ intra-airway concentration profile is little changed between the end of inspiration and the capnogram convected out of the mouth on expiration. Preliminary measurements suggest that Equation (32.5) might be approximated in the form:

$$A(V) \approx \sqrt{\frac{K\dot{Q}c}{D\dfrac{\partial c}{\partial V}}}, \tag{32.6}$$

where the last two terms in the bracket under the square root sign in Equation (32.5) are replaced by the constant K (Scherer *et al.*, 1983).

III The CO_2 exchange between the FRC and the V_T by molecular diffusion during inhalation shown in the SPM calculation in Figure 32.4 above suggests that one could compute the resistance $\bar{R}$ to this exchange or to the similar but oppositely directed O_2 exchange by evaluating the double integral:

$$\bar{R}_{O_2} = \frac{1}{\bar{G}_{O_2}} = \frac{1}{a}\int_0^a\left[\int_0^x \frac{\mathrm{d}\zeta}{AD_{O_2}}\right]\mathrm{d}x. \tag{32.7}$$

In Equation (32.7), $A(\zeta)$ is the Weibel's (1991) trumpet bell airway $A(x)$ function shown in Figure 32.2, D_{O_2} is the molecular diffusivity of an O_2–air mixture, a is the length of the Weibel's (1991) acinus (~8.0 mm), and $\bar{G}$ is the average trumpet bell acinar airway diffusive conductance for O_2. If the integrals in Equation (32.7) are evaluated, for the Weibel's $A(x)$ function, one obtains:

$$\bar{R}_{O_2} \approx 0.411\,\text{mmHg min/ml},$$

which is more than an order of magnitude higher than ($1/D_{L_{O_2}}$ (lung diffusing capacity for O_2) $\approx$ 0.0333 mmHg min/ml) (Weibel, 1989). This suggests that the diffusive resistance to O_2 or CO_2 transfer between the V_T and FRC during inspiration is much higher than that across the alveolar membrane, contrary to current assumption in respiratory physiology.

IV Finally, a possible future use of the capnogram might be in lung volume reduction surgery which has been performed on a trial basis over the last several years in an attempt to ameliorate the debilitating effects of severe emphysema (Ware, 2003). Figure 32.11 above indicates that capnograms in healthy and severe emphysematous (COPD) lungs show several characteristic differences. The COPD capnogram typically has a much steeper sloping phase III and contains much less CO_2 in the area under the curve. This difference in shape suggests that it might be possible and/or desirable to use the capnogram either intra-operatively or pre- and post-operatively to determine to what extent the surgery has succeeded in restoring airway gas transport to a more normal or healthy state. Of course, obtaining capnograms intra-operatively during lung surgery presents many technical problems and may prove to be not possible or advisable.

Conclusion

The SPM provides a powerful and flexible method for investigating the effect of many anatomical and physiological parameters on the shape of the time or volume-based capnogram. As discussed above, several studies have been done to date which compare SPM predictions with physiological measurements obtained from the capnogram. In most cases, the comparisons show the SPM to be quite accurate. In addition, the SPM can be used to predict data such as intra-airway CO_2 concentration profiles that cannot be measured experimentally. In the future, it is likely that progress will be made though an iterative combination of SPM numerical simulation suggesting new experimental measurements while the results of these measurements in turn suggest further refinements of the SPM.

Acknowledgment

The authors acknowledge many valuable discussions with Dr. Gordon R. Neufeld.

References

Farmery, A.D. (1995). Volumetric capnography and lung growth in children: a simple model validated. *Anesthesiology*, **83**: 1377–1379.

Gobran, S.R. (1991). Numerical modelling of respiratory and inert gas exchange in healthy human lungs. Ph.D. Dissertation, University of Pennsylvania, Philadelphia.

Haefeli-Bleuer, B. & Weibel, E.R. (1988). Morphometry of the human pulmonary acinus. *Anat. Rec.*, **220**: 401–414.

Huang, J.W. (2000). Non-invasive estimation of cardiac output and mixed venous PCO_2 using the single path model of gas exchange. Ph.D. Dissertation, University of Pennsylvania, Philadelphia.

Huang, J.W., Yang, G.C., Scherer, P.W. & Neufeld, G.R. (2000). Airway cross section strongly influences alveolar plateau slope of capnograms for smaller tidal volumes. *Respir. Physiol.*, **119**: 51–55.

Neff, J.D. (1996). Applications of the single path convection diffusion model of the human respiratory system. Ph.D. Dissertation, University of Pennsylvania, Philadelphia.

Neufeld, G.R., Gobran, S., Baumgardner, J.E., Aukburg, S.J., Schreiner, M. & Scherer, P.W. (1991). Diffusivity, respiratory rate and tidal volume influence inert gas expirograms. *Respir. Physiol.*, **84**: 31–47.

Neufeld, G.R., Schwardt, J.D., Gobran, S.R., Baumgardner, J.E., Schreiner, M.S., Aukburg, S.J. & Scherer, P.W. (1992). Modelling steady state pulmonary elimination of He, SF_6 and CO_2: effect of morphometry. *Respir. Physiol.*, **88**: 257–275.

Paiva, M. (1972). Computation of the boundary conditions for diffusion in the human lung. *Comput. Biomed. Res.*, **5**: 585–595.

Ream, R.S., Schreiner, M.S., Neff, J.D., McRae, K.M., Jawad, A.F., Scherer, P.W. & Neufeld, G.R. (1995). Volumetric capnography in children. Influence of growth on the alveolar plateau slope. *Anesthesiology*, **82**: 64–73.

Scherer, P.W., Shendalman, L.H. & Greene, N.M. (1972). Simultaneous diffusion and convection in single breath lung washout. *Bull. Math. Biophys.*, **34**: 393–412.

Scherer, P.W., Neufeld, G.R., Aukburg, S.J. & Hess, G.D. (1983). Measurement of effective peripheral bronchial cross section from single-breath gas washout. *J. Biomech. Eng.*, **105**: 290–293.

Scherer, P.W., Gobran, S., Aukburg, S.J., Baumgardner, J.E., Bartkowski, R. & Neufeld, G.R. (1988). Numerical and experimental study of steady-state CO_2 and inert gas washout. *J. Appl. Physiol.*, **64**: 1022–1029.

Schreiner, M.S., Leksell, L.G., Gobran, S.R., Hoffman, E.A., Scherer, P.W. & Neufeld, G.R. (1993). Microemboli reduce phase III slopes of CO_2 and invert phase III slopes of infused SF_6. *Respir. Physiol.*, **91**: 137–154.

Schwardt, J.D. (1992). Influence of airway structure on gas expirograms. Ph.D. Dissertation, University of Pennsylvania, Philadelphia.

Schwardt, J.D., Gobran, S.R., Neufeld, G.R., Aukburg, S.J. & Scherer, P.W. (1991). Sensitivity of CO_2 washout to changes in acinar structure in a single-path model of lung airways. *Ann. Biomed. Eng.*, **19**: 679–697.

Schwardt, J.D., Neufeld, G.R., Baumgardner, J.E. & Scherer, P.W. (1994). Noninvasive recovery of acinar anatomic information from CO_2 expirograms. *Ann. Biomed. Eng.*, **22**: 293–306.

Ware, J.H. (2003). The National Emphysema Treatment Trial – how strong is the evidence? *New Engl. J. Med.*, **348**: 2055–2056.

Weibel, E.R. (1963). *Morphometry of the Human Lung*. Springer-Verlag, Berlin.

Weibel, E.R. (1989). Lung morphometry and models in respiratory physiology. In: Chang, H.K. & Paiva, M. (eds) *Respiratory Physiology an Analytical Approach*. Marcel Dekker, Inc., New York.

Weibel, E.R. (1991). The lung. In: Crystal, R.G. & West, J.B. (eds) *Scientific Foundations*. Raven Press, Ltd., New York; pp. 715.

Whiteley, J.P., Turner, M.J., Baker, A.B., Gavaghan, D.J. & Hahn, C.E. (2002). The effects of ventilation pattern on carbon dioxide transfer in three computer models of the airways. *Respir. Physiol. Neurobiol.*, **131**: 269–284.

Appendix: list of symbols

$A(z)$	Total airway cross-sectional area at generation z (cm^2)
$c(z, t)$	CO_2 gas concentration in generation z at time t (volume of gas of interest/unit volume total gas in airway, dimensionless)
C_B	Mixed venous CO_2 gas concentration in equilibrium with pulmonary arterial blood (dimensionless)
C_{ME}	Mixed expired CO_2 gas concentration (dimensionless)
D_{mol}	Molecular diffusivity of CO_2 gas in air ($D_{CO_2} = 0.17\,cm^2/s$)
$\bar{G}$	Average diffusive conductance AD/l of alveolar airways for CO_2
$l(z)$	Airway length per generation at generation z (cm)
N_A	Number of alveoli per generation at generation z (dimensionless)
NS	Normalized phase III slope of the capnogram, $((dc/dV)/c_{ME})$ (l^{-1})
N_T	Total number of alveoli in Weibel lung (dimensionless)
$\dot{Q}(z, t)$	Airway volume flow rate in generation z at time t (cm^3/s)
$\dot{Q}_B$	Total cardiac output (cm^3/s)
$\bar{R}$	Average resistance to acinar airway gas exchange between the V_T and FRC (mmHg min/ml)
$S(z, t)$	Alveolar capillary source term (s^{-1})
t	Time (s)
$V(z)$	Airway volume per generation at generation z (cm^3)
$V_A(z, t)$	Alveolar volume per generation at generation z and time t (cm^3)
$\dot{V}CO_2$	Volume of CO_2 gas evolved from alveolar capillary blood or exhaled at mouth per minute (ml/min)
V_{Daw}	Airways (Fowler) dead-space (cm^3)
V_T	Tidal volume (cm^3)
$\dot{V}_T(t)$	Tidal volume flow rate at mouth (cm^3/s)
z	Generational coordinate (dimensionless)
λ	CO_2 gas solubility in blood (volume gas dissolved/unit volume of blood/fractional concentration of gas over blood, dimensionless)

HISTORICAL PERSPECTIVES

PART 3

HISTORICAL PERSPECTIVES: INTRODUCTION 33

M.B. Jaffe

The history of time and volumetric capnography is closely intertwined with the developments in respiratory physiology and medicine. We have attempted to capture this with an overview of the key historical developments of carbon dioxide (CO_2) and the gas laws as well as the measurement of CO_2 and its volume, both chemical and physical methods.

We are fortunate to be able to include contributions from two of the pioneers in capnography. Prof. Dr. Bob Smalhout, an early proponent of clinical capnography and an author of the *Atlas of Capnography* published in 1975, describes the tumultuous introduction of capnography in The Netherlands. Dr. Roger Fletcher in his thesis and series of papers on the single breath test for CO_2 helped bridge the gap between physiology and clinical practice and present in a unified form the concepts of CO_2 elimination and dead space. He helped to increase the clinical understanding of gas exchange and served as a catalyst for the use and understanding of the clinical value of volumetric capnography. He describes how technology in the form of the Siemens Model 930 analyzer coupled with the need to address clinical problems helped to dramatically increase the recognition of volumetric capnography's potential as a valuable diagnostic and monitoring tool.

Advances in technology often drive clinical developments. This linkage can be seen in an interview with Max Liston, one of the early developers of gas measurement technology, Liston describes how research often takes the most unexpected turns, which send developments in directions not anticipated.

BRIEF HISTORY OF TIME AND VOLUMETRIC CAPNOGRAPHY

34

M.B. Jaffe

Carbon dioxide and the gas laws

Carbon dioxide (CO_2) is now the fourth most abundant gas (after nitrogen, oxygen and argon) on earth. Several billion years ago, before O_2 assumed its present position, CO_2 was much more plentiful. Today we worry that its modest concentration in the atmosphere might rise a little over its current level of some 0.04%.

For most of its history, no one had heard of CO_2. However, even in antiquity people knew of evil airs, for example in the famous Grotto del Cane (Naples) where a poisonous gas lingered at the floor of the grotto so that dogs (and cats and chicken) would be overcome by a gas while people could survive a trip into the grotto as long as they would stay upright – and as long as they kept their noses well above the CO_2 seeping out of cracks in the bottom of the cave.

Jan Baptista Van Helmont (1579/80–1644) was the first to recognize the formation of CO_2 gas during fermentation and the burning of wood. He called it gas sylvestre (Sylvester, a spirit of the woods). But that title it had to surrender when in 1755 J. Black named it fixed air because he had discovered it as a constituent in carbonated alkali. The gas finally yielded to chemical analysis when Antoine-Laurent de Lavoisier (1743–1794) showed it to be an oxide of carbon. It took many years before the gas could be measured in the exhalation or in the blood of man and beast.

Before measurements of CO_2 gas became possible, measurements involving gases had to be developed. Thus, we must mention Guericke (1602–1686), who had held many posts, among them mayor in the city of Magdeburg, the capital of Saxony-Anhalt in Germany. The University of Magdeburg now calls itself the Otto-von-Guericke University, in recognition of its famous son. Around 1650, Guericke had managed to evacuate air from two matching hemispheres, which thus emptied off much of the air resisted separation. Many think of him as having introduced us to the concept of barometric pressure but in doing so he also showed us how to aspirate gas by means of a vacuum pump.

Next we must mention Robert Boyle (1627–1691), an aristocrat-experimenter who taught in Oxford and London and who published several scientific treatises describing his experiments, among them one on New Experiments … touching the Spring of the Air (Boyle, 1660). Again, vacuum pumps played a role. We now remember Boyle's law, which states that pressure = k/volume, an important fact when gases are exposed to different pressures during measurements. One of Boyle's assistants at Oxford, Robert Hooke (1635–1703), had built a vacuum pump for Boyle. This was not Hooke's most memorable accomplishment, of which there were many, but an important one for our account.

If pressure affects the volume of gas, so does temperature, a fact compressed into $V = kT$ by the French balloonist-scientist Jacques Alexander César Charles (1746–1823). Joseph Louis Gay–Lussac (1778–1850), another French balloonist-scientist contributed details by describing the relationship between pressure and temperature when volume and amount are held constant, that is: $P/T = k$.[1] In 1834 Émile Clapeyron (1799–1864) combined the laws of Boyle, Charles and Gay–Lussac into the first formulation of the ideal gas law as $PV = R(T + 267)$ (temperature in degrees celsius).[2]

At this point we can break with the string of French balloonists and turn to the British Isles and Professor William Thomson (1824–1907) who later would be knighted in 1892 as Lord Kelvin of Largs and is now known as Lord Kelvin. He proposed an absolute scale of temperature in 1848 and wrote the ideal gas law in the well known form $PV = nRT$, where n is the number

[1]The law expressing this relationship (isovolumic) was named after Charles at the suggestion of Gay–Lussac and intended to give credit to the unpublished work of Charles performed in 1787.

[2]Note later work revealed that the number should actually be 273.2, giving: $PV = R(T + 273.2)$.

of moles of gas present, R is the universal gas constant and T is absolute temperature in degrees Kelvin. This terse, mathematical summary, the result of many empirical observations and insight, states that the product of the pressure (P) and volume (V) of an ideal gas is proportional to its absolute temperature (T) and to the number of molecules in it. In 1873 the Dutch physicist Johannes van der Waals (1837–1923) modified the ideal gas law and derived another gas law to account for the behavior of real fluids. The van der Waals equation is commonly expressed as $(P + a/V^2)(V - b) = RT$, where the values for the constants a and b are different for real gases.

The current frequently used infrared spectrometry of CO_2 owes thanks to William Herschel (1738–1822) known primarily as the astronomer who discovered Uranus (1781), but he also discovered infrared radiation (1800). He passed sunlight through a prism, holding a thermometer just beyond the red end of the visible spectrum, and observed the temperature increase. From this observation Herschel concluded that there must be an invisible form of energy (Herschel, 1800).

Pierre Bouguer(1698–1758) in 1729 first expressed the relationship between the absorption of radiant energy and the absorbing medium. Noting: "In a medium of uniform transparency the light remaining in a collimated beam is an exponential function of the length of the path in the medium" (from the French) (Gillispie, 1980). Johann Heinrich Lambert (1728–1777) considered as the founder of the theory of light measurement published the classic tome "Photometria" in Latin (Lambert, 1760) in which he described the logarithmic law of the absorption of light, now often known as Beer–Lambert law (after August Beer (1825–1863)) or Lambert–Beer law. Later Angström (1889) described pressure broadening and observed that by increasing the size of the sample cell with a constant amount of gas, the infrared absorption was reduced contrary to that predicted by Lambert–Beer's law (Cormack & Powell, 1972).

John Tyndall (1820–1893) studied the radiative properties of various gases and constructed the first ratio spectrophotometer, which he used to measure the absorption of gases, such as water vapor, "carbonic acid" (now known as CO_2), ozone, and hydrocarbons. He also observed the large differences in the abilities of "perfectly colorless and invisible gases and vapors" to absorb and transmit radiant heat, and noted that oxygen, nitrogen, and hydrogen are almost transparent to radiant heat but that water vapor, CO_2, and ozone are the very good absorbers of heat radiation, and that "even in small quantities, these gases absorb much more strongly than the atmosphere itself" (Burchfield, 1981). Tyndall is also credited making some of the first measurements of expired CO_2 in humans (Tyndall, 1865). He notes in his Rede Lecture "the presence of the minutest quantity of carbonic acid (carbon dioxide) may be detected by its action on the rays from the carbonic oxide (carbon monoxide) flame ... Radiant heat may indeed be employed as a means of determining practically the amount of carbonic acid expired from the lungs."

August Krogh (1874–1949) working in the Laboratory of Medical Physiology under Professor Christian Bohr was intrigued with problems connected with the gas exchange of the living organism. With his wife, Dr. Marie Krogh, he undertook a series of experiments and concluded, contrary to the views held at the time by Bohr and J.S. Haldane, that diffusion alone was sufficient to explain the gas exchange in the lungs. Krogh's results were later confirmed by others and have become widely accepted. Additionally, Krogh made a number of contributions to the development of physiological instrumentation including a recording spirometer, an electromagnetic bicycle ergometer, and improved methods for gas analysis (Rehlberg, 1951).

Measurement of CO_2 and its volume

Chemical

John Scott Haldane (1860–1936), amongst his many contributions, had described the 1st version of a gas analyzer using chemical absorption. For many years thereafter it was considered *the* reference method for CO_2 subsequently known as the Haldane method (Haldane, 1912). The principle of Haldane's method of gas analysis was to draw a known volume of gas (10 ml) into a graduated burette by raising and lowering a reservoir of mercury held underneath. The gas was then exposed to a series of absorbents (i.e. sodium or potassium hydroxide for CO_2), and the diminution of volume was recorded, while the gas was kept at a constant temperature and pressure. The volume of CO_2 in the original sample was computed as the ratio of the change in volume divided by the total volume.

Lloyd (1958) modified the Haldane apparatus and improved its accuracy to within 0.02% vol/vol. However, the method was considered complex, very slow and highly dependent upon operator skill. Campbell (1960) described a simpler version of Haldane's apparatus that was judged to be sufficiently accurate for clinical work. Similarly, a smaller version of the Haldane apparatus described by Scholander (1947) used 0.5 ml samples instead of 10 ml. Apparatus for gas analysis with gas sample sizes ranging from 35 ml to a fraction of 1 ml and accuracy of 0.005% to 2% taking from several minutes to hours to analyze have

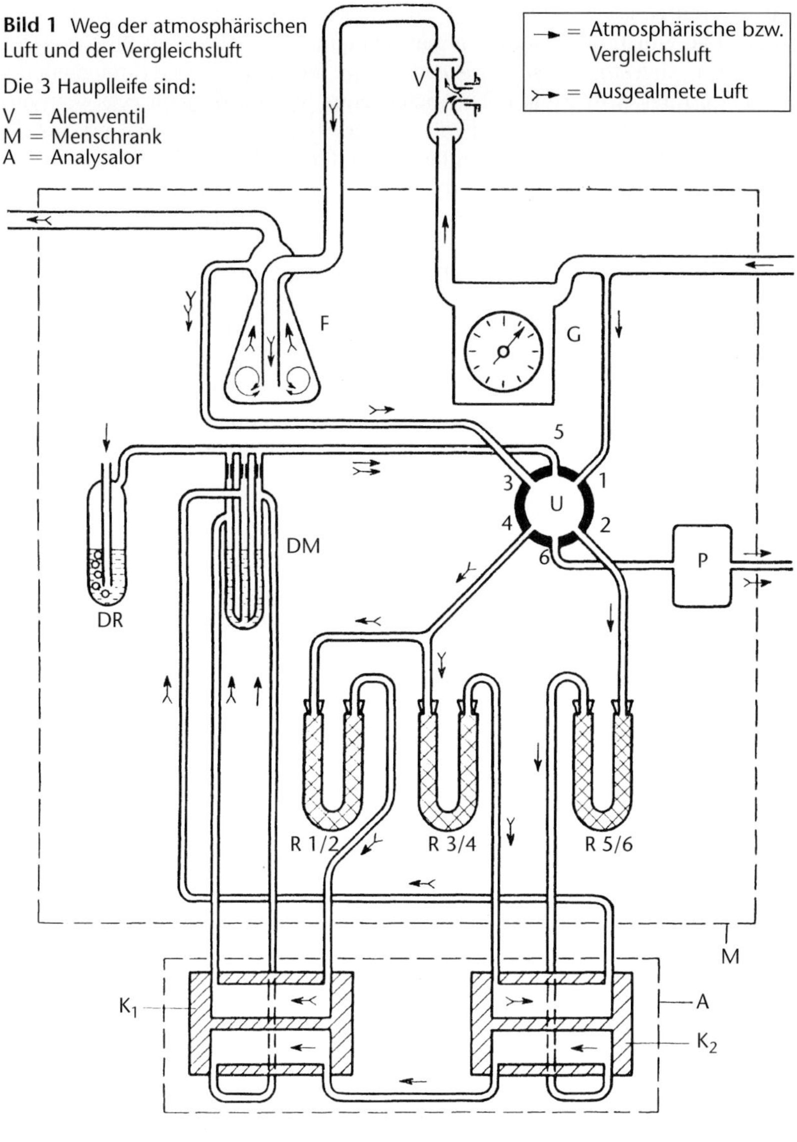

Figure 34.1 Resting metabolic rate device from Hartmann & Braun (1952). (Reproduced with permission from Institut für Stadtgeschichte Frankfurt a. M.: Hartmann & Braun-Archiv. (W1/25 Nr. 5750-5800)). The single parts: G: breath volume meter (tidal volume device); F: mixing chamber; U: pneumatic switch; P: membrane pump (diaphragm pump); R 1/2: dry and absorption tube for O_2 measurement; R 3/4: drying tube for CO_2 measurement; R 5/6: drying tube for reference gas; DM: triple manometer; DR: pressure controller; K_1: measurement block for CO_2 free respiratory air with O_2 deficit; K_2: measurement block for CO_2 containing breathing gas.

been described (Comroe, 1950). A variety of modifications to simplify the method as well as to account for errors, such as those due to the presence of nitrous oxide (N_2O) have been reported (Nunn, 1958). The Van Slyke apparatus (Van Slyke & O'Neill, 1924), well known to many by now mature clinicians is similar to the Haldane and Scholander apparatus, and was primarily used clinically for blood gas analysis.

Various investigators sought to extend these discrete chemical absorption-based measurement methods to "continuous" analysis. Rein (1933) combined the chemical method with a hot-wire flowmeter to obtain a continuous recording of gas concentration by measuring the "imbalance" between two chambers; in one, the gas is absorbed and in the other it is not. Bezinger (1938) introduced a rubber bag of 2–3 l capacity between subject and measuring device to buffer peaks in flow velocity. Hartmann and Braun of Frankfurt am Main Germany, offered a device in the 1950s that automated this analysis (Figure 34.1).

Physical

August Herman Pfund (1879–1949) developed an early gas analyzer in 1939 that was used at Johns Hopkins Hospital in Baltimore to measure CO and CO_2 (Pfund, 1940; Pfund & Gemmill, 1940). Pfund described this thermal method of CO_2 measurement as "mak(ing) possible continuous analysis without disturbing the mixture" in contrast to chemical methods that destroy the material under test. An electrically heated spiral of nichrome wire and silvered concave mirror served as the radiation source. The radiation passed through an absorption cell and into a detector. The detector consisted of "three bakelite rings with 36 brass studs to which thin wires of iron and constantan (a copper–nickel alloy with high electrical resistance and a low temperature coefficient) are attached to form a thermopile of 33 junctions in series." The detector cell was filled with a mixture of 3% CO_2 and 97% dry air. If no CO_2 was present in the absorption cell, the radiation would be absorbed in the detector cell and the increase in temperature would be measured by the thermopile. The presence of CO_2 in the absorption cell would cause less radiation to be absorbed in the detector cell, and therefore a smaller rise in temperature.

Karl Friedrich Luft (1909–1999) is often credited with developing the infrared technology using a balanced condenser microphone detector consisting of sealed cells containing pure CO_2 separated by a diaphragm. This kind of detector, now known as the Luft cell, can be traced to the photo-acoustic effect first observed by Alexander Graham Bell and later demonstrated by Bell at the Paris Exposition in 1880. Bell (1880) exposed a test tube containing cigar smoke to chopped sunlight – this was the photo part. The test tube was connected to a hearing tube from which emanated sound – the acoustic part. The pitch of the sound waves was controlled by the frequency of the chopped sunlight. John Tyndall (1881) and Wilhelm Röntgen (1881) performed similar experiments after learning of Bell's discovery.

In 1937 Luft joined BASF where he was confronted with a measurement problem (Luft *et al.*, 1993). The method of fabrication of plastic resulted in a highly explosive mixture of butane and air. In order to avoid the creation of such mixture a method to measure low concentrations of butane was sought. It was observed that this chemical has strong absorption in infrared band but that known photometric methods of the time failed since they were too strongly affected by interfering gases in the mixture, such as CO_2 and water vapor. Luft came up with an idea that the gas could be a "radiation receiver" and by doing that have the necessary selectivity required. He discussed this with Lehrer who had just successfully developed a recording infrared spectrophotometer. This discussion led to collaboration and development of a device. The superiority of the new device over existing electrochemical devices soon even convinced the factory chemists who were skeptical about using a device based on physical principles. This device known as the URAS (ultrarot absorptions-Schreiber – infrared absorption writer) consisted of the three main components (power supply, optics, and amplifiers) packaged in separate off-the-shelf electrical switching boxes that were bolted together. Despite using common components, their supply problems that started shortly before the war continued throughout the war. The manufacture of these detector cells was considered to be a very tedious and delicate process. In 1943 Luft's often-referenced paper on these cells was published in Zeitschrift für Technische Physik (Luft, 1943). He and Lehrer were awarded a patent (filed in 1938) on the technology (Lehrer & Luft, 1943). Despite all of the problems, BASF was able to manufacture several hundred units that were mostly used in I.G. Farbenindustrie chemical factories although a number of these devices were destroyed during air bombardments (Luft *et al.*, 1993). Additionally, the technique was used for environmental monitoring in submarines. A large number of manufactured devices that were moved into the salt mines were confiscated by the occupational powers and moved to the US and England after the war (Luft *et al.*, 1993). At the end of 1952, Hartmann and Braun acquired the URAS trademark and license to manufacture and distribute the URAS device from BASF (Luft *et al.*, 1993). The Luft detector is shown in Figure 34.2 and is described as in the original German patent.

Concurrently, Veingerov (1938) at the State Optical Institute of Leningrad under A.A. Lyebyedyev (1893–1969) built early IR-radiation detectors and opto-acoustical gas analyzers to study infrared absorption in gases.

Concerns about the environment in the 1960s stimulated exploration of photo-acoustic spectroscopy especially when coupled with new light sources and highly sensitive microphones. The technology promised to help with the identification and quantitation of trace amounts of atmospheric pollutants. Today, expansion of the technology to measure several gases simultaneously is available.

Just as absorption of infrared energy can increase rotational and vibrational activity of molecules, so can absorption of visible or ultraviolet radiation. Predicted by Smekal (1923) and confirmed by Raman and Krishnan (1928), the phenomenon is called Raman scattering. Radiation scattering can occur in several ways. For example, sunrays become visible beams when airborne dust dances in their path. In this case, the particles are large compared to the wavelength of light (Tyndall effect). When the scattered particles are small (molecules), two kinds of scattering occur. One is an absorption–re-emission phenomenon in which the wavelength does not change; it occurs instantaneously, within 10–12 s (Rayleigh scattering). Although wavelength does not change, shorter wavelengths are scattered more efficiently. This explains why the sky

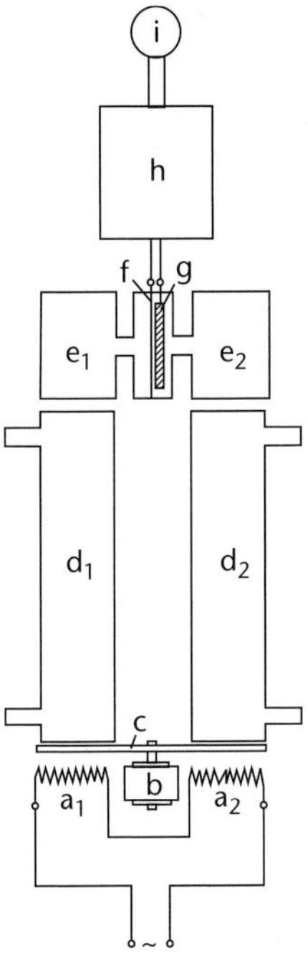

Figure 34.2 Luft's device – (The radiation coming from the sources a_1 and a_2 is periodically interrupted through a shutter wheel c that is driven by motor b. The shutter wheel c has slits in such a way the radiation from both sources can pass through at the same time (or is interrupted at the same time). Behind shutter wheel c the radiation runs through the pipes d_1 and d_2, where d_1 contains the gas to be measured and d_2 is filled with a reference gas (*at half atmosphere*). Following that the radiation enters the chambers e_1 and e_2, which contain – as a "reception layer" – the gas that is to be determined. Both chambers are separated (in an almost gas-tight fashion) from each other through a thin (metal) membrane f; this membrane forms with the insulated counter plate g an electrical capacitor. If the gas mixture contains the component that is to be determined, chamber e_1 receives a weaker radiation than e_2; as a consequence and corresponding to the interruptions by the shutter wheel c there is a periodic pressure difference between the chambers e_1 and e_2 which can – through membrane f – be transformed in changes of capacitance. The membrane capacitor is followed by an amplifier h, which allows a readout at the measuring instrument i of the capacitance variations and thereby the concentration of the gas that is to be determined". (Translated from German) (Lehrer & Luft, 1943).

appears blue; the shorter blue wavelengths in sunlight are preferentially scattered, which increases the intensity of that wavelength as it reaches earth.

A second kind of absorption–re-emission scattering can cause a wavelength change. This implies that some of the absorbed radiation is retained, increasing the amplitude of molecular vibrations. The remaining energy is remitted at a longer, or slightly shifted wavelength (lower frequency) as is required by conservation of energy.

By definition, both the Raman and Rayleigh transitions produce scattered light, and so, must be measured off the path of incident light, usually at right angles. The intensity is usually very low. A rule of thumb is that only 0.1% of the incident light is scattered. Of that, only 0.1% experiences a Raman shift; therefore, about one in a million photons is scattered with a change in wavelength. Consequently, continuous Raman monitoring requires the high photon densities obtainable from lasers and efficient separation of the relatively high intensity Rayleigh scattering from the low intensity Raman scattering. Early investigators used mercury vapor lamps and long exposures of fast photographic emulsions. These have given way to high intensity coherent lasers and extremely sensitive photon detectors.

An additional method of clinical relevance of quantifying gas concentrations is mass spectroscopy. The idea of separating charged particles (ions) by their mass was first proposed and practically applied by J.J. Thompson and F.W. Aston (Hill, 1966), who used the technique in isotope research. The technical evolution of that idea from a laboratory tool useful in many fields of research to a practical clinical instrument required 50 years of experience, the prodding and support of the National Aeronautics and Space Administration (NASA), and the vision of early medical users who recognized its potential.

Researchers through the 1950s and 1960s were quick to take advantage of the mass spectrometer to measure several gases simultaneously and to explore basic questions in respiratory physiology (Fowler, 1969). NASA supported the development of mass spectrometry as the appropriate technique for monitoring respiratory gases, planetary atmospheres, and closed environments in outer space. In medicine, mass spectrometry was first used for monitoring in the intensive care unit (ICU), because the gases to be monitored were relatively simple. In the operating room (OR), detecting N_2O and CO_2 presented a problem because both gases have almost identical masses. A mass spectrometer with the resolving power to separate them was considered too expensive. Measuring anesthetic vapors presented several challenges. Techniques had to be developed to accommodate the relatively large mass of the agents to spectrometers with lower mass ranges. In addition, reducing pressure, from atmospheric to very low pressure, required for mass spectrometers was difficult. By the early 1980s, the sampling and detection problems were resolved and reliability was improved; in 1981 mass spectrometry became established as a cost-effective and reliable monitor for OR use (Ozanne *et al.*, 1981). In recent years, the enhanced capabilities of infrared devices have challenged what was once the unique position of mass spectrometry as a multi-gas monitor.

Early clinical applications

John Hutchinson (1811–1861) published a paper about a water spirometer and the measurements made with it (Hutchinson, 1846) (Figure 34.3). Hutchinson recorded the vital capacities of over 4000 persons with his spirometer and classified them in such categories as "paupers", "first Battalion grenadier guards", "pugilists and wrestlers", "giants and dwarfs", "girls", "gentleman", and "diseased cases". He demonstrated the linear relationship of vital capacity to height and also showed that that vital capacity does not relate with weight at any given height (Petty, 2002). Volume measuring devices similar to one originally described by Hutchinson are still in use today with only minor alterations. However, volume may be easily obtained from the integration of flow. This led to development of devices based upon the pressure drop across capillary tubes (Fleisch, 1925) and screens (Silverman, 1946; Lilly, 1950).

The first "portable" metabolism apparatus was devised by Nathan Zuntz (1847–1920) (Figure 34.4) (Zuntz & Loewy, 1920; Fenn & Rahn, 1964). In 1892 Zuntz's student Magnus-Levy applied this apparatus at the bedside and undertook pioneering investigations of metabolism in patients with a variety of medical conditions including myxedema, hyperthyroidism, obesity, and pregnancy (Lusk, 1933).

Since the early 1900s, gas exchange was most often clinically measured by the "gold standard" Douglas bag method (Douglas, 1911) or Tissot spirometer (Tissot, 1904). In fact it was noted that Douglas as part of the preparations for an expedition to Pike's Peak in Colorado, developed the bag method for collection of expired gases (Douglas *et al.*, 1913). The Douglas bag required the collection of exhaled air in large, impermeable canvas bags (50 l), and subsequent sampling and analysis of the collected gas to measure the mixed gas fractions and the total expired volume by manual "squeezing" the entire content of the bag through a spirometer. Problems noted with Douglas bag technique include faulty technique and loss of CO_2 through pores in the bag. Shepard (1955) suggested filling the bag to near capacity within 15 min in order to minimize loss by diffusion while Balchum *et al.* (1954) recommended using synthetic bags with lower permeability to CO_2, realizing that the solubility coefficient of rubber with respect to the respiratory gases was the primary problem. With the Tissot type spirometer, the subject breathes through a two-way respiratory valve, passing all expired gas into a calibrated cylinder, which is sealed, from the outside by a water seal in a

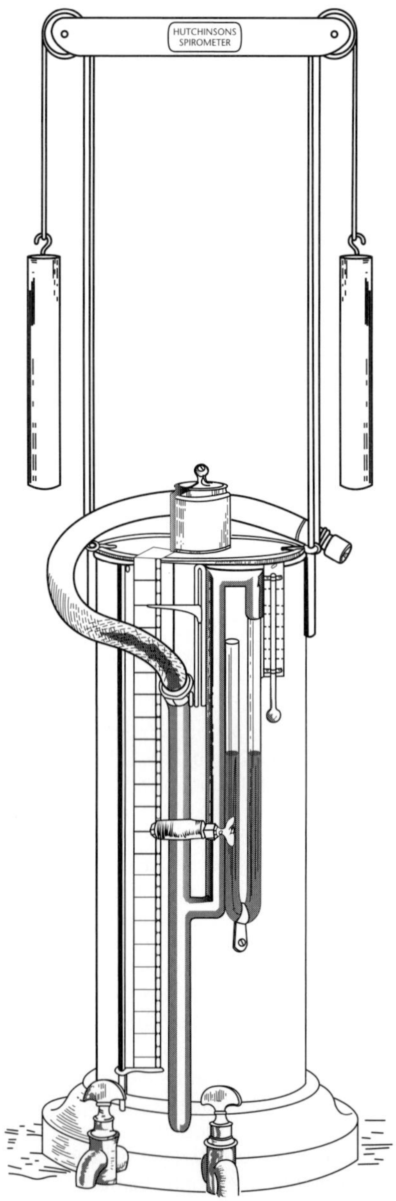

Figure 34.3 Improved spirometer with which John Hutchinson in 1846 measured the subdivisions of the lung volumes in over 4000 subjects, thereby laying the foundation for modern tests of ventilatory function. (From Hutchinson, 1846).

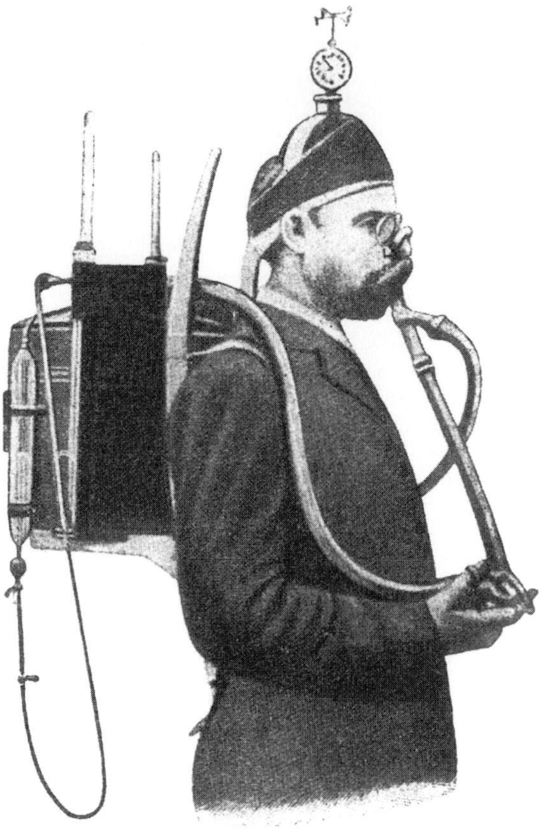

Figure 34.4 Nathan Zuntz and his portable metabolism apparatus. (From Zuntz, 1920.)

second cylinder. Ventilation is determined by recording the total volume of gas, time of collection period, calibration constant, temperature of the gas and barometric pressure (Consolazio *et al.*, 1963).

In the 1960s, with the development of the Parkinson-Cowan dry gas meter, the measurement of inspired minute ventilation also became commonplace. The complexity and manual nature of these measurements led to the development of semi-automated methods (Wilmore & Costill, 1974). In this approach the measurement of the expired mixed gas fractions was initially achieved by sampling gas from a mixing chamber into 2-l latex bags for subsequent analysis. It included drawing a continuous sample of exhaled air from a mixing chamber directly into electronic gas analyzers. The voltage output of these gas analyzers and the inspired ventilation meter was converted to digital form and the calculations for O_2 consumption and CO_2 elimination performed by a microcomputer. The time lag between the process of drying and the analysis of the gas and the measurement of volumes made it necessary to make timing adjustments.

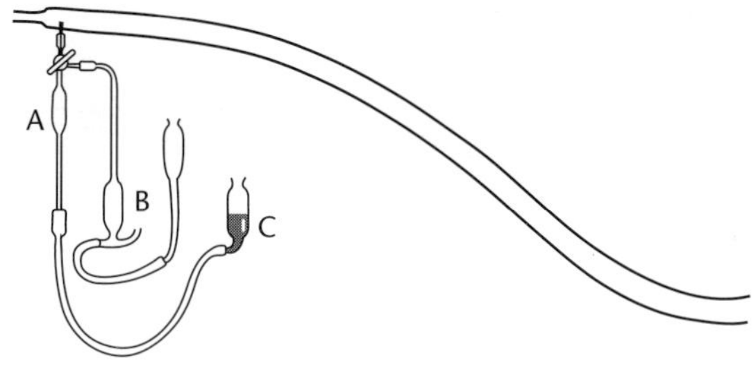

Figure 34.5 Apparatus for obtaining and analyzing alveolar air. (Reproduced with permission from Haldane, J.S. & Priestley, J.G. (1935). *Respiration*, 2nd edition. Oxford, London.)

The concept of dead-space was first clearly described by Zuntz in 1882 (Haldane & Priestley 1935). In 1890 Christian Bohr (1891) introduced his equation for calculating respiratory dead-space in terms of concentrations of alveolar and expired gases (Figure 34.5). Enghoff (1938) later substituted arterial values to approximate the alveolar values. The earliest description in the literature of the volumetric capnogram and a method to determine "airway" dead-space is that of Aitken and Clark-Kennedy (1928) (Figure 34.6). Fowler (1948) describing the single breath test for nitrogen (SBT-N_2) curve sought to use uniform terminology to clarify the "meaning of dead-space" and thus divided this curve into four phases: I, II, III, and IV. He also desired to better understand the magnitude and constancy of the dead-space. This happened shortly after the controversy between Krogh and Linhard and Haldane and Priestley over the size of dead-space. Krogh and Linhard (1913) measured dead-space and found it to vary over a narrow range (and confirmed by others) whereas Haldane and Priestley suggested that dead-space might increase as much as 800 ml during a maximal inflation.

Krogh (1923) developed an improved kymographic method using a spirometer chamber with CO_2 and moisture absorbants. Krogh (1923) recognized that the look-up tables for estimating basal metabolism advanced by Harris and Benedict (1919) had "nothing to do with the biological laws which must be supposed to govern the relations between the metabolism and sex, weight, height, and age, respectively". Instead, he suggested actual measurements of metabolism as they are still practiced today.

Different methods to sample "alveolar" CO_2 gas were developed (Fowler & Comroe, 1950) including single breath methods requiring forced expirations at the end of a normal expiration or inspiration and the collection of gas for analysis and multiple breath methods. Continuous analysis permitted gas from "a single expiration to be 'fractionated' into many successive samples" (Fowler & Comroe, 1950, p. 221). It was

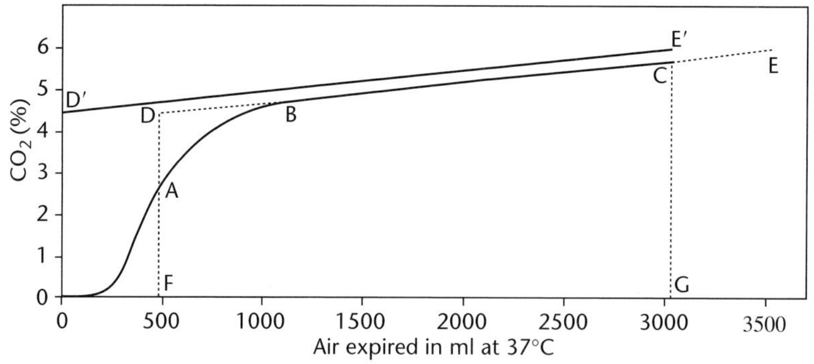

Figure 34.6 Diagram to show the method of deducing the alveolar CO_2 curve and the dead-space from the experimental CO_2 curve. The flat part BC of the experimental curve OABC is prolonged to the left to D until the area FDCG equals the area OABCG, DF, and CG being perpendicular to OG. OF then represents the volume of the dead-space. DC is prolonged to the right to E, over a distance equal to OF (when measured horizontally). The whole line DE then represents the changing concentration of alveolar CO_2 throughout expiration. (Reproduced with permission from Aitken, R.S. & Clark-Kennedy, A.E. (1928). On the fluctuation in the composition of the alveolar air during the respiratory cycle in muscular capacity. *J. Physiol.*, **65**: 389–411.)

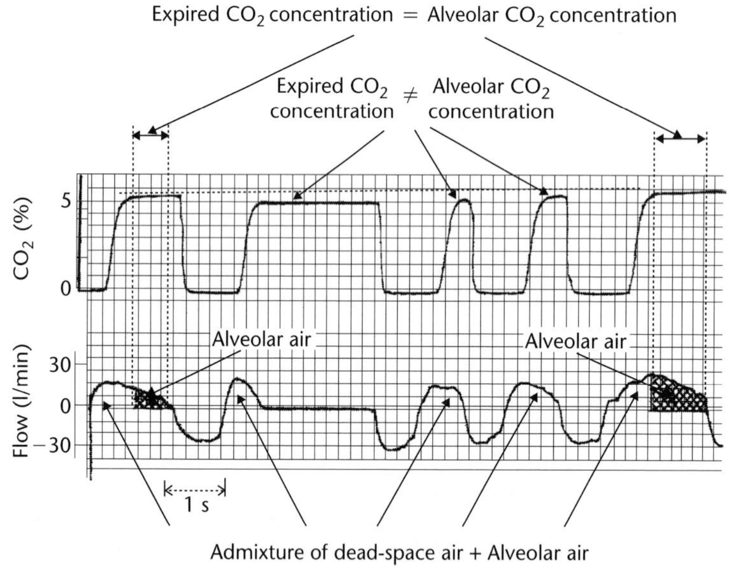

Figure 34.7 Simultaneous CO_2 and flow curve showing criteria for reading alveolar concentration of CO_2 from recorded plateau. (Reproduced with permission from Elam, J.A., Brown, E.L. & Ten Pas, R.H. (1955). Carbon dioxide homeostasis during anesthesia. I. Instrumentation. *Anesthesiology*, **16**: 876–885.)

recognized that continuous analysis was relevant to the measurement of intrapulmonary gas mixing and ventilation–perfusion relationship (Fowler & Comroe, 1950, p. 222) and "enhanced by simultaneous analysis of gas volumes" but that these instruments "are rather complex and are not generally available."

Elam and colleagues working on the problem of CO_2 elimination from closed circuit anesthesia systems under US Army support published early pioneering work in the field. They were first to publish capnographic profiles of human respiration in the anesthesiology literature (Peppriell *et al.*, 1991; Sands & Bacon, 1998). Their work on CO_2 homeostasis published in a series of four papers (Elam & Brown, 1955; 1956a, b; Elam *et al.*, 1955) included both normal and abnormal characteristics of the capnographic profile and measurements of dead-space and alveolar ventilation. "As part of this work, Elam built a machine to 'mimic' human respiration which resulted in an early prototype of a ventilator that worked in either volume or pressure modes" (Figure 34.7). (Peppriell *et al*, 1991) Additionally, the advent of commercial air travel with pressurized passenger compartments propelled the development of technology to measure CO_2 (Clamans, 1952).

Smalhout (1967) and Smalhout and Kalenda (1981) popularized the use of the terms capnography, capnograph and capnogram. The publication of their atlas of strip chart recordings of capnograms helped to illustrate many of the applications of capnography.[3] However they noted that this "represent(ed) little more than the surface of a deep pool" (Smalhout & Kalenda 1981). (For an account of the early days of time capnography see Chapter 35.) Weingarten (1990) summarized their contributions by noting that:

> "Under their direction, capnography survived a stormy gestational period as it reached maturity in The Netherlands. It was introduced in the US at a small private meeting sponsored by a major instrument manufacturer held in conjunction with the World Congress on Intensive Care Medicine in Washington DC, in May 1978. Five anesthesiologists attended the meeting, two of whom concluded that capnography would prove to be of very little value."

While single breath curves for CO_2 appeared as early as 1961 in the literature (Berengo & Cutillo, 1961) it was not until Fletcher in his doctoral thesis (1980) and later as various publications (Fletcher & Jonson, 1984) presented the concepts of dead-space and CO_2 elimination in a unified framework. His presentation became widely known as the SBT or single breath CO_2 ($SBCO_2$) curve (i.e. the expiratory portion of the volumetric capnogram). (For an account of the early days of volumetric capnography see Chapter 36.)

Commercial – time and volumetric

In 1950, Max Liston founded the Liston-Becker Company, whose principal products were side-stream sampling non-dispersive infrared (NDIR) analyzers (Liston, 1954) including the Models 16, 28, and 30. The Liston-Becker Gas Analyzer and its successor designs consisted of a "pickup" unit and "control" unit. The pick-up unit, located near the patient's head, was sealed and could be pressurized with up to 5 lbs air pressure to make it safe for use with explosive anesthetic gas mixtures (Siebecker *et al.*, 1954). This company had developed a capacitance-based photometer for measuring CO_2 and other heteroatomic gases. The instruments were adapted for medical use and were also installed on American and NATO nuclear submarines to monitor internal atmospheric CO_2 levels. In 1955, Beckman Instruments acquired the Liston-Becker Company. Beckman Instruments continued development of NDIR gas analyzers with Max Liston remaining as a director of engineering until 1965 (for more details see the excerpts from an interview with Max Liston) Representative Beckman capnographs included the Beckman Model LB-1 and Beckman LB-2 analyzers.[4]

Representative systems using the Luft detector included Hartmann and Braun URAS series of instruments, and Godart capnographs (Table 34.1) (Blackburn & Williams, 1980), a modification of the URAS 4 (Cormack & Powell, 1972). These systems were widely used for CO_2 measurement in the 1960s and 1970s (Hill & Powell, 1968).

In the early 1970s, exercise researchers developed their own systems to automate the tedious steps associated with Douglas bags. This led to the development of commercial metabolic carts with first and second generation mixing chambers based on the Beckman metabolic measurement cart (MMC). It used a Monroe calculator for computation and printout (Beckman Instruments, 1981) and Beckman MMC Horizon System with an Intel 8085 microprocessor with 64 KB of memory with two floppy disk drives for program and data storage (Beckman Instruments, 1983). Side-stream gas was sampled from the mixing chamber and measured by an infrared CO_2 analyzer (Beckman LB-2 head) and polarographic O_2 analyzer (Beckman OM-11 bench). Flow was measured at the exit port of the mixing chamber using a turbine flowmeter. CO_2 elimination and O_2 consumption was determined using the Haldane equation, which assumes a net N_2 change of zero. While initially developed for studies of exercise physiology these devices were later

[3] Termed infrared CO_2 meters from the 1950s and into the early 1970s, the term capnograph derive from the Godart Capnograph.

[4] Beckman Model LB-1 originally marketed by the Spinco (centrifuge) division in Palo Alto, CA eventually ended up with the advanced technology operations (ATO) division in Anaheim, CA, which was primarily responsible for government contracts including placing the technology on-board the US nuclear submarine fleet. The ATO divisions focus changed and in the 1970s became the physiological measurement operations (PMO) division which was divested by the company shortly after its acquisition by Smithkline in 1982 and became a separate company called Sensormedics. The LB-1 was originally intended for use in ORs in which ether and cyclopropane were commonly used anesthetics. This accounts for the separation of the sample head from the rest of the instrument. The head was pressurized (with a bicycle pump) to avoid any in-leakage of ambient gases and included a pressure switch which disabled power to the head if the pressure dropped. The LB-1 was sold with a separate sample pump, which was also to be used outside the OR (Allen Norton, 2003, personal communication).

Table 34.1 Representative commercial infrared CO_2 analyzers used clinically (from 1950s through present)

Manufacturer (location)	Model	Features of interest
	1950s, 1960s and 1970s	
Hartmann & Braun (Frankfurt, DE)	URAS 1	Side-stream, Luft cell detector
Liston-Becker (Springdale, CT)	16	Total sampling (i.e. main-stream) using 7/8 inch tubing with 90% response time of 50 ms
Godart-Statham (Utrecht, Holland)	Capnograph Mark I	Side-stream, Luft cell detector, sampling rate 0.25–3 l/min
Beckman Instruments[1] (Pasadena, CA)	LB-1, LB-2, LB-3	Side-stream, different detectors for CO_2, halothane and N_2O
	1980s	
Hewlett-Packard (Waltham, MA)	M14360A	Main-stream, solid-state source, chopper wheel on detector
Siemens-Elema (Solna, Sweden)	Model 930	Main-stream integrated with 900 series ventilators
Criticare Systems (Waukesha, WI)	Poet®	Side-stream
Cascadia Technology Corp.[2] (Redmond, WA)	Capnostat®	Main-stream, all solid-state design with thick film source
	1990s	
Andros Analyzers (Berkeley, CA)	Breathwatch™ Model 4210	Main-stream design with IR lamp source
BCI (Waukesha, WI)	Capnocheck® Model 8200	Side-stream
Novametrix Medical Systems (Wallingford, CA)	Capnostat® II, III	Main-stream, smaller versions of previous generations
Pryon Corp[3] (Menomonee Falls, WI)	SC-300	Main-stream, all solid-state design
Oridion Systems (Needham, MA/Jerusalem, Israel)	MicroCap®	Low flow side-stream (50 ml/min)
	2000s	
Respironics-Novametrix (Wallingford, CA)	LoFlo™	Low flow side-stream (50 ml/min), sample cell part of sample set
Respironics-Novametrix (Wallingford, CA)	Capnostat®V	Main-stream, all signal processing in on-airway sensor head

[1] In 1950 National Technical Laboratories, Pasadena, CA was changed to Beckman Instruments.
[2] Acquired by Novametrix Medical Systems, Inc.
[3] Acquired by Protocol Systems and Protocol acquired by Welch-Allyn.
Notes: model name may list either the monitor name or sensor name (if main-stream), also ordering within decades approximate to year of product introduction, sources include Medical Electronics, various years, medical literature and company product literature. Trademarks are property of their respective owners.

adapted for bedside nutritional studies. Macfarlane (2001) recently published an extensive review of the devices for exercise.

In 1988, a Raman scattering instrument was introduced for clinical use. The RAman SCattering AnaLyzer (RASCAL) monitor was originally developed by a group of researchers from the University of Utah who formed a medical instrumentation company (Albion Instruments) to commercialize a laser-based Raman scattering technology. This company was subsequently bought by Ohmeda (Louisville, CO). Both the RASCAL and its successor RASCAL II monitors were online side-stream monitors for O_2, CO_2, N_2, N_2O and the three anesthetic vapors, halothane, enflurane, and isoflurane (Westenskow *et al.*, 1989). It used eight discrete optical channels to both identify and quantitate all gases. Each channel employs collection optics to gather the scattered radiation, a rejection filter to eliminate the unshifted Rayleigh light, and a Raman line filter, a narrow band-pass dielectric interference filter, which isolates the waveband intensity that quantitates the gas. A photo-multiplier tube monitors radiation intensities. However, this device is no longer marketed.

Early main-stream infrared devices (as those used by Elam) were physically large, cumbersome and

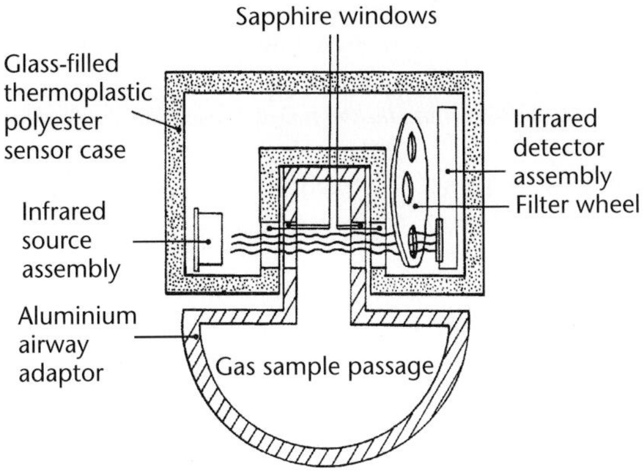

Figure 34.8 Cross-sectional view of a mechanical main-stream sensor (HP47210A). (Reproduced with permission from Kinsella, S.M. (1985). Assessment of the Hewlett-Packard HP47210A capnometer. *Br. J. Anaesth.*, **57**: 919–923.)

impractical for clinical use. Advancements in both main-stream and side-stream technology decreased the size of these devices to allow their inclusion in clinical monitors. However, it was not until the introduction of devices such as the Hewlett-Packard 47210A (Figure 34.8) that main-stream devices began to be used in the clinical environment (Solomon, 1981; Kinsella, 1985). Its airway adapter consisted of a hollow aluminum casting with sapphire windows. The sensor comprised an infrared source (heated broad-band black body radiator) and a detector assembly consisting of a rotating filter wheel, a band-pass filter and a lead–selenide detector. Siemens-Elema's introduced a main-stream CO_2 sensor add-on for the Servo ventilator 900 series of ventilator, the CO_2 Analyzer 930 (1981) (Table 34.1). It used a single detector with a filter specific for CO_2 and a chopper on the detector side. It interfaced with the ventilator and combined the measurements of flow and CO_2, and measured "CO_2 tidal production" as well as end-tidal CO_2. It introduced in a commercial product the concepts of effective and ineffective ventilation.

Innovations in main-stream gas sensors of the late 1980s eliminated the mechanical chopper of earlier designs resulting in smaller more robust main-stream CO_2 sensors included pulsed thick film infrared sources (Knodle *et al.*, 1994) and increased the robustness due to window contamination by the use of a coaxial optical design (Knodle *et al.*, 1990).

In the early 1990s volumetric capnography sensors appeared combining main-stream flow and CO_2 into an integrated airway adapter (Kofoed *et al.*, 1998) and also main-stream flow and side-stream CO_2 (Merilainen *et al.*, 1992). Technological advances in side-stream systems continue with newer source designs (Rosenfeld & Boasson, 1988) and novel configurations with removable sample cells (Rich *et al.*, 2003) as well as main-stream designs using digital signal processors and miniaturized optics. Future technological improvements promise greater robustness, adaptability and performance.

References

Aitken, R.S. & Clark-Kennedy, A.E. (1928). On the fluctuation in the composition of the alveolar air during the respiratory cycle in muscular capacity. *J. Physiol.*, **65**: 389–411.

Balchum, O.J., Hartman, S.A., Slonim, N.B., Dressler, S.H. & Ravin, A. (1953). The permeability of the Douglas type bag to respiratory gases. *J. Lab. Clin. Med.*, **41**: 268–280.

Beckman MMC Operating Instructions Beckman Instruments (1981). *Physiological Measurements Operations*, 2nd edition. Anaheim, CA.

Beckman MMC Horizon Systems Operating Instructions, Beckman Instruments (1983). *Physiological Measurements Operations*. Anaheim, CA.

Bell, A.G. (1880). Upon the production of sound by radiant energy. *Am. J. Sci.*, **20**: 305–324.

Berengo, A. & Cutillo, A. (1961). Single breath analysis of carbon dioxide records. *J. Appl. Physiol.*, **16**: 522–530.

Bezinger, T. (1938). Untersuchungen uber die Atmung und den Gasstoffwechel, insbesondere bei Suerstoffmangel und unterdruck, mit fortlaufend unmittelbar aufzeichnenden Methoden. (Studies on respiration and gas exchange with continuous direct recording methods.) *Ergebnisse der Physiologie.*, **40**: 1–52.

Blackburn, J.P. & Williams, T.R. (1980). Evaluation of the Datex CD-101 and Godart Capnograph Mark II infra-red carbon dioxide analysers. *Br. J. Anaesth.*, **52**: 551–555.

Bohr, C. (1891). Über die Lungenathmung. *Skand. Arch. Physiol.*, **2**: 236–268.

Boyle, R. (1660). New experiments physico-mechanical, touching the spring of the air and its effects, Oxford.

Burchfield, J.A. (1981). John Tyndall – a biographical sketch. In: *John Tyndall, Essays on a Natural Philosopher*. Royal Dublin Society.

Campbell, E.J.M. (1960). Simplification of Haldane's apparatus for measuring CO_2 concentration in respired gases in clinical practice. *Br. Med. J.*, **1**: 457–458.

Clamans, H.G. (1952). Continuous recording of oxygen, carbon dioxide and other gases in sealed cabins. *J Aviat. Med.*, **23**: 330–333.

CO_2 Analyzer 930-operating manual. (1981). *CO_2 Analyzer 930-Operating Manual*, 2nd edition. Siemens-Elema AB Ventilator Division, S-17195, Solna Sweden.

Comroe Jr, J.H. (1950). V measurements of composition of respired gases. *Methods in Medical Research*, Vol. 2. The Year Book Publishers, Inc., Chicago; pp. 122–131.

Consolazio, C.F., Johnson, R.E. & Pecora, L.J. (1963). *Physiological Measurements of Metabolic Functions in Man*. McGraw-Hill Book Company, New York.

Cormack, R. & Powell, J.N. (1972). Improving the performance of the infra-red carbon dioxide meter. *Brit. J. Anaesth.*, **44**: 131–141.

Douglas, C.G. (1911). A method for determining the total respiratory exchange in man. *Proc. Phys Soc.*, **xviii**: 17–18.

Douglas, C.G., Haldane, J.S., Henderson, Y. & Schneider, E.C. (1913). Physiological observations made on Pike's Peak, Colorado, with special reference to adaptation to low barometric pressures. *Phil. Trans. Roy. Soc. (Lond.), Ser. B*, **203**: 185–318.

Elam, J.A. & Brown, E.L. (1955). Carbon dioxide homeostasis during anesthesia. II. Total sampling for determination of dead space, alveolar ventilation, and carbon dioxide output. *Anesthesiology*, **16**: 886–902.

Elam, J.A. & Brown, E.L. (1956a). Carbon dioxide homeostasis during anesthesia. III. Ventilation and carbon dioxide elimination. *Anesthesiology*, **17**: 116–128.

Elam, J.A. & Brown, E.L. (1956b). Carbon dioxide homeostasis during anesthesia. IV. An evaluation of the partial rebreathing system. *Anesthesiology*, **17**: 129–134.

Elam, J.A., Brown, E.L. & Ten Pas, R.H. (1955). Carbon dioxide homeostasis during anesthesia. I. Instrumentation. *Anesthesiology*, **16**: 876–885.

Enghoff, H. (1938). Volumen inefficax. *Uppsala Läkaref. Förhand.*, **44**: 191.

Fenn, W. & Rahn, H. (1964). *Handbook of Physiology – Section 3: Respiration* Vol. 1.

Fleisch, A. (1925). Pneumotachograph: apparatus for recording respiratory flow. *Arch. F. d. ges. Physiol.*, **209**: 713–722.

Fletcher, R. (1980). The single breath test for carbon dioxide (Thesis). Lund, Sweden.

Fletcher, R. & Jonson, B. (1984). Deadspace and the single breath test for carbon dioxide during anesthesia and artificial ventilation. *Br. J. Anaesth.*, **56**: 109–119.

Fowler, W.S. (1948). Lung function studies. II. The respiratory deadspace. *Am. J. Physiol.*, **154**: 405.

Fowler, W.S. & Comroe Jr, J.H. (1950). Alveolar gas. *Methods in Medical Research*, Vol. 2.. The Year Book Publishers, Inc., Chicago. 219–226.

Fowler, K.T. (1969). The respiratory mass spectrometer. *Phys. Med. Biol.*, **14**: 185–199.

Gillispie, C.C. (ed.) (1980). *Dictionary of Scientific Biography* (multi-volume). Macmillan Publishing Co, New York.

Haldane, J.S. (1912). *Methods of Air Analysis*. Griffin, London.

Haldane, J.S. & Priestley, J.G. (1935). *Respiration*, 2nd edition. Oxford, London.

Harris, J.A. & Benedict, F.G. (1919). *A Biometric Study of Basal Metabolism in Man*. Carnegie Publications, No. 279, 129.200.

Herschel, W. (1800). Investigation of the powers of the prismatic colours to heat and illuminate objects. *Phil. Trans.*, 255.

Hill, N.C. (1966). *Introduction to Mass Spectrometry*. Jeyden, London.

Hill, D.W. & Powell, T. (1968). Non-dispersive infra-red gas analysis in science, medicine and industry. Plenum Press, New York.

Hutchinson, J. (1846). On the capacity of the lungs, and on the respiratory functions, with a view of establishing a precise and easy method of detecting disease by the spirometer. *Medico-Chirurg. Trans. (Lond.)*, **29**: 137–161.

Kinsella, S.M. (1985). Assessment of the Hewlett-Packard HP47210A capnometer. *Br. J. Anaesth.*, **57**: 919–923.

Knodle, D., Graham, P.K. & Labuda, L.L. (1994). Infrared source. US Patent 5,369,277, 29 November.

Knodle, D.W., Mace, L.E. & Labuda, L.L. (1990). Gas analyzers. US Patent 4,914,720, 3 April.

Kofoed, S.A., Orr, J.A., & Rich, D.R. (1998). Multiple function airway adapter. US Patent 5,789,660, 4 August.

Krogh, A. (1923). Determination of standard (basal) metabolism of patients by a recording apparatus. *Boston Med. Surg. J.*, **189**: 313–317.

Krogh, A. & Lindhard, J. (1913). The volume of the "dead space" in breathing. *J Physiol.*, **47**: 30–44.

Lambert, J.H. (1760). Photometria sive de Mensura et Gradibus Luminis, Colorum et Umbrae. Augsbourg, Widow of E. Klett.

Lavoisier, A. (1862). Oeuvres de Lavoisier. Publiees par les soins de son excellence le ministre de l'instruction publique et des cultes. Tome 2, Memoires de chimie et de physique. Paris, Imprimerie Imperiale.

Lehrer, E. & Luft, K. (1943).Verfahren zur Bestimmung von Bestandteilen in Stoffgemischen mittels Strahlungsabsorption. Patentschrift (Process for determining the components of mixtures through radiation absorption) Nr. 730,478. Ausgegeben am 14 Januar.

Lilly, J.C. (1950). Flow meter for recording respiratory flow of human subjects. *Methods in Medical Research*, Vol. 2. The Year Book Publishers, Inc., Chicago. 113–121.

Liston M.D. (2003). Interviews by David C. Brock and Gerald E. Gallwas at Irvine, California and Fullerton, California, 19 February 2002 and 22 January 2003 (Philadelphia: Chemical Heritage Foundation, Oral History Transcript 0252).

Liston, M.D. (1954). Apparatus for the analyzation of mixtures. US Patent 2,698,390, Issued 28 December .

Lloyd, B.B. (1958). A development of Haldane's gas analysis apparatus. *J. Physiol.*, **143**: 5–6.

Luft, K. (1943). Über eine neue Methode der registrierenden Gasanalyse mit Hilfe der Absorption ultraroter Strahlen ohne spektrale Zerlegung. *Ztschr.f. Techn. Phys.*, **24**: 97–104.

Luft, K.F., Schaefer, W. & Wiegleb, G. (1993). "50 Jahre NDIR-Gasanalyse" (50 years NDIR gas analysis). *Tm. Technisches. Messen.*, **60**: 363–371.

Lusk, G. (1933). Clio Medica Ser. *Nutrition*, **10**: Hoeber, New York.

Macfarlane, D.J. (2001). Automated metabolic gas analysis systems. *Sports Med.*, **31**: 841–861.

Merilainen, P.T., Eskelinen, K. & Hanninen, H.E. (1992). Gas flow restricting and directing device intended for flow measurement. US Patent 5,088,332, 18 February.

Nunn, J.F. (1958). Respiratory measurements in the presence of nitrous oxide. *Br. J. Anaesth.*, **30**: 254–263.

Ozanne, G.M., Young, W.G., Mazzei, W.J. & Severinghaus, J.W. (1981). Multi-patient anesthetic mass spectrometry: rapid analysis of data stored in long catheters. *Anesthesiology*, **55**: 62–70.

Peppriell, J.E., Bacon, D.R., Lema, M.J., Ament, R. & Yearley, C.K. (1991). The development of academic anesthesiology at the Roswell Park Memorial Institute. James O. Elam, MD, and Elwyn S. Brown, MD. *Anesth. Analg.*, **72**: 538–545.

Petty, T.L. (2002). John Hutchinson's mysterious machine revisited. *Chest*, **121**: 219S–223S.

Pfund, A.H. (1940). Apparatus for detecting and measuring heteroatomic gases. US Patent 2,212,2111, 20 August.

Pfund, A.H. & Gemmill, C.L. (1940). An infrared absorption method for the quantitative analysis of respiratory and other gases. *Bull. Johns. Hopkins Hosp.*, **67**: 61–65.

Raman, C.V. & Krishnan, K.S. (1928). A new type of secondary radiation. *Nature*, **121**: 501.

Rehlberg, P.B. (1951). *August Krogh. Yale J. Biol. Med.*, **24**: 83–102.

Rein, H. (1933). Gas exchange recorder. Attempts at continuous registration of respiratory gas exchange in man and animals. Arch *f. exper. Path. U. Pharmkol.*, **171**: 363.

Rich, D.R., Pierry, A.T., Fudge, B.M., Sandor, J.L., & Triunfo, J.A. (2003). Side-stream gas sampling system with detachable sample cell. Patent Cooperation Treaty Publication, 60/370,002 16 October.

Röntgen, W.C. (1881). Über Tone, welche durch intermittirende Bestralung eines Gases entstechen. *Annalen Der Physik und Chemie.*, **12**: 155–159.

Rosenfeld, E.Z. & Boasson, H. (1988). Gas analyzer and a source of IR radiation therefor. US Patent 4,755,675 July 5.

Sands, R.P. & Bacon, D.R. (1998). An inventive mind: the career of James O. Elam, M.D. *Anesthesiology*, **88**: 1107–1112.

Scholander, P.F. (1947). Analyzer for accurate estimation of respiratory gases in one-half cubic centimeter samples. *J. Biol. Chem.*, **167**: 235–250.

Shepard, R.J. (1955). A critical examination of the Douglas bag technique. *J. Physiol.*, **127**: 515–524.

Siebecker, K.L., Mendenhall, J.T. & Emanuel, D.A. (1954). Carbon dioxide in anesthetic atmospheres as measured by the Liston-Becker (infra-red absorption) gas analyzer. *J Thorac. Surg.*, **27**: 468–476.

Silverman, L. (1946). Respiratory air flow characteristics and their relation to certain lung conditions occurring in industry. *J. Indust. Hyg. Toxicol.*, **28**: 183.

Smalhout, B. (1967). Capnografie (Thesis), University of Utrecht, The Netherlands. A. Oosthoek Publ. Co., Utrecht, The Netherlands.

Smalhout, B. & Kalenda, Z. (1981). *An Atlas of Capnography*, 2nd edition. Kerckebosche Zeist, The Netherlands. p. 163.

Smekal, A. (1923). Naturwiss II. 873.

Solomon, R.J. (1981). A reliable, accurate CO_2 analyzer for medical use. *Hewlett-Packard J..*, **32**: 3–21.

Tissot, J. (1904). Nouvelle méthode de mesure et d' inscription du débit et des mouvements respirtoires de l'homme et des animaux. *J. Physiol. Pathol. Gén.*, **6**: 688–700.

Tyndall, J. (1865). On Radiation. The "Rede" Lecture delivered in the Senate-House before the University of Cambridge on Tuesday, May 16, Longman, Green, Longman, Roberts & Green, London. 62 pages.

Tyndall, J. (1881). Action of an intermittent beam of radiant light upon gaseous matter. *Pro. Roy. Soc.*, **31**: 307–317.

Van Slyke, D.D. & O'Neill, J.M. (1924). The determination of gases in blood and other solutions by vacuum extraction and manometric measurement. *J. Biol. Chem.*, **61**: 523–529.

Veingerov, M.L. (1938). Eine Methode der Gasanalyse beruhend auf dem optisch-akustischen Tyndall-Röntgeneffekt. *Dokl. Akad. Nauk SSSR*, **19**: 687–688.

Weingarten, M. (1990). Respiratory monitoring of carbon dioxide and oxygen: a ten-year perspective. *J. Clin. Monit.*, **6**: 217–225.

Westenskow, D.R., Smith, K.W., Coleman, D.L., Gregonis, D.E. & VanWagenen, R.A. (1989). Clinical evaluation of a Raman scattering multiple gas analyzer for the operating room. *Anesthesiology*, **70**: 350–355.

Wilmore, J.H. & Costill, D.L. (1974). Semiautomated systems approach to the assessment of oxygen uptake during exercise. *J. Appl. Physiol.*, **36**: 618–620.

Zuntz, N. & Loewy, A. (eds) (1920). Lehrbuch der Physiologie des Menschen. Leipzig, F.C.W. Vogel.

THE FIRST YEARS OF CLINICAL CAPNOGRAPHY 35

B. Smalhout

The clinical use of capnography had its beginning in the Second World War. The German Navy had excellent submarines, which could remain submerged for a long time. There was oxygen enough on board, but the problem was to get rid of the enormous quantities of carbon dioxide (CO_2) produced by the crew. Each submarine was equipped with CO_2 absorbers, but their capacity was limited. We have to realize that an average crew of 60 men produced, in 24 h, at least 44,000 l or nearly 10,000 US gallons of pure CO_2, making a longer stay inside the hull of the ship very uncomfortable.

That is why the German bio-engineer Karl Luft was invited to investigate this problem. Luft was already well known for his work on CO_2 detection based on infrared absorption. He had constructed a useful apparatus named the URAS, the abbreviation of Ultra Rot Absorptions Schreiber (infrared absorption writer). At first, the machine was only used as a measuring device for CO_2. In our terminology, a capnometer. Later, a one-channel recorder was added. From that moment on, the changes in CO_2 contents of the respiratory cycle could be studied online, turning the capnometer into a real capnograph.

After the war, this instrument became available for clinical use, although at first mainly for scientific purposes. Holland was one of the first countries where the capnograph was used as a monitoring device for patients with respiratory problems. My first experience with a capnograph was in 1957, when I was working as a young medical officer in the Central Military Hospital of Utrecht, The Netherlands. A comatose soldier with severe brain trauma needed artificial ventilation. In those years, no ventilators were available in the hospital, so the patient was ventilated day and night by hand. While squeezing the bag, we had to observe the small indicator of the capnometer. The CO_2 contents of the expirated air had to be between 4% and 5% (equivalent to 32 and 40 mmHg). Working in eight 3-h shifts a day, we kept the soldier alive for many weeks, until he recovered and resumed his spontaneous respiration.

Two years later, I worked as a Resident in Anaesthesiology in the University Hospital of Utrecht. At that time, it was already known that there was a relationship between the partial pressure of CO_2 (PCO_2) and the intracranial pressure. So, the neurosurgical clinic had the first operation theater equipped with a capnograph of the famous brand Hartmann & Braun. It was a typically German instrument: heavy, indestructible, but very reliable. It needed a warming-up time of about 2 h. Therefore, we kept the capnograph connected to the wall plug continuously, day and night. It worked faultlessly for nearly 20 years (Figure 35.1).

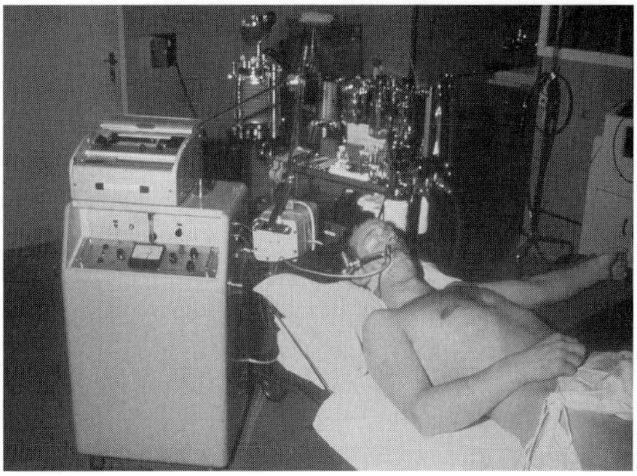

Figure 35.1 The first capnograph in the Central Military Hospital, Utrecht, The Netherlands (1962). On top the one-channel Omniascriptor. Photo: Ltn. Klunder.

By means of a one-channel recorder, the Omniascriptor, mounted on top of the machine, an online capnogram could be recorded on paper tape. Two paper speeds were possible. At low speed, the paper was running 25 mm/min. The high speed was 30 times faster: 25 mm in 2 s. The sampling flow was roughly 500 ml/min, via a side-stream system. Figure 35.2 shows an example of such a recording. Every peak represents one respiration. It allows to measure the respiratory rate by counting the peaks in 1 min.

The high-speed recording at the right side shows the classical shape of the capnogram, starting the expiration at R, rapidly rising to its alveolar plateau QR. This plateau is slightly sloping upwards to the right.

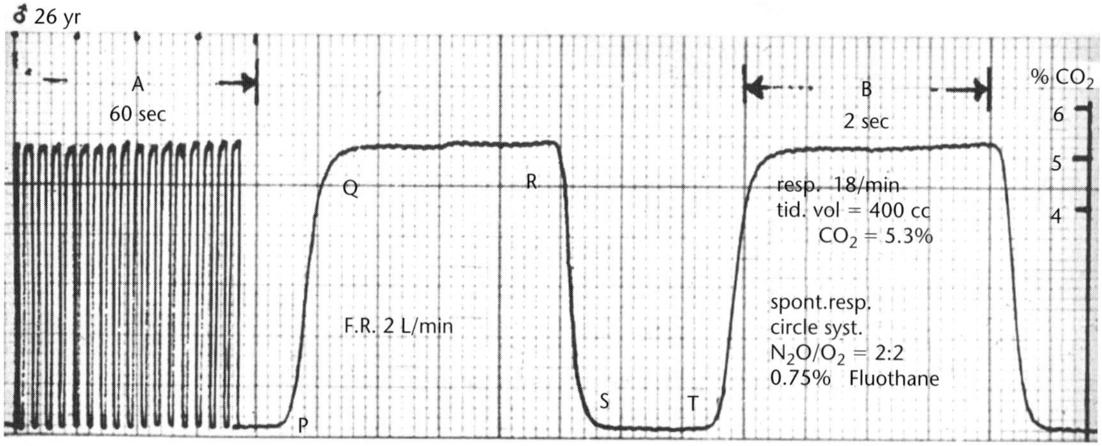

Figure 35.2 The normal capnogram, recorded on the original paper tape of the Omniascriptor (1962).

From the point where the alveolar plateau reaches its highest level, the so-called end-tidal CO_2 ($ETCO_2$) can be measured. Under optimal conditions in a patient with an adequate blood circulation, patent airways and a normal lung function, the $ETCO_2$ is more or less equivalent to the arterial PCO_2 (P_aCO_2).

The next inspiration begins at R. The curve drops steeply downwards and the segment ST represents the remaining part of the inspiration. Because mostly the inspiratory gas mixture contains practically no CO_2, the capnogram has to return to the zero- or baseline. If not, this fact is probably caused by rebreathing, just as in the submarines studied by Karl Luft.

There is only one normal shape of the capnographic waveform. But there are lots of variations possible. At first, little attention was paid to these variations, and the capnograph was mainly used as a capnometer. But once appointed as a neuro-anesthesiologist, I started to run the Omniascriptor continuously at low speed during every operation. After every 10 min, one or two respirations were recorded at high paper speed, to study the capnographic waveform. So I used about 2.5 m or 7.5 feet of paper tape per hour. Very lengthy neurosurgical operations sometimes took more than 8 h, and during that time the Omniascriptor produced about 20 m of paper tape. But every respiration of the patient during the whole anesthetic and surgical procedure was documented.

During 7 years I collected and studied about 6000 capnographic recordings with a total length of 20 km. On the paper tape were always mentioned the clinical data and the surgical events of the patient. So, I learned that there were many variations in the shape of the capnogram, but that all of them had a clinical meaning. They were significant for specific physiological, technical or pathological conditions or events. These variations enabled the anesthesiologist to make diagnoses, to detect discrepancies, to prevent calamities, and to judge the clinical condition of the patient. In 1967, these findings resulted in a Ph.D. thesis, entitled *Capnography – its importance in diagnosis, operation and after-treatment of neurosurgical patients*. It was written in Dutch with a summary in English. In 450 pages, the interpretation of the capnographic waveform in dysregulation of respiration and blood circulation, and its role in monitoring neuro-anesthesia was described.

Based on this publication, *An Atlas of Capnography* (Smalhout & Kalenda, 1975) was published in 1975. A second, revised edition was printed in 1981. From that year on, more than 100 lectures on capnography were given by me in more than 50 cities throughout the US and Canada. Up to that time, capnography was hardly known in North America.

But although in those years the principle of capnography was known better in Europe, most hospitals in European countries did not use it as a routine in clinical practice. After hundreds of lectures in nearly all the European countries, from Spain to Sweden and from Great Britain to Russia, the firm of Hewlett Packard made it possible for me to publish a small booklet for daily use in operation theaters. It was printed on plastic pages, so it could be washed and cleaned if blood was spilt on the contents. The title was *A Quick Guide to Capnography and Its Use in Differential Diagnosis* (Smalhout, 1981). This booklet was distributed all over the world, in several languages, including Japanese and Chinese.

In 1978, the Health Council of the Netherlands published an *Advisory Report on Anaesthesiology* (162 pages), concerning all the facets of this specialty. In the chapter about monitoring equipment, the routine use of a capnograph in combination with a recording device was stated as mandatory. Since that time, all operation theaters in The Netherlands are equipped with capnographs.

The analysis of the capnogram

The capnogram has to be studied for five qualities:

1 *The frequency* gives us information about the respiratory rate or the frequency of the ventilator.
2 *The maximum height* of the CO_2 wave, indicating the $ETCO_2$.
3 *The rhythm* that can be seen on the slow recording. Especially in spontaneous respiration, it is important to see if the patient's breathing is regular, irregular or periodic. Many types of irregularity are typical for a dysfunction of the brainstem, for example, the Cheyne–Stokes breathing. In case of an artificially ventilated patient, the capnogram offers a perfect technical control of the ventilator.
4 *The shape* of the capnographic curve. The waveform enables the anesthesiologist to make a differential diagnosis between a multitude of medical or technical airway problems.
5 *The baseline*, or zero-line. The capnogram has to return to this baseline after every expiration. If not, the patient is probably rebreathing his own CO_2.

The origin of the capnogram

The expired CO_2 that is analyzed and recorded as a waveform has passed through the following stages inside and outside the body:

1 *Production:* CO_2 is produced in the body cells. The quantity varies with the metabolism. If the patient is cooling down, the metabolism and hence the production of CO_2, is diminished. If the ventilation remains stable, as in artificial respiration, the $ETCO_2$ is going down. On the other hand, if the body temperature is rising, the level of the expired CO_2 is going up. In this way, the capnogram is the earliest warning system for malignant hyperthermia.
2 *Transport:* Once the CO_2 is produced, it has to be transported to the lungs by the blood stream. So, the level of the capnogram is also dependent of the quality of the circulation. If the ventilation and the body temperature are kept stable, the $ETCO_2$ follows closely the variations in blood pressure, or, rather, the perfusion. If there is no blood pressure or perfusion, as in cardiac arrest, then no CO_2 is transported to the lungs and the low-speed capnogram shows a rapid washout pattern. On the other hand, the efforts and effectiveness of resuscitation attempts are also immediately recorded.
3 *Elimination:* After having arrived in the lungs, the CO_2 has to be eliminated. This elimination depends on the state of the lungs, the airways, the respiratory mechanism and the condition of the technical devices used in anesthesia and intensive care.

Capnographic possibilities

So, capnography enables monitoring of the:

1 Metabolism
2 Circulation
3 Lung perfusion
4 Lung diffusion
5 Position of the endotracheal (ET) tube
6 Patency of the ET tube
7 Quality of the spontaneous respiration
8 Patency of the airways
9 Functioning of the ventilator
10 State of the connecting tubing
11 Activity of the CO_2 absorber
12 Effect of drugs used in anesthesia
13 Position of the patient on the operating room (OR) table.

Some examples of all these possibilities will be given.

The capnograph as a monitor of the metabolism

If a patient is cooling down, for instance during a medical intervention, or as a result of an accident (nearly drowned in ice-cold water), the metabolism becomes lower than normal. If such a patient is ventilated with a respiratory minute volume, according to his age or weight, he will certainly be hyperventilated, which can endanger his brain function. If the body temperature decreases from 37°C to 30°C, the $ETCO_2$ is falling from 5% (40 mmHg) to 3% (24 mmHg), assuming that the ventilation is unchanged. The $ETCO_2$ can be a reliable indication for the correct respiratory volume. So, in studying the capnogram, it is always necessary to know the body temperature.

Another cause for an increased metabolism is muscular activity. A very good example is an epileptic fit. Such an event is shown in Figure 35.3. The patient was a 26-year-old woman who underwent brain surgery under general anesthesia with muscular relaxation. A three-channel recording is to be seen. From top to bottom, the electrocardiograph (ECG), the plethysmogram

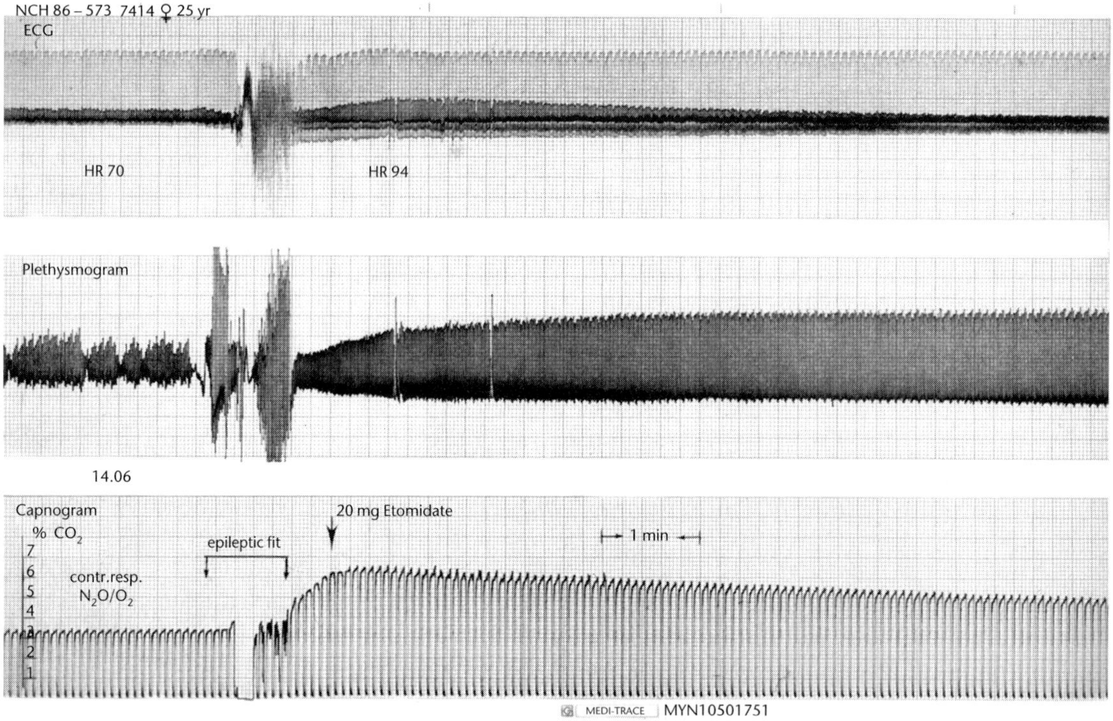

Figure 35.3 ECG, plethysmogram and capnogram during an epileptic fit (1986).

(taken from a fingertip) and the capnogram. Paper speed: 25 mm/min. $ETCO_2$: 3.2%. The patient was connected to a ventilator and slightly hyperventilated to lower the intracranial pressure. Suddenly, the very regular pattern was interrupted by an epileptic fit (indicated by arrows). The ECG and the plethysmogram were suddenly disturbed by the uncontrolled contractions of all the muscles, despite an estimated adequate dose of muscle relaxants. During the 12 s of the tonic phase of the attack there was no ventilation at all. But immediately after that, the capnogram was rising rapidly. Within 1 min, the $ETCO_2$ was increased twofold, because of the muscle contractions. After the epileptic fit, it took some considerable time before the CO_2 production returned to normal. As can be seen, the plethysmographic amplitude was also increased. This is caused by vasodilatation as a consequence of the higher P_aCO_2.

The capnograph as a monitor of the ventilation: There are at least 10 important ventilatory complications possible in a patient on an operation table:

1. Disconnection of the tubing
2. Leakage in the ventilating system
3. Ventilator failure
4. Hypoventilation
5. Hyperventilation
6. Obstruction of the ET tube
7. Obstruction of the airways
8. Rebreathing
9. Residual curarization
10. ET tube in esophagus.

Figure 35.4, a recording from 1964, shows two fragments from a capnogram of a 3-year-old boy, who was breathing spontaneously under general anesthesia with halothane. On the left side a capnogram is recorded during breathing a gas mixture with 0.25% halothane (fluothane). The capnographic waveform is perfectly normal. The plateau is nearly horizontal, the $ETCO_2$ is 4.8% (38.4 mmHg), and the respiratory rate is 25. After increasing the halothane concentration to 2%, the capnographic wave changed completely within 15 min. The alveolar plateau had become much shorter, because in the meantime the patient had developed a tachypnea. The $ETCO_2$ had risen to 7% (56 mmHg), indicating a serious respiratory depression. This diagnosis can be made at a glance.

Figure 35.5 shows a three-channel high-speed recording of a 61-year-old man with a serious cardiopulmonary disease (COPD). There is no real alveolar plateau. The oblique curve slopes upwards to about 6.4%, and then drops at the next inspiration. The CO_2 level cannot be considered as end-tidal,

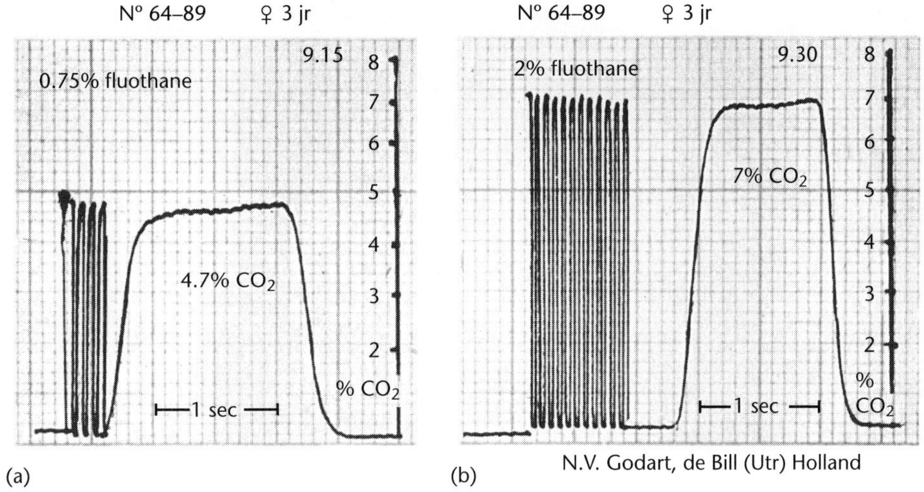

Figure 35.4 Capnogram of normal respiration (a) and during respiratory depression (b). (1964), Godart capnograph.

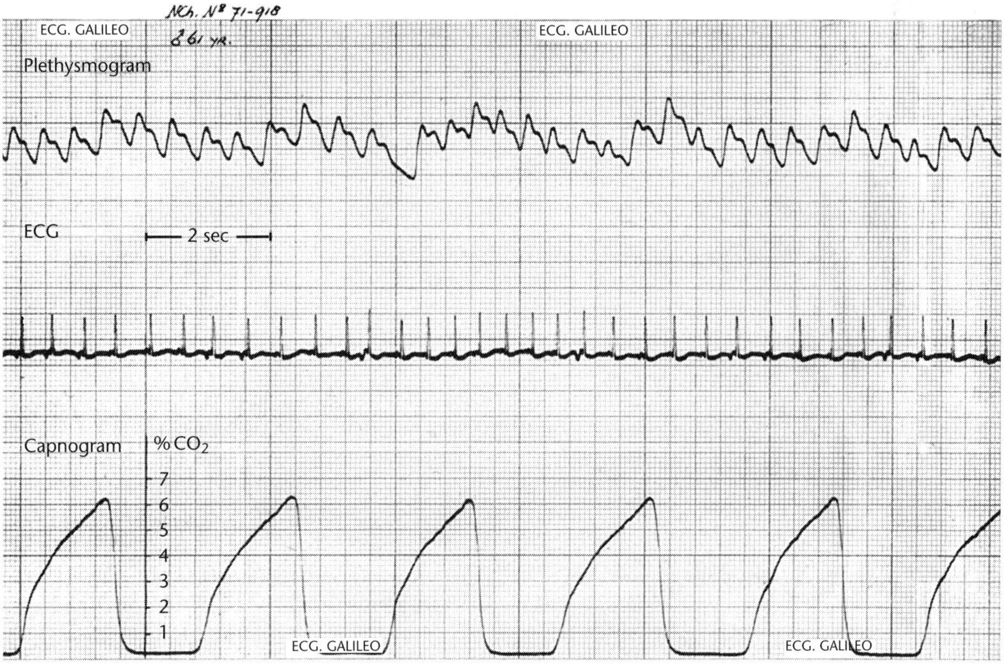

Figure 35.5 Plethysmogram, ECG and capnogram of a man aged 61 years with COPD (1971).

because an alveolar plateau is lacking. Such patients mostly have a considerable alveolar–arterial CO_2 difference. The shape of the capnogram is typical for an expiratory problem.

Figure 35.6, made in 1981, shows the high-speed three-channel recording of a 13-year-old girl, suffering from cystic fibrosis. The capnogram was taken when the spontaneously breathing girl was just falling asleep. The sampling tube was carefully placed in the nasopharynx.

On the left side, four capnographic curves are to be seen. They are completely lacking an alveolar plateau and look like alligators' teeth. The CO_2 concentration is seemingly low, about 4%, but the respiratory rate is very high, about 65 per minute. But when compressing the thoracic cage manually, the capnographic curve sloped slowly upwards and reached a horizontal plateau of more than 10% (80 mmHg!). This was the real $ETCO_2$, two and a half times higher than expected

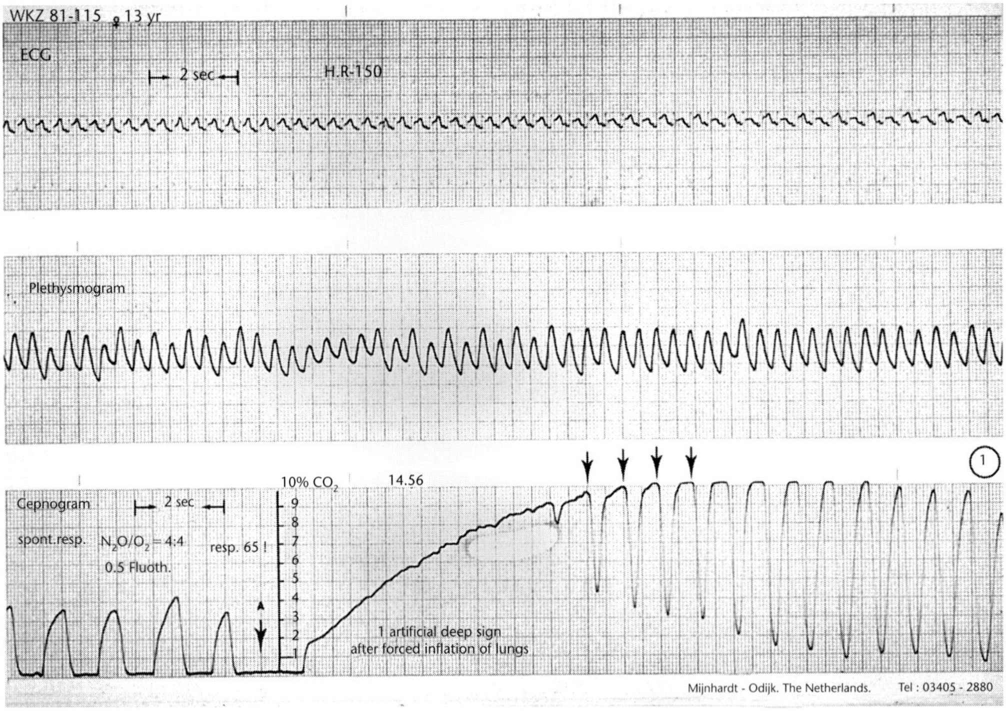

Figure 35.6 ECG, plethysmogram and capnogram of a 13-year-old girl with cystic fibrosis (1981). Left: spontaneous respiration; Right: during forced expiration.

before. As visible, the alveolar plateau is interrupted in a regular way (indicated by arrows). This is caused by the respiratory attempts of the child, while her thoracic cage was still compressed. In this way, in nearly every patient who has an expiratory problem, a real $ETCO_2$ can be obtained.

The effect of muscle relaxants

Often, when a patient is emerging from an anesthetic, it is still possible that he/she is still under the influence of muscle relaxants which are used during the anesthetic procedure. Of course, nowadays this can be detected by means of electromyography and by obtaining the so-called "train of four". Still, the "residual curarization", as it was called formerly, when curare was used as a muscle relaxant, remains a potential danger. But already in the early 1960s, it was possible to capnographically judge the patient's respiratory efforts. Even in patients who are awake postoperatively and even can breathe and talk, a respiratory disaster caused by muscle relaxants can develop in the recovery room.

The typical shape of the capnogram in such a patient is to be seen in Figure 35.7, recorded in 1966. It is derived from a 63-year-old man breathing spontaneously for more than 2 h after one single dose of 20 mg curare. The first fragment shows the high-speed recording of two consecutive respirations. The curve starts nearly normal with an alveolar plateau of about 5.4% (43.2 mmHg). But in the second half of this plateau, a deep incision or cleft can be seen. This cleft is caused by the fact that the thoracic respiratory muscles are more paralyzed than the much stronger diaphragm. So, the recording consists of two different capnograms. The biggest one is caused by the diaphragm, and the little one by the thoracic muscles. Both waves are partially covering each other.

Such a highly specific capnogram is an absolute indication to administer an antidote. In this case, 0.5 mg prostigmine was given. The effect of this treatment can be seen in the second fragment. The capnographic waveform immediately became normal.

The same type of "curare" capnogram can be seen in spontaneously breathing patients suffering from a (fresh) cervical transverse lesion. They are also breathing mainly with their diaphragm. Of course, these patients do not react to antidotes, but as soon as their sternal bone is stabilized mechanically the typical cleft in the capnographic plateau disappears.

Since 1970s, most capnograms in the Institute of Anaesthesiology of the University Hospital of Utrecht were recorded on multi-channel paper, which was running continuously during the entire anesthetic and

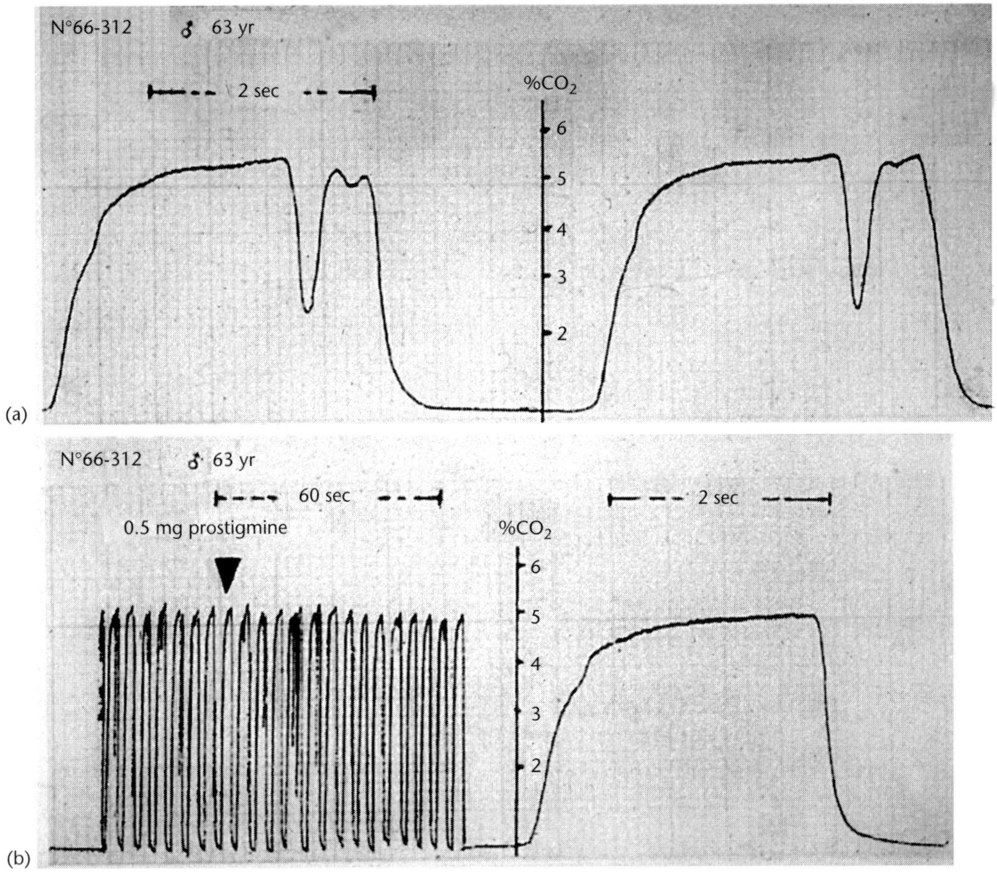

Figure 35.7 (a) "Curare-capnogram" of spontaneous respiration of a 63-year-old man. Effect of residual muscle relaxants. (b) The effect of an antidote (prostigmine) (1966).

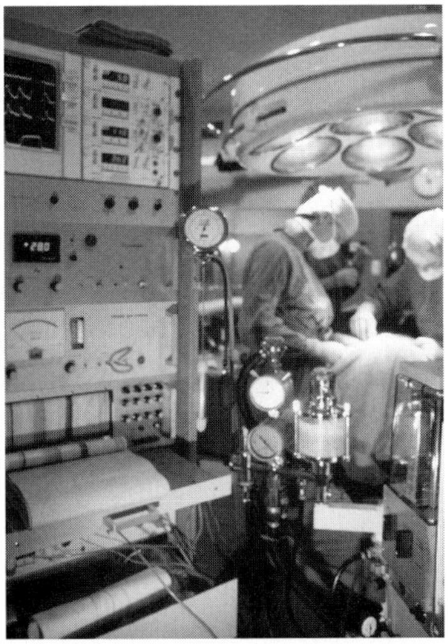

Figure 35.8 Monitor unit of the Institute of Anaesthesiology, with continuously running four-channel recording on paper tape. University Hospital of Utrecht, The Netherlands (1981). Photo: C.F. Timmers.

surgical procedures (Figure 35.8). All monitors were built into one large unit. Such a unit was available in every OR or induction room.

Cardiogenic oscillations

The following two figures show the effect of an anesthetic drug on the capnographic waveform. Figure 35.9 displays the capnogram and the plethysmogram of a 13-year-old healthy girl. Her capnogram is excellent, with a beautiful alveolar plateau, and a normal $ETCO_2$ of 5.2% (41 mmHg). But, after having received 50 μg of fentanyl, this pattern quickly changed. This can be seen in Figure 35.10. There are fewer respirations, because of a lower respiratory rate. The beautiful plateau has disappeared, and in its stead secondary peaks are visible, synchronic with the beating of the heart. The $ETCO_2$ has risen to about 6.5% (52 mmHg), which is much too high. There are less capnographic curves, because of the lower respiratory rate. The secondary peaks, indicated by arrows, are called cardiogenic oscillations.

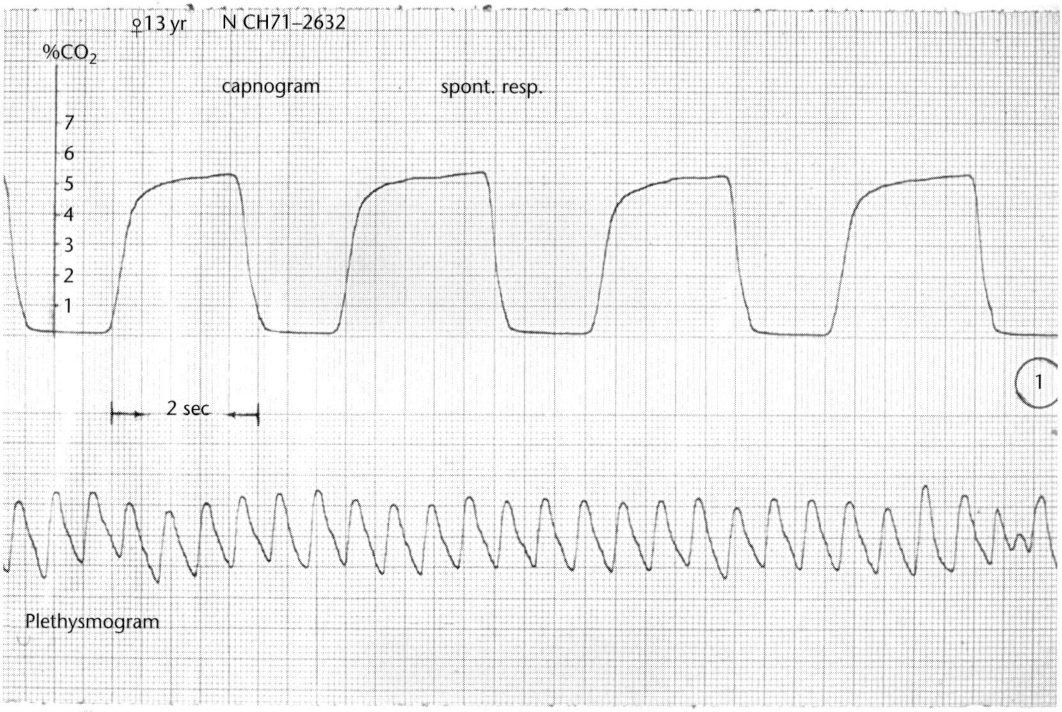

Figure 35.9 Capnogram and plethysmogram of a girl aged 13. Spontaneous respiration (1971).

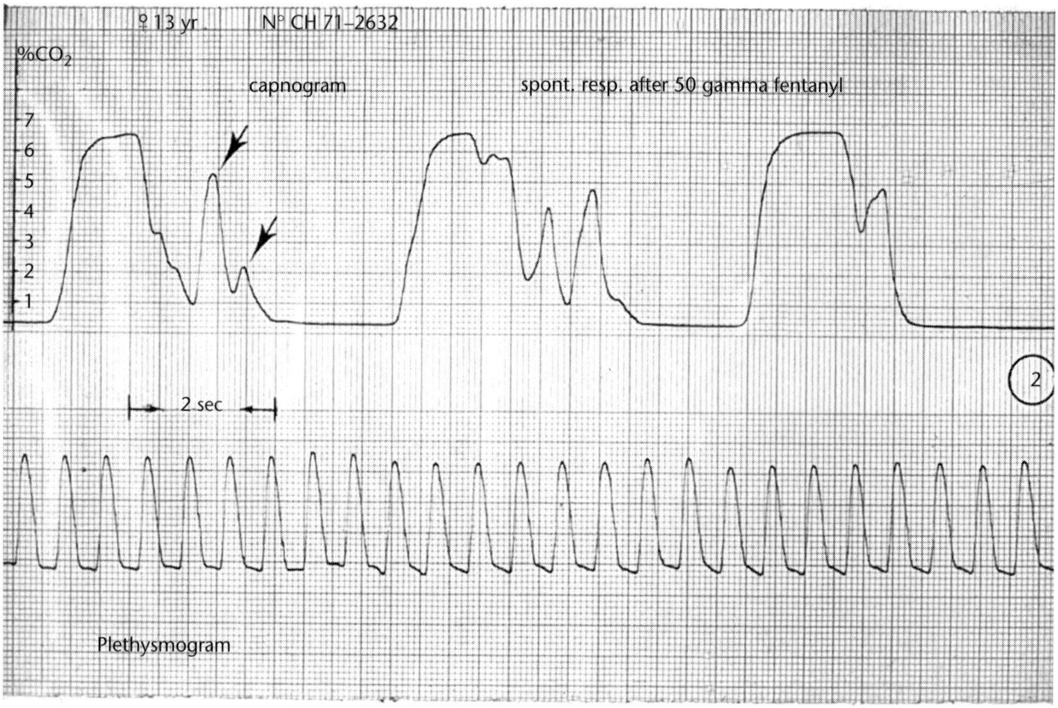

Figure 35.10 *Idem.*, but after 50 μg of fentanyl. Cardiogenic oscillations.

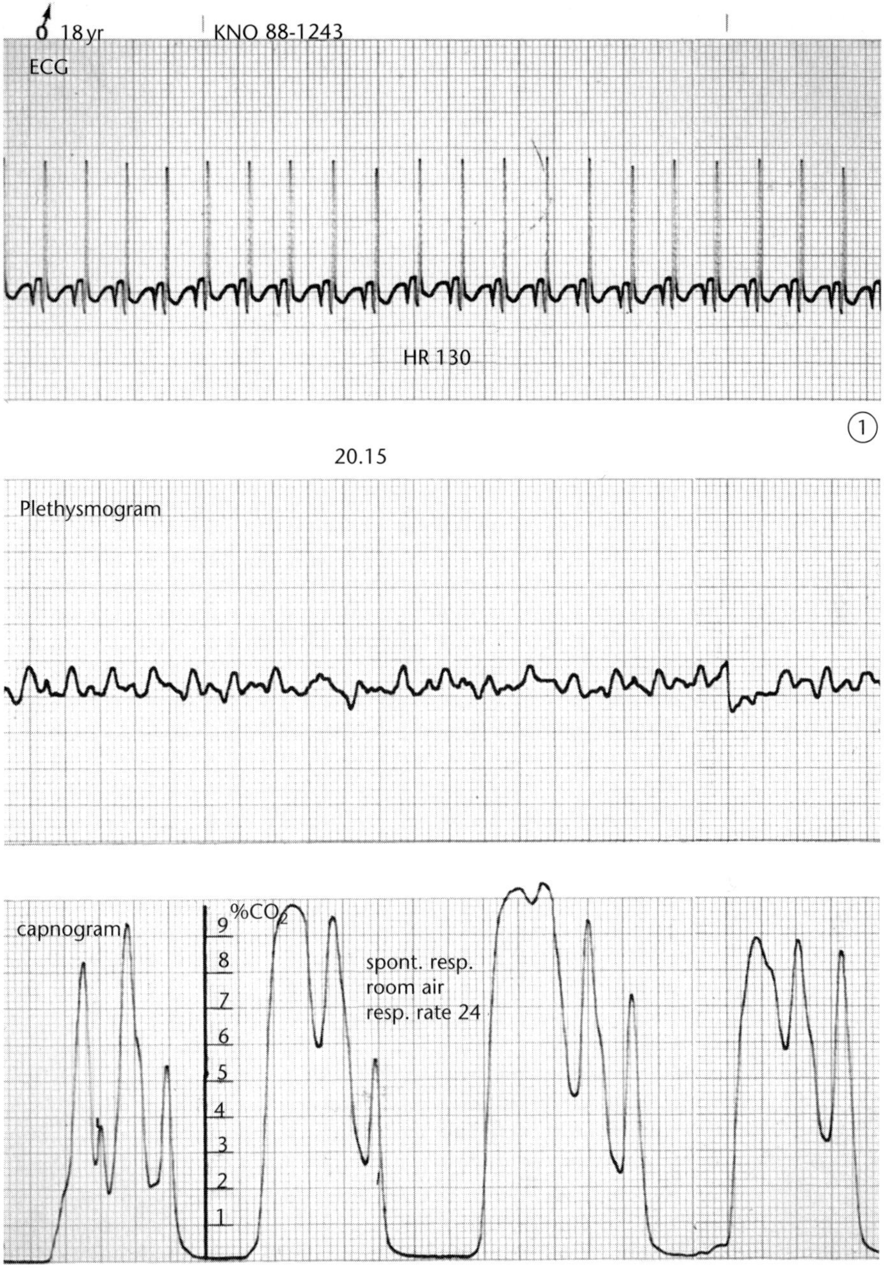

Figure 35.11 ECG, plethysmogram and capnogram of 18-year-old boy with Duchenne disease (1988). Spontaneous respiration. Multiple cardiogenic oscillations. Very high $ETCO_2$.

They are caused by the beating of the heart against the lungs. This can only be seen when either the respiration is very slow, or the tidal volume is small. Cardiogenic oscillations always mean that the respiration is inadequate.

This can clearly be seen in a 18-year-old boy with a severe Morbus Duchenne (progressive muscular atrophy). Figure 35.11 displays the high-speed three-channel recording of his capnogram, ECG and plethysmogram, when he was still breathing spontaneously. The respiratory rate was 24, and his capnogram mainly showed very high cardiogenic oscillations that reached a top level of more than 10% (80 mmHg) CO_2. Such a capnogram is an absolute indication for artificial or assisted respiration.

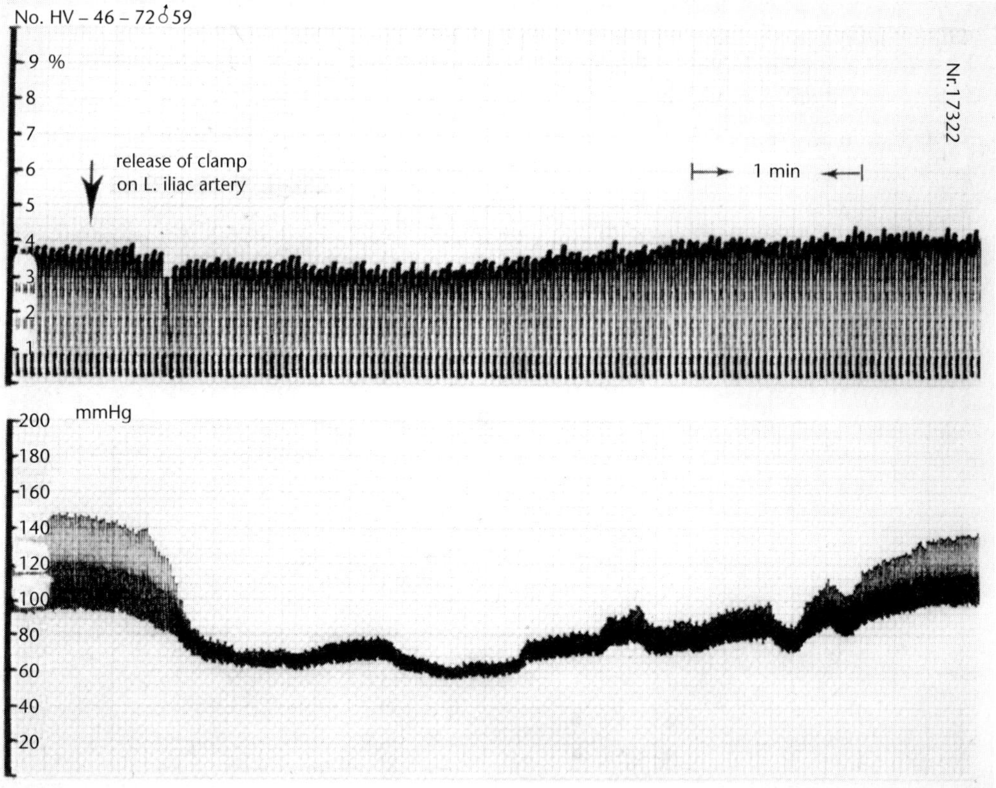

Figure 35.12 Capnogram and arterial blood pressure of a man aged 59. Effect of hypotension on the capnogram (1972).

The capnograph as a monitor of the circulation

The most important circulatory complications are:

1 Hypotension
2 Cardiac/circulatory arrest
3 Air embolism
4 Hypertension.

When the ventilation is kept stable by means of a ventilator, running with a constant speed, volume and pressure, and the body temperature of the patient remains unchanged, then the $ETCO_2$ follows closely the variations in blood perfusion. The clinical use of this phenomenon was described for the first time by Leigh (1957, 1961).

Figure 35.12 shows a two-channel slow recording of the capnogram and the direct arterial pressure in a man 59 years of age. The fragment covers a period of about 3 min. The patient underwent an operation for an abdominal aortic aneurysm. At the moment indicated by an arrow, the clamp on the left iliac artery was released. Within half a minute, the systolic blood pressure dropped from 145 to 70 mmHg and was restored after 3 min. The capnogram descended in the same way, falling from 3.8% to 3%. When the blood pressure started to rise again, the capnogram was going up simultaneously and even exceeded the original level. The explanation is that when the circulation increased, all the CO_2 which was stored in the tissues during the period of hypotension, was quickly transported to the lungs by the improved perfusion.

The variations in the height of the capnogram are mostly not as impressive as those of the blood pressure. This is caused by the fact that even at a low blood pressure, the blood perfusion to a great extent can remain sufficient. It offers the opportunity to judge whether a certain hypotension is life threatening or not. This is beautifully illustrated in the next two cases.

The first one was a man, 76-year old. After a right-sided lung resection complications occurred, making a re-intervention inevitable. During this operation, the surgeon accidentally ruptured the right pulmonary artery, causing massive bleeding. In order to stop the hemorrhage, he put a finger in the hole. A typical Dutch habit, as is known worldwide. But every time when he withdrew his finger in an attempt to close the hole surgically, a gush of blood spurted out of the

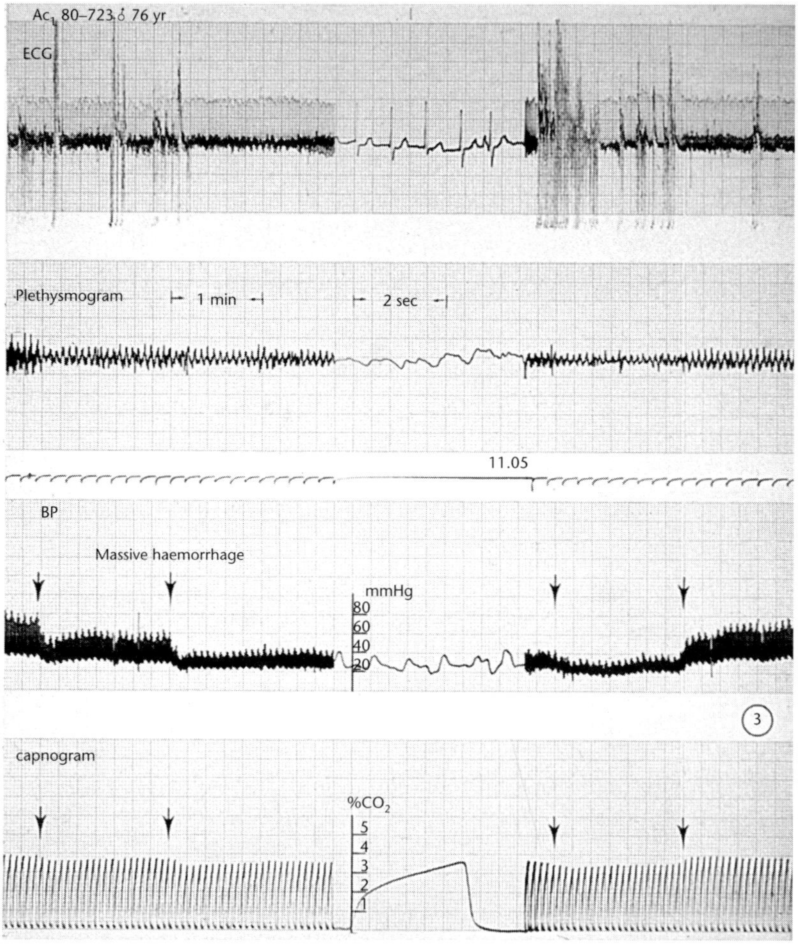

Figure 35.13 ECG, plethysmogram, blood pressure and capnogram of 76-year-old man during pulmonectomy, right. Severe loss of blood. Effect on capnogram (1980).

artery. So, the blood pressure went down stepwise. On the four-channel recording this is indicated by arrows (Figure 35.13). The capnogram showed the same stepwise fall. The lowest blood pressure was 40/20 mmHg, which is very low indeed for a man aged 76. But still a reasonable capnogram was visible, not lower than 3.8% (30.4 mmHg). This meant that the blood perfusion was still sufficient to sustain life. So there was, at that moment, not a life-endangering situation. At the right side is to be seen that the blood pressure was rising again, due to massive blood transfusion. Also, this improvement is visible on the capnogram.

In the next case, Figure 35.14, of a 45-year-old man, with a large kidney tumor that had grown through the diaphragm into the right lung, the hemorrhage was so abundant that the blood pressure fell below 20 mmHg! Clearly to be seen is that below the systolic pressure of 40 the capnogram also collapsed. That means that the patient was in mortal danger. But, as soon as the blood pressure, due to the transfusion, was rising a little (only up to 40 mmHg), the $ETCO_2$ went up. By means of such documentation, it can be proven that the most dangerous period of hypotension (between A and B) lasted no longer than a few minutes.

Cardiac arrest and resuscitation

Figure 35.15 probably shows the first capnographic recording in the world of a cardiac arrest and the resuscitation in a man 55 years of age. This capnogram was recorded in 1962, with the one-channel Omniascriptor and a Hartmann & Braun capnograph. The patient was breathing spontaneously. At the left the washout curve, which is so typical for a circulatory arrest, is clearly visible. One minute later, external cardiac massage was started. The effect on the capnogram is visible, but showed the massage to be insufficient. In the meantime, the patient was intubated and ventilated manually. A thoracotomy was performed (indicated by an arrow) 150 s after the moment of the cardiac arrest. The effect of open cardiac massage can be seen on the

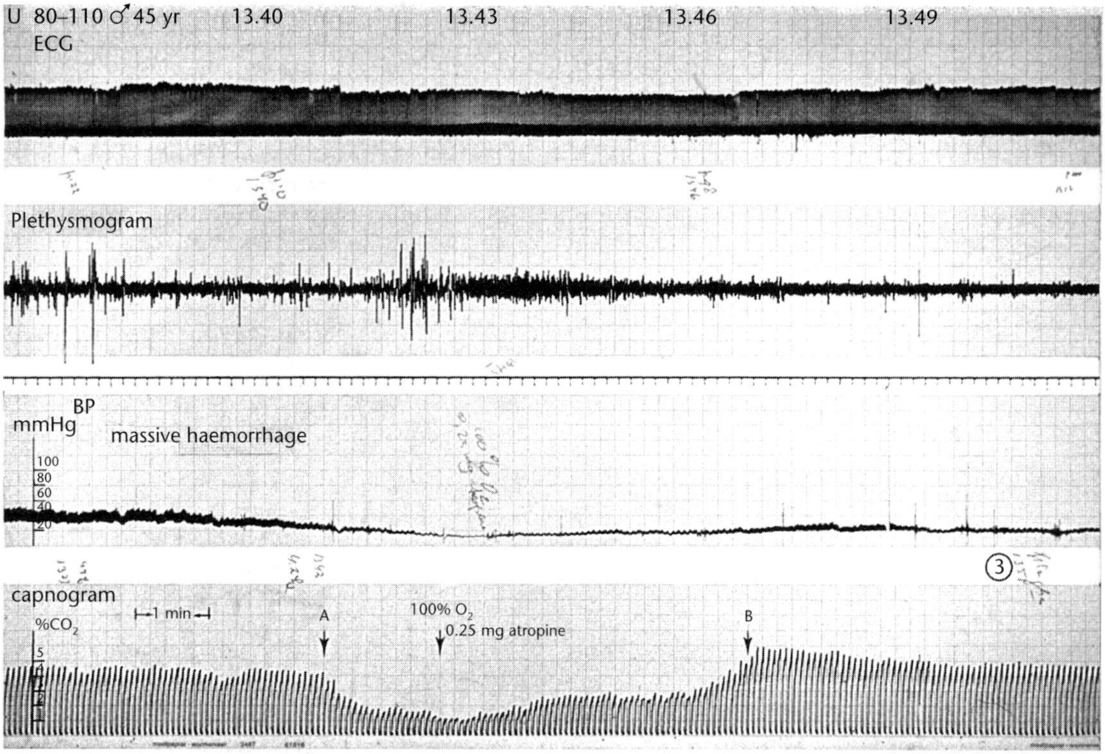

Figure 35.14 ECG, plethysmogram, blood pressure and capnogram of a 45-year-old man, during removal of a large kidney tumor, right. Extreme loss of blood. Systolic blood pressure lower than 20 mmHg. Effect on capnogram.

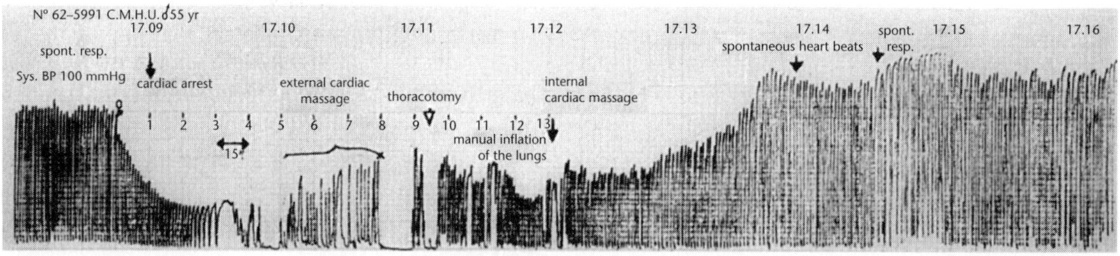

Figure 35.15 The first capnographic recording of a cardiac arrest and resuscitation of a man, aged 55. Central Military Hospital, Utrecht (1962).

capnogram. The CO_2 was rising rapidly, and soon the heart resumed its spontaneous activity.

From the recording can be learned that the whole procedure, from diagnosis to recovery, took exactly 5 min. So, in 1969 it was already clear that capnographic documentation of such events was very precise and legally very important in cases where doubt was cast on the medical conduct.

So, since 1970s, resuscitations in the Institute of Anaesthesiology of the University Hospital of Utrecht were, whenever possible, monitored with at least a capnograph. An example is to be seen in Figure 35.16, a low-speed two-channel recording of the cardiac resuscitation of a 50-year-old man, in 1971. The patient was ventilated mechanically with a constant frequency, tidal volume and pressure. So, all the variations in $ETCO_2$ were caused by changes in blood perfusion of the lungs. External cardiac massage was performed and that kept the CO_2 and, hence, the lung perfusion, on an acceptable level. But every one or 2 min, the resuscitator stopped a moment to look on the screen of the ECG

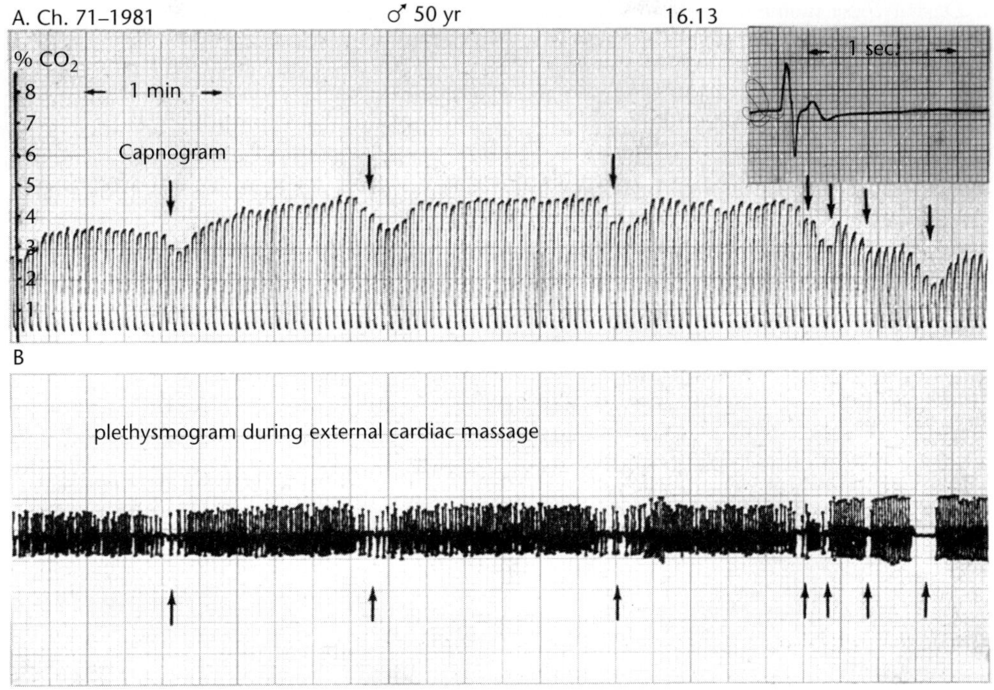

Figure 35.16 Capnogram and plethysmogram of a man aged 50 years, during external cardiac massage. At the right, the resuscitator becomes exhausted (1981).

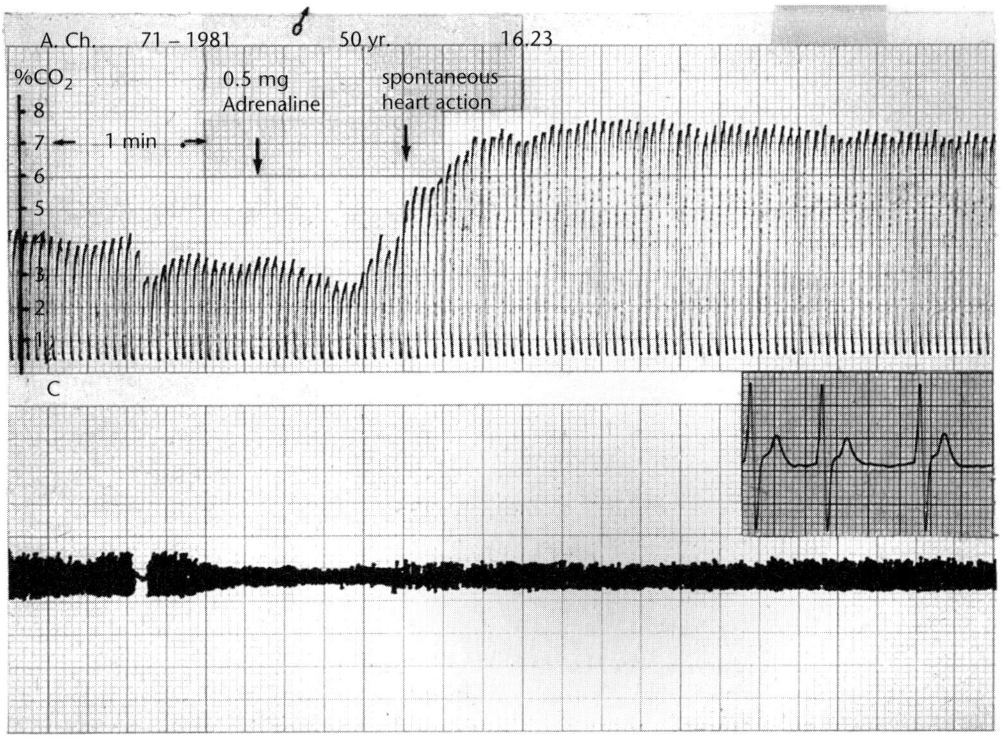

Figure 35.17 The capnographic recording of the successful resuscitation (1981).

monitor. During these moments there was no blood circulation, and immediately the capnogram started to descend, while the plethysmogram showed no pulsations. As soon as the cardiac massage was resumed the CO_2 was climbing again. These moments, indicated by arrows, are clearly to be seen. But at the right side of the recording, the average level of the $ETCO_2$ was falling down gradually. That meant that the resuscitator became exhausted and needed to be replaced. The successful effect of a fresh resuscitator can be seen in Figure 35.17.

So, the capnograph proved to be an excellent and reliable device to judge the efficiency of the resuscitation

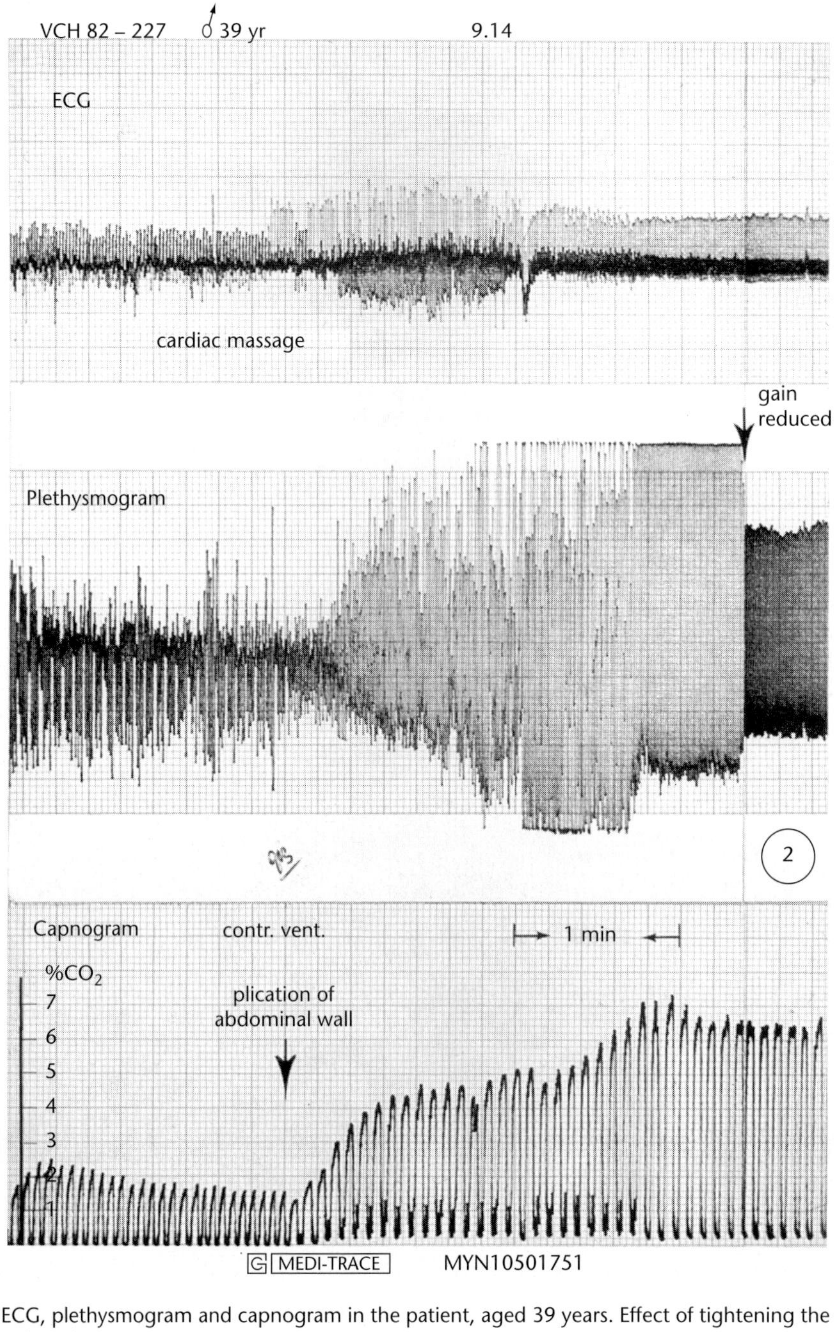

Figure 35.18 ECG, plethysmogram and capnogram in the patient, aged 39 years. Effect of tightening the abdominal wall. Successful external cardiac massage.

technique. The next case, recorded in 1981, is a beautiful illustration of this statement. It concerned a 39-year-old man who had undergone many laparotomies for nephrectomies and kidney transplants. His transplanted kidney showed signs of rejection and had to be removed. Directly after induction of the general anesthesia, an asystole developed. External cardiac massage was started immediately, but the effect was poor. No blood pressure could be measured and the average level of the $ETCO_2$ during mechanical ventilation was not higher than 2% (16 mmHg). His pupils became wide and were not reacting to light. His abdominal wall represented an old battlefield of surgical scars, and was extremely flabby. When pushing the sternum downwards during the cardiac massage, the abdominal wall was bulging forwards, displaying a huge abdominal hernia. On the assumption that the heart escaped our attempts of compression by moving downwards in the direction of the flabby belly, we tried to make the anterior abdominal wall as tight as possible by grasping the skin and the underlying muscles in our hands and folding them in creases. The dramatic effect was clearly visible on the capnogram as well as on the plethysmogram and the ECG. So, guided by the capnogram, the patient could be resuscitated successfully (Figure 35.18).

The capnograph as a monitor of technical defects

Technical defects in anesthesia machines, connecting tubes, ventilators, valve housings, ET tubes, etc., are life endangering. Already in the 1960s it became clear that the capnograph was an early warning device and could prevent disasters. A few examples will be shown. In Figure 35.19, a fragment of the three-channel recording is to be seen of a 71-year-old lady who underwent plastic surgery. She was mechanically ventilated. Her capnogram was absolutely perfect, as can be seen on the high-speed recording at the left. Suddenly the regular capnographic pattern was interrupted (indicated by an arrow) and the high-speed capnographic recording at the right shows the typical shape of an expiratory problem, as in, for example, COPD (see Figure 35.5). Because it is impossible to develop a COPD in a few seconds, the underlying problem can either be a sudden bronchial spasm, or a kinking of the ET tube. A quick inspection showed that it was indeed the tube and the problem could be solved on the spot.

Other technical problems are, for example, leakages, disconnection of corrugated tubes, or saturation of

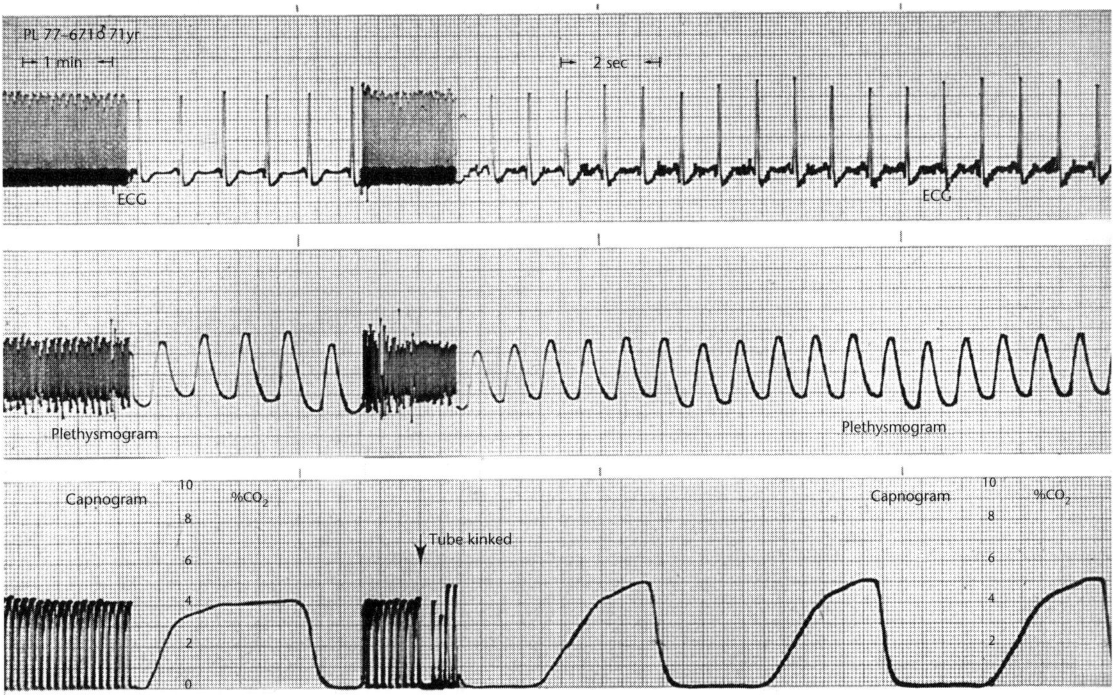

Figure 35.19 ECG, plethysmogram and capnogram of a 71-year-old woman. Effect on the shape of the capnogram by kinking of the ET.

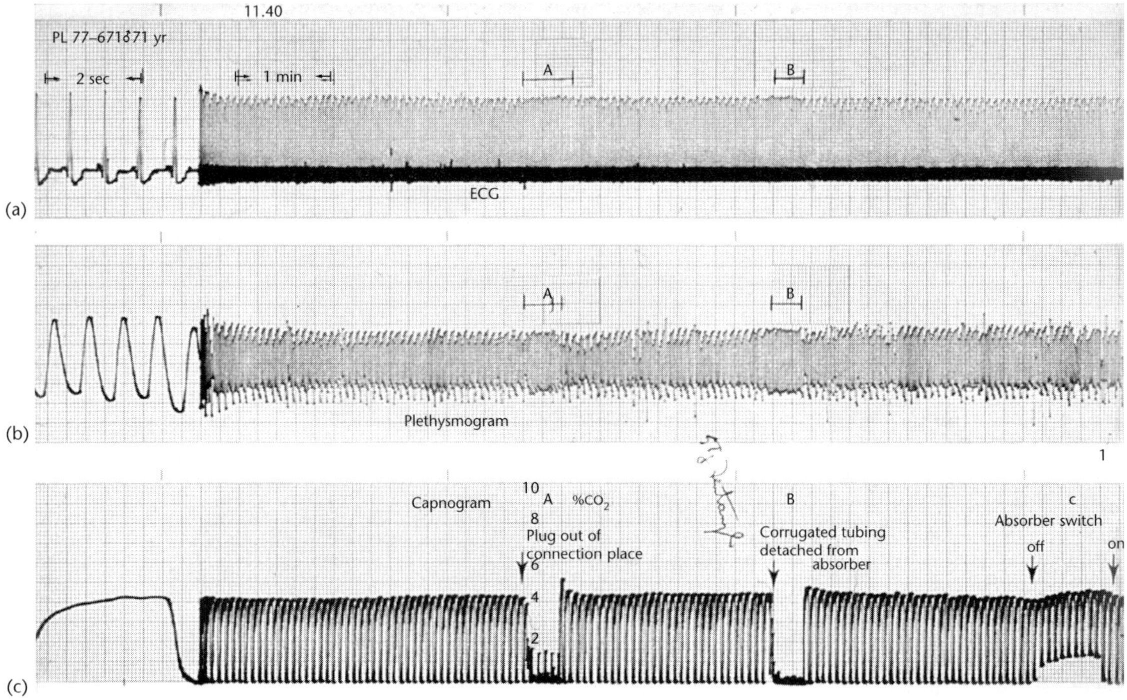

Figure 35.20 The capnographic recording of a leakage (a), a disconnection (b) and switching off and on the sodalime absorber (c).

the CO_2 absorbers. All this can be seen in Figure 35.20. Leakages and disconnections cause sudden interruptions of the CO_2 pattern, and inactivity of the CO_2 absorber (recorded on the right) makes the baseline rise, returning to zero as soon as a fresh absorbent canister has been switched on.

The capnograph as a monitor of medical errors

Medical errors are still important factors that can cost the life or the health of a patient. Therefore, it is desirable that such catastrophes can be recorded in an objective way, comparable with the data flight-recorder (the so-called black box) in a commercial airplane. This is not only important for legal reasons, but also for the analysis and reconstruction of anesthetic or surgical accidents. The capnograph offers such a possibility provided that the device is running continuously during the whole medical procedure.

Nearly fatal pain stimulus

Figure 35.21 shows a 5 min long fragment of a 21-year-old four-channel recording of a 58-year-old woman. She was suffering of a highly dangerous intracranial aneurysm of the arterial communicans anterior. Awaiting the start of the operation, she was already under anesthesia and mechanically ventilated, being paralyzed by muscle relaxants. She was slightly hyperventilated to an $ETCO_2$ of 3.7% (29.6 mmHg) to diminish the intracranial pressure. The blood pressure was lowered to 60/30 mmHg to prevent spontaneous rupture of the aneurysm during the neurosurgical intervention. Because already 40 min had passed since the induction of the anesthesia, the patient needed a new dose of the analgesic fentanyl before the start of the operation. But without any warning or consulting the anesthesiologist, the surgeon suddenly made a deep incision in the patient's head. That moment is indicated on the left side by an arrow. The woman reacted violently to this painful stimulus. Although she did not move because of the muscle relaxants, her blood pressure rose within 1 min from 60/30 to 170/90 mmHg, creating a mortally dangerous situation. A fatal rupture of the aneurysm could be expected every moment. The plethysmogram disappeared practically for about 10 s by extreme capillary vasoconstriction. This was caused by the adrenalin from the adrenal glands. After that, the plethysmographic oscillations increased fourfold, by the rise in blood pressure. The capnogram rose from 3.7% (29.6 mmHg) to 5.2%

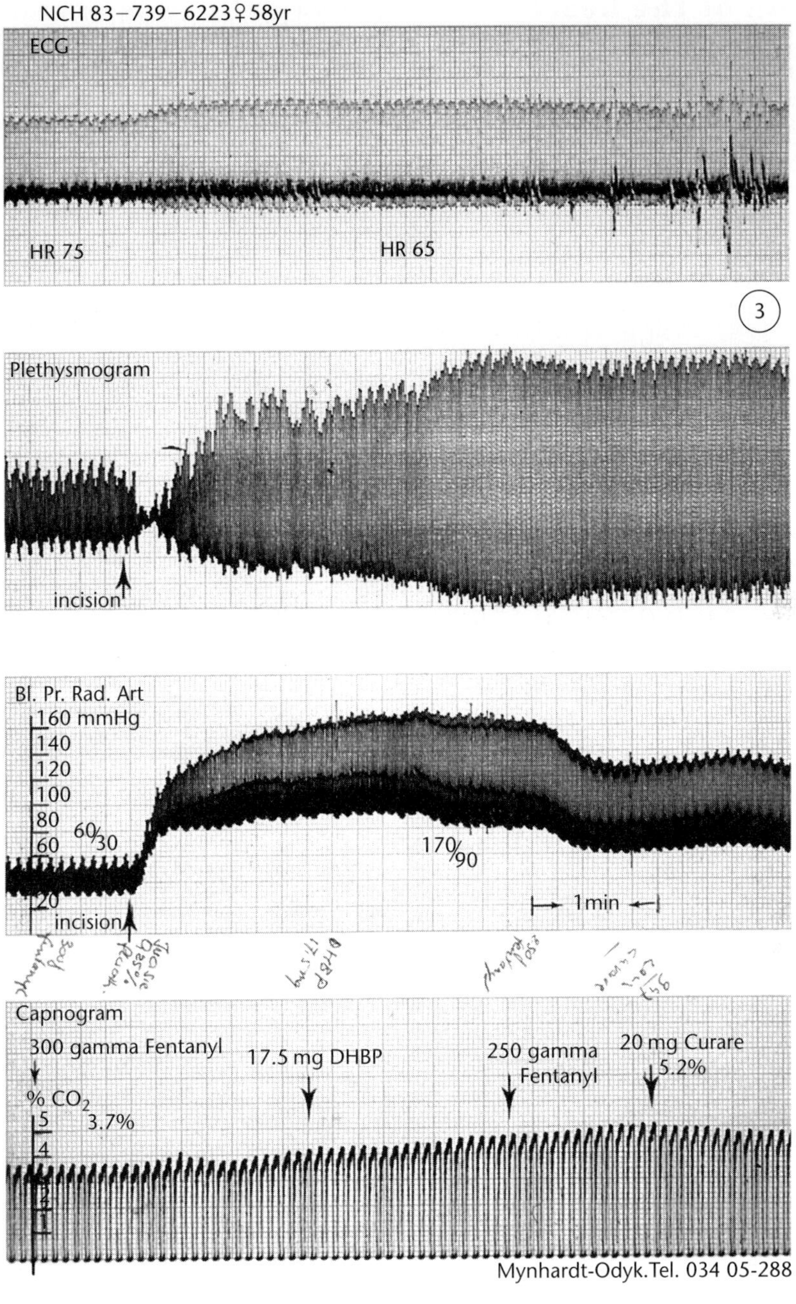

Figure 35.21 ECG, plethysmogram, blood pressure and capnogram of a 58-year-old woman (1983). The nearly fatal effect of a painful stimulus.

(41.6 mmHg). It was a hell of a job to normalize the blood pressure again. Fortunately, no intracranial hemorrhage occurred.

But suppose that the uncoordinated action of the neurosurgeon had resulted in a calamity, then certainly he would have accused the anesthesiologist for the fatal outcome, because he would state that no patient could die from a simple skin incision. So, probably, something must have gone wrong with the anesthesia, and he would blame the anesthesiologist. With the recording shown above in his hands, the anesthesiologist could have proved his innocence and indicated the real guilty party.

Compression of the heart

A surgical team performs a lobectomy of the right lung. The thoracic surgeon is busy closing the bronchial stump with staples. His assistant has two hands in the open chest of the patient. At that moment, Figure 35.22 was recorded. As can be seen, indicated by the first arrow, the ECG suddenly changed, the capnogram narrowed considerably, the blood pressure fell from 130/70 to 45/30 mmHg. The capnogram closely followed the variations of the blood pressure and fell from 4.5% (36 mmHg) to 1% (8.5 mmHg). This combination is typical for a mechanical compression of the heart. There were simply too many hands and instruments in the thoracic cavity. The surgeons were urgently requested to withdraw as soon as possible, which they did immediately, knowing that everything was being recorded. The favorable effect can be seen directly after

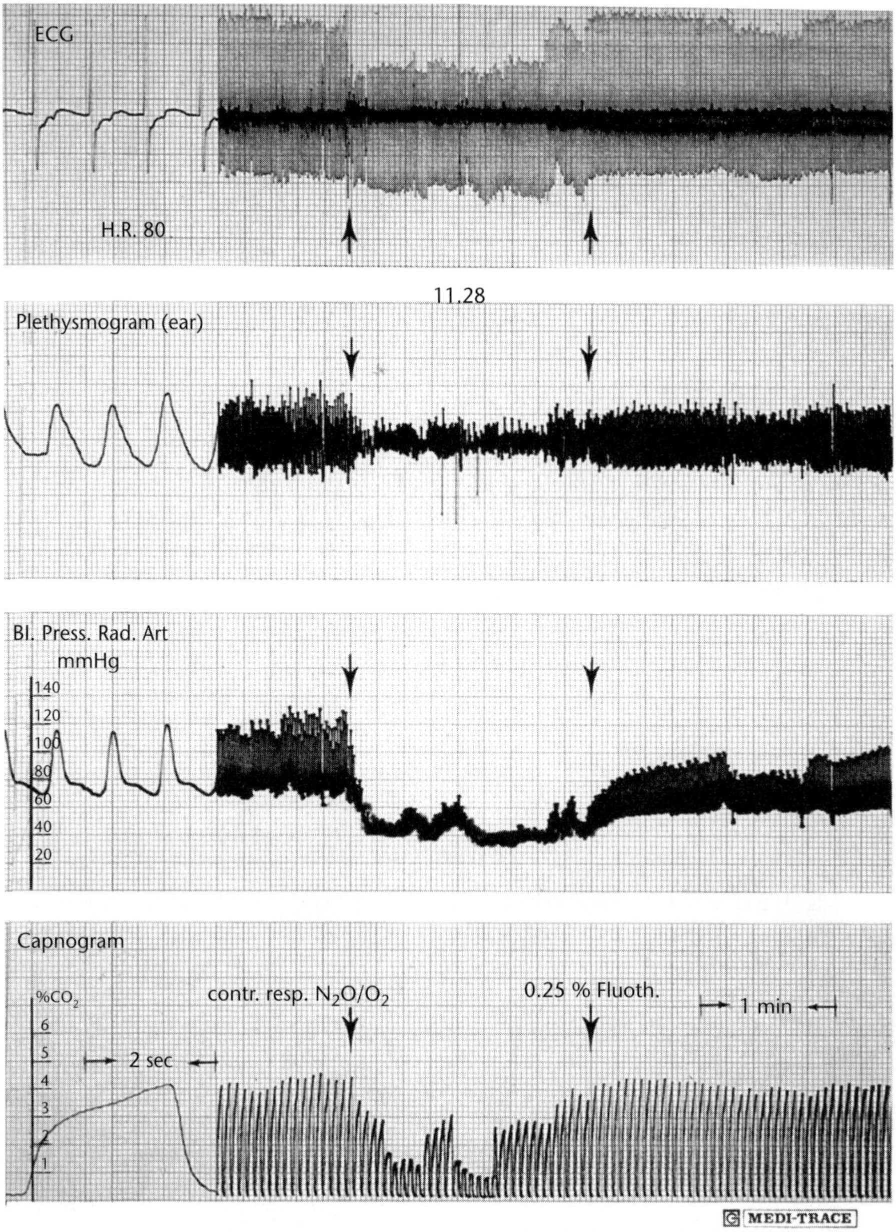

Figure 35.22 ECG, plethysmogram, blood pressure and capnogram of a patient during lung resection. Effect on all the vital parameters of compression of the heart, followed by withdrawal of hands and instruments.

the second arrow. The life-endangering situation had lasted exactly 108 s.

Air embolism

Air embolism is a very dangerous complication and the diagnosis is often too late. The classic symptom of the so-called "mill-wheel murmur" can only be heard after a considerable amount of air is collected in the heart – and then the situation is already nearly fatal. The capnogram has proved to give a very reliable and early warning. Even a small bubble of air can be detected immediately. Figure 35.23 shows the four-channel recording of such an event in a 20-year-old man during an orthopedic operation. Typical for air

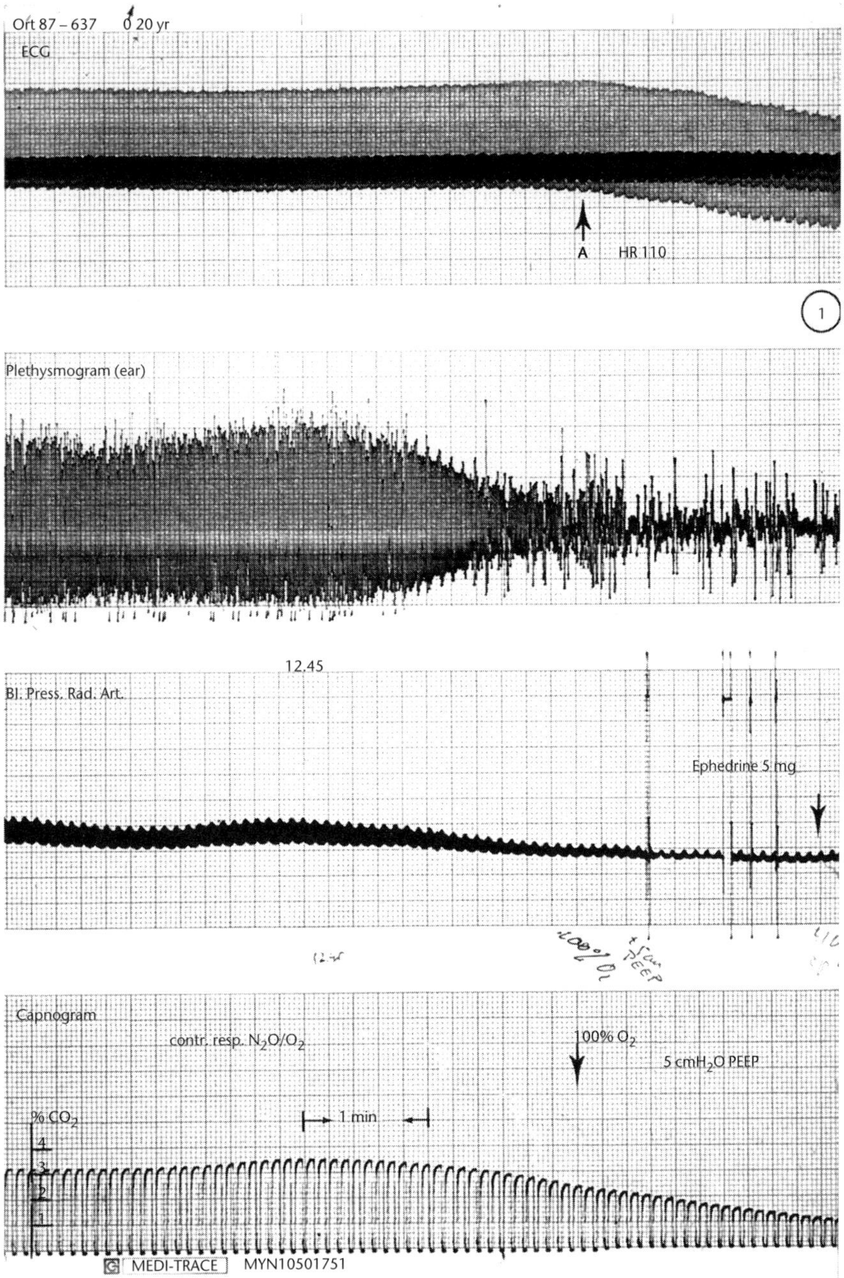

Figure 35.23 ECG, plethysmogram, blood pressure and capnogram during air embolism (1986). Man, 20 years of age.

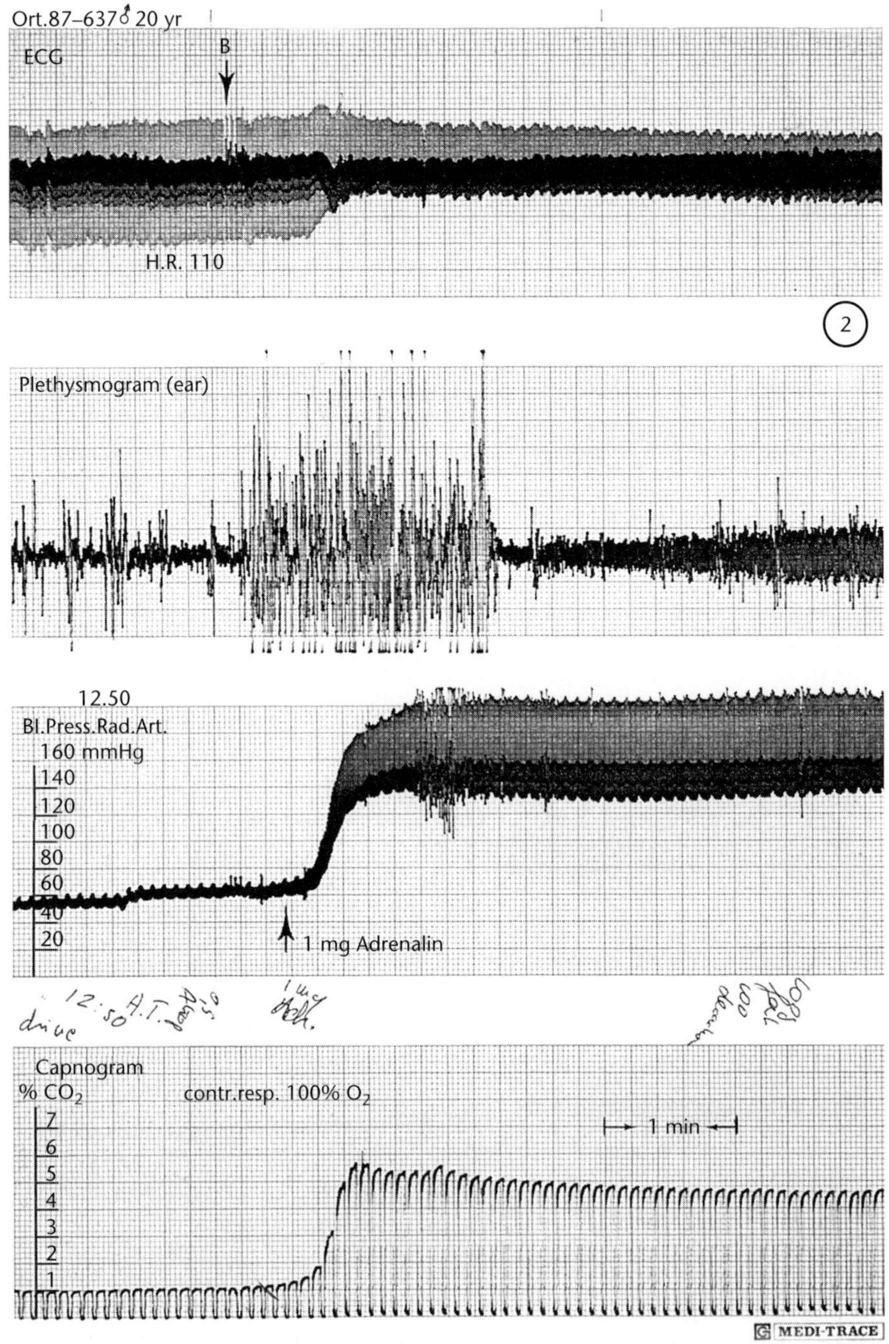

Figure 35.24 The resuscitation of the patient in Figure 35.23.

embolism is that the ECG during the first minutes remains unchanged. But the plethysmogram narrows immediately, while the capnogram is gradually descending, synchronous with the blood pressure. When only a few small air bubbles enter the blood stream, the capnogram shows little dips. Air bubbles cause severe vasoconstriction in the lung capillaries, diminishing the lung perfusion and by doing so lowering the expired CO_2 contents. And just as in the case of a cardiac arrest, the effect of the treatment or resuscitation can clearly be seen on the capnogram (Figure 35.24).

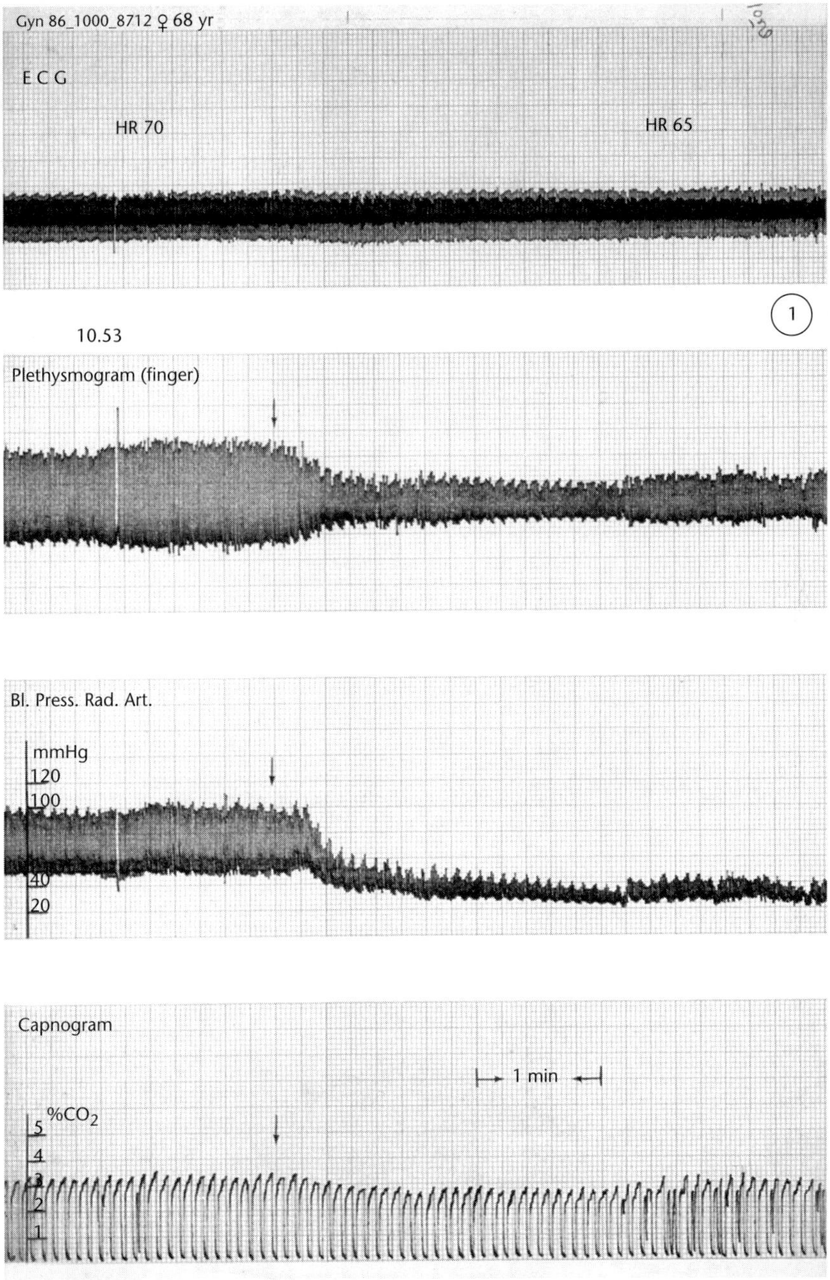

Figure 35.25 ECG, plethysmogram, blood pressure and capnogram of a patient during the filling of the abdominal cavity with gauzes in order to keep the bowels away, a woman aged 68 years. Effect on the plethysmogram, the blood pressure and the capnogram of compression of the vena cava inferior.

Compression of the inferior cava vein

During a laparotomy of a 68-year-old woman, for debulking an ovarian carcinoma, the gynecologists used a vast amount of towels and gauze to keep the bowels out of sight from the operation field. Suddenly an impressive change was to be seen on the four-channel low-speed recording (Figure 35.25). While the ECG did not change, oscillations of the plethysmogram diminished in size, the blood pressure fell from 100/50 to 50/20 mmHg, and at the same moment the $ETCO_2$ was going down. In principle, there were three diagnostic possibilities:

1 severe sudden loss of blood
2 air embolism
3 compression of the inferior cava vein, preventing the venous return to the heart.

Since there was no blood loss and the possibility of air embolism was negligible, the most probable diagnosis was compression of the cava vein by the towels and the gauzes. The gynecological team was urgently requested to remove all the gauzes from the abdominal cavity as soon as possible. This improved the clinical situation immediately, as can be seen in Figure 35.26. Because of the continuous recording, the life-threatening complication could be detected, diagnosed and solved within a few minutes. The reasonable capnographic $ETCO_2$ which was never lower than 3% (24 mmHg) proved

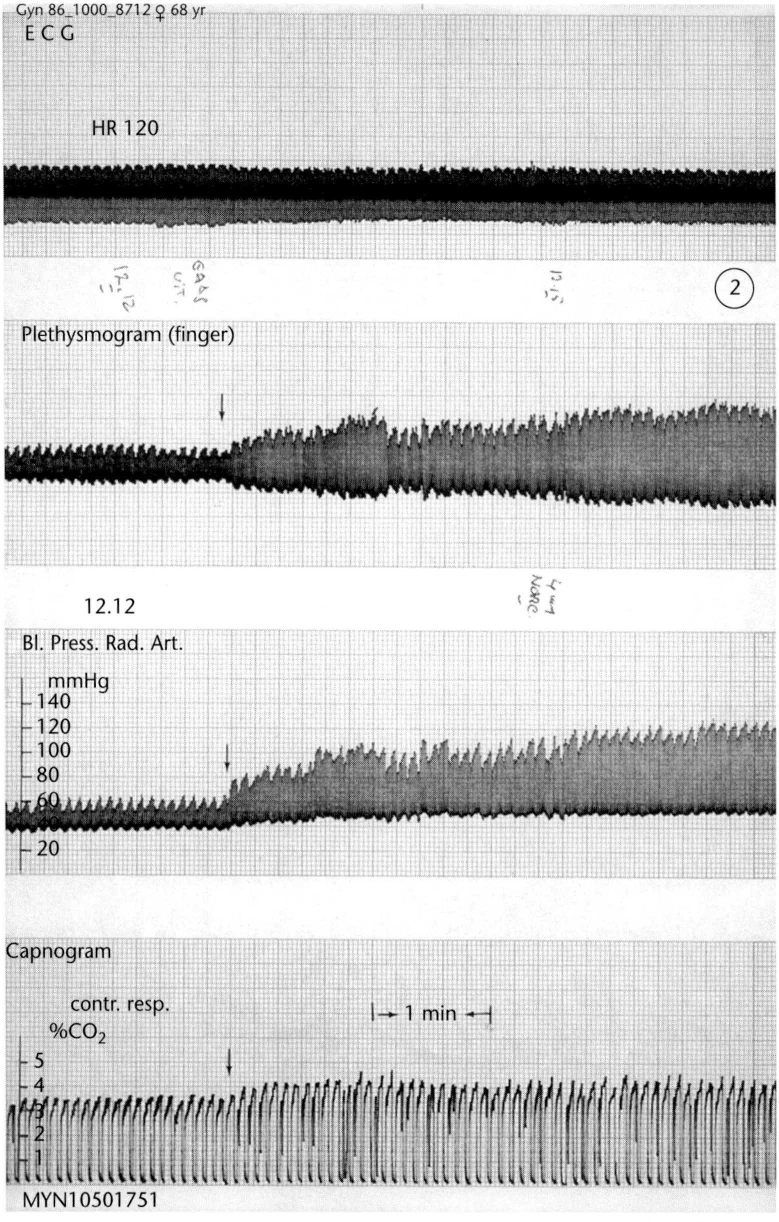

Figure 35.26 Recovery of the vital parameters in the same patient, after removal of all the gauzes and towels out of the abdominal cavity.

that the blood perfusion during the event was never insufficient.

Is a certain hypotension dangerous or not?

Always the question arises whether a certain fall in blood pressure becomes life threatening. The clinical experience in more than 40 years of capnography taught us that as long as the $ETCO_2$ during a period of hypotension is not lower than about 2.5% (20 mmHg), the perfusion of the lung is more or less comparable with that in the other organs, especially kidneys, heart and brain. Sometimes the capnogram even indicates that during a certain hypotension the perfusion can be improved. In Figure 35.27 this is to be seen in a 66-year-old male neurosurgical patient. He underwent

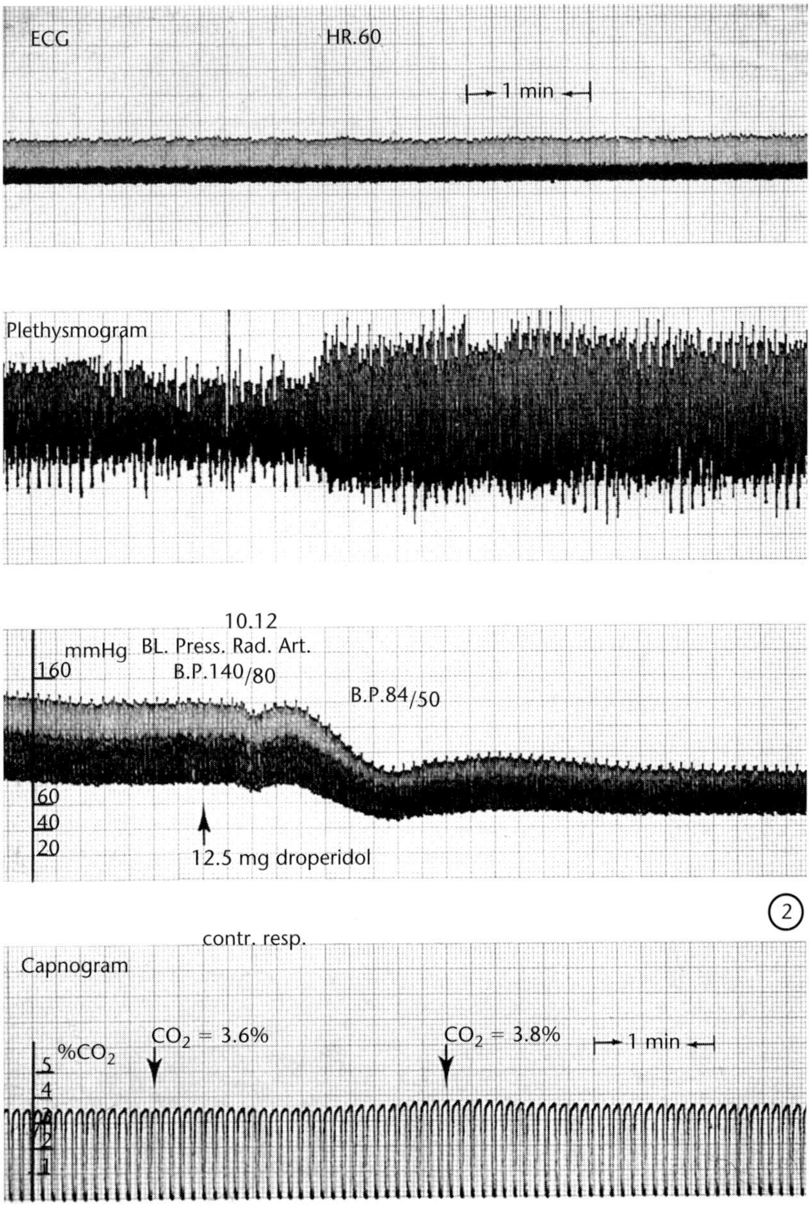

Figure 35.27 ECG, plethysmogram, blood pressure and capnogram of a man, 66 years of age. Lowering the blood pressure after 12.5 mg DHBP or droperidol. But the broadening of the plethysmogram and the rising of the capnogram indicate an improved perfusion.

an extra–intracranial bypass operation. His blood pressure of 140/80 was purposely lowered to 84/50 by means of 12.5 mg dehydro-benzperidol (DHBP). This is a low dose for a man of this age. But the plethysmogram, was broadening considerably, indicating vasodilatation and the capnogram rose from 3.6% (28.8 mmHg) to 3.8% (30.4 mmHg). This proved that although the blood pressure was low, the perfusion even had improved.

Central neurologic disturbances of the spontaneous respiration

Already in the 1950s, it became clear that the capnograph was an excellent instrument for recording and studying spontaneous respiration, especially in patients with intracranial pathology. There are many variations of the respiratory rhythm, caused by neurological disturbances in the brain or the brainstem.

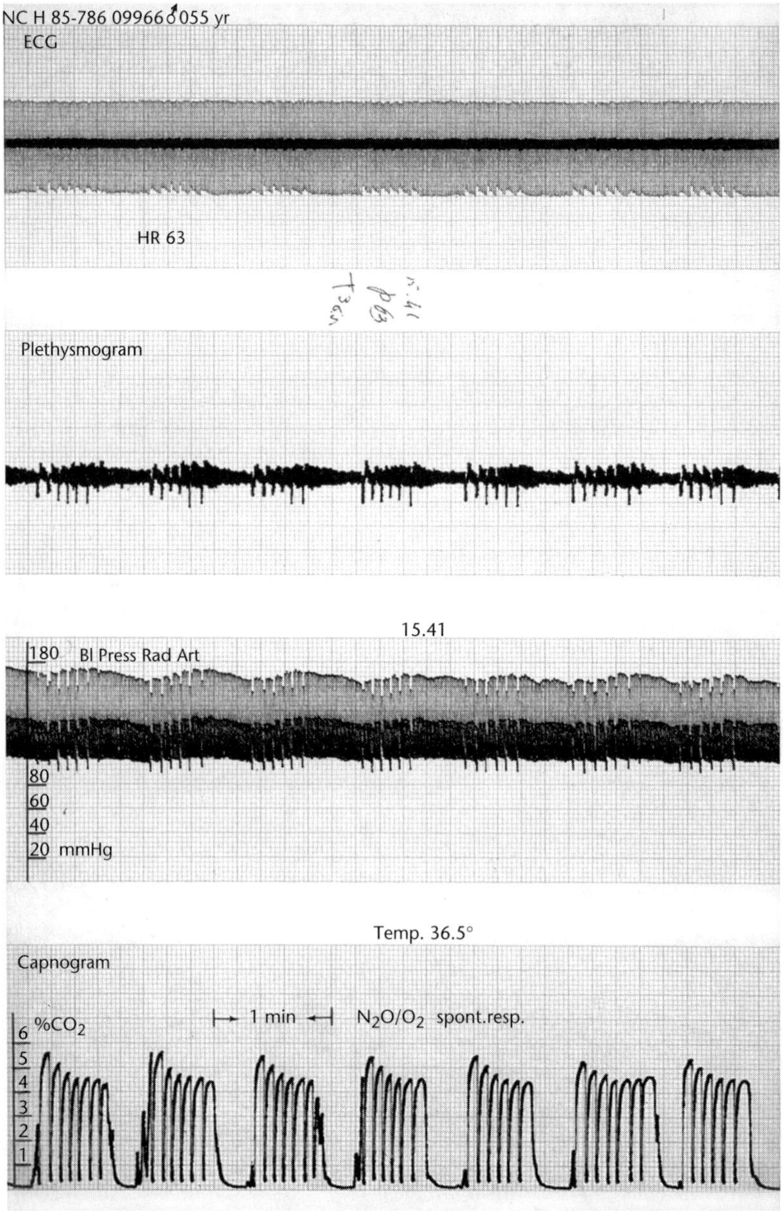

Figure 35.28 ECG, plethysmogram, blood pressure and capnogram of a 55-year-old man after a craniotomy. Spontaneous respiration. Typical Cheyne–Stokes breathing.

Strange enough, they are less well known than the cardiac arrhythmias. This book is not the place to describe them all. That is already extensively done by Frowein (1963).

But one example is perhaps enough to illustrate the exceptional value of the capnograph in recording and studying central respiratory problems; Figure 35.28 shows the capnogram of the spontaneous respiration, together with the ECG, the blood pressure and the plethysmogram of a 55-year-old man. He was just recovering from an intracranial operation on the trigeminel nerve. Clearly to be seen is the typical pattern of the classical Cheyne–Stokes breathing, indicating a brainstem disturbance. It is striking that the periodical rhythm of the respiration is also visible in the other vital systems.

Summary

More than 40 years of clinical capnography have shown that the capnograph is one of the most useful monitors in anesthesiology and intensive care. Its high value is only comparable with that of the ECG and the pulse-oximeter. Nearly all the clinical possibilities of the capnograph were already discovered in the years between 1950s and 1970s. All the recordings shown in this chapter are made by the author himself. Coming from his personal archives, and recorded between 1962 and 1982. they reflect the increasing importance of the CO_2 infrared monitor in the first decades of clinical capnography. During the recent World Congress of Anaesthesiology, which took place in April 2004 in Paris, a Canadian anesthesiologist told the audience that in his country the insurance companies have lowered the insurance premiums for medical liability with 80% for anesthesiologists who monitor their patients with a capnograph.

Conclusion

The history of clinical capnography has proven that the measuring and recording of expired CO_2 can prevent catastrophic events. There are only two conditions: the recording must be (a) continuous and (b) simultaneous with other vital parameters. In so doing, the monitor acts like a flight data-recorder in commercial aviation. The recording can be documented on paper tape or electronically on a compact disk (CD). The paper tape has the advantage that it is easy to write down very quickly additional information, and the whole anesthetic conduct of even many hours can be overlooked on the spot. The disadvantage is the considerable amount of paper tape that has to be stored in the archives. During an 8-h operation, about 20 m (60 feet) of paper tape can be collected. But the safety of the patient and the judicial security of the anesthesiologist are improved in an impressive way that was never possible before. So the hell of the German submarine warfare between 1940 and 1945 unexpectedly gave birth to the incredible blessing of capnography that still saves and protects millions of lives all over the world.

References

Digby Leigh, M., Jenkins, L.C., Benton, M.K. & Lewis, J.B. (1957). Continuous alveolar carbon dioxide analysis as a monitor of pulmonary blood flow. *Anesthesiology*, **18**: 878.

Digby Leigh, M., Jones, J.C. & Motley, H.L. (1961). The expired carbon dioxide as a continuous guide of the pulmonary and circulatory systems during anaesthesia and surgery *J. Thorac. Cardiovasc. Surg.*, **41**: 597.

Frowein, R.A. Zentrale Atemstörungen bei Schädel-Hirn Verletzungen und bei Hirntumoren (1963) Springer-Verlag, Berlin, Göttingen, Heidelberg.

Health Council of the Netherlands – *Advisory Report on Anaesthesiology. Part I: Recent developments in Anaesthesiology* Government Publishing Office, The Hague (1978, 1980).

Smalhout, B. *Capnography* – Its importance in diagnosis, operations and after treatment of neurosurgical patients. The interpretation of the capnogram in dysregulation of respiration and blood circulation, and its role in monitoring neuro-anaesthesia. Oosthoek's Publishing Co., Utrecht, The Netherlands (1967) Ph.D. thesis, University of Utrecht.

Smalhout, B. & Kalenda, Z. (1975). *An Atlas of Capnography*. Kerckebosch Publications, Zeist, The Netherlands.

Smalhout, B. (1981). *A Quick Guide to Capnography and its use in Differential Diagnosis*. Hewlett Packard, Böblingen, Germany.

VOLUMETRIC CAPNOGRAPHY: THE EARLY DAYS

36

R. Fletcher

In 1975, I was a trainee at the Department of Anaesthesia in the University Hospital, Lund, Sweden, when the Siemens-Elema CO_2 Analyzer 930 was newly installed in the cardiac surgery operating rooms. The compact and user-friendly 930 was said to owe its technology to the space exploration programme. It could only work in conjunction with the Servo ventilator, from which it drew power and timing signals. The rapid response of its Ge–As sensor gave it a vastly superior performance to the previous generation of capnographs. The 50% response time (12 ms) of the original model meant that the CO_2 signal was only slightly delayed compared to the Servo's flow signal (4 ms) (Fletcher, 1980). The flow signal made possible volumetric capnography; that is, not only the measurement of expired CO_2 partial pressure or fraction, but also the minute expired CO_2 volume, $\dot{V}CO_2$. However, CO_2 measurement was affected by the presence of N_2O, which in practice meant that 930s used in anaesthesia and intensive care had to be separately calibrated.

My mentor was Lars Nordström, a cardiac anaesthetist, who had already written his MD thesis on use of the Servo ventilator. He coupled the device to an eight-channel writer, so that in addition to electrocardiography (ECG), arterial and venous pressure, we had expired partial pressure of CO_2 (PCO_2), volume of CO_2 expired per breath, and also airway flow and pressure. This was the advanced stuff for the 1970s, for I do not believe that capnography in any form was in regular clinical use at this time anywhere outside the Netherlands, where Smalhout had pioneered it, certainly not in any cardiac theatres of which I was aware.

The revolution that the 930 brought about in our clinical practice and our understanding of gas exchange depended on two aspects of its function. Firstly, by measuring $\dot{V}CO_2$, it became simultaneously a metabolic monitor (What better measure of metabolic activity?), and a monitor of cardio-respiratory integrity; any interruption in the transport of CO_2-rich blood from the tissues to the airway, whether in perfusion or ventilation, is detected. Secondly, the ability to plot expired CO_2 against expired volume allowed us to present CO_2 single breath tests (SBT-CO_2; Figure 36.1), which

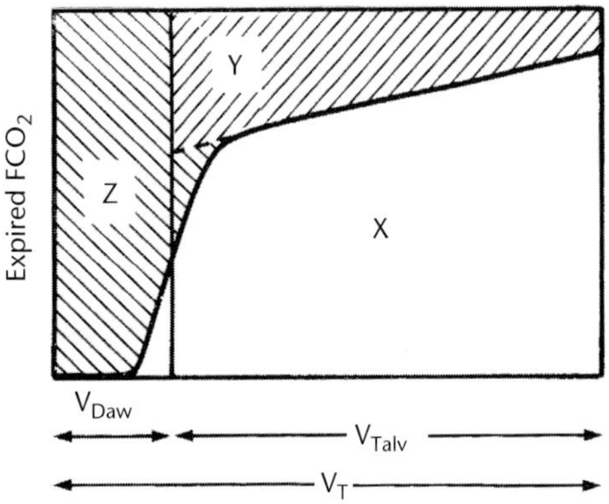

Figure 36.1 Schematic single breath test. F_aCO_2 represents the FCO_2 of a gas in equilibrium with arterial blood. Area X represents the volume of CO_2 in the breath. Area Y represents the alveolar deadspace. The alveolar deadspace fraction is given by Y/(X + Y). V_{Talv} is the alveolar tidal volume. The physiological deadspace fraction is represented by areas (Y + Z)/(X + Y + Z). Note that fractions are used, rather than partial pressures, in order that the areas may represent CO_2 volumes, actual or notional.

yield diagnostic information. Many pulmonary conditions produce characteristic changes, giving further insight into the gas exchange process. We were able to reconstruct intra-operative events from this information, for instance, protamine anaphylaxis (Nordström *et al.*, 1978).

My doctorate was supervised by Prof. Björn Jonson, a pulmonary clinical physiologist, who had also been involved in the development of the Servo ventilator. We obtained data from patients with lung fibrosis, emphysema, obstructive disease, sarcoidosis and even pulmonary embolism. An existing computer program was adapted by Lisbet Janson to print out SBT-CO_2.

We quantified the single breath tests using Jonson's term *efficiency*, which compares the volume of CO_2 eliminated per breath to what would be eliminated by a theoretical, square wave, ideal breath (Figure 36.2). Thus the mean *efficiency* of patients with lung fibrosis

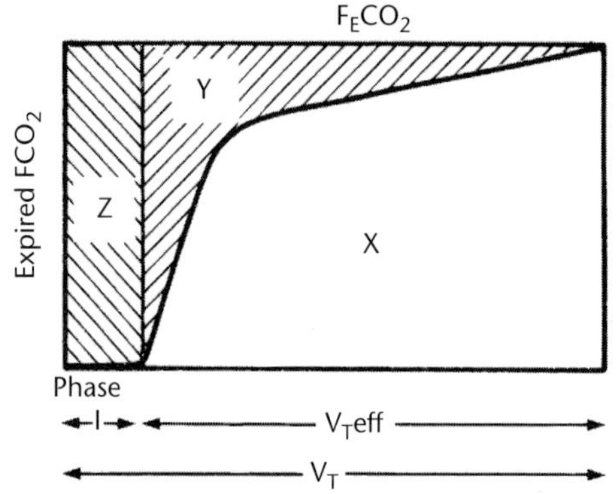

Figure 36.2 Definition of *efficiency*. The breath is divided into phase I, the ineffective part, and V_{Teff}, the effective part (which contains phases I and II). *Efficiency* is calculated from 100 times area X divided by areas (X + Y). In effect, efficiency is a non-invasive measure of ventilatory efficiency.

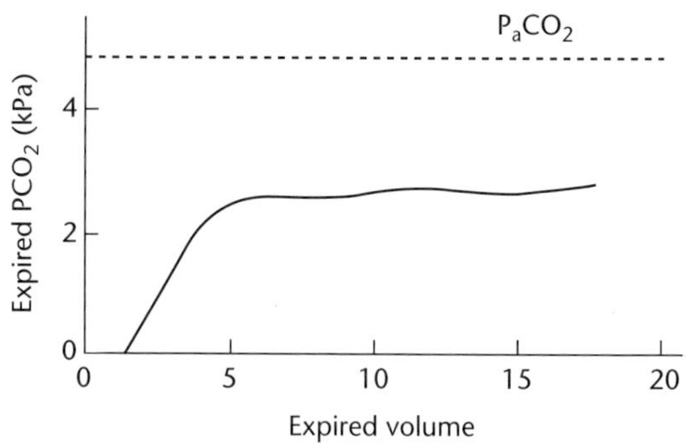

Figure 36.3 CO_2 single breath test obtained from a patient with pulmonary embolism. There is a large alveolar deadspace, creating a large arterial–ETCO$_2$ difference. The fluctuations in alveolar CO_2 are known as cardiogenic oscillations; on the time plot, they can be seen to have the same frequency as the heart rate. A similar picture is seen during a carcinoid flush (see text).

was 82%, whereas emphysema gave 75%. Gross obesity gave a fourth phase to the tracing, one we ascribed to the influence at end expiration of slowly emptying low ventilation/perfusion ($\dot{V}/\dot{Q}$) basal areas. The tests could be combined with an inserted value for arterial blood CO_2 (Figure 36.1). Thus pulmonary embolism (Figure 36.3) gave a striking picture; a flat single breath test with a massive alveolar deadspace, a truly "parallel" deadspace. There were marked "cardiogenic oscillations", which we ascribed to cardiac activity affecting the filling and emptying of lung regions with greatly different $\dot{V}/\dot{Q}$ ratios. Capnography is used today in Lund as a diagnostic test for pulmonary embolism. A similar picture, captured intra-operatively, was seen during a carcinoid flush. It was the first time I had seen such sudden reductions in $\dot{V}CO_2$ and end-tidal PCO_2 ($P_{et}CO_2$), which were too sudden to be due to metabolic changes. At first I assumed, there had been an equipment malfunction, but the recorded data showed a picture very like that in Figure 36.3.

Gordon Cumming, then at Midhurst Medical Institute, Sussex, England, suggested we plot CO_2 cumulative volume against expired volume, as he was doing in his studies with Keith Horsfield on O_2 and nitrogen. Cumming regarded the S-shaped increase in expired CO_2, phase II, as the recruitment of transit times for the different unit pathways. His method gave us an alternative to that of Fowler for measuring "series", anatomical or airway deadspace, $V_D$aw, our preferred term. It was preferred because it was clear that "anatomical" deadspace varied much more than could be accounted for on purely anatomical grounds; time, flow rate and ventilatory pattern greatly affected it, as exemplified by Nordström's term "mean distribution time". However, it became clear that Cumming's method for $V_D$aw was subject to the same constraints as Fowler's. Particularly in obstructive lung disease, it became necessary to find another way of identifying the midpoint of the fresh gas/alveolar gas interface, such as the "point of inflexion" in phase II.

I recorded CO_2 single breath tests from anaesthetised, ventilated patients at frequencies of 15–20 (mean tidal volume 0.45 l) and 9 breaths/min (mean tidal volume 0.74 l), and compared the efficiency of gas exchange. Inspiration occupied 25% of cycle, and the end-inspiratory pause was 10% of cycle. $V_D$aw was the same at both settings, probably due to more time for the interface to diffuse proximally at the slower rate. The alveolar deadspace fraction and the arterial–end-tidal difference were always much less at the large tidal volumes, which we ascribed to more even spatial distribution of inspired gas. There were no differences in calculated venous admixture, however (Fletcher & Jonson, 1984). As a result of these observations, we published an article describing our concept of deadspace (Fletcher *et al.*, 1981).

Twenty-five years ago, the importance of avoiding hypothermia during anaesthesia and surgery was still not well appreciated. Some patients coming to our recovery unit, still intubated after major surgery, were hypothermic and starting to shiver. The 930 showed us that shivering can double CO_2 production, which explained why the patients became hypertensive, tachycardic and hypercapnic. Clearly, their hypertension could not be fully managed until the shivering and hypercapnia had been treated. Without the 930, these metabolic consequences would have not been picked up until later, exposing the patient to an unnecessary period of instability.

Capnography was an essential part of our monitoring for patients susceptible to malignant hyperpyrexia (MH). An unusual case presented itself: an infant with a myopathy developed MH, and there were repeated episodes of increased temperature and CO_2 elimination post-operatively, which responded to dantrolene (Fletcher *et al.*, 1982).

In severe lung disease, the 930 reduced the amount of guesswork involved in setting the ventilator. When transferring a patient from volume- to pressure-controlled ventilation, it makes more sense to aim for a given $\dot{V}CO_2$ rather than a particular minute ventilation. Pressure control was more always effective at removing CO_2 for any given peak pressure, as mean distribution time was increased. With the 930, it was also possible to immediately ascertain the effect on $\dot{V}CO_2$ of extending the inspiratory phase, or increasing positive end-expiratory pressure (PEEP). Allied with pulse oximetry, this greatly simplified setting the ventilator in severe lung disease. Internationally, the received wisdom at the time favoured large tidal volume, low rate ventilation. However, my colleagues and I argued, from first principles, that smaller tidal volumes at greater rates, and with a generous PEEP, would better avoid collapse of unstable units and also avoid high peak pressures. Experimentation with the 930 showed that such ventilatory patterns were indeed possible without hypercapnia. I was able to show (Fletcher and Stannard, 1999) that when compliance is low, as during laparoscopy in the head down position, the ratio "$\dot{V}CO_2$: peak airway pressure" was greater at 15 and 20 breaths/min than at 10 breaths/min.

The 930 became essential monitoring for cardiac surgery. I used it to get a picture of CO_2 elimination as cardiopulmonary bypass was started, producing a family of curves, resembling pulmonary embolism (Fletcher, 1987). When surgery for congenital cardiac disease expanded in Lund, I turned my attention to gas exchange in infants, and in particular the pattern of CO_2 elimination in intra-cardiac right–left (R–L) shunting. As expected, normal children, and those with atrial septal defects, had very little alveolar deadspace and a zero arterial–$P_{et}CO_2$ difference (Fletcher *et al.*, 1986). Congenital cyanotic heart disease was associated with a lower CO_2 production, reflecting a lesser metabolic rate (Fletcher, 1988). However, I realised I had not fully understood the problem when writing my thesis. If one rewrites the shunt equation using CO_2 instead of O_2, it becomes clear that R–L shunting causes a significant "apparent" or "virtual" alveolar or parallel deadspace, and thus a significant arterial–end-tidal CO_2 (ETCO$_2$) difference. This effect appeared to be overlooked in the literature; the explanation usually offered for the increased arterial–ETCO$_2$ difference in R–L shunting was "alveolar hypoperfusion". In fact the shunt equation makes it clear that it is not necessary to postulate this mechanism in order to explain much of the alveolar deadspace observed, although later work (Short *et al.*, 2001) suggested that alveolar hypoperfusion might occur.

With the help of Andrew Black, I demonstrated the theoretical relationship between the arterial–ETCO$_2$ difference and arterial PO_2 (P_aO_2) (Fletcher, 1989). When pulse oximetry became clinically available, my colleague Olof Werner suggested I demonstrate the theoretical relationship between the arterial–$P_{et}CO_2$ difference and arterial saturation (Fletcher, 1991). Depending on haemoglobin concentration and arterial PCO_2 (P_aCO_2), there is a more or less straight-line relationship between the two.

There were many practical applications in cardiothoracic anaesthesia. Work done by Werner and his colleagues in Lund had already shown the benefits of volumetric capnography in pulmonary surgery (Werner *et al.*, 1984a, b). After surgery designed to palliate cyanotic lesions, $\dot{V}CO_2$ and expired PCO_2 were greater when the circulation was restored. In lung transplantation, the use of two ventilators and two capnographs showed what proportion of the total respiratory load each lung was performing. Giving sodium bicarbonate always produced a sharp increase in $\dot{V}CO_2$.

It is a matter of personal regret that promotion and production of the Siemens-Elema 930 ceased without a successor in view; however, the gauntlet has been taken up elsewhere. The technology will become more sophisticated, and the sensors more compact and robust. Innovative anaesthesiologists will find new applications for the information offered by volumetric capnography! Its benefits are the ability to measure $\dot{V}CO_2$, a measure of metabolism or of cardio-respiratory function and secondly presentation of the CO_2 single breath test (i.e. expired CO_2 plotted against expired volume) as a diagnostic tool. Clearly, the most interest will be in the fields of intensive care and in cardiothoracic surgery, but no doubt other novel applications will add themselves to those already discovered.

References

Fletcher, R. (1980). The single breath test for carbon dioxide. Thesis, University of Lund, Sweden.

Fletcher, R. (1987). Lung function during reduced pulmonary perfusion. *Br. J. Anaesth.*, **59**: 652P.

Fletcher, R. (1988). Carbon dioxide production in cyanotic children during anaesthesia with controlled ventilation. *Br. J. Anaesth.*, **56**: 109–119.

Fletcher, R. (1989). The relationship between alveolar deadspace and arterial oxygenation in children with congenital heart disease. *Br. J. Anaesth.*, **62**: 168–176.

Fletcher, R. (1991). The relationship between the arterial to end-tidal PCO_2 difference and hemoglobin saturation in congenital heart disease. *Anesthesiology*, **75**: 210–215.

Fletcher, R. & Jonson, B. (1984). Deadspace and the single breath test for CO_2 during anaesthesia/IPPV. *Br. J. Anaesth.*, **56**: 109–119.

Fletcher, R. & Stannard, L. (1999). Best ventilator setting for major gynaecological laparoscopic surgery. *Br. J. Anaesth.*, **83**: 184P.

Fletcher, R., Jonson, B., Cumming, G. & Brew, J. (1981). The concept of dead space with special reference to the single breath test for CO_2. *Br. J. Anaesth.*, **53**: 77–88.

Fletcher, R., Blennow, G., Olsson, A.-K., Ranklev, E. & Törnebrandt, K. (1982). Malignant hyperthermia in a myopathic child. Prolonged postoperative course requiring dantrolene. *Acta Anaesthesiol. Scand.*, **26**: 435.

Fletcher, R., Niklason, L. & Drefeldt, B. (1986). Gas exchange during controlled ventilation in children with normal and abnormal pulmonary circulation. *Anesth. Analg.*, **65**: 645–652.

Nordström, L., Fletcher, R. & Pavek, K. (1978). Shock of anaphylactoid type induced by protamine, a continuous cardiorespiratory record. *Acta Anaesthesiol. Scand.*, **22**: 195–201.

Short, J.A., Paris, S.T., Booker, P.D. & Fletcher, R. (2001). Arterial to end tidal carbon dioxide tension difference in children with congenital heart disease. *Br. J. Anaesth.*, **86**: 349–353.

Werner, O., Malmkvist, G., Beckman, A., Stahle, S. & Nordstrom, L. (1984a). Carbon dioxide elimination from each lung during endobronchial anaesthesia. *Br. J. Anaesth.*, **56**: 995–1001.

Werner, O., Malmkvist, G., Beckman, A., Stahle, S. & Nordstrom, L. (1984b). Gas exchange and haemodynamics during thoracotomy. *Br. J. Anaesth.*, **56**: 1343–1349.

EXCERPTS FROM AN INTERVIEW WITH MAX LISTON* 37

Interviewed by D.C. Brock & G.E. Gallwas

On how Max Liston got into the gas analyzer business ...

"Dr. [James] Elam and Dr. George Saxton, two of the doctors that I worked with on the Oximeter during the war, and some of the other doctors had been down in Atlantic City at a convention, got into an argument. All of them had experienced some cardiac arrests on the operating table. These were anesthesiologists. They thought it was due to CO_2 (carbon dioxide) accumulation. So they got me out of bed at two o'clock in the morning and in my weakened condition at that time, talked me into building a CO_2 analyzer for them so they could resolve this concern.

That's how I happened to get into the gas analyzer business. I had just left Perkin-Elmer at the time so I was looking for something to do.... The first CO_2 analyzer was sent to Dr. Drinkard's lab under Dr. Whittenberger at Harvard University. That became known as the capnograph, or, Model 16.

It turned out, rather interestingly, that the doctors were right. The anesthetic machines then used what they called a "Q-circuit". This circuit recirculated the gas, adding oxygen and removing the CO_2 by a sodium hydroxide canister. The gases they were using were explosive and they did not want to vent them out into the room.... What they found after receiving the instrument was that the patient was inhaling high levels of CO_2. This was caused by the gas taking the path of least resistance, which was frequently in the center of the canister. So the outside color indication did not change. But the two main manufacturers of anesthetic machines had the same problem. The CO_2 levels on the inhalation side got up as high as 5 percent. As soon as that was known, they put in baffles and cured the desiccant problem.

Then the next thing they discovered was that the flapper valve they used to keep the flow going in one direction would stick when it got wet, and stay open. So there was re-breathing due to that. When those two problems were cured, much of the cardiac arrests went away, and so in a sense, I worked myself out of a job. [Laughter] But it was still useful research. The next big break we got was that the polio foundation decided to equip all their polio centers with our analyzer, and that was quite successful. In fact, their cure rate doubled after they started. What they had been doing with these Drinkard-type, what the press called, "Iron Lungs" is adjusting them for normal title volumes for their weight. When they'reparalyzed, their metabolism is way down, so they were blowing all of these patients into alkalosis. When they got the analyzer, they could control the CO_2 and keep it to normal levels. Their success rate with patients and time in the iron lungs dropped in half and the death rate dropped in half. So that was a very successful program.

On the design of the CO_2 analyzer ...

The basic concept was not mine; I don't want to take credit for it. Dr. Pfund had conceived and patented the positive and negative types. The positive type used the gas of interest to charge the detector. This gas of interest absorbs the energy at the wavelengths where it has molecular resonance. By measuring the expansion we can produce a detector that responds only at wavelengths of analytical interest. By placing a sample cell preceding the detector and placing the unknown gas in the sample cell, it will weaken the energy seen by the detector. This weakening is a measure of the quantity of the unknown gas present. To implement this principle we employed two beams: one containing the sample cell and the second, a dummy cell that is charged with a non-absorbing gas. Two detector chambers were used. One was to receive the energy from each

*Excerpted with permission from Max Liston and the Chemical Heritage Foundation. Liston M.D. (2003). Interviews by David C. Brock and Gerald E. Gallwas at Irvine, California and Fullerton, California, 19 February 2002 and 22 January 2003 (Philadelphia: Chemical Heritage Foundation, Oral History Transcript 0252).

of the two beams with a sensitive diaphragm separating them. A stationary electrode is placed near the diaphragm to form a capacitor. Changes in the capacitance thereby produce a signal that is a function of the unknown in the sample cell. In order to eliminate the effects of ambient temperature and radiation, a mechanical chopper was employed to product energy pulses.

The negative type also employs two beams and two thermocouple detectors. However, in this case one of the beams has a filter cell to remove the energy where the unknown absorbs. The gas is then passed through both beams. Since the energy in the absorption energy of the unknown has been largely removed from one beam, absorption is little changed by the unknown sample. The other beam has no attenuation of the regions of interest. Therefore, the energy in this beam is changed by the absorption of the unknown. The thermocouples are connected in opposition, so the net signal is a function of the quantity of the gas of interest present in the sample cell.

Dr. Pfund had difficulty in measuring the expansion in the positive type analyzer. He and Dr. Williams of Leeds & Northrup heard about the GM Amplifier. This was my first introduction to non-dispersive IR. Dr. Pfund's analyzer was used by the Army Chemical Center during World War II to develop the flame throwers that were so successful in the Italian conflict. After the war, Leeds & Northrup offered this analyzer for commercial sale, but it was not too successful in that it operated DC, so that it was extremely sensitive to temperature changes.

On the birth of non-dispersive IR ...

Oh, yes, definitely. I had occasion to read a review paper a number of years ago on non-dispersive IR, which prompted me to do a literature search. Of all things, I found a reference dating back to Lord Kelvin [William Thomson] in a paper that he read before the Philosophical Society of London back in the 1800s. He described an experiment where he took a tube, pointed it at the sun and interrupted the sun's radiation at a high-frequency using a multichannel disc and put his ear down to a hole at the other end of this tube. When he put in what he called "lamp damp" which was, I assume, methane, he could hear a tone at the chopping rate of the blade. So this really dates back.

Well, in any event, another thing that I didn't mention is that I was doing some work for the Naval Research Labs. This was actually while I was still with Perkin-Elmer. I was visiting down there and the scavengers that go into Germany had brought back some instruments, and they didn't know what they were. They looked like analytical instruments. They took me around and showed me one, and immediately I recognized it as a positive IR analyzer that was identical to what Pfund had patented in this country, developed by Luft. But these were extremely crude. They had rock salt windows attached to a glass tube with clay. He did suggest that this might be used for measuring gasses in mines. They were used extensively in Germany during World War II, even though it took a Ph.D. to run them!

On non-dispersive IR technology – changes from the early days ...

Well, there have been several major changes, I'd say, but the main one is in the early stages, all of us were using a capacitor diaphragm, very delicate. In fact, the ones we did, we made the diaphragm out of gold leaf. [So when it moved,] it changed the capacity. It had a stationary electrode next to this piece of gold leaf, which was so thin you could see through it. In fact, if you couldn't see through it, we wouldn't use it. It was too heavy. ... It would move as the gas heated up, see, it had this selective absorption, so it absorbed energy at the wave length of interest, and then this would vibrate and you measured that motion by the change in capacity. ... Now, the original ones of Luft, and actually some of the others, used an electrometer approach, which I didn't like because that meant working at 10,000 megaohms or higher which humidity or dirt or anything else could mess up. So, I used an RF [radio frequency] approach in all my instruments, and that was one of the things that we contributed to the early stages of the development.

Here's one aside that was interesting to me because it demonstrated the power of measurement, which was not prevalent in the medical field at this early stage. Drs Elam and Saxton were commissioned by the Army Chemical Center to study methods of resuscitating subjects who had been exposed to nerve gas. One of the early and lethal effects of nerve gas is to paralyze the respiratory drive. In 1 week using our Model 16 capnograph, they were able to develop data, which convinced both the Boy Scouts and the Red Cross to discontinue their physical chest manipulations and teach the mouth-to-mouth resuscitation, which is still the preferred method today."

TECHNOLOGICAL PERSPECTIVES

PART

4

TECHNOLOGICAL PERSPECTIVES: INTRODUCTION

38

M.B. Jaffe

Even though the book's principal focus is on clinical issues we thought it was important to include a section that highlights technical issues. We hope this section helps clinicians to interpret product specifications and to understand the role standards play in shaping the products manufacturers offer. We have also sought to provide a general understanding of the principles of the different technologies used to measure carbon dioxide (CO_2) and flow. However, we have reviewed only those technologies that have been employed in commercial devices used clinically. We include a chapter illustrating how technical and clinical issues are intertwined and examining the issues related to combining the waveforms of CO_2 and flow.

TECHNICAL SPECIFICATIONS AND STANDARDS 39

D.E. Supkis

Introduction

The performance specifications of a capnograph are discussed in the context of the ISO 21647 standard for respiratory gas monitors (RGMs). Additionally, alarm systems are discussed with reference to the Alarm Standard (IEC 60601-1-8, 2003).

Standards

Clinicians use standards in every aspect of daily life; from which side of the road their automobiles travel on to how pharmaceuticals are prescribed. A standard is defined by Merriam-Webster as: "something established by authority, custom, or general consent as a model or example". Standards govern the equipment used during various clinical situations (i.e. surgical anesthesia), and how the information provided by the equipment is used. These standards are clinical practice guidelines developed by various clinical organizations, such as the American Society of Anesthesiologists, American Association for Respiratory Care and others. Equipment standards will be the focus in this section, and clinical practice guidelines are addressed elsewhere in this book.

There are two main developers of standards – governmental agencies, such as the Food and Drug Administration (FDA) and standards development organizations (SDOs) (i.e. American Society for Testing and Materials (ASTM), Comité Européen for Normalisation (CEN), British Standards Institute (BSI), International Electrotechnical Commission (IEC) and International Organisation for Standardisation (ISO)) For a standard to be written by an SDO there first has to be a need expressed. This need can be identified by manufacturers, governmental bodies or by users (clinicians). Typically, manufacturers identify the need for a standard. This usually occurs when the device or technology that is the subject of the standard becomes accepted by the clinicians and is widely used. In addition since multiple manufactures or providers of the technology, compete in the marketplace, if a new manufacturer wants to provide the technology, then a widely accepted standard is extremely useful. The standard acts as a guideline for development of their product. And, with documentation of conformance to the standard, then approval by governmental regulatory agencies is expedited. This is especially true if the governmental regulatory agency recognizes the standard.

After the need for a new standard is assessed, usually by a formal balloting process, a standard development organization will host a working group consisting of clinicians, manufacturers and interested parties (including representatives of governmental regulatory agencies). While specific details of the standards development process may differ slightly between different SDOs, the overall process is the same. The working group of clinicians, manufacturers and interested parties develop a working draft of the standard. The working group will ballot the working draft among the members of the working group. Once the draft has matured and has been affirmed by the working group ballot process, the draft standard is balloted to the subcommittee in charge of the standard (e.g. for capnography in the US it is F29 of ASTM). The committee will discuss the standard and will conduct a formal ballot of the draft standard. Most SDOs have strict voting regulations. One of the most important regulations is the requirement that the total number of voting manufacturers cannot out number the total number of voting users and interested parties. The draft standard rarely passes on the first ballot and will need to be balloted several times before passing. The working group reviews the negative votes and the draft standard is modified as needed. Once the committee has approved the draft standard, then the draft standard is submitted for society (e.g. ASTM) balloting. This is a perfunctory step and is rarely disapproved. The entire process of identifying a need to final approval of the standard is extremely slow. It is common to take 2–5 years to get a standard approved. The other problem is that the standard process has its own vocabulary and unique procedures. For a newcomer to the world of standards this new parlance and approach can be quite daunting. It is difficult for users and interested parties to participate in the development of standards. This is due to the limited amount of time they can be away from their primary jobs and their limited travel budget. Hence, there are many manufacturers serving as members of the committee but only a few have voting status. Once the standard is approved by the society, then governmental agencies may adopt the standard. Other SDOs will usually use the approved standard as a basis for their own standard. They often will often adopt the standard or use that standard as a base for their own equipment standard.

Performance measures

Equipment standards are consensus-based standards for minimum safety and performance of medical equipment. They do not address how and where the equipment is to be used. The how and where the equipment is to be used are covered by clinical practice standards. Equipment standards normally focus on how the equipment is to react in the clinical environment; therefore these standards are not aimed at the clinicians and users, these standards are written for manufacturers and for governmental regulatory organizations. For example, in the US, the FDA would adopt a consensus standard and use that standard as a basis for pre-market approval of medical electrical devices. The FDA may choose and usually does add additional requirements to the consensus standards.

Before we discuss performance measures, a few definitions (ISO/FDIS 21647, 2003) are in order. Note that standards attempt to define terms in clear and unambiguous language as possible often using other defined terms as part of the definition. One has to realize that the definitions will be translated into many languages, and even though the "official" language of standards is English, there many variants of English. While it might seem obvious, what constitutes a RGM must be defined.

An RGM is defined as:

> *medical electrical equipment intended to measure the gas level(s) or partial pressure(s) in respiratory gases NOTE: The RGM consists of a complete monitor including accessories, sensor, and sampling tube (in the case of a diverting RGM) specified by the manufacturer in the accompanying documents for the intended use of the RGM. (Definition 3.15.)*

This definition is somewhat incomplete in that the scope of this IEC/ISO standard limits the device to use with humans and to continuous monitoring. It does not address spot check devices, such as those that use colorimetric techniques to measure carbon dioxide (CO_2).

By definition there are only two types of RGMs:

1. Where the sensor or detector is placed within the respiratory gas stream. There is an electronic cable connecting the sensor and to the supporting electronics. These devices are commonly known as a main-stream RGM. For purposes of the standard, a main-stream RGM is defined as a non-diverting RGM.
2. The other types of RGMs are the side-stream or diverting monitors. The diverting monitors removes a portion of the respiratory gas from the breathing circuit and transport the respiratory gasses via a tube to the sensor, which is located within the housing of the RGM. The standard clearly defines the distinction between what are commonly known as side- and main-stream gas monitors as well as the terms used to define each of these monitor types.

Another important definition is "sampling site". There may be some confusion about the "sampling site". For non-diverting monitors it is clear that the sample site is the location in the respiratory circuit of sensor. The confusion is for diverting monitors. Is the sampling site in the housing of the RGM, or could it be the location of where the respiratory gasses are sampled by a diverting RGM? The defined location of the "sampling site" for a diverting RGM is the "location at which respiratory gases are diverted for measurement to a remote sensor in a diverting RGM".

Measurement accuracy

Measurement accuracy is the ability for a RGM to determine what is actually in respiratory gas mixtures. This sounds fairly easy, but it turns out to be fairly difficult. There are many complicating factors here that the RGM has to take into account.

First, the composition of respiratory gases is not a binary or a two-part gas mixture (oxygen, O_2 and nitrogen) or even a three-part gas mixture, (O_2, nitrogen and CO_2). There are many different gases. There can be acetone (diabetic ketoacidosis), ethanol, methane (bowel obstruction) and the ever present, water vapor. Water vapor is disruptive to all current technologies for measuring respiratory gases. Diverting or side-stream RGMs are especially susceptible to interference by water. The gas sample with the water vapor is transported via the sampling tube (which is usually several feet long) from the sample site to the sensor. The water vapor will cool and start to condense. The condensate can cause obstruction to the flow of respiratory gases in the RGM or contaminate the sample site resulting in inaccurate respiratory gas measurements.

O_2 analyzers can be a very simple device used to measure the fraction inspired O_2 (F_IO_2 meter). There are several technologies that are currently used that are quite adequate, robust and inexpensive. There are other O_2 analyzers that can measure expired O_2 concentration on a breath-by-breath basis. The technology used in these O_2 analyzers is quite different than the simple F_IO_2 meter. The goal of the standard was not to render the simple, but adequate O_2 analyzers obsolete. Measurement accuracy is specified by the ISO/IEC standard is given in Table 39.1.

The next major difficulty in measurement accuracy is how does one take into account the actions of other gases present in the respiratory gas mixtures? Most equipment standards try to emulate clinical situations in their testing procedures. Trying to emulate clinical conditions is technically difficult. There are many different clinical conditions. Equipment standards try to develop testing apparatus and test procedures that are representative of clinical situations. Otherwise, the testing becomes difficult and subject to interpretation. The gas mixtures called for in the standard for measuring accuracy use nitrogen as the carrier gas. Most test gases do not contain O_2. The presence of O_2 degrades the shelf life of the test gases; the O_2 reacts with the halogenated agents and the walls of the containment vessel. Therefore, over time the O_2 concentration in the test gas mixtures changes. The test gases were also chosen so that they could be easily obtained in reasonable quantities and could be transported by routine methods. Certain combinations of halogenated agents in an O_2 mixture are not stable or potentially explosive. The accuracy requirements for halogenated anesthetic agents and nitrous oxide are broad. This is done purposely for two reasons: (a) halogenated agents are chemically very similar to each other and (b) historical.

Table 39.1 Measurement accuracy (from ISO/DIS 21647, 2003)

Gas	Measurement accuracy (gas levels in % volume fraction)
Halogenated agent	±(volume fraction of 0.2% + 15% of gas level)
CO_2	±(volume fraction of 0.43% + 8% of gas level)
Nitrous oxide	±(volume fraction of 2.0% + 8% of gas level)
O_2	±(volume fraction of 2.5% + 2.5% of gas level)

Another problem in the measurement of accuracy can be illustrated through accuracy statements for CO_2. In the previous standard, third iteration (ASTM F1456-01), the accuracy of CO_2 was stated in confusing language. The accuracy requirements were in a different format than other RGMs, that is, anesthetic agents and O_2 analyzers. The accuracy for CO_2 was referred as CO_2 plus or minus (by in fraction of 0.14% plus 8% of the gas level) gas levels in volume fraction %.

Measurement accuracy has been defined as the "quality which characterizes the ability of an RGM to give indications approximating to the true value of the quantity measured". The maximum inaccuracy for a capnograph has been defined in the standard as: CO_2 plus or minus (volume fraction of 0.43% plus 8% of gas level) gas levels in volume fraction %.

The offset provided some tightening of the specifications around 0, but not clinically or technically insurmountable and a little bit of loosening around the physiological that range again clinically not significant. A graphic illustration of the old (ISO 9918, 1993) and new (ISO/DIS 21647, 2003) statements is presented in Figure 39.1.

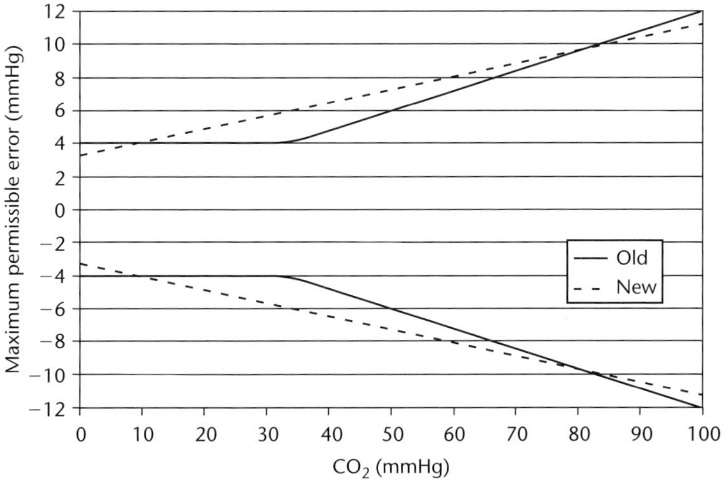

Figure 39.1 Maximum inaccuracy specification per ISO RGM standards.

Measurement range

Capnometers for clinical use must be able to detect CO_2 in the range of 0–10% or 76 mmHg. An extended range to 100 mmHg and greater can be useful for detection of gross hypercapnia.

Measurement drift

An RGM is usually left on for extended periods of time and may not be turned off for weeks or months at a time. When an electronic device such as a capnograph is initially powered on there is an interval of time where the device "warms up". After the "warm up" period the device can be used. If the device is used for an extended interval of time the calibration of the device may wander outside of normal operation. This wandering over an interval of time is called drift. A capnograph should be able to hold its calibration for a reasonable period of time. The capnograph should not have to be recalibrated or have its calibration checked every few hours – needed in the first generation machines. The standard of the current RGM addresses as drift of measurement. The monitor is set up in normal operating mode and allowed to stabilize for at least 6 h. At the beginning of the test the RGM is tested for accuracy. It is then tested for accuracy after operating for 6 h, then at 3 h intervals thereafter to ensure the accuracy has been maintained and there is not significant drift of measurement. The test gases try to mimic clinical situations. The test gases used in accuracy testing consist of CO_2, nitrous oxide, O_2 and anesthetic vapors with a balance of nitrogen. Since test gases that contain O_2 and anesthetic vapors are inherently unstable, this testing is kept to a minimum.

Response time

One of the most important features for the clinician is the total system response time. Basically, when there is a change in patient condition, when is the clinician notified of that change? The standard defines total system response time as the time from the step function change in gas levels at the sampling site to achieve a 90% of a final gas reading. This is often further subdivided into delay time and rise time. Delay time is sometimes called lag or transit time. Delay time depends on sampling flow rate, diameter and length of sampling tube, and sample viscosity. In general, faster flows, shorter tubes with larger lumens, and lower viscosity result in shorter delay time. Rise time can be characterized in a number of ways. All relate to the assumption that the 0–100% response is exponential and lengthy. In most applications we are not interested in how long it takes to obtain 100% response: 90% or 95% is usually satisfactory (see Figure 39.2). By subjecting a measuring system to an instantaneous change, that is, a change that is very fast compared with the response of the system being measured, we

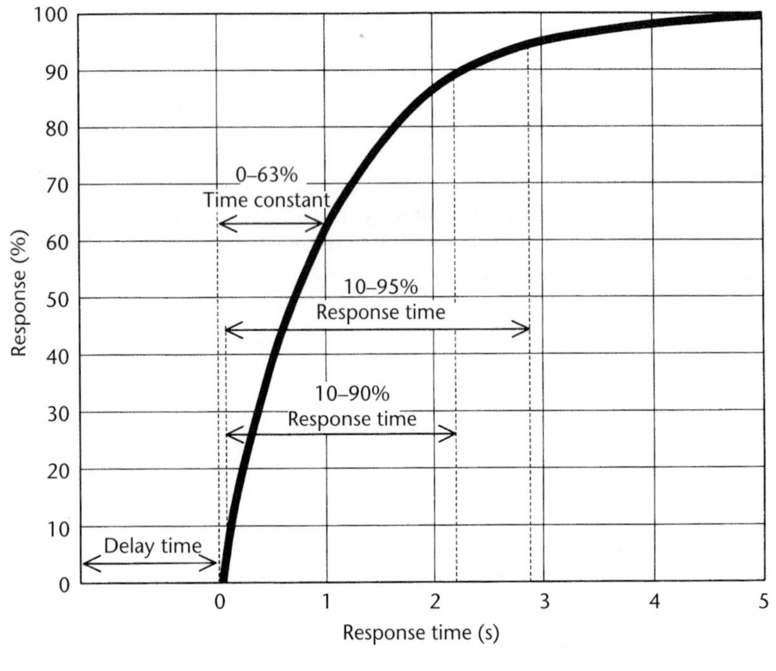

Figure 39.2 For side-stream sampling, total response time is equal to the delay or transit time in the sampling catheter plus the measurement rise time which is expressed different ways. (Reproduced from Gravenstein, J.S., Paulus, D.A. & Hayes, T.J. (1989). *Capnography in Clinical Practice,* 2nd edition. Butterworth-Heinemann, Boston.)

can measure the true response characteristics of the system. This is sometimes referred to as a step change. The manufacturers are to disclose the total response time to the clinician so that the clinicians can make a reasonable comparison between varieties of manufacturers. Non-diverting capnographs have an advantage in this area, as there is no delay time.

For main-stream or non-diverting RGMs, the total system response time is primarily a function of how fast the respiratory gas starts flowing past the sensor. The RGM standard standardizes the flow of gases as specific velocity so that manufacturers with different sample size cells have a level of playing field of about total system response time. It is now possible to compare performance of pediatric and adult RGMs. For diverting or side-stream RGMs, the manufacturer must list the total system response time for each sample flow rate that the RGM is designed to operate with. This way the clinician can begin to compare a variety of diverting RGMs because the total system response time is highly dependent on the sample flow rate. For example, with a neonatal respiratory circuit, it would be inappropriate for a sample rate to be 250 ml/min; this sample flow rate would be the little flow left for mechanical ventilation of the infant and render mechanical ventilation inadequate. But the total system's response time would be quite good. On the other hand, a 10 ml/min sample rate on an adult patient would have an inadequate total system response time.

What response time is necessary? The answer to that question has two parts. First, response time must be fast enough to measure both end-tidal and inspiratory gas concentrations accurately. Second, response time should also be fast enough to provide a high-fidelity display of the concentration waveform. Interpretation is valid only when the waveform accurately represents the profile, or at least, accurately enough to detect the events for which the patient is being monitored.

Interfering gas and vapor effects

The quantitative effects (if any) on gas readings caused by the interfering gases given by the gas levels listed in Table 39.2 shall be disclosed in the instructions for use (e.g. users or service manual). The capnometer can and usually encounters unexpected gases as well as new anesthetic and therapeutic gases. It is the intent of the standard to require the manufacturer to disclosure the effects of these gases on the measurement of CO_2. These unexpected gasses may cause the capnometer to display falsely low or high readings.

Table 39.2 Test gas levels of interfering gases and vapors (from ISO/FDIS 21647, 2003)

Gas or vapor	Gas level (% volume fraction)
Nitrous oxide	60[a]
Halothane	4[a]
Enflurane	5[a]
Isoflurane	5[a]
Sevoflurane	5[a]
Xenon	80[b]
Helium	50[c]
Metered dose-inhaler propellants	Specified by the manufacturer
Desflurane	15[a]
Ethanol	Specified by the manufacturer
Isopropanol alcohol	Specified by the manufacturer
Acetone	Specified by the manufacturer
Methane	Specified by the manufacturer

Test gas levels shall be ±20 % of the specified level.
[a] If intended for use with inhalation halogenated agents.
[b] If intended for use with xenon.
[c] If intended for use with helium.

Commonly occurring interfering gases include ethanol, acetone (e.g. diabetic ketoacidosis) and methane (e.g. bowel obstruction). Isopropanol, primary ingredient in "alcohol wipes", is used as a cleaning agent for medical equipment. During the cleaning of medical equipment capnographs may inadvertently sample vapors of isopropanol resulting in a prolonged inaccuracy of capnograph, depending on the technology used. Xenon, a relatively new anesthetic vapor primarily utilized in a research environment, has some major technology problems to over come before becoming widely used. Helium O_2 mixtures (i.e. heliox) are now quite commonly used in patients with upper respiratory airway obstruction to help bridge the patient with an obstructed airway until definitive management can completed. The propellants used in metered dose inhalers and frequently in the operating room, intensive care and emergency room settings can cause interference in RGMs.

Units

As international organizations, both the ISO and IEC normally require all units of measurement to be expressed in the metric system. Unfortunately, medicine has not completely adapted or converted over to the metric system. It is common and easier to use the traditional non-metric units of measure for certain

Table 39.3 RGM alarm priorities (from ISO/FDIS 21647, 2003)

Gas	Alarm condition priority	
	Low gas level	High gas level
Inspired halogenated anesthetic agent	Low priority[a]	Medium priority
Exhaled CO_2	Medium priority	Medium priority
Inspired CO_2	–	Medium priority
Inspired nitrous oxide	Low priority[a]	Medium priority[a]
Inspired O_2	Medium priority	Medium priority[a]
Inspired $O_2 < 18\%$	High priority	–
Multiple halogenated anesthetic agents present[b]	Medium priority	Medium priority
Multiple halogenated anesthetic agents value <3MAC[c]	Low priority	Low priority
Multiple halogenated anesthetic agents value >3MAC[c]	medium priority	Medium priority

The priorities listed are the minimum priority. Exhaled gas level alarm conditions may also be provided.
[a] This alarm condition is optional.
[b] When the RGM is capable of detecting but not capable of quantifying and displaying the mixture of halogenated anesthetic agents.
[c] When the RGM is capable of detecting, quantifying and displaying the mixture of halogenated anesthetic agents.

measurements, such as volume percent to express the concentration of anesthetic gases and vapors[1] and mmHg for the measurement of CO_2.

Alarm systems

There has been a lot of work recently with medical alarms with new definitions of alarm conditions, and alarm signals which has been published as IEC 60601-1-8 (2003). The equipment manufacturers typically had to develop alarms as needed and saw fit. It is common to have a variety of alarm protocols in one operating room and these different protocols differ from room to room, to post-anesthetic care unit (PACU), and to intensive care unit (ICU). Large manufacturers could have different protocols with different product lines. This standard has been through many lively discussions, heated drafts and contentious voting cycles. It has unified the clinical alarm protocols in a single document. Basically, three different types of alarm conditions are defined: high, medium and low priority with a variety of alarm signals mandated by the alarm condition. To simplify it, low-priority alarm condition triggers a low-priority alarm which is just notification, usually a blinking light. A medium-priority alarm condition signals a medium-priority alarm, which is a beep and a flashing light. A high-priority alarm condition results in a high-priority alarm signal, usually flashing lights and beeping sirens. The respiratory gas alarm condition priorities are listed in Table 39.3. The only high-priority alarm listed in the entire table is for when the fracture inspired O_2 is less than 18%. This is life-threatening and could be caused by a mechanical failure and usually is not the result of a clinical intervention. For anesthetic agents there is a two-tiered alarm system based upon if the RGM can quantitate a mixture of anesthetic agents.

Luer connections

The Luer connector is the most common connector in the entire hospital. It connects every single piece of intravenous (i.v.) tubing, every single needle and a variety of other devices together. The Luer connector is defined as a 6% conical taper by international standard (ISO 594-1, 1986; ISO 594-2, 1998). The Luer connector is a compact, secure and easily manufactured connector. This has given rise to its ubiquity within the hospital. Unfortunately, it has created some problems. In Europe there is a report of cross-connects between i.v. and enteral feeding systems and several medication errors have been linked to Luer connectors. The European Committee for Standardization, CEN commissioned a report by the CEN Healthcare Sector Forum (CEN/CHeF) to examine if there was a problem with the use of Luer connectors. The investigative committee was tasked with reviewing the world's medical literature involving Luer connectors and cross-connects. After an extensive search of the world's literature, they found

[1] The standard does provide that anesthetic vapors be converted over to MAC values, minimum alveolar concentration values. The manufacturer must either use the standard MAC values of a healthy 40-year-old adult male patient which is published in the package insert mandated by the US FDA or disclose how MAC values are derived.

about a dozen reports of cross-connects. These cross-connects occurred mainly in two categories: (1) enteral feeding devices being connected to the i.v. systems and (2) pneumatic powered devices being connected to i.v. systems. Several of the cross-connects was the result of patients themselves mistakenly connecting one system to the other system. The CEN/CHef recommended that Luer connectors be limited to the i.v. systems only and sought to develop new connectors for all other systems, such as respiratory, gastrointestinal, urinary and neuroaxial. The task of developing new connector systems has now been given to the CEN BTTF Task Force. They are currently in the process of trying to develop new series of connectors for these other systems. The risk assessment for harm to the patient as it relates to RGMs is solely related to cross-connect of the exhaust port of diverting (i.e. side-stream) monitors. Note that the current standard mandates that the exhaust port shall not be a Luer connector and as such significantly decreases the risk of the exhaust port being connected to an i.v. system thereby causing harm to the patient. Cross-connects of the inlet port to the diverting or side-stream RGMs present no hazard to the patient. The sample tube connection to the breathing circuit is usually a female Luer connection. This is clinically important because dose-inhaler bronchodilator medications are given through this port as well as resuscitative drugs. Unfortunately, an i.v. or feeding tube can also be attached to this port, but there is a large disparity in size of i.v. tube connections and it is quite obvious that this is not to be connected to either enteral or i.v. fluids. The manufacturers of enteral feedings are aggressively pursuing new connections through the CEN BTTF Task Force and are independently working to eliminate cross-connects with Luer fittings.

The current standard

The current ISO/IEC RGM standard is a combination of individual standards of O_2 analyzers, capnographs and anesthetic agent monitors. This is at least the third generation of each of these individual standards and prior to this, each individual standard had flaws where the manufacturer could not meet the standard or meet the other standard that affected his integrated RGM. The RGM is primarily written for manufacturers to ensure that all RGMs act the same way in the clinical environment and for regulators to have a basis of accepting or rejecting new RGMs. For clinicians, the standard serves as a basis for comparison of RGMs, ensuring that all RGMs work in a similar function.

Electromagnetic interference and radiation

Noise is unwanted signal. It has as its cause factors that are both external and internal to the measuring system. Noise cannot only interfere with our ability to get accurate quantitative information but also, in gas analysis, may obscure some details of waveform that may be important. External sources include electromagnetic radiation in the radio frequency range. Radio transmitters, oscillators and power lines, for example, transmit noise in a narrow band. Wide-band sources include radiation from the stratosphere, and discharges from various electrical equipment (X-ray, motors, pumps, lighting, etc.). An electrical conductor can act as an antenna for the reception of this type of signal. Interference can be greatly reduced by proper shielding, which involves enclosing the critical conductors in a conductive material that is grounded. Therefore standards have been developed to test medical equipment for their immunity to electromagnetic interferences as well as to assure that they do not emit electromagnetic interference that might interfere with other equipment. A collateral standard, IEC 60601-1-2 (2001) has been developed and describes these tests.

Calibration

Long-term stability is an important criterion and determines the frequency of calibration. Even if calibration is automatic, it requires time and may interrupt monitoring. Indeed, to attain the full benefits of capnography, for example, monitoring must be continuous. Automatic zeroing during the inspiratory phase is particularly troublesome because inspiratory gas occasionally contains CO_2 (e.g. when an expiratory valve fails or the CO_2 absorber is exhausted). As a practical matter, lengthy procedures for calibration should be required infrequently and brief ones no more than once a day. Most modem infrared capnographs are stable for at least 1 month, and perhaps longer; some claim 1 year. There are various ways to confirm the accuracy of end-tidal values of CO_2 when an instrument generates data that do not match clinical expectations. An optical filter, a beam occluder, or a sample cell containing CO_2 or gas from a cylinder, all produce signals that can confirm the operation of the instrument.

End note

The tables in this chapter are from ISO/DIS 21647 with permission of the American National Standards Institute

References

ASTM F1456-01 (2001). Standard specification for minimum performance and safety requirements for capnometers.

Gravenstein, J.S., Paulus, D.A. & Hayes, T. (1995). *Gas Monitoring in Clinical Practice*, 2nd edition. Butterworth-Heineman, Newton, Massachusetts.

ISO 9918 (1993). Capnometers for use with humans-requirements.

ISO/DIS 21647 (2003). Medical electrical equipment – particular requirements for the basic safety and essential performance of respiratory gas monitors.

IEC 60601-1 (1988). Medical electrical equipment. Part 1: General requirements for safety. December.

IEC 60601-1-2 (2001). Medical electrical equipment. Part 1–2: General requirements for safety – collateral standard: electromagnetic compatibility–requirements and tests. September.

IEC 60601-1-8 (2003). Medical electrical equipment. Part 1–8: General requirements for safety – collateral standard: general requirements, tests and guidance for alarm systems in medical electrical equipment and medical electrical systems. August.

ISO 594-1 (1986). Conical fittings with a 6% (Luer) taper for syringes, needles and certain other medical equipment. Part 1: General requirements.

ISO 594-2 (1998). Conical fittings with 6% (Luer) taper for syringes, needles and certain other medical equipment. Part 2: Lock fittings.

CARBON DIOXIDE MEASUREMENT 40

M.B. Jaffe

In this chapter we review technical aspects of carbon dioxide (CO_2) measurement techniques currently available – infrared (IR), acoustic, colorimetric, and mass spectrometry with a focus on IR-based approaches. The interesting Raman method is no longer commercially available and therefore not discussed. We are also comparing mainstream and sidestream approaches. Before discussing the technologies, some interesting properties of CO_2 will be reviewed.

CO_2 and its physical properties

Interest in the critical role of CO_2 in such essential phenomena as metabolism, photosynthesis, combustion, and environmental temperature control, has furthered the development of a number of methods to detect and quantify CO_2. Carbon dioxide's well-documented physical properties are the key to understanding the relevant analytic techniques (Table 40.1).

At normal temperatures and pressures, CO_2 is a colorless, odorless gas. Its concentration in air is so small (0.03%) that air is usually treated as if the partial pressure of CO_2 (PCO_2) were zero. This may not be so in some poorly ventilated rooms or encapsulated spaces (submarines) where the PCO_2 can rise above 1% of ambient pressure.

CO_2 has a molecular weight of 44, is very soluble in polar solvents such as water, and reacts with water to form carbonic acid, a weak acid. Also, this molecule is easily fragmented and ionized to form charged species. It has optical absorption bands in the IR spectrum. There is a remarkable similarity between some of the physical properties of CO_2 and nitrous oxide (N_2O). Both deviate from the ideal gas law to the same degree, as indicated by their mole volumes of 22.25 l instead of the ideal mole volume of 22.4 l. Both are soluble in water, which is an advantage physiologically but a disadvantage with on-line methods of

Table 40.1 Selected CO_2 devices used clinically

Technology	Type	Manufacturer	Model(s)**	References of interest
IR	Mainstream	Respironics-Novametrix (Wallingford, CT)	Capnostat® III,V	Knodle *et al.*, 1990, 1994
	Mainstream	Protocol (Pryon) (MenomoneeFalls, WI)	SC-300	Knodle & Clary, 1997
	Sidestream	Respironics-Novametrix (Wallingford, CT)	LoFlo™	Rich *et al.*, 2003
	Sidestream	Oridion (Needham, MA; Jerusalem, IL)	Microstream®	Coleman & Krauss, 1999
Colorimetric	Indicator-metacresol purple	Nellcor Puritan-Bennett (Pleasanton,CA)	EasyCap® II	Fehder, 1988
Photoacoustic	–	Innova AirTech Instruments (Ballerup, Denmark)	Model 1312	Nexo *et al.*, 1989
Mass Spectroscopy	Quadrupole	Centronic Limited (Croydon/UK)	MGA 200	–

**Monitor or sensor technology/name.

analysis in wet systems where out-gassing in a rapidly changing concentration can be a problem. N_2O also has absorption bands in the IR spectrum, some of them close to those of CO_2.

Measuring gas concentration in a respired gas requires a continuous, fast response and the ability to distinguish different gases from each other. This technology is very different from that used to measure CO_2 in a sample of gas or blood. The technologies that have been successful rely on the asymmetric modes of molecular vibration to enable CO_2 to absorb IR light; the symmetric modes of vibration to enable CO_2 scatter light (Raman) and the ability of the molecule to be charged in an electron beam to enable the use of mass spectrometry.

The electromagnetic spectrum can be described by wavelength (λ), wave number ($1/\lambda$), and frequency ($v = c/\lambda$), where c is the velocity of light. IR spectroscopists use wave number because it is proportional to energy:

$$E = hv = hc/\lambda,$$

where h is Planck's constant. This relationship is a reminder that higher energy quanta have higher frequencies, higher wave numbers, and shorter wavelengths. Some of these frequencies have enough energy to ionize molecules (roentgen and ultraviolet), some are absorbed and cause chemical reactions (ultraviolet and visible), and some influence the vibration and rotation of molecules (IR). The IR spectrum begins just beyond the red part of the visible spectrum (0.4–0.8 μm) and extends to approximately 40 m. (10^{-6} m = 1 μm) The near ultraviolet begins at 0.2 μm and extends up to the visible. The far ultraviolet (less than 0.2 μm) and the X-ray region involve high-energy quanta. Generally, the last two have not been practical nor suitable for on-line clinical gas monitoring because of safety concerns.

Infrared

General description

The IR part of the spectrum has some distinct advantages for medical monitoring. IR energy is safe because it causes no permanent changes in the molecule. The absorption of IR light increases molecular rotation and vibration, which increases temperature and pressure, but only modestly. Therefore, IR technology can be used on-line to measure respiratory gases. Blackbody radiators heated to moderate temperatures can be used to radiate IR energy, which can be detected by a host of solid-state devices. Materials that can transmit IR energy are readily available for

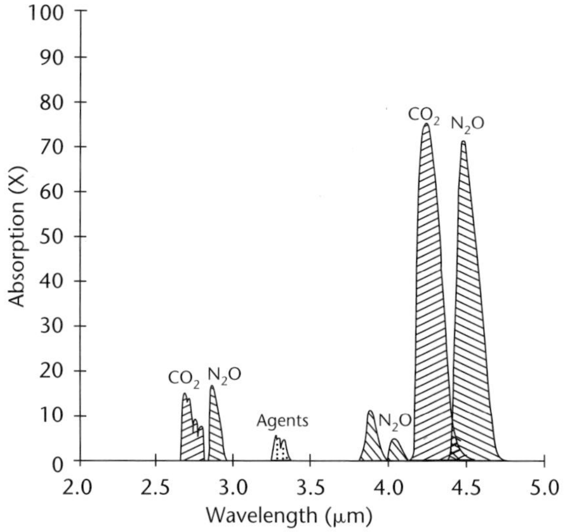

Figure 40.1 The IR absorption spectrum for the gases CO_2 and N_2O and the volatile anesthetic agents (from Raemer & Calalang, 1991). (Reproduced with permission from Raemer, D.B. & Calalang, I. (1991). Accuracy of end-tidal carbon dioxide tension analyzers. *J. Clin. Monit.*, **7**: 195–208.)

sample cell windows and filters. In other words, IR instruments are simple and relatively inexpensive.

CO_2 has a strong absorption band in the near IR region (4.26 μm), which lies between two strong bands for water vapor and yet is separated enough from the main bands of most other potentially interfering molecules (Figure 40.1).

IR absorption requirements

In order to absorb IR radiation, a molecule must be both asymmetric and polyatomic. Atoms or molecules such as helium, argon, hydrogen, oxygen, and nitrogen do not satisfy these requirements and, therefore, do not absorb IR radiation. CO_2, N_2O, and water do. However, molecular asymmetry does not simply mean that different atoms exist in the same molecule. It also means that allowed IR vibrations will cause centers of electrical charge to be displaced; in other words, an allowed vibration will alter the molecule's dipole moment. A dipole consists of two equal and opposite electrical charges that are slightly separated. Its moment is the product of charge and distance. CO_2 serves as a good example of the principles involved because it has both symmetric and asymmetric vibrations. The frequency with which these vibrations occur depends on the masses of the atoms as well as the strength of the bond holding the atoms together. These vibrations occur at frequencies on the order of 1013 per second. This corresponds to frequencies found within the IR part of the spectrum. Absorption of IR energy simply increases the amplitude of these vibrations but does not change their frequencies. As a linear molecule with n atoms has $3n - 5$ fundamental vibrations, CO_2 ($n = 3$) must have four fundamental vibrational modes. For CO_2, two IR-active fundamental vibrations are predicted and two are found: one at 2349 cm^{-1} (4.26 μm) and the other at 667 cm^{-1} (14.99 μm). Fortunately, the high-intensity waveband for CO_2 at 4.26 μm lies between two intense bands for water. With carefully characterized, narrow-band pass optical filters, CO_2 can be measured with little interference either from water vapor or from the neighboring band for N_2O! (Alpert *et al.*, 1970).

Pressure broadening

As we have seen, IR absorption is a measure of the vibrational frequencies of atoms within a molecule. Associated with these vibrational absorptions bands are a number of other lines related to the rotation of the molecule. These energy transitions are usually small and are sometimes called rotational or sidebands. Overall then, the IR spectra of gases are due to a combination of transitions involving both vibrational and rotational energy levels, which combine to produce a band structure. These transitions depend on factors both internal and external to the molecule. Internally, the vibrational frequencies depend on the strength of the bond between atoms and their relative masses. Rotation depends on their moments of inertia. Externally, temperature, spatial arrangement of atoms, intermolecular forces, and collisions between molecules influence these transitions. This external relationship results in absorptions that depend on the other molecules in the gas mixture as these influence intermolecular forces. Collisional dependence can be seen empirically because sidebands widen as the pressure increases. As pressure decreases (either due to changes in total pressure or the PCO_2), less intermolecular collisions occur and the bandwidth narrows. Similarly, as the pressure increases, more collisions occur and the bandwidth widens (Bergman *et al.*, 1958). This dependence on pressure is recognized in the usual terminology-collision or pressure broadening and tends to be not device-specific (Kennell *et al.*, 1973). It is a complex function of the total pressure and the presence of other gases. In effect, the absorption band is spread out and the use of narrow-band sources or filters fail to correct for this effect. System software using nominal values typically compensates for this effect.

Consequently, a calibration curve depends not only on total pressure but also on the constituents of the gas mixture. Change the constituents and the curve changes. Correction for this effect is perhaps most important for CO_2 because CO_2 is usually present in relatively low concentrations (5%) along with other gases that can vary greatly and reach high concentrations. In the intensive care unit (ICU), for example, CO_2 will be measured in expired gas and in a wide variety of O_2 concentrations; in the operating room (OR), measurements will be made in the presence of high concentrations of N_2O and O_2 as well as low concentrations of volatile anesthetic agents. It is not expected that the accuracy of measurement of N_2O, present in high concentrations will be much influenced by relatively small amounts of CO_2 and volatile anesthetic agents. Correction for the significant concentrations of O_2, however, has not been reported; the effect is probably small and the accuracy requirements for N_2O is not great.

The measured absorption of CO_2 can be altered by cross-interference and collision broadening due to the presence of gases such as N_2O and O_2. Cross-interference, the overlapping of absorption bands of other gases, can occur from N_2O due to the presence of strong absorption bands that slightly overlap both edges of the CO_2 band (Figure 40.1). The impact of this effect can vary significantly between devices. However, the use of narrow-band sources or narrow-band filters in front of the detector with sufficiently small half power bandwidths can effectively eliminate the effect of cross-interference.

Lambert–Beer law

All IR instruments consist of a radiation source, a cell through which samples of gas flow, and a detector that produce a signal related to the intensity of the radiation that is detected. The quantitative aspects of photometric measurement are stated by the Lambert–Beer law as:

$$A = \log(I_0/I) = \varepsilon I_c$$

Under carefully controlled conditions at a select absorption band, the absorbance of a sample (A) is proportional both to the concentration of sample (c) and the depth of the absorbing layer (I). The molar extinction coefficient (ε) is a wavelength-dependent constant characterizing the sample. I_0 is the intensity of radiation with no sample in the beam and I the intensity with a sample. For solutions, absorbencies are additive. Absorbance then can also be written as minus the log of the transmittance ($A = -\log T$), which denotes that the relationship between concentration and transmittance is non-linear. Transmittance approaches zero as concentration approaches infinity.

However, there is a part of the range that is close to linear.

In the IR region, gases do not follow the Lambert–Beer law because of the pressure-broadening effect. Both total pressure and diluent gases influence the sidebands and, thus, the amount of radiation absorbed. However, under controlled conditions, calibration curves can be constructed, the influence of perturbations studied, and quantitations made.

Non-dispersive IR monitors

IR absorption methods of gas measurement can be sensitive and selective as well as provide a continuous, accurate, precise, and rapid response that is not saturated nor damaged by high concentration of the "target" gases such as CO_2. Most continuous monitors of respiratory gases are of the non-dispersive IR (NDIR) type; there is no provision for dispersing the radiation into its component wavelengths as in dispersive types (i.e. spectrometers). The "essentials" of nearly all IR gas analyzer are (a) a source of IR radiation with an emission spectrum that includes the absorption bands of the gases to be measured; (b) a sample cell fitted with windows "possessing" suitable transmission properties; (c) an optical or gas filter to limit the wavelength range measured by the detector; (d) a means, either physical in the form of a rotating chopper disk or an electronic circuit, to modulate the IR radiation from the source; and (e) a detector to convert the IR radiation into an electrical signal (Hill & Powell, 1968). NDIR-type devices can be classified into two categories based upon whether or not the device uses a selective or non-selective detector. A selective detector would use a narrow-band filter so that only light within that band would be measured whereas a non-selective design would not use such filtering. NDIR-type devices can be further divided into double-beam-in-space or double-beam-in-time (i.e. single path, dual wavelength) (Hill & Powell, 1968). The primary components of an IR system, the source, the detector, and chopper will be described in greater detail.

Sources

The source of IR radiation may be broad- or narrow-band. It may be electronically pulsed or constant and chopped mechanically. It may be filtered with narrow-band filters either at the source or the detectors. For narrow-band emission, some sidestream monitors use an electric discharge source consisting of a hermetically sealed glass tube containing a gas. The gas is excited by the application of a high voltage, radio frequency electromagnetic field. This results in the emission of a narrow IR spectrum. Benches with broad-band sources also utilize reliable and stable narrow-band interference filters in front of the detectors to measure in-band signal for CO_2 and separately out-of-band signal as a reference channel. Thus, one can select only a portion of the CO_2 band effectively eliminating any interference from water vapor or even closer bands of N_2O. The absorption of the IR radiation by CO_2 is non-linear, affected by the presence of other gases and proportional to gas concentration, path length, and absorption coefficient of the particular gas. The non-linearities, path length, and specifics of the bench design are compensated for with data from an empirical lookup table that translates the measured signals to a value in CO_2 which is then corrected by most manufacturers for the effects of gases such as O_2 and N_2O.

Detectors

Detectors can be a microphone or solid state. Microphone-type detectors are filled with IR absorbing gas, which is heated by the radiation it receives and expands as a consequence. The microphone detector can have a single chamber or a dual chamber. The single-chamber type is also called the Veingerov design (Veingerov, 1938), and the dual-chamber type is called the Luft design (Luft, 1943). In the Luft design the diaphragm separates the two chambers. The single-chamber design has less drift but is more sensitive to vibration. The position of the diaphragm can be detected by capacitance techniques or by measuring the gas flow from one chamber to the other. Another way of designing a respiratory gas detector, common to nearly all current commercial devices, is to use solid-state sensors that have broad-spectral sensitivity and an optical filter that transmits radiation in the appropriate region. These filters can be made with bandwidths that are quite narrow, 5% of the peak wavelength at 50% transmission. An excellent detector for gases such as CO_2 with strong absorption peaks in the near IR range is lead selenide because of its broad-spectral response in the near IR region. It is sometimes thermoelectrically cooled to improve signal-to-noise ratio. One limitation of the solid-state detector is lower sensitivity (relative to the microphone types of the same path length) when the measured concentrations are low. The disadvantages of the microphone designs include vibration sensitivity and higher cost.

Chopper

The use of a chopper, either mechanical or electronic, permits a common source and detector in the double-beam-in-time types but has the added advantage of producing and alternating signals, one from the sample beam and the other from the reference beam. The PCO_2 is then calculated using the difference of the transmittance of the two measured signals. Also a chopper can be used to modulate the IR source and a beam splitter used so that half of the light is seen by a detector with a filter selective to a strong absorption band for CO_2 and the other half seen by a detector with a filter selective to a region of the IR spectrum where little or no IR radiation is absorbed by CO_2. The PCO_2 is then calculated using the ratio of the transmittance of the two measured signals.

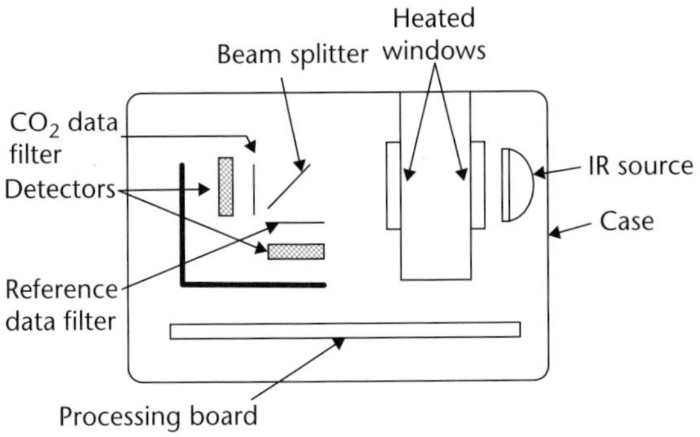

Figure 40.2 Cross-section of representative solid-state mainstream coaxial design.

Some analyzers use a single beam with a rotating filter wheel. This has the advantage of combining the signal modulation produced by the chopper with multi-gas monitoring, as well as source and sample cell monitoring with a reference cell. Appropriate optical filters are mounted in the wheel along with a reference cell. Each revolution provides the necessary optical information to calculate gas concentrations. For greater detail on IR spectroscopy and IR instrumentation consult any of the excellent references books (Kruse *et al.*, 1962; Alpert *et al.*, 1970) (Figure 40.2).

Other methods

Photoacoustic spectroscopy

Photoacoustic spectroscopy (PAS) combines pulsed excitation of the gas by IR energy and acoustic detection of the pressure changes by a sensitive microphone (Rosencwaig, 1980). Photoexcitation is accomplished by intermittently exposing the gas sample to filtered IR radiation. In this regard, it is much like transmission IR spectrometry in which one needs a source, filter, chopper, and detector (Figure 40.3). The benefits of a chopper in transmission IR technique have been discussed. Here, however, the chopper serves a different function. It is an essential part of the signal, not part of a detection strategy. IR energy causes changes in the vibrational and rotational energy of the molecule.

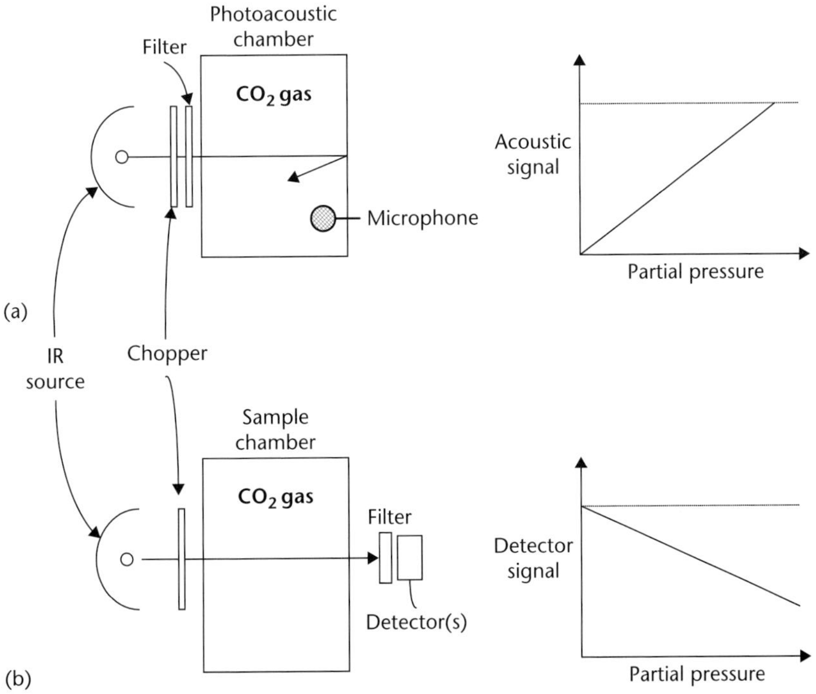

Figure 40.3 Contrast of two methods (a) photoacoustic spectroscopy and (b) transmission IR spectroscopy.

This energy can be transferred to neighboring molecules through collisions, which increases their translational (kinetic) energy. This results in an increase in collisional frequency, or, in other words, an increase in pressure. All of this occurs very quickly, so that during the dark periods, the collisional frequency decreases and the pressure drops. A microphone detects this cyclical change in pressure. The system is designed so that the frequency of the pressure (sound) wave differs for each gas. The sequence for PAS is

light → absorption → heating → thermal expansion → pressure wave → acoustic detection,

whereas for transmission IR spectrometry it is instead:

light → absorption → photo-optical detection.

Colorimetric

Chemical sensors trace their roots to observations made in 1916 and to basic chemistry. The influence of CO_2 on pH is well described by the Henderson–Hasselbalch equation. Increasing CO_2 concentration in an aqueous medium causes the concentration (activity) of the hydrogen ion to increase and consequently the pH decreases. This relationship describes the underlying mechanism of the Stow–Severinghaus P_aCO_2 electrode, which is part of every blood gas analyzer.

In addition to electrometric detection involving pH electrodes, a change in pH can be followed by a change in color of a dye solution. The yellow–red color change of a phenol sulfonphthalein solution, for example, occurs over a pH range of 6.6–8.0, making it useful for acid–base titrations. Marriott (1916) first explored carbon dioxide's visual detection for medical purposes. Draper (1938) later suggested using bromoscresol purple in a calcium carbonate solution to detect rebreathing. Later, Berman and associates (1984) advocated a cresol red, phenolphthalein solution to confirm placement of the endotracheal tube.

These suggestions did not receive wide acceptance because the methods were inconvenient, requiring the placement of an aqueous solution in the breathing circuit and they are not fast enough for breath-to breath detection. In general, an acceptable device should include a stable dye that does not produce toxic fumes, low air-flow resistance and dead-space so as not to compromise the work of breathing and a color change that is fast and not red–green so as not to eliminate 8% of the population that is color blind. Also it should be easily incorporated into the breathing circuit. A number of colorimetric devices have been available over the last several years. Table 40.2 presents the specifications of two representative devices. These disposable detectors, when placed at the endotracheal tube, makes possible the viewing of the color of a mesh substrate coated with an indicator dye. Surrounding each detector area is a color chart.

In general, the color change should be observed for at least several breaths before interpreting results. They are not generally affected by N_2O, volatile anesthetic agents, and short exposures to water vapor. The color fades after a period of use measured in hours, so it is not intended for long-term use. Shelf life up to 24 months is claimed for some devices if the foil package is unopened. Investigators report generally good performance of colorimetric devices but they note its

Table 40.2 Representative colormetric devices

Device name/ manufacturer	CO_2 color changes		Dead-space (ml)	Flow resistance, weight, recommended patient size max usage time
EASY CAP® II[1] Nellcor Inc.	Purple "A" – slight change in color "B" – light purple to tan "C" – hues of yellow	"room" air 0.03 to <0.5% 0.5 to <2% 2–5	25	3 cmH_2O at 60 LPM 20 g >15 kg Up to 2 h
StatCO2™ Mercury medical	Blue Green Yellow	No CO_2 present 1–2% CO_2 >5%	25	3 cmH_2O at 60 LPM 22 g >15 kg Up to 24 h

[1] Introduced to the market as the forced mid-expiratory flow (FEF) end-tidal CO_2 detector by Fenem Inc and later acquired by Nellcor Inc.

Sources: Nellcor Puritan Bennett Inc. EASY CAP II brochure, 1997 and Mercury Medical StatCO2 brochure 2003.

problems include that they are semi quantitative, have no alarms, difficult to read in the dark, and have suggested their use only if quantitative capnometry is not available (Petroianu *et al.*, 1998). Additionally, Puntervoll *et al.* (2002) compared capnography to a colorimetric device and noted that it may falsely indicate correct tracheal intubation when the tube is in fact in the esophagus due to the device's sensitivity to low CO_2 values.

Mass spectroscopy

Two types of mass spectrometers have been important medically: the magnetic sector with fixed detectors and the quadrupole. Each has been used either as a dedicated instrument providing continuous monitoring of single patients or as a shared instrument (multiplexed) providing discontinuous monitoring of several patients in sequence.

Magnetic sector-fixed detector

In the same way that light can be separated into its component wavelengths using a prism or diffraction grating, so too can a gas mixture be separated into its component parts by a combined electric and magnetic field. Sample gas is aspirated into a vacuum chamber and, there, is ionized by an electron beam. The charged fragments are accelerated by an electric field into a dispersion chamber where they are separated according to mass by an orthogonal magnetic field. Discrete detectors in the focal plane measure the component gases.

Quadrupole mass filter

The magnetic sector and quadrupole instruments are similar in that both require a high vacuum because the mean free path (distance traveled between collisions) must be long compared with the chamber dimensions and because the separation scheme requires that the particles be charged (Barrington, 1963). The principles used for separation, however, are quite different. The quadrupole is really a mass filter that depends on the influence of a combined direct current (DC) and radio frequency field (Figure 40.4). Four parallel rods are designed so that the tuning of the combined fields will result in particles of only one type traversing the longitudinal axis and ending up at the ion collector. The trajectory of all others is such that they strike one of the four rods and are removed from the ion beam. Changing the voltages in a controlled way makes it possible to scan the mass spectrum. This can be done in a few milliseconds. Sampling the collector output at appropriate times in the scan makes it possible to measure the component masses. Scanning and sampling repetitively provide continuous monitoring.

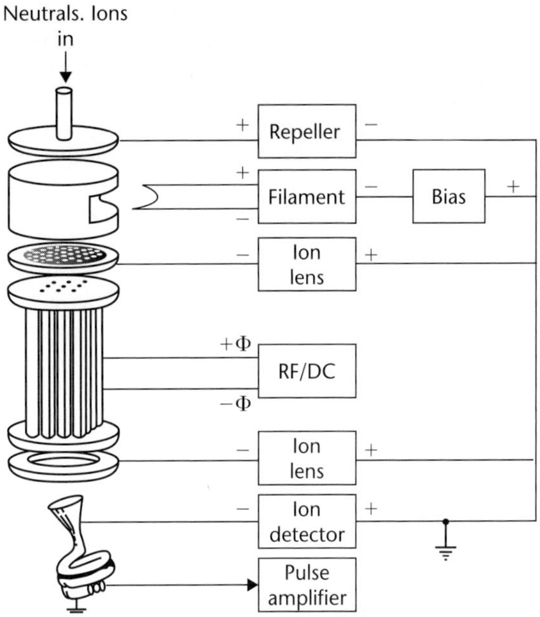

Figure 40.4 Instrumental design of a miniature linear quadrupole array, showing a miniature ionization source, the quadrupole rod array and ceramic jigs for positioning, and an electron multiplier detector. Each quadrupole rod is 25 mm long and has a radius of 1 mm. (From Orient *et al.*,1997.)

Technical challenges

A mass spectrometer presents interesting design challenges. In part, these involve moving a gas sample at atmospheric pressure to a distant measurement chamber, which is at a low pressure–and doing so without altering the relative concentrations of the component gases. It turns out that gas flow at high and low pressures are influenced by different relationships. These relationships must be understood and appropriate measurement strategies implemented to get reliable results. In the ionization chamber, gas molecules will be charged and split into fragments. These must be identified and traced to their parent molecule. Some overlap of fragments is to be expected and corrections must be formulated. Similarly, CO_2 and N_2O present a problem, as each has a molecular weight close to 44. In addition, agents with large molecular weights may be beyond the mass range of most spectrometers; therefore, their fragments must be measured.

Advances have been made on the miniaturization of the various component systems of a variety of the mass spectrometer types including the sample introduction,

ion source, mass analyzer, ion detection, data acquisition, and vacuum systems (Badman & Cooks, 2000). They note that miniaturization benefits types of all mass analyzers because the mean free path of the ions is reduced due to the reduction in the distance of travel and the number of collisions with background gases, relative with a larger sized device operated at the same pressure. The most common miniature mass analyzers are linear quadrupole type (Figure 40.4), which is being driven by demands for size and the desire for an instrument that can operate effectively at relatively high (millitorr range) pressures (Badman & Cooks, 2000).

Mainstream and sidestream capnography

A capnometer, by definition is either diverting (i.e. sidestream) or non-diverting (i.e. mainstream). A diverting capnometer transports a portion of the respired gases from the sampling site, through a sampling tube, to the sensor whereas a non-diverting capnometer does not transport gas away from the sampling site (ISO, 1993; 2003; McArthur, 2003). The measurement of the partial pressure of a gas significantly distant from the sampling site requires that a number of "laws of physics" issues be addressed including (1) water removal, (2) different conditions at the sampling site and sample cell in terms of temperature and humidity, (3) mixing of the sample gas as it is drawn through the cell, (4) variable pressure drop across the tubing and the possible misrepresentation of the partial pressure values due to the above and other effects and (5) dynamic distortions to the waveform. While some of these effects can be compensated for or corrected by other measurements or by the assumption of nominal values, other effects cannot.

With mainstream devices, the sensor consisting of the sample cell and IR bench is placed at the airway. This location results in a "crisp" capnogram that reflects in real time the PCO_2 within the airway. On the other hand, sidestream devices aspirate a sample of gas from the breathing circuit through a six to eight foot long small bore tube. This sample is then often passed through a water trap and drying tubing prior to being analyzed in a sample cell. Using a remote location results in a delay time of up to several seconds and a rise time distortion of perhaps greater than 200 ms.

Mainstream devices with their limitations on size and weight have to date only offered measurement of a single gas such as CO_2 whereas sidestream devices can offer measurement of all of the respiratory and anesthesia gases. However, technological developments have seen the recent availability of mainstream devices with CO_2 and O_2 as well as anesthetic agents in lightweight devices.

Water vapor effects can cause cross-interference (absorption band overlap) and collision broadening but the band at 4.26 μm is relatively free from any water vapor absorption effects and shows minimal collision broadening effects. Partial pressure dilution effects on the other hand are of concern. Mainstream IR analyzers, when located near the patient connection, measure gas near body temperature and pressure, saturated (BTPS) conditions. Water vapor condensate on the windows of the airway adapter has been effectively minimized in mainstream systems by heating its windows above body temperature or by using coatings. How close the exact water vapor pressure is to BTPS conditions depends on factors including the presence and type of humidification, fresh gas flow, length of time in use, and ambient temperature (Raemer & Calalang, 1991). Normally, exhaled gas is fully saturated and/or slightly less than 37°C. This results in a water vapor pressure of 47 mmHg. In sidestream systems the temperature of the sampled gases decreases toward room temperature during its transit from the patient connection to the monitor. This results in condensate forming on the walls of the tubing and a resulting decrease in the partial pressure of water vapor from the BTPS value of 47 mmHg. With the inclusion of water permeable tubing, such as Nafion® brand tubing, the water vapor pressure in the tubing will tend to equilibrate with the water vapor pressure in the room.[1] This decrease in water vapor pressure can cause a small apparent increase in CO_2 concentration (Fletcher *et al.*, 1983). Mainstream capnometers will correctly read the PCO_2 at the conditions in the breathing circuit typically at or near BTPS. Sidestream devices compensate with software for water vapor removed and as a result may introduce errors if assumed conditions are very different from actual conditions (Severinghaus, 1989), which may change over time. The use of water traps, particularly in anesthesia, can easily lead in some designs to partial failure or blockage of the trap causing dramatic changes in waveforms and end-tidal values. This is particularly significant in systems that do not show the capnogram.

The limitations of the technologies and design choices and their performance in the different clinical environments and patient populations that they may be used on must be considered. Capnography as a "front-line" monitor is well established (Williamson *et al.*, 1993). The different technologies have been evaluated in the literature (Raemer & Calalang, 1991; Lauber *et al.*, 1995). Aspects of each technology will be reviewed (Table 40.3).

[1] Note that the driving force here is that water vapor pressure gradient, not the total pressure.

Table 40.3 Comparison of mainstream and sidestream CO_2 analyzers*

Feature	Mainstream	Sidestream
Airway connections		
Location of IR analysis unit ("bench")	At the airway connector	In the monitor
Weight of airway connection	Medium (<2 oz)	Light
Location of airway connector	End of endotracheal tube	End of endotracheal tube (may replace "angle" connector)
Gases available?	CO_2 (O_2, N_2O, agents available in technology in development)	CO_2, O_2, N_2O, agents
Use on non-intubated patients?	Yes but only with a facemask or mouthpiece. Possible dilution of sample with significant loss of seal	Yes with nasal adapter or oxygen prongs. Probable dilution of sample.
Connecting tube or cable?	Cable	Sample tube
Required components to "sample" gas	Airway adapter and bench	Airway adapter, sample tube, filters, water trap, water permeable tubing
Cost of replacing airway connector	Bench expensive to replace; airway adapter inexpensive to moderately expensive	Very inexpensive on a per sensor basis – but on very wet patients may require hourly changes
Sample volume drawn	None	Less than 250 ml/min; newer systems use 50 ml/min
Dead-space added to airway connector	Small (<1 ml in neonates)	Minimal
Zeroing and calibration		
Zeroing	Manual – user may use gas cell or zero on airway adapter if needed	Automatic – requires internal valving and sometimes external gas tanks
Accuracy of zeroing	Accurate; may use separate ref cell in place of airway adapter	Accurate; uses sample tubing and adapter that will be used during monitoring
Response and signal fidelity		
Delay between sampling and waveform display	None	Less than 3 s
Bench 10–90% rise time	Typically <70 ms	Typically >200 ms
Accuracy of waveform shape	Excellent. No affect due to variable pressure drop	Variable – Depends upon factors including sample rate, mixing, sample cell design etc.
Moisture and contamination		
Changes in water vapor pressure	Not affected	Affected due to condensation and drying of sample
Moisture handling	Bench at airway adapter contains a means to prevent condensation, water droplets may condense on window but usually clear rapidly	Water trap – modern water traps can be extremely efficient but tend to clog (some use Nafion tubing which equilibrates with ambient humidity)
Potential of cross-contamination between patients	None – Disposable or reusable airway adapter can be sterilized and then reused at no risk of contamination	None – airway adapter and sample tubes can be disposed at low cost or sterilized and reused at no risk of contamination provided no purging or return of gas to patient breathing circuit
Gas scavenging required (with anesthetic agents)?	No	Yes
Compensations		
Airway pressure compensation	Not required	Pressure fluctuations due to sample rate compensated with measurement of pressure

*Adapted from Respironics, Inc., Murrysville, PA, with permission.

Mainstream capnography: overview

The sample cell, referred to as the cuvette, serves as the airway adapter and is located in the respiratory gas stream obviating the need for gas sampling and scavenging. It interfaces directly to the IR bench. A source emits IR radiation that includes the absorption band for CO_2. Photodetectors, typically located on the other side of the airway adapter, measure the transmitted radiation. A multi-conductor lightweight, flexible cable transmits the amplified detected signals to the monitor from which the PCO_2 is calculated and displayed graphically in the form of a capnogram. The monitor has traditionally contained only the electronics associated with control and measurement functions of the IR bench. Newer designs incorporating advancements in electronics packaging and components have moved these electronics into the measurement head.

Many of the disadvantages of mainstream sensors presented by some authors in the past are primarily technological in nature and often relate to prior generations of that technology. These disadvantages are often listed in older reviews (Hess, 1990; Block & McDonald, 1992) of the technology while more recent reviews note otherwise (Ward & Yealy, 1998). This includes possible damage during handling, increased mechanical dead-space, issues of weight on airway, and use limited to only intubated patients. For example, the mainstream IR benches have been in the past termed "vulnerable to costly damage." While earlier IR benches were vulnerable primarily due to the use of moving parts such as chopper or filter wheels, some newer mainstream IR benches utilize all solid-state designs that have been shown to be robust enough to survive repeated drops onto hard floors and have been in use in high impact areas such as the emergency room, ambulances, and transport for well over a decade. Historically, the primary concerns of mainstream-based systems related to size and weight. However, the reductions in both size and weight have alleviated these concerns. Current generation mainstream devices, besides being relatively light, and low in dead-space have generally demonstrated better performance than conventional sidestream system in terms of signal fidelity and end-tidal measurements particularly at higher respiratory rates in small children (Pascucci *et al.*, 1989). Careful airway adapter design and advances in technology have reduced the concerns for dead-space and weight. As with any airway adapter used for gas monitoring (either mainstream or sidestream), improper connection to other breathing circuit elements can cause artifacts in the capnogram. For example, a partial disconnection of a mainstream adapter can mimic a "curare-cleft" capnogram (Tripathi, 1998) but is easily recognizable.

Condensed water or water-like mixtures can affect the windows of the airway adapter. If droplets appear within the cuvette optical path, severe scattering and absorption can occur. However, devices using approaches such as a single-beam ratiometric design can compensate for the contamination if scattering/absorption effects are not spectrum dependent. Dust particles and optically opaque particles do not appreciably affect system precision.

Sidestream capnography: overview

Sidestream gas analyzers utilize a long sampling plastic tube connected to an adapter in the breathing circuit (such as a T-piece at the endotracheal tube or mask connector) or a nasal catheter. The sample gas is continuously aspirated from the breathing circuit through the sampling tube and into the sample cell within the monitor (Figure 40.5) at sample flow rates ranging from 50 to 250 ml/min.

The location of the sampling port varies and may range anywhere from an elbow connected to an endotracheal tube to the "Y". For example, it may be placed on the ventilator or patient side of an in-line filter or heat moisture exchanger (HME). Placement on the ventilator side results in a drier sampling tube

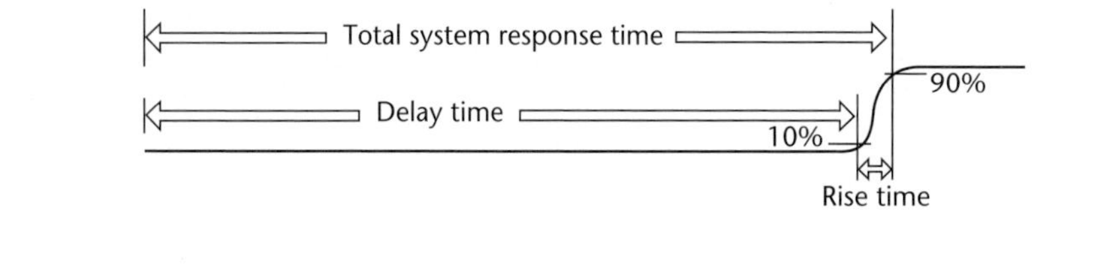

Figure 40.5 Physical components of a gas sampling system with total system response time, delay time, and rise time illustrated. (Image courtesy of Respironics, Inc., Murrysville, PA.)

with the inherent risk of distortion of the capnographic waveform and lower end-tidal values (Hardman *et al.*, 1997; Goodman & Johnson, 2001), whereas placement of the patient side can result in the accumulation of condensate and patient secretions in the sampling system. The sampled gas that is withdrawn from the patient may contain anesthetic gases and as such this gas should be routed to a gas scavenging system or returned to the patient breathing system to avoid pollution of the OR environment (Lawson & Jelenich, 1985), costs associated with greater usage of anesthetic (Boldt *et al.*, 1998) gases and possible exposure risks in under ventilated areas (NIOSH ALERT, 1994; Smith, 1998).

Condensation from humidified sample gas in combination with patient secretions occasionally can block and contaminate the sampling line. To protect the sample cell from condensate, the distal end of the sampling tube is often connected to a water trap and water vapor permeable tubing such as Nafion® tubing. Water trap and filter designs effectiveness vary between manufacturers. Additionally, sources of leaks external to the monitor such as loose fittings (Zupan *et al.*, 1988), cracked or slit sampling tubes (Skeehan & Biebuyck, 1991; Tripathi & Pandey, 2000), cracked sample filters (Body *et al.*, 2000) and cracked airway adapters (Ti & Dhara, 1998) along with sources of leaks internal to the monitor such as partial disconnection (Healzer *et al.*, 1995) have been reported as possible causes of artifact in the capnogram. Leaks as well as obstructions can occur at connection points and tubes within the sidestream sampling system. More recent designs of airway adapters for sidestream systems have reduced the likelihood of aspirating secretions by the use of sampling ports that are located in the center of the adapter rather than at the wall and have reduced the effect of leaks by including a removable sample cell as part of the sample set.

Even with no leaks or obstructions in the sampling system, significant distortion of the capnogram can occur under some conditions. At the sample tubing-airway interface, expired gas may be diluted with entrained ambient air whenever the gas flow rate falls below the "constant" sample flow rate (Epstein *et al.*, 1980). The design of the sampling tube and its positioning within the breathing circuit or nares (if a nasal catheter is used) can affect the quantity of surrounding air that is entrained along with the expired gas. Within the sample tube itself dispersion may occur due to the effects of velocity profile and diffusion (Epstein *et al.*, 1980). Additionally, the sample flow rate may vary significantly as a function of a number of factors including the sample tube length (Schena *et al.*, 1984), airway pressure, and the presence of an exhaust line occlusion (Hussain & Raphael, 1997). Some monitors compensate by either increasing the sampling flow or attempt to purge the sample tubes when an increased pressure drop is sensed across a flow restriction. In spite of the presence of water traps and water permeable tubing, liquids may be aspirated into the monitor's internal components.

Conventional sidestream capnographs may not be accurate in neonatal and pediatric patients because they aspirate a significant portion of the patient's total ventilation (Gravenstein, 1989). Older sidestream designs used sample rates as high as 250 ml/min but newer designs have reduced the flow rate, the diameter of the sampling tube (1 mm ID) and sample cell. This tradeoff decreases the ventilation levels that can be monitored and extends the operating life of the filter and/or water trap while at the same time potentially increasing the possibility of occlusion.

Artifacts in sidestream CO_2 waveforms can take on many forms. For example, excessive damping of the response (Figure 40.6) can occur. In some circumstances the artifact may resemble physiologic changes which may be characteristic of diseases such as some forms of restrictive or obstructive lung disease (Pascucci, 1989). For example, Pascucci notes that "a falsely low value for end-tidal CO_2 may incorrectly assure the clinician that alveolar ventilation is adequate when, in fact, it is not." He further notes that

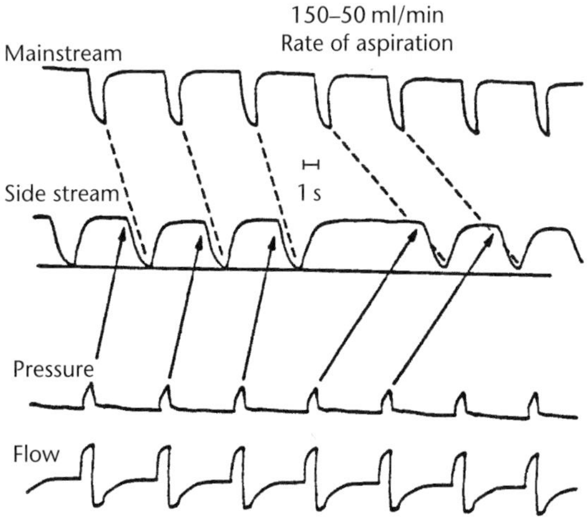

Figure 40.6 Relationship between capnogram (both mainstream and sidestream) and other "pneumatic" parameters of pressure and flow. Note the time delay and dampening effects from reducing the sample flow rate in the sidestream system. (Reproduced with permission from Gravenstein, J.S., Paulus, D.A. & Hayes, T.J. (1989). *Capnography in Clinical Practice*, 2nd edition. Butterworth-Heinemann, Boston.)

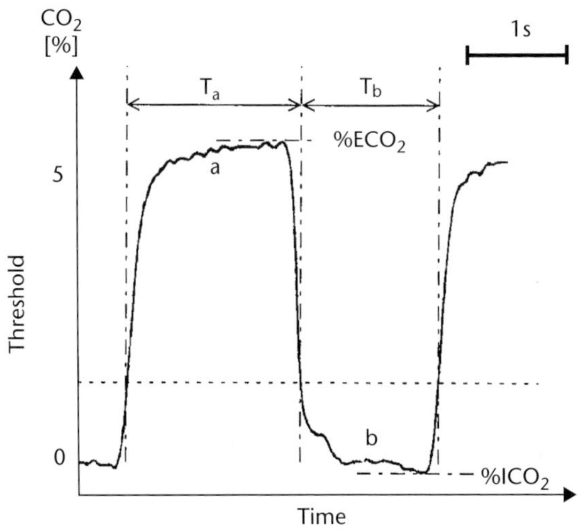

Figure 40.7 Normal capnogram. During expiration, exhaled CO_2 causes a peak in the capnogram at a. During the inspiratory phase, fresh gas or room air is sampled, and the capnogram returns to its baseline at b. Breaths may be counted and timed by the use of a simple thresholding technique; each crossing of the threshold by the capnogram is noted, allowing calculation of parameters describing each breath. % ECO_2 is the end-tidal level and $\%ICO_2$ is the inspired level. (Reproduced with permission from Smith, T.C., Green, A. & Hutton, P. (1994). Recognition of cardiogenic artifact in pediatric capnograms. *J. Clin. Monit.*, **10**: 270–275.)

"the inability of the capnogram to return to zero baseline on inspiration, a common artifact sidestream recordings, may suggest rebreathing of CO_2 and prompt unnecessary changes in fresh gas flow or modifications of the patient circuit" (Pascucci, 1989).

The use of conventional sidestream monitoring requires that careful attention be paid both to the physical setup external and internal to the monitor. The recent introduction of more robust devices has lessened some of these concerns.

Algorithmic issues

End-tidal CO_2

The specifics of each manufacturer's algorithm for end-tidal measurements such as averaging windows, breath-to-breath averaging and its definition of end-tidal must be considered when interpreting data. This is particularly important if no waveform is displayed. Unfortunately, whether the reported end-tidal value is the PCO_2 at the end of expiration or the largest value during the "expiratory" period defined by the capnogram (which can be elongated by rebreathing) or something entirely different depends upon the manufacturer, and often is not disclosed.

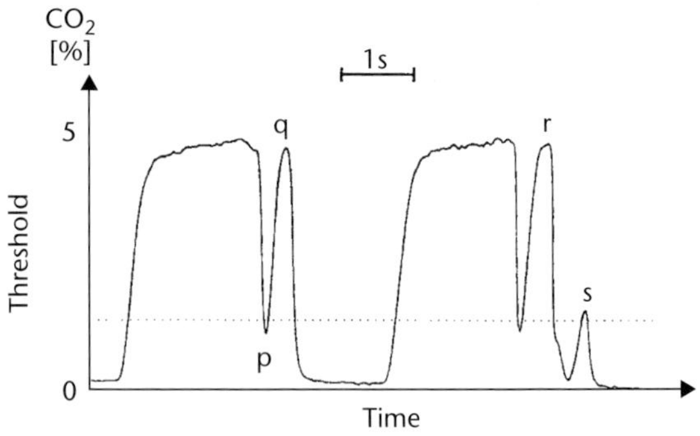

Figure 40.8 Capnogram representing two breaths that could be misclassified as representing five by a simple thresholding algorithm. A cardiogenic oscillation at the end of the first expiration crosses the threshold at p, causing peak q to be misclassified as a new expiratory phase. Similarly, oscillation artifacts r and s are also misclassified. Simultaneous recordings of chest and abdominal movement using respiratory inductance plethysmography was used in this figure to exclude non-cardiogenic causes. (Reproduced with permission from Smith, T.C., Green, A. & Hutton, P. (1994). Recognition of cardiogenic artifact in pediatric capnograms. *J. Clin. Monit.*, **10**: 270–275).

Breath-detect

Algorithms to detect and delineate breaths using capnograms often are solely based upon simple thresholds (Figure 40.7). However, such approaches are susceptible to brief swings due to cardiogenic oscillations and noise (Figure 40.8). More sophisticated and robust approaches may use multiple signals such as flow, pressure, and CO_2 waveforms (Govindarajan & Prakash, 1990) and/or additional criteria.

References

Alpert, N.L., Keiser, W.E. & Szymanski, H.A. (1970). *IR Theory and Practice of Infrared Spectroscopy*, 2nd edition. Plenum Press, New York.

Badman, E.R. & Cooks, R.G. (2000). Miniature mass analyzers. *J. Mass Spectrom.*, **35**: 659–671.

Barrington, A.E. (1963). *High Vacuum Engineering*. Englewood Cliffs, NJ. Prentice Hall.

Bergman, N.A., Rackow, H. & Frumin, M.J. (1958). The collision broadening effect of nitrous oxide upon infrared analysis of carbon dioxide during anesthesia. *Anesthesiology*, **19**: 19–26.

Berman, J.A., Furgiuele, J.J. & Marx, G.F. (1984). The Einstein carbon dioxide detector. *Anesthesiology*, **60**: 613–614.

Block, Jr. F.E. & McDonald, J.S. (1992). Sidestream versus mainstream carbon dioxide analyzers. *J. Clin. Monit.*, **8**: 139–141.

Body, S.C., Taylor, K. & Philip, J.H. (2000). Dual-plateau capnogram caused by cracked sample filter. *Anesth. Analg.*, **90**: 233–234.

Boldt, J., Jaun, N., Kumle, B., Heck, M. & Mund, K. (1998). Economic considerations of the use of new anesthetics: a comparison of propofol, sevoflurane, desflurane, and isoflurane. *Anesth. Analg.* **86**: 504–509.

Coleman, Y., & Krauss, B. (1999). Microstream capnography technology: a new approach to an old problem. *J. Clin. Monit. Comput.* **15**: 403–409.

Draper, W.B. (1938). Means of indicating presence and relative amounts of carbon dioxide in gases for breathing. US Patent 2,136,236, issued 8 November.

Epstein, R.A., Reznik, A.M. & Epstein, M.A.F. (1980). Determinants of distortions in CO_2 catheter sampling systems: a mathematical model. *Resp. Physiol.*, **41**: 127–136.

Fehder, C.G. (1988). Carbon dioxide indicator device. US Patent 4,728,499, issued 1 March.

Fletcher, R., Werner, O., Nordstrom, L. & Jonson, B. (1983). Sources of error and their correction in the measurement of carbon dioxide elimination using the Siemens-Elema CO_2 analyzer. *Br. J. Anaesth.*, **55**: 177–185.

Goodman, E. & Johnson, P.A. (2001). End-tidal carbon dioxide tracing configuration depends on sampling size. *Anesth. Analg.*, **92**: 1357–1358.

Govindarajan, N. & Prakash, O. (1990). Breath detection algorithm in digital computers. *Int. J. Clin. Monit. Comput.*, **7**: 59–64.

Gravenstein, J.S., Paulus, D.A. & Hayes, T.J. (1989). *Capnography in Clinical Practice*, 2nd edition. Butterworth-Heinemann, Boston.

Gravenstein, N. (1989). Capnometry in infants should not be done at lower sampling flow rates. *J. Clin. Monit.*, **5**: 63–64.

Hardman, J.G., Curran, J. & Mahajan, R.P. (1997). End-tidal carbon dioxide measurement and breathing system filters. *Anaesthesia*, **52**: 646–648.

Healzer, J.M., Spiegelman, W.G. & Jaffe, R.A. (1995). Internal gas analyzer leak resulting in an abnormal capnogram and incorrect calibration. *Anesth. Analg.*, **81**: 202–203.

Hess, D. (1990). Capnometry and capnography: technical aspects, physiologic aspects, and clinical applications. *Respir. Care*, **35**: 557–573.

Hill, D.W. & Powell, T. 1968. *Non-dispersive Infra-red Gas Analysis in Science, Medicine and Industry*. Plenum Press, New York.

Hussain, S. & Raphael, D.T. (1997). Analysis of a straight-line capnographic waveform. *Anesth. Analg.*, **85**: 465.

ISO 9918 (1993). Capnometers for use with humans – requirements.

ISO/FDIS 21647 (2003). Medical electrical equipment – particular requirements for the basic safety and essential performance of respiratory gas monitors.

Kennell, E.M., Andrews, R.W. & Wollman, H. (1973). Correction factors for nitrous oxide in the infrared analysis of carbon dioxide. *Anesthesiology*, **39**: 441–443.

Knodle, D.W. & Clary, T.R. (1997). Nondispersive infrared radiation source. US Patent 5,602,398, issued 11 February.

Knodle, D.W., Graham, P.K. & Labuda, L.L. (1994). Infrared source. US Patent 5,369,277, issued 29 November.

Knodle, D.W., Mace, L.E. & Labuda, L.L. (1990). Gas analyzers. US Patent 4,914,720, issued 3 April.

Kruse, D.W., McGlauchlin, L.D. & McQuistam, R.B. (1962). *Elements of Infrared Technology – Generation, Transmission and Detection*. John Wiley & Sons, Inc., New York.

Lauber, R., Seeberger, B. & Zbinden, A.M. (1995). Carbon dioxide analysers: accuracy, alarm limits and effects of interfering gases. *Can. J. Anaesth.*, **42**: 643–656.

Lawson, D. & Jelenich, S. (1985). Capnographs: a new operating room pollution hazard? *Anesth. Analg.*, **64**: 378.

Luft, K. (1943). Über eine neue Methode der registrierenden Gasanalyse mit Hilfe der Absorption ultraroter Strahlen ohne spektrale Zerlegung. *Ztschr. f. Techn. Phys.*, **24**: 97–104.

Marriott, W.M. (1916). Determination of alveolar carbon dioxide tension by a simple method. *J. Am. Med. Assoc.*, **66**: 1594–1596.

McArthur, C.D. (2003). AARC clinical practice guideline. Capnography/capnometry during mechanical ventilation – 2003, revision and update. *Respir Care.*, **48**: 534–539.

Nexo, S.A., Christensen, J. & Jorgensen, I.E. (1989). Photoacoustic gas analyzer US Patent 4,818,882, issued 4 April.

NIOSH ALERT (1994). Controlling Exposures to Nitrous Oxide. DHHS (NIOSH) Publication No. 94–100.

Orient, O.J., Chutjian, A., Garkanian, V. (1997). Miniature, high-resolution, quadrupole mass-spectrometer array. *Rev. Sci. Instrum.*, **68**: 1393–1397.

Pascucci, R.C., Schena, J.A. & Thompson, J.E. (1989). Comparison of a sidestream and mainstream capnometer in infants. *Crit Care Med.*, **17**: 560–562.

Petroianu, G.A., Maleck, W.H., Bergler, W.F., Altmannsberger, S. & Rufer, R. (1998). Preliminary observations on the Colibri CO_2-indicator. *Am. J. Emerg. Med.*, **16**: 677–680.

Puntervoll, S.A., Soreide, E., Jacewicz, W. & Bjelland, E. (2002). Rapid detection of oesophageal intubation: take care when using colorimetric capnometry. *Acta Anaesthesiol. Scand.*, **46**: 455–457.

Raemer, D.B. & Calalang, I. (1991). Accuracy of end-tidal carbon dioxide tension analyzers. *J. Clin. Monit.*, **7**: 195–208.

Rich, D.R., Pierry, A.T., Fudge, B.M., Sandor, J.L. & Triunfo, J.A. (2003). *Sidestream Gas Sampling System with Detachable Sample Cell*. Patent Cooperation Treaty Publication, 60/370,002 16 October.

Rosencwaig, A. (1980). *Photoacoustics and Photoacoustic Spectroscopy*. John Wiley and Sons, New York, NY.

Schena, J., Thompson, J. & Crone, R.K. (1984). Mechanical influences on the capnogram. *Crit. Care Med.*, **12**: 672–674.

Severinghaus, J.R. (1989). Water vapor calibration errors in some capnometers: respiratory conventions misunderstood by manufacturers? *Anesthesiology*, **70**: 996–998.

Skeehan, T.M. & Biebuyck, J.F. (1991). Erroneous mass spectrometer data caused by faulty patient sampling tube; case report and laboratory study. *J. Clin. Monit.*, **7**: 313–319.

Smith, D.A. (1998). Hazards of nitrous oxide exposure in healthcare personnel. *AANA J.*, **66**: 390–393.

Smith, T.C., Green, A. & Hutton, P. (1994). Recognition of cardiogenic artifact in pediatric capnograms. *J. Clin. Monit.*, **10**: 270–275

Ti, L.K. & Dhara, S.S. (1998). Another cause of a prolonged downstroke on the capnograph. *Anesthesiology*, **89**: 801–802.

Tripathi, M. (1998). A partial disconnection at the main stream CO_2 transducer mimics "curare-cleft" capnograph. *Anesthesiology* **88(4)**: 1117–1119.

Tripathi, M. & Pandey, M. (2000). Atypical "tails-up" capnograph due to breach in the sampling tube of side-stream capnometer. *J. Clin. Monit. Comput.* **16**: 17–20

Veingerov, M.L. (1938). Eine Methode der Gasanalyse beruhend auf dem optisch-akustischen Tyndall-Röntgeneffekt. *Dokl. Akad. Nauk. SSSR.*, **19**: 687–688.

Ward, K.R. & Yealy, D.M. (1998). End-tidal carbon dioxide monitoring in emergency medicine, Part 1: Basic principles. *Acad. Emerg. Med.* **5**: 628–636.

Williamson, J.A., Webb, R.K., Cockings, J. & Morgan, C. (1993). The Australian Incident Monitoring Study. The capnograph: applications and limitations – an analysis of 2000 incident reports. *Anaesth. Intens. Care*, **21**: 551–557.

Zupan, J., Martin, M. & Benumof, J.L. (1988). End-tidal CO_2 excretion waveform and error with gas sampling line leak. *Anesth. Analg.* **67**: 579–581.

FLOW MEASUREMENT 41

M.B. Jaffe

The importance of flow

Gas measurements are becoming routine in both the operating room (OR) and the intensive care unit (ICU). At present, most of the technologies provide breath-by-breath information presenting expiratory values and inspiratory minimum values for each of the gases. In addition, the shape of the waveform has been of great value when monitoring carbon dioxide (CO_2). The addition of simultaneous measurement of flow adds important information to the measurement of exhaled CO_2.

Volume

In its simplest terms, measuring flow makes possible the online determination of inspired and expired volumes. Assuming constant flow (as with an inspiratory square wave common to many ventilators), and knowing the time during which the flow occurs, enables the determination of volume. However, expiratory flow (in contrast to inspiratory flow) is normally not constant, and volume must be expressed as integral of flow. Calculations of flow make use of integration methods, such as trapezoidal rule or higher order methods. If we perform this integration for both inspiratory and expiratory flow, we can compare results and detect breathing circuit leaks. This determination could be made over a single breath, over several breaths, or over a time (e.g. 1 min for minute volume). A second application might be to display gas concentration versus volume instead of time as is conventional today in volumetric capnography.

Clinical issues: overview

The clinical measurement of respired gas flow on patients, particularly during mechanical ventilation, requires attention to sensor(s) location, gas composition, gas temperature, inlet conditions, humidity, dead-space, effective resistance of breathing circuit, and operating range of flow sensor. When comparing flow measured by two different devices all of these considerations must be taken into account. Additionally, the bandwidth of the flow signal must also be considered. For non-intubated, resting, adult tidal breathing, a bandwidth of at least 4 Hz is required (Lemen *et al.*, 1982). Others have suggested higher bandwidths particularly for infants (Turner *et al.*, 1993). Recent clinical guidelines suggest sampling rates of 100 or 200 samples/s depending on integration methods used to obtain values sufficiently accurate for research purposes in infants (Frey *et al.*, 2000). Various technologies have been used clinically to measure airway flow. Many of these techniques were originally developed strictly for precise short-term laboratory measurements. These applications require meticulous attention to detail including calibration and operator attendance at all times.

A continuous, bi-directional airway flow measurement used in the clinical environment demands simplicity, reliability, ease of use, and the ability to work in wet, circuits without operator intervention. The devices should be relatively inexpensive, have minimal dead-space, work over wide flow ranges and require minimal or no calibration. Devices typically designed for the pulmonary function testing environment will generally not work well in continuous monitoring applications.

Continuous, accurate, and reliable flow measurements under clinical conditions have been a major technical challenge. The number of solutions proposed gives a measure of the difficulty of the problem. Solutions can be catalogued under principles involving ultrasound detection, hot-wire anemometry, and differential pressure measurements.

Factors affecting flow readings

A number of factors that can affect the flow measured independent of the technology used should be considered including sensor location, gas conditions, gas composition and temperature, inlet conditions, resistance, dead-space, humidity effects, and operating ranges. Additionally, factors such as lung compliance,

Table 41.1 Flow sensor location

Ventilator	Flow sensor	Site
Bear 5	Vortex shedding	Distal to exhalation valve
Bird 6500ST	Variable orifice	At exhalation valve outlet
Hamilton veolar	Variable orifice	Proximal airway
Puritan-Bennet 7200a	Hot-wire	Distal to exhalation valve
Siemens servo 900c	Screen	Proximal to exhalation valve for expiratory and inspiratory limb for inspiratory

Reproduced with permission from Tobin, M.J. (1994). *Principles and Practice of Mechanical Ventilation.* McGraw-Hill, Inc., New York.

presence and nature of secretions, and leak (endotracheal tube, ETT type) (cuffed versus uncuffed and degree of inflation of cuff) should be considered.

Sensor location

Proximal flow measured at the patient's airway can be substantially different from flow measured inside of or at the ventilator, particularly if not adequately compensated. Many ventilators measure flow, not at the proximal airway, but close to the ventilator. (Table 41.1) This can result in a substantial difference between the flow that is delivered to the patient and flow that the ventilator reports as delivered due to the wasted compression volume and differences due to humidification. This wasted portion of the tidal volume, that is compression volume, does not ventilate the patient's lungs, remains within the breathing circuit, and tends to elongate and distend the breathing circuit tubing. The compression volume is related to the internal volume of the ventilator, volume of the humidifier (if present), volume and compliance of circuit tubing, and volume of other components of the breathing circuit, such as heat moisture exchangers (HMEs). The volume due to compression loss that does not reach the patient becomes increasingly important as pressures increase and volume decreases. During the inspiratory portion of a ventilator-delivered breath, compression occurs throughout the breathing circuit, and the breathing tubing distends and elongates. During the expiratory portion of a ventilator-delivered breath, the compressed gas, and stored energy in the distended and elongated breathing tubes is released; and this additional volume is measured by sensors at the exhalation port of the ventilator. Unless volume measurements are made directly at the patient's airway the exhaled volume displayed by the ventilator can overestimate the patient's actual tidal volume by the compressible volume (Tobin, 1994). Some ventilators allow for a correction factor (i.e. compression factor) of the measured volume for circuit compression volume. The factor, calculated as compression volume over the corresponding ventilation pressure, allows a compressible volume to be estimated by multiplying this factor by the peak pressure less positive end-expiratory pressure (PEEP). Even with this correction applied, precise estimation of the compression volume is difficult due to variations between individual breathing circuits, use of humidifiers, HMEs, and other circuit components. Failure to account for the wasted compression volume could result in hypoventilation in ventilator supported patients. Studies of several ventilators found that the discrepancy between displayed and proximally measured volume was as high as 23% (Gammage *et al.*, 1988) and varied significantly on the same ventilator with different manufacturer's breathing circuits (Bartel *et al.*, 1985).

Gas conditions

Gas volumes may be expressed at different conditions and differences between these conditions has often led to confusion. Conventionally, ventilation is reported at BTPS (body temperature of 37°C, ambient pressure, and saturated with water vapor) while gas volumes associated with CO_2 elimination ($\dot{V}CO_2$) and oxygen (O_2) consumption ($\dot{V}O_2$) are often reported in STPD (standard temperature 0°C, pressure 760 mmHg and dry). To convert between the different conditions, the ideal gas law, $PV = nRT$ (where P is pressure in absolute terms, V is volume, n moles of non-water molecules, R is 62.3656 l mmHg/mol degree, and T is temperature in absolute terms) is applied at these two conditions. Note that the total pressure consists of the partial pressures of the gases and water vapor. Applying this relationship where 47 mmHg is the water vapor pressure at 37°C (body temperature), and 0 and 760 mmHg are the standard temperature and pressure, respectively, one obtains:

$$V_{\mathrm{STPD}} = \frac{(P_{\mathrm{B}} - 47)(V_{\mathrm{BTPS}})(273)}{760(273 + 37)} = \frac{(P_{\mathrm{B}} - 47)(V_{\mathrm{BTPS}})}{863},$$

Using these expressions, one can calculate the volumes at different conditions and demonstrate differences in measured volumes at different points in the breathing circuit.

The effect of humidification on the measurement of volume is often a point of confusion. Within the airways, the respiratory gases can be considered to be effectively saturated with water vapor. As such, the vapor pressure of water depends entirely on temperature. To calculate water vapor pressure for a saturated system, different equations have been developed including a precise equation consisting of a logarithmic function (Goff & Gratch, 1946) and a quadratic equation that provides a reasonable degree of accuracy. Relative humidity, a measure of saturation for moist air, is calculated as the ratio of partial pressure of water (P_{H2O}) over the vapor pressure of water (P_{vapor}) at the same temperature. Here we have not considered aspects of cooling, rain out and the associated temperature gradients, and humidity changes that occur in breathing circuits. For more detail, please consult reviews on inspired gas conditioning (Shelly, 1992) and humidification and mechanical ventilation (Branson, 1999). It should be noted that when inspired gas is less than 100% saturated, or has a temperature that is less then body temperature, expired tidal volume will be larger than inspired tidal volume because of the water vapor that is added in the lungs.

Gas composition/temperature

Accurate flow measurement requires that the nominal values for the inspiratory and expiratory gas composition and temperatures be often considered. For some devices the user can choose typical ambient values for O_2, CO_2, and nitrogen if one is testing with a calibration syringe or typical clinical values. Compensations for additional gases such as nitrous oxide, helium, or an anesthetic agent are often available. The effect of not properly compensating for the gas concentrations can result in a significant change in the reported flow value, depending on the flow measurement technology. Gas composition correction assumes the viscosity can be computed as the linear combination of the product of each individual viscosity and its gas fraction. Gas flow sensors that are based on thermal measurements such as hot-wire, or hot-film, anemometers are sensitive to the heat capacity of the measured gas.

Inlet conditions

Flow sensors should be designed to be insensitive to changes in inlet conditions and should be carefully considered independent of the measurement technology. For example, changing the proximal connections from a direct ETT connection to a connection via an elbow markedly changes the cross-sectional profile of the flow entering the flow sensor. A robust flow sensor design should have little change on the measured flow

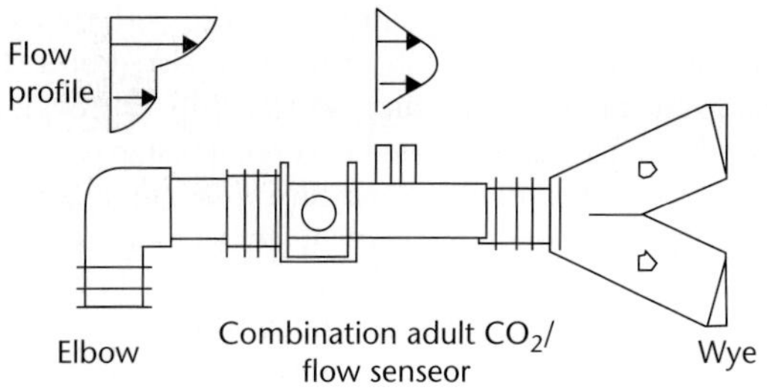

Figure 41.1 Expiratory flow velocity profiles at exit of elbow and at differential pressure sensor illustrating the effect of entrance length. (Image courtesy of Respironics, Inc., Murrysville, PA.)

regardless of the type and geometry of upstream devices. Even small changes in the geometry of the breathing circuit tubing relative to the flow sensor can have significant effect on the measured flow. For example, it has been demonstrated that Fleisch pneumotachographs connected between the wye ("Y") piece and ETTs can exhibit a flow-rate-dependent error in measured flow up to 10% (Kreit & Sciurba, 1996). If sufficient entrance length is provided in the flow sensor then laminar flow and a consistent flow velocity profile can be achieved. However this is usually not practical so entrance length to a flow sensor must be traded off against the design requirement of minimal dead-space (Figure 41.1). Thus a balance must be sought between low dead-space and insensitivity to changes in inlet conditions. Inlet flow conditioners can be designed into the flow sensor to mitigate the effects of unknown upstream geometry.

Humidity

Flow sensors should be designed to be insensitive to moisture accumulation on the flow sensing/measurement portion of the sensor. With differential flow sensors, the measurement and generation of the flow-dependent pressure drop can be affected by the presence of moisture on the walls of the flow sensor. The same applies for hot-wire and ultrasonic flow sensors. However, proper breathing circuit maintenance and avoiding gravity dependent positions within the breathing circuit is still required to avoid pooling of water and sputum in the flow sensor.

Resistance

The addition of a flow sensor to a breathing circuit should have minimal impact on the measured quantity – flow. Typically, resistance of a flow meter in product specifications and standards for pulmonary function testing is stated in terms of a pressure drop or resistance at a particular flow rate. When reading resistance specifications it is important to consider both the flow rate at which the pressure drop is reported and the nature of the flow–pressure relationship. For devices that do not have an inherent linear relationship consider the relationship of flow–pressure over the expected flows and pressures. For such devices a more relevant measure would be a flow–pressure plot or a better figure of merit that reports the added work of breathing due to the device under specified conditions rather than the pressure drop at a particular flow rate.

Operating range of flow sensor/choosing the right sensor

While the operating range for flow is constrained by the range of the sensors and associated measurement electronics, the operating range of derived parameters, such as volume must be considered in light of the flow sensor's range and of physiological limits. As with all of the measurement technologies, no single sensor will work over the range spanning from neonate to adult. To span this wide range, most manufacturers have used two or more different sensors. The criteria for selecting which sensor to use should include consideration of ETT size, age of the patient, flow/volume values, and the acceptable levels of dead-space and resistance.

The use of volume measurements in breathing circuits must consider the effects of gas conditions, compression volumes and location of the flow sensors so that the values may be properly interpreted. If possible, proximal flow sensors should be used to minimize the problems associated with gas conditions and compression.

Flow measurement technologies

For relatively dry gas, laboratory quality airflow measurements, great attention is placed upon accuracy, calibration, repeatability, and precision. Flow meters that perform suitably in these environments include Fleisch and Lilly style pneumotachometers, hot-wire, and hot-film, anemometers, rotating vane spirometers, and ultrasonic flow meters. Hot-wire anemometers (also known as thermal dissipation devices), based upon the convective cooling by the flowing gas, often use heated (>300°C) platinum or a platinum alloy. As such these devices are considered inappropriate when flammable gases are present (Yoshiya *et al.*, 1979). Rotating vane spirometers (which will not be discussed) tend to underestimate at low flows and overestimate at high flows due to friction and inertia of the turbine (Hsley *et al.*, 1993; Yeh *et al.*, 1987). Overall, in respiratory research the most widely used flow measurement device used is the Fleisch type differential pressure with a heated screen orifice. Differential pressure sensors, hot-wire anemometers, and ultrasonic sensors will each be discussed.

Differential pressure flow sensors

Differential pressure flow sensors incorporate some type of restriction (point orifice, variable flap, vena constriction, annular obstruction, target or linear flow restrictor) that generates a pressure difference across the sensor. Flexible tubing, attached to either side of the flow obstruction, transmits the differential pressure signal to a sensitive pressure sensor located inside a monitor at the bedside. Factors that influence the measurement of flow for this type of sensor include the gas molecular weight, temperature, and airway pressure (Turner *et al.*, 1989; Sullivan *et al.*, 1984).

Fleisch type

The popular Fleisch pneumotachograph (Fleisch, 1925) uses a bundle of capillary tubes that provides a small but fixed resistance to airflow and is based on Poiseuille's law in which the laminar flow in a thin tube is proportional to the pressure loss per unit length. This design ensures laminar flow through the sensor body thereby producing a nearly linear relationship between flow and differential pressure. The pressure drop across these capillaries is calibrated in terms of flow and is measured continuously by a differential pressure transducer. A family of pneumotachs is needed to cover the complete physiological range. The Fleisch pneumotach is calibrated to work over a range in flows that are laminar. This means that attention needs to be paid to breathing circuit details, so that turbulent flow is not inadvertently introduced, which could cause error. While it is an excellent device for short-term monitoring, it is easily contaminated by sputum and water condensate, which may change the flow characteristic of the device. As such heated pneumotachs are available. Also due to its relatively large surface area (dead-space) it is often not suited for continuous respiratory monitoring. In addition, it is heavy, costly, and difficult to clean.

Silverman modification/Lilly

In the 1940s Silverman and Whittenberg (1950) (and also Lilly (1950)) suggested a modification to the above, which was intended to reduce the condensation problem. This pneumotach uses a small, fixed resistance, provided by a fine metal mesh (400 mesh wire screen) that provides airflow resistance protected by

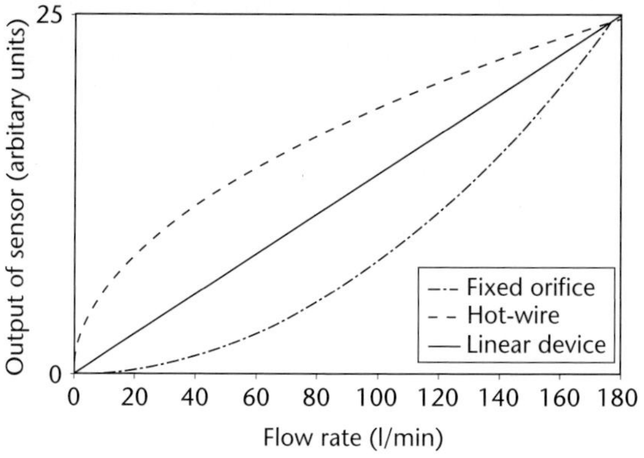

Figure 41.2 Flow versus "output" for a "linear" device (i.e. Fleisch pneumotachograph) and "non-linear" devices (fixed orifice flow sensor) and hot-wire anemometer over the adult flow range. (Image courtesy of Respironics, Inc., Murrysville, PA.)

two lower-mesh screens on either side. These protective screens condense water vapor, collect particulates, improve laminar flow at high frequencies, and lower dead-space. However, water vapor remains a problem even with the advent of heaters and the problem monitoring continuous proximal airway flows, as with the Fleisch pneumotach, was not completely solved.

Variable orifice type

The variable orifice type flow sensors have become popular in the long-term critical care monitoring environment due to their improved immunity to artifactual flow signals caused by moisture and secretions in the breathing circuit (Osborn, 1978, 1978a) (Figure 41.3). These flow sensors use a flexible sheet material (plastic or stainless steel) to create an opening that is small when flow is low and wide as flow increases. This dynamically changing orifice results in a more linear relationship between differential pressure and flow, allowing a larger range of flows to be measured accurately than is traditionally allowed by a fixed orifice type of device. The variable orifice flow meter works quite well under conditions of moisture and mucous. The variable orifice type flow meter's accuracy depends, however, upon the consistent stress-strain characteristics of the variable orifice flap, which can be degraded by inter-device variations created during manufacturing or intra-device changes due to fatigue during long-term use. In order to solve this problem, some manufacturers offer sensors with device specific factory pre-calibration parameters stored within a memory chip attached within the flow meter connector. Variable flap flow meters can be very susceptible to changes in flow patterns generated by different breathing circuit adapters (inlet configurations) placed immediately before the flow meter.

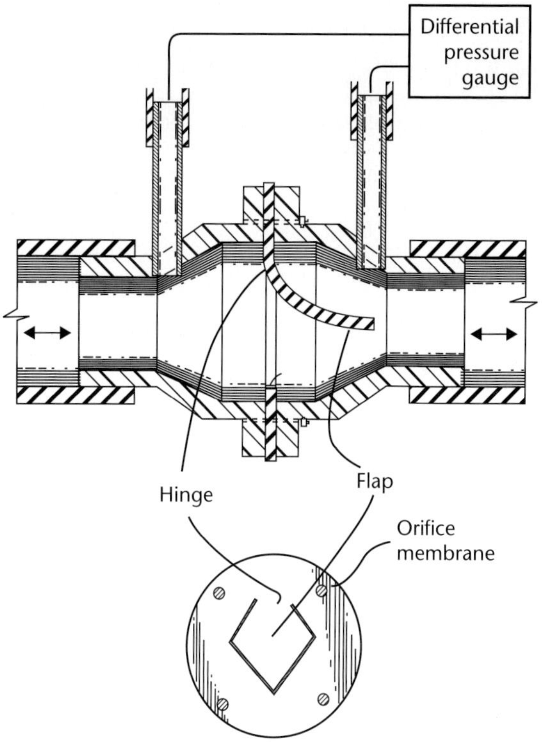

Figure 41.3 Variable orifice pneumotachograph. (Adapted from Osborn, 1978, 1978a.)

Fixed orifice type

The pressure drop across a fixed orifice flow sensor is, in general, proportional to the square of the flow. The relationship between the measured differential pressure to flow (l/min) can be described by the equation.

$$\frac{P_m T_{std}}{P_{std} T_m} K\sqrt{\Delta P},$$

where P_m, P_{std}, T_m, and T_{std} are the measured and standard pressures (in mmHg) and temperatures (in °K), respectively; K is a correction factor that includes gas composition and other factors and ΔP is the differential pressure (in mmHg). The $P_m T_{std}/P_{std} T_m$ is the ideal gas law correction of calculated flow to standard conditions. Microprocessors can be programmed to store the parameters of these flow sensors and compensate for this non-linear pressure–flow relationship. In addition, recent advances in differential pressure sensor technology have made it possible to measure the very low flows reliably. Some fixed orifice flow sensors use pitot tubes to measure the velocity of

Table 41.2 Representative commercial flow sensors used clinically

Technology	Type	Manufacturer	Model	Reference
Differential	Screen	Hans Rudolph	3830/4830 adult pneumotach	Rudolph, 1991
	Variable orifice	Bicore	Varflex® flow transducer	Stupecky, 1991
	Variable orifice	Bird	Partner® IIi volume monitor	Guillaume *et al.*, 1991
	Fixed orifice (target)	Respironics-Novametrix	Series 3 flow sensors	Kofoed & Orr, 1996
	Fixed orifice (pitot)	Datex-Ohmeda	D-lite® flow sensor	Merilainen *et al.*, 1993
	Fixed orifice (pitot)	Medical Graphics	Prevent™ pneumotach	Porszasz *et al.*, 1994
Hot-wire	CTA	Bear	NVM-1 (neonatal volume monitor)	Cutler, 1993
Ultrasonic	Time of flight	NDD	Easyone™ spirometer	Harnoncourt *et al.*, 1996; Buess *et al.*, 1986; 1989

All trademarks are the property of their respective holders.

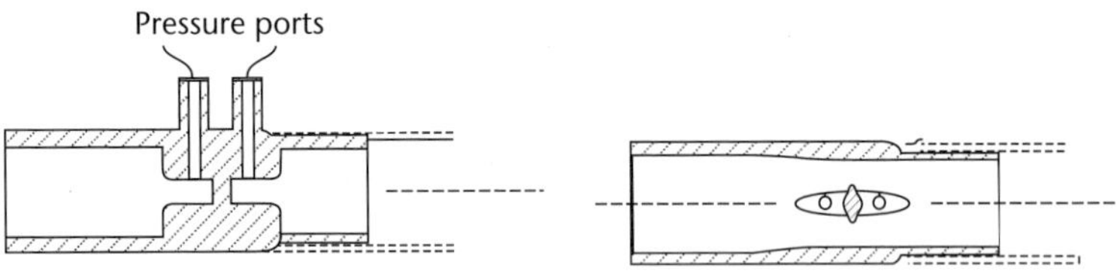

Figure 41.4 Fixed orifice target flow sensor. (Adapted from Kofoed, S.A. & Orr J.A., 1996.)

gas flow, and as such are based upon different measurement principles than target flow meters that measure the disk drag force produced by the reduced annular area. Figure 41.4 illustrates a commercial device

Turbulent flow meters

Elliott *et al.* (1977) pursued resistive flow concepts and investigated a turbulent air flow meter. Fleisch type pneumotachs produce linear responses over a range of laminar flows and are dependent on gas viscosity. Turbulent flow meters, however, have a power law relationship depending on dimensions, length and diameter, as well as viscosity and density. The major advantages of this type of flow meter are that it is relatively uninfluenced by the wet airways usually found in breathing circuits and less influenced by changing gas composition. Its major disadvantages are its accuracy at low flows and its relatively high-pressure drop at high flows. Turbulent flow meters typically have a higher resistance to flow when compared with laminar type flow meters. The turbulent flow approach was further pursued by Saklad *et al.* (1979). Instead of creating turbulence in a tube, this group created turbulence across a fixed orifice. They claimed as major advantages insensitivity to temperature changes and water vapor.

Hot-wire flow sensors

Earlier studies of heat transfer from a heated wire by Boussinesq (1905) were extended by King (1914) who sought to experimentally verify his theoretical results (Stainback & Nagabushana, 1993). The basic "heat balance" relationship can be written as:

heat stored = electrical power in − aerodynamic heat transfer out,

or mathematically as

$$\frac{\mathrm{d}c_w}{\mathrm{d}t} = P - Q,$$

where c_w is the specific heat of the wire.

From this basic relationship King obtained an equation for the hot-wire heat loss:

$$Q = L(k_t) + 2\sqrt{(\pi k_t c_p \rho u r_w)}(T_w - T_{adw}),$$

where Q is the heat loss per unit time (forced convective heat transfer), T_w the wire temperature, T_{adw} temperature adiabatic wall condition, L characteristic length, k_t heat conductivity at specified temperature, c_p specific heat at constant pressure, ρ density of flowing medium, r_w radius of the wire, and u magnitude of the velocity.

It can observed from the above equation that the heat loss is a function of the properties of the wire including its dimensions and heat conductivity and properties of the fluid including its specific heat and density. Additionally, note that nature of the equation is such that lower flow rates sensitivity increases and at higher flow rates it decreases. Thus, the hot-wire sensor tends to be more accurate at low flow rates, but less accurate at high flow rates. Also note that hot-wire anemometers are insensitive to the direction of flow and as such two heated wires need to be placed in series so that the flow direction can be determined.

The two types of hot-wire anemometers primarily used are the constant current anemometer (CCA) and the constant temperature anemometer (CTA). Both designs usually use a bridge circuit (such as the Wheatstone bridge) with one of the legs the hot-wire. By passing a current through the wire ("resistor") its temperature increases and it becomes a "hot-wire." The resistance of a wire (e.g. platinum) is generally proportional to its temperature over the operating range. With the constant current type of hot-wire anemometer, the gas flows past the hot-wire, the wire is cooled, and the altered resistance of the wire is measured to indicate the flow rate of the gas passing the hot-wire resistor. With this type of sensor the current level is usually low, such that the sensor does not become heated.

CTAs are designed to maintain the temperature, as reflected by the resistance of the hot-wire anemometer constant. The resistance level is chosen to be higher than the sensor resistance at ambient conditions, consequently the temperature of the sensor will be higher than ambient. As the resistance of the wire resistor changes in response to gas flow, the current through the platinum wire resistor is adjusted to keep its temperature, and hence its resistance, constant. The resulting voltage drop across the resistor is the indication of the flow rate of the gas (Table 41.2).

In general hot-wire sensors are typically used for measurements in air and other electrically non-conducting fluids. For clinical use the advantages that have been cited include high linearity, wide dynamic range, practically negligible influences of temperature and vapor pressure with humidified gases, capability of measuring bi-directional airflow and ease of operation (Yoshiya *et al.*, 1975, 1979). Problems that have limited its clinical applicability include calibration difficulties, influences of barometric pressure, influences of the composition of gases including anesthetic agents, stability with time, use with nebulizers, hot-wire burning,

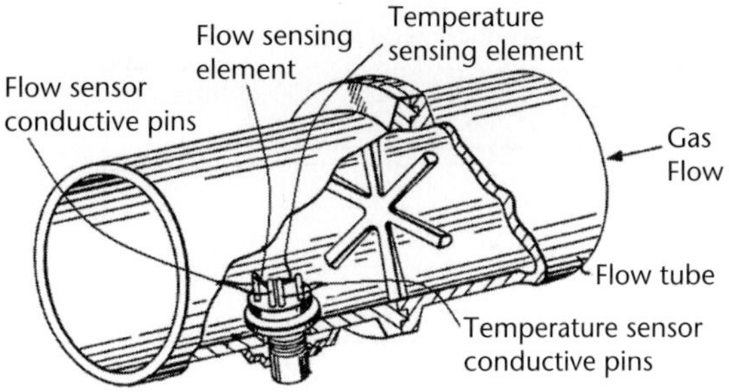

Figure 41.5 Hot-wire sensor assembly mounted in a flow tube. (Adapted from Cutler, 1993.)

possibility of producing nitrogen oxides by the catalytic action of the hot-wire, interchangeability of transducers, sterilization, vulnerability to damage (i.e. handle with care), and flammability (Yoshiya *et al.*, 1979). Stability may be impaired with foreign materials such as sputum, dust or water droplets adhering to the hot-wire altering its temperature coefficient. Designs have been improved performance, however, the influences of gas composition and barometric pressure are unavoidable. Figure 41.5 illustrates a commercial hot-wire device.

Ultrasonic flow sensors

An ultrasonic sensor, such as that proposed by Blumenfeld *et al.* (1974, 1975) does not depend on a Doppler shift in ultrasound frequency but simply measures the influence of gas flow on the transmission times of pulses between two crystals. The transit time principle is based on opposite sending and receiving transducers used to transmit signals through the flow. The signal travels faster when moving with the flow stream rather than against the flow stream. The difference between the two transit times is used to calculate the flow rate. Thus the transmission time (t_d) is decreased in the direction of flow (downstream) and increased (t_u) in the opposite direction (upstream). It can be shown (Buess *et al.*, 1986) that,

$$t_d \cong t_u - t_d = \frac{2Lu \cdot \cos(\beta)}{c^2},$$

where $u << c$, u = mean flow velocity along the sound path, c = velocity of sound, L = the length of the sound transmission path, β is the angle between the transducer and flow axis (Table 41.2).

Although the mathematical relationships are clear, the potential variability of L and c can introduce considerable complexity. The ultrasound velocity depends on temperature and humidity. The speed of sound, c,

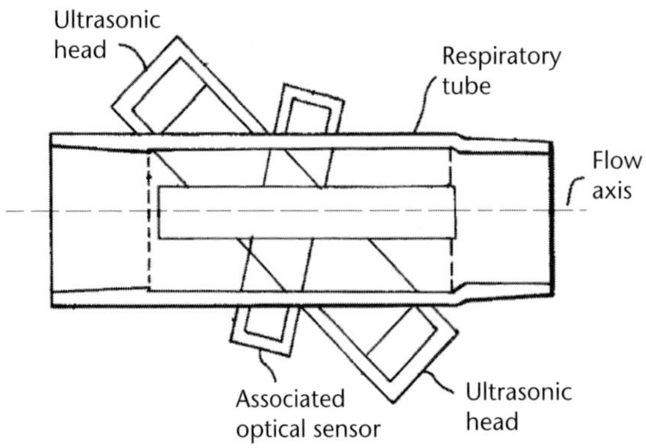

Figure 41.6 Ultrasonic flow sensor. (Adapted from Harnoncourt, 1996.)

also depends on the fractional composition and densities of the gases as well as their specific heats at constant pressure and constant volume. Buess *et al.* (1986) notes that during air-breathing the maximal changes in c^2 term is limited to $\pm 3\%$. Also, the measured average flow velocity between acoustic sensors does not always represent the required average flow velocity. The bottom line is that composition, temperature, and water vapor dependence require careful control in order to implement corrections that provide accurate flow measurements. Additionally, costs associated with the measurement circuitry have traditionally made ultrasonic sensors costly. However, with the development of application specific integrated circuits (ASICs) for these sensors costs have been reduced. Figure 41.6 shows in schematic form a time of flight device.

Summary

Advances in technology have impacted all of the methods described. Increased performance of piezoresistive pressure sensors has improved the low-end performance characteristics of differential pressure flow methods. Novel approaches in hot-wire have overcome some of its shortcomings. Advances in microelectronics such as the use of ASICs have decreased the costs of ultrasonic flow sensors. Even while technology has permitted cost and performance improvements to be made on all fronts, the correct sensor type for each application depends on a careful evaluation of each product and how its fits the particular needs.

References

Bartel, L.P., Bazik, J.R. & Powner, D.J. (1985). Compression volume during mechanical ventilation: comparison of ventilators and tubing circuits. *Crit. Care Med.*, **13(10)**: 851–854.

Blumenfeld, W., Turney, S.Z. & Denman, R.J. (1975). A coaxial ultrasonic pneumotachometer. *Med. Biol. Eng.*, **13(6)**: 855–860.

Blumenfeld, W., Wilson, P.D. & Turney, S. (1974). A mathematical model for the ultrasonic measurement of respiratory flow. *Med. Biol. Eng.*, **12(5)**: 621–625.

Boussinesq, J. (1905). An equation for the phenomena of heat convection and an estimate of the cooling power of fluids. *J. Mathematiq.*, **1**: pp. 285–332, also *Comptes Rendus*, **133**: p. 257.

Branson, R.D. (1999). Humidification for patients with artificial airways. *Resp. Care.*, **44(6)**: 630–641.

Buess, C., Guggenbuhl, W. & Koller, E.A. (1989). A pulsed diagonal-beam ultrasonic airflow meter. *J. Appl. Physiol.*, **67(6)**: 2639.

Buess, C., Pietsch, P., Guggenbuhl, W., Koller, E.A. (1986). Design and construction of a pulsed ultrasonic air flowmeter. *IEEE. Trans. Biomed. Eng.*, **33(8)**: 768–774.

Cutler, C.W. (1993). Flow sensor system and method. US Patent 5,263,369, issued 23 November.

Elliott, S.E., Shore, J.H., Barnes, C.W., Lindauer, J., Osbom, J.J. (1977). Turbulent airflow meter for long-term monitoring in patient-ventilator circuits. *J. Appl. Physiol.*, **42(3)**: 4561160.

Fleisch, A. (1925). Pneuomotachograph: apparatus for recording respiratory flow. *Arch. ges. Physiol.*, **209**: 713–722.

Frey, U., Stocks, J., Coates, A., Sly, P., Bates, J. (2000). Specifications for equipment used for infant pulmonary function testing. ERS/ATS Task Force on standards for infant respiratory function testing. European Respiratory Society/American Thoracic Society. *Eur. Respir. J.*, **16(4)**: 731–740.

Gammage, G.W., Baner, M.J., Blanch, P.B., Kirby, R.R. (1988). Ventilator displayed tidal volume: what you see may not be what you get. *Crit. Care Med.*, **16**: 454 [abstract].

Goff, J.A. & Gratch, S. (1946). Low-pressure properties of water from − 160 to 212 deg F. *Trans. Am. Soc. Heat. Vent.*, **52**: 95–122.

Guillaume, D.W., Norton, M.G. & DeVries, D.F. (1991). Variable orifice flow sensing apparatus. US Patent 4,993,269., issued 19 February.

Harnoncourt, K., Guggenbuhl, W., Schlegelmilch, R.M., Buess, C. (1996). Apparatus for measuring the paramters of respiratory gases. US Patent 5,503,151, April 2.

Hsley, A.H., Hart, J.D., Withers, R.T. & Roberts, J.G. (1993). Evaluation of five small turbine-type respirometers used in adult anesthesia. *J. Clin. Monit.*, **9**: 196–201.

King, L.V. (1914). On the convection of heat from small cylinders in a stream of fluid, *Phil. Trans. of Roy. Soc. (Lond.), Ser. A*, **214(14)**: pp. 373–432.

Kofoed, S.A. & Orr, J.A. (1996). Differential pressure sensor for respiratory monitoring. US Patent 5,535,633, issued 16 July.

Kreit, J.W. & Sciurba, F.C. (1996). The accuracy of pneumotachograh measurements during mechanical ventilation. *Am. J. Respir. Crit. Care Med.*, **154**: 913–917.

Lemen, R.J., Gerdes, C.B., Wegmann, M.J., Perrin, K.J. (1982). Frequency spectra of flow and volume events for forced vital capacity. *J. Appl. Physiol.*, **53(4)**: 977–984.

Lilly, J.C. (1950). Flow meter for recording respiratory flow of human subjects. In: *Methods in Medical Research*, Vol. 2. The Year Book Publishers, Inc., Chicago; pp. 113–121.

Merilainen, P., Hanninen, H. and Tuomaala, L. (1993). A novel sensor for routine continuous spirometry of intubated patients, *J. Clin. Monit.*, **9**: 374–380.

Osbom, J.J. (1978a). A flow meter for respiratory monitoring. *Crit. Care Med.*, **6**: 349–351.

Osborn, J.J. (1978). Variable orifice gas flow sensing head. US Patent 4,083,245, issued 11 April.

Porszasz, J., Barstow, T.J. & Wasserman, K. (1994). Evaluation of a symmetrically disposed pitot tube flowmeter for measuring gas flow during exercise. *J. Appl. Physiol.*, **77**: 2659–2665.

Rudolph, K.A. (1991). Pneumotach. US Patent 5,060,655, issued 29 October.

Saklad, M., Sullivan, M., Paliotta, J., Lipsky, M. (1979). Pneumotachography: a new low deadspace, humidity independent device. *Anesthesiology*, **51**: 149–153.

Shelly, M.P. (1992). Inspired gas conditioning. *Resp. Care*, **37(9)**: 1070–1080.

Silverman, L. & Whittenberg, J.L. (1950). *Methods in Medical Research*, Vol. 2; p. 104.

Stainback, P.C. & Nagabushana, K.A. (1993). Review of Hot-Wire Anemometry Techniques and the Range of their Applicability for Various Flows. *Electron. J. Fluid. Eng., Trans. ASME*, **167**: 1–54.

Stupecky, J. (1991). Variable area obstruction gas flow meter. US Patent 4,989,456, issued 5 February.

Sullivan, W.J., Peters, G.M. & Enright, P.L. (1984). Pneumotachographs: theory and clinical application. *Respiratory Care*, **29**: 736–749.

Tobin, M.J. (1994). *Principles and Practice of Mechanical Ventilation*. McGraw-Hill, Inc., New York.

Turner, M.J., Davies, V.A., De Ravel, T.J., Rothberg, A.D., MacLeod, I.M. (1993). Bandwidths of respiratory gas flow and pressure waveforms in mechanically ventilated infants. *Physiol. Meas.*, **14**: 419–431.

Turner, M.J., MacLeod, I.M. & Rothberg, A.D. (1989). Effects of temperature and composition on the viscosity of respiratory gases. *J. Appl. Physiol.*, **67(1)**: 472–477.

Yeh, M.P., Adams, T.D., Gardner, R.M. & Yanowitz, F.G. (1987). Turbine flowmeter vs Fleisch pneumotachometer: a comparative study for exercise testing. *J. Appl. Physiol.*, **63**: 1289–1295.

Yoshiya, I., Nakajima, T., Nagai, I., Jitsukawa, S. (1975). A bidirectional respiratory flowmeter using the hot-wire principle. *J. Appl. Physiol.*, **38(2)**: 360–365.

Yoshiya, I., Shimada, Y. & Tanaka, K. (1979). Evaluation of a hot-wire respiratory flow-meter for clinical applicability. *J. Appl. Physiol.*, **47**: 1131–1135.

COMBINING FLOW AND CARBON DIOXIDE 42

M.B. Jaffe & J. Orr

Introduction

The combination of flow and carbon dioxide (CO_2) gas concentration makes possible the continuous assessment of CO_2 production. If CO_2 gas concentration and flow were constant, multiplying the two would provide information on CO_2 elimination for each breath. For example, if the exhalation phase lasts 2 s:

$$\begin{aligned} CO_2\ \text{(elimination)} &= \text{concentration} \times \text{flow} \times \text{time} \\ &= 0.04\ \text{(i.e. 4\%)} \times 250\,\text{ml/s} \times 2 \\ &= 20\,\text{ml/breath.} \end{aligned}$$

Gas uptake could be reckoned in a similar way using the differences between inspiratory and expiratory values. In the clinical situation, these measurements do not change instantaneously and are not constant. Therefore, these multiplications must be made over short periods and the results added. The challenge is to integrate concentration and flow signals in such a way that the temporal relationship between the two variables is accurate. Time constants become a major consideration.

Volume of carbon dioxide defined

During normal conditions the lung will excrete CO_2 at the same rate as the total body production rate and there will be no net change in body CO_2 stores. Volume of carbon dioxide ($\dot{V}CO_2$), CO_2 elimination (often incorrectly referred to as CO_2 production) is the net volume of CO_2 measured at the mouth or airway, and calculated as the difference between expired and inspired CO_2 normalized to a minute. $\dot{V}CO_2$ is computed either by taking integral of the dot product of the flow and CO_2 waveforms over the breath cycle. $\dot{V}CO_2$ is usually reported at Standard Temperature and Pressure Dry (STPD) conditions. For breath-by-breath measurements it is calculated as:

$$\dot{V}CO_2 = \sum_{\text{breath}} FCO_2(t) * V(t) * \Delta t,$$

where $FCO_2(t)$ and $V(t)$ are the sampled individual values of the CO_2 and flow waveforms summed over the entire breath and Δt is the sampling interval. When present, inspired CO_2, if not accounted for could result in an error in the calculation of $\dot{V}CO_2$ of several percent (Breen, 1996). However, in anesthesia and in intensive care, components such as filters, heat/moisture exange filters (HMEs), connecting tubes, elbows, airway adapters and suction adapters are placed between the endotracheal tube connector and "Y" causing partial rebreathing and therefore inspired CO_2. Placement of the sampling site more proximal will potentially allow the end-tidal CO_2 ($ETCO_2$) value to better reflect the alveolar concentration. Placement of the sampling site adapter as close to the inspiratory limb (or "Y") as possible will not eliminate the apparatus deadspace due to the volume of the adapter and connectors (Breen, 1996). If the inspiratory CO_2 volume is ignored, the overestimation of $\dot{V}CO_2$ will increase with decreases in tidal volume (V_d/V_t) and/or increases in apparatus deadspace. Note this discussion applies to both side-stream and mainstream devices. Also consider that the last part of the alveolar plateau of the capnogram which is normally considered to be the end-tidal partial pressure of carbon dioxide (PCO_2), is also the PCO_2 of the alveolar gas in the apparatus deadspace that is rebreathed in the next inspiration and does not contribute to the overall pulmonary CO_2 elimination. Placement of the flow/CO_2 sensor in the expiratory limb removes the need to measure inspired CO_2 or account for rebreathing; however, standard capnometry is not possible when only expired gas is analyzed.

Figure 42.1 illustrates the cross multiplication process with the plot of an actual waveform flow and CO_2 versus time of a mechanical breath delivered in a volume control mode. Note that due to apparatus deadspace from the mainstream sensor, "Y" and other circuit components, a small volume of end-expiratory CO_2 (from the previous breath) is rebreathed upon the initiation of inspiration. Note that in this patient, the expiratory CO_2 waveform rises rapidly to a plateau and the CO_2 volume curve follows that of the expiratory portion of the flow waveform. $\dot{V}CO_2$ would then be the difference between the expiratory and inspiratory areas of the cross products. Now if we plot PCO_2

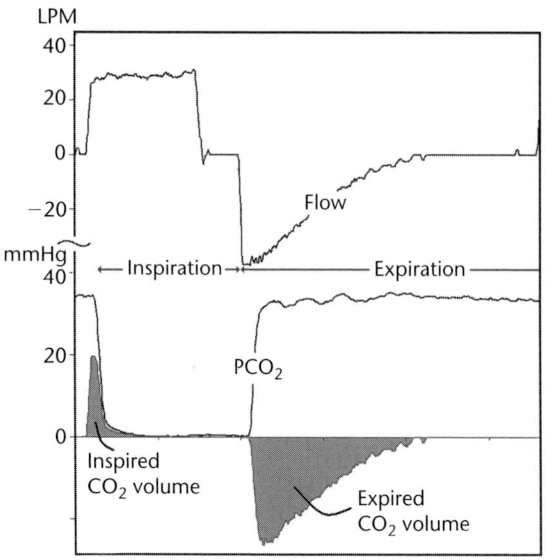

Figure 42.1 Plot of flow and CO_2 waveforms for an individual ventilator delivered breath with cross product showing inspired and expired CO_2 volumes. LPM: liters per minute.

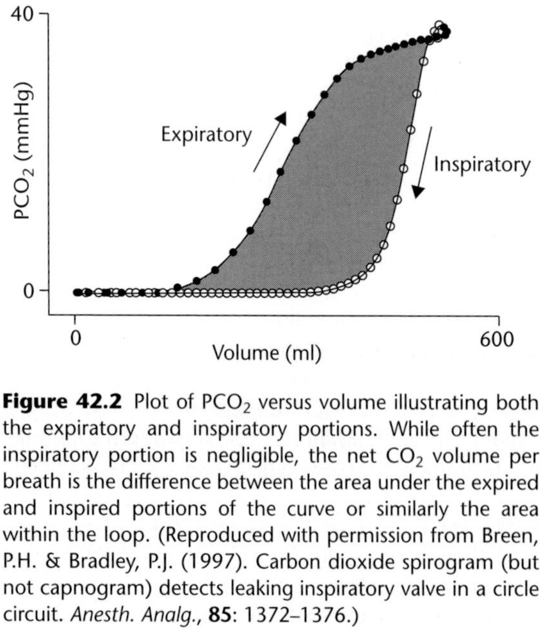

Figure 42.2 Plot of PCO_2 versus volume illustrating both the expiratory and inspiratory portions. While often the inspiratory portion is negligible, the net CO_2 volume per breath is the difference between the area under the expired and inspired portions of the curve or similarly the area within the loop. (Reproduced with permission from Breen, P.H. & Bradley, P.J. (1997). Carbon dioxide spirogram (but not capnogram) detects leaking inspiratory valve in a circle circuit. *Anesth. Analg.*, **85**: 1372–1376.)

and volume instead, CO_2 elimination ($\dot{V}CO_2$), the net volume of CO_2 eliminated can be viewed as the area between the expiratory and inspiratory curves (Figure 42.2). With no rebreathing, the volume of CO_2 eliminated during a breath is the area under the volumetric capnogram. However, the presence of inspiratory CO_2 must be accounted for when reporting and interpreting $\dot{V}CO_2$ (Breen, 1996).

$\dot{V}CO_2$ does not accurately reflect the underlying physiology when there are leaks in the collecting system or where conditions exist such that all the gas that is considered part of the alveolar ventilation volume cannot be measured; that is, pneumothorax with leak or endotracheal tube cuff leaking on exhalation. Due to the complex interaction between V_d/V_t, physiological dead space and alveolar ventilation the volume of CO_2 excreted by each breath is variable. The results of several breaths are often averaged in an attempt to decrease the effect of normal breath-to-breath changes in volume. Depending on how $\dot{V}CO_2$ is used (metabolic versus ventilator adjustments), different averaging interval may be required and include a range of averaging intervals such as 1 breath, 8 breaths, 1 min, 3 min and longer.

During steady-state conditions the lung will excrete CO_2 at the same rate as the total body production rate, and there will be no net change in body CO_2 stores. In this case $\dot{V}CO_2$ is representative of total body production and is proportional to metabolic rate. Because the body stores a large amount of CO_2 relative to the rate at which CO_2 is produced, eliminated CO_2 can be different from metabolically produced CO_2 for a long time (up to 1 h) following a change in ventilation. However, changes in $\dot{V}CO_2$ can provide an instantaneous indication of the change in alveolar ventilation (Taskar, 1995).

Signal processing issues

Fletcher (1983) evaluated the effects of a number of "potential and real sources of error" for the Siemens-Elema CO_2 Analyzer 930 which computed expired CO_2 volume using a mainstream CO_2 analyzer and a flow sensor in the expiratory limb of the ventilator. Some of these effects will be considered in a more general context:

- *Rebreathing of gas in the tubing* will cause $\dot{V}CO_2$ to be overestimated if not considered.
- *Effects of other gases* on the measurement depends upon the both measurement method for flow and CO_2.
- *Delay in CO_2* analysis is more of a consideration with sidestream systems but proper frequency matching of the signals must be considered.
- *Non-linearity of CO_2* and flow sensors are a function of how well the sensor has been characterized by the manufacturer and how well the sensor follows that characterization and how well the calibration corrects for any error.
- *Variations in temperature and vapor content of expired gas* affecting volume correction and $FECO_2$ is

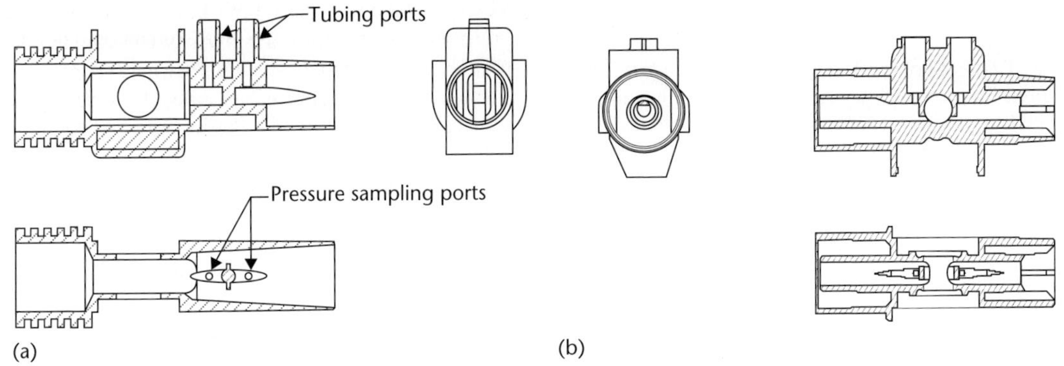

Figure 42.3 (a) Combination adult and (b) combination neonatal CO_2/flow sensors: side, top and end sections. (Image courtesy of Respironics, Inc., Murrysville, PA.)

more of an issue with sidestream systems and mainstream systems, which measure CO_2 and flow at different points.

In order to avoid the undesirable effect of aliasing, an anti-aliasing filter (i.e. low pass) is employed before the analog to digital converter. However, it is necessary to know the bandwidth of the signal of interest so that the filter's cutoff frequency is sufficiently high. For example, an anti-aliasing filter with a bandwidth of 10 Hz can be applied to the signal to effectively remove a 13 Hz noise component. Butterworth filters commonly used for anti-aliasing are used for its maximally flat response in the transmission passband, minimal passband ripple and is best suited for applications requiring preservation of amplitude linearity in the passband region. Methods for determining the frequency response of the flow and gas analyzers have been published (Jackson & Vinegar, 1979). The reader may wish to review these and other references for more detailed discussions on the subject. Note that since integration of the dot product of the flow and CO_2 signals over an entire breath generates a significant low-pass filter, there is little need to further low-pass filter the input signals prior to integration.

Additionally it is important that the signals be properly matched in frequency. Different sensors have different frequency responses and the frequency response of the flow and CO_2 signal must be suitably matched. With both mainstream sensors for flow and CO_2 located at or very close to the same point in the gas stream the principal issues is matching the frequency response of the two sensors. Figure 42.3 illustrates a commercial airway adapter with flow and CO_2 located adjacent (adult design) and not on top of each other using a split fixed orifice design. If the sensors are separated, as with a mainstream CO_2 sensor and separate flow sensors in the inspiratory and expiratory limb of the ventilator, the additional problems of correcting for the effects of different gas characteristics (temperature and humidity) and calibration issues associated with using separate sensors for inspiratory and expiratory flow. When trying to combine a mainstream flow sensor with a sidestream CO_2 signal, the issues become much more complicated. Investigators have pursued approaches ranging from first order corrections (Noguchi *et al.*, 1982; Yamamoto *et al.*, 1987) to higher order non-linear approaches that have characterized the step response of the gas analyzer for each gas of interest and corrected the measured signal with an inverted form of this function (Farmery & Hahn, 2000). Additionally approaches have also been pursued using impulse line model to correct for time compression due to effects of airway pressure on sample flow rate in positive pressure breathing systems (Farmery & Hahn, 2001).

Calibration issues

The accuracy of these devices can be verified using a simple bench procedure. The procedure requires establishing a bench model of a mechanically ventilated lung. A known flow of pure CO_2 (i.e. 200 ml/min) is infused into a mechanical lung simulator (i.e. Training Test Lung, Michigan Instruments, Grand Rapids Michigan) using a precision gas flow controller. When the $\dot{V}CO_2$ measurement device under test is connected to the test lung, the measured CO_2 elimination should match the CO_2 infusion rate (Orr, 1989). Care should be taken to ensure that the flow controller used to determine the injection of CO_2 is accurate and is not affected by the pressure change in the lung. This type of simulation can be used to test the effect of signal alignment, and frequency matching of the signals, as well as compensation of inspired CO_2 and other effects.

References

Breen, P.H., Serina, E.R. & Barker, SJ. (1996). Measurement of pulmonary CO_2 elimination must exclude inspired CO_2 measured at the capnometer sampling site. *J. Clin. Monit.*, **12**: 231–236.

Breen, P.H. & Bradley, P.J. (1997). Carbon dioxide spirogram (but not capnogram) detects leaking inspiratory valve in a circle circuit. *Anesth. Analg.*, **85**: 1372–1376.

Farmery, A.D. & Hahn, C.E. (2000). Response-time enhancement of a clinical gas analyzer facilitates measurement of breath-by-breath gas exchange. *J. Appl. Physiol.*, **89**: 581–589.

Farmery, A.D. & Hahn, C.E. (2001). A method of reconstruction of clinical gas-analyzer signals corrupted by positive-pressure ventilation. *J. Appl. Physiol.*, **90**: 1282–1290.

Fletcher, R., Werner, O., Nordstrom, L. & Jonson, B. (1983). Sources of error and their correction in the measurement of carbon dioxide elimination using the Siemens-Elema CO_2 analyzer. *Br. J. Anaesth.*, **55**: 177–185.

Jackson, A.C. & Vinegar, A. (1979). A technique for measuring frequency response of pressure, volume, and flow transducers. *J. Appl. Physiol.*, **47**: 462–467.

Noguchi, H., Ogushi, Y., Yoshiya, I., Itakura, N. & Yamabayashi, H. (1982). Breath-by-breath VCO_2 and VO_2 required compensation for transport delay and dynamic response. *J. Appl. Physiol.*, **52**: 79–84.

Orr, J.A., Westenskow, D.R. & Bauer, A. (1989). A prototype gas exchange monitor for exercise stress testing aboard NASA Space Station. *J. Appl. Physiol.*, **66**: 492–497.

Taskar, V., John, J., Larsson, A., Wetterberg, T. & Jonson, B. (1995). Dynamics of carbon dioxide elimination following ventilator resetting. *Chest*, **108**: 196–202.

Yamamoto, Y., Takei, Y., Mokushi, K., Morita, H., Mutoh, Y. & Miyashita, M. (1987). Breath-by-breath measurement of alveolar gas exchange with a slow-response gas analyser. *Med. Biol. Eng. Comput.*, **25**: 141–146.

APPENDIX: PATTERNS OF TIME-BASED CAPNOGRAMS

Examples of some frequently observed capnographic patterns. The added explanations are not exhaustive. For details, please consult relevant chapter in the book.

Normal waveforms and nomenclature*

The "normal" capnogram is a waveform that represents the varying carbon dioxide (CO_2) levels throughout the respiratory cycle.
Waveform characteristics:

- A–B baseline
- B–C Expiratory upstroke
- C–D Expiratory plateau
- D End-tidal concentration
- D–E Inspiration begins

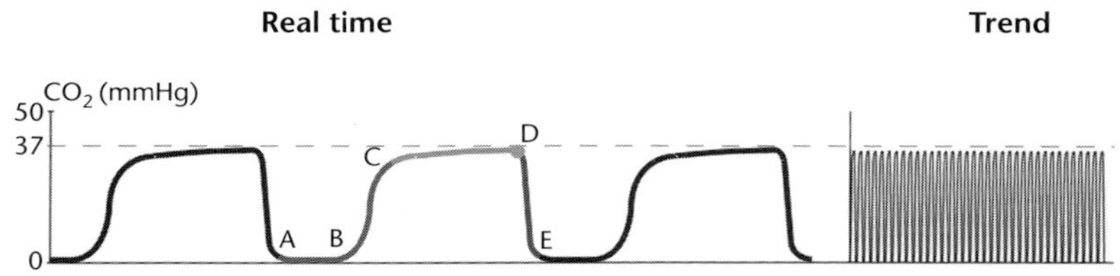

Typically, the time scale (abscissa) for the capnogram is 12.5 mm/s and that of the trend plot 25 mm/min). The ordinate can be calibrated in CO_2 percent (of ambient pressure) or in mmHg, torr, a kPa where 1 kPa = 7.5 mmHg and 1 torr = 1 mmHg.

Time capnogram nomenclature – inspiratory segment (Phase 0) and expiratory segment (divided into phases I, II, & III), α angle, angle between phase II and III; β angle, angle between phase III and descending limb of phase 0 (inspiration). With permission from Kodali, B.S. & Philips, J. (2000). Defining segments and phases of a time capnogram. *Anesth. Analg.*, **91**: 973–977.

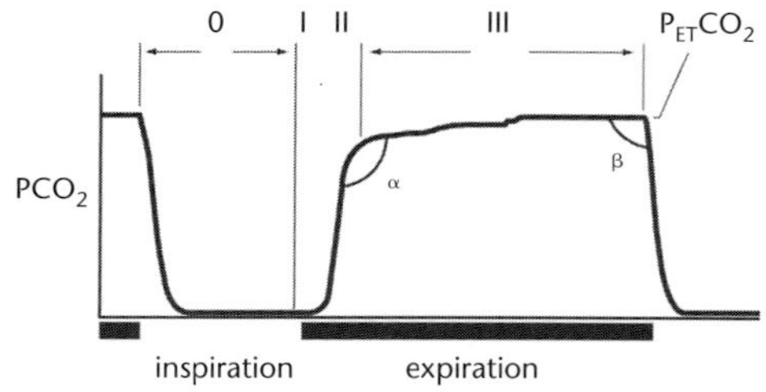

Waveforms (real time and trend)*

Hypoventilation

Elevated plateau (phase III) and end-expiratory values of the capnogram, as seen, for example, with hypoventilation. Check for malignant hypothermia. Observe the extended inspiratory slope. Check inspiratory value.

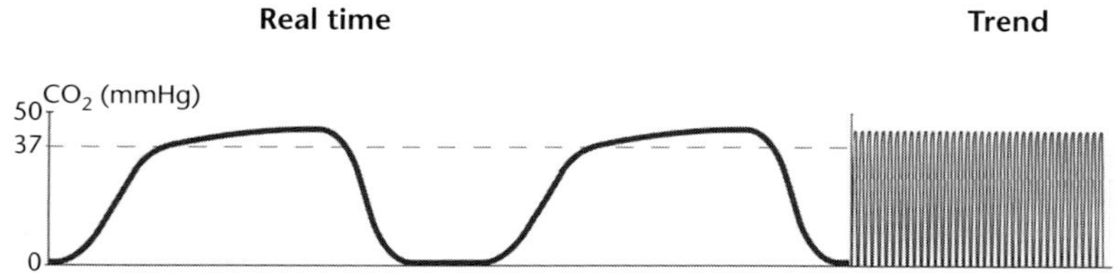

* All images used in this appendix except those with references already listed derived from Respironics, Inc., Murrysville, PA, Publications.

Rapidly increasing partial pressure of CO_2 (PCO_2) at end-tidal ($P_{et}CO_2$) as might occur with the addition of CO_2 to blood (bicarbonate infusion or laparoscopic CO_2 insufflation) or with improving perfusion of the lungs after a period of low cardiac output. Sepsis and malignant hyperthermia raise CO_2 production, but end-tidal levels increase more slowly than shown here.

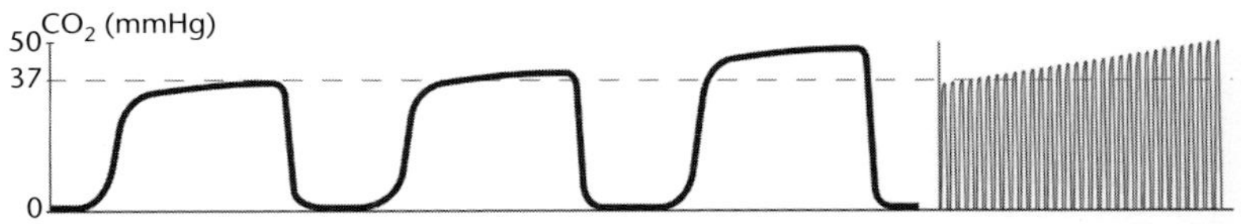

Hyperventilation

Decreasing $P_{et}CO_2$ as might be seen with hyperventilation or decreasing delivery of CO_2 to the lungs with falling cardiac output or pulmonary embolism.

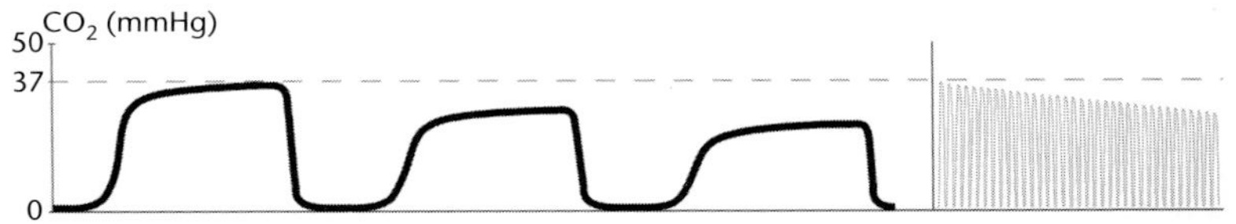

Non-diagnostic

Damped capnograms (poorly defined phases, no obvious $P_{et}CO_2$) is difficult to interpret as it might be seen with high fresh gas flows in a spontaneously breathing patient during pre-oxygenation by face mask. It does not enable an estimation of the adequacy of breathing or of arterial PCO_2 (P_aCO_2).

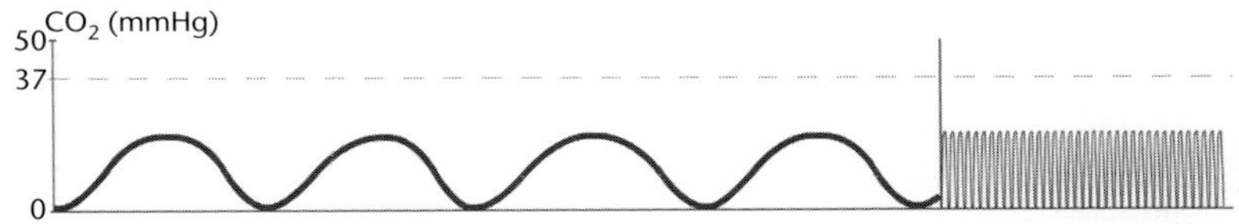

Rebreathing

Increasing levels of inspired CO_2 as might be seen with the addition of deadspace to the endotracheal tube or exhausted CO_2 absorber.

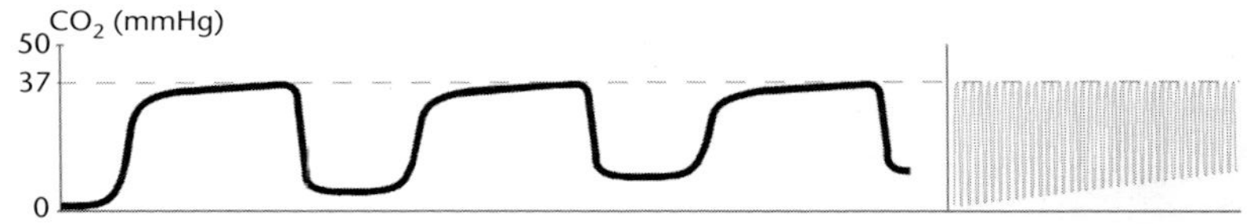

Sudden loss of expiratory CO_2

Cessation of ventilation as might occur with disconnection, extubation, kinking or obstruction of endotracheal tube.

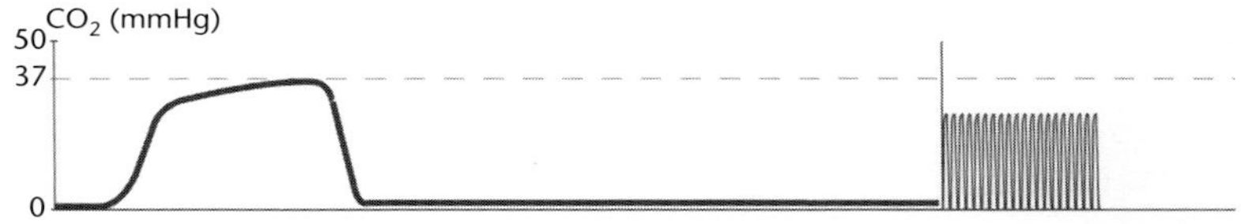

Spontaneous breathing during mechanical ventilation

Interruption of plateau phase of capnogram by a spontaneous breath with a tidal volume large enough to reach zero PCO_2 as might be seen in a patient who takes breaths during mechanical ventilation of the lungs.

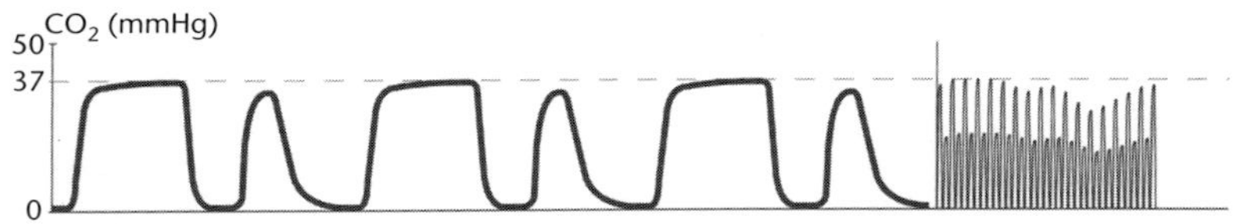

Muscle relaxants (i.e. curare cleft)

The plateau phase of the capnogram is interrupted by small inspiratory efforts of the patient as might be seen in patients on mechanical ventilation. If the patient's P_aCO_2 is high enough to trigger the respiratory center and if the center is not depressed, a patient weakened by neuromuscular blockade might attempt to take a breath. Other explanations: In a weakened patient a hiccup or pain (very light anesthesia) might produce these inspiratory efforts. Smalhout calls these "curare clefts" – see relevant chapter in this book. Compression of the chest (e.g. by the surgeon) can also cause irregularities of the plateau (both up and down).

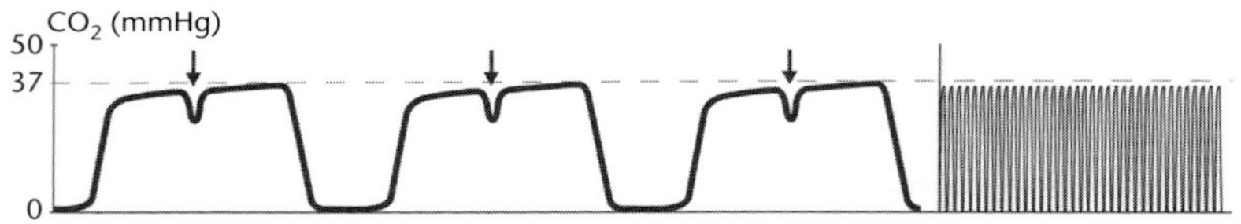

Faulty ventilator circuit valve

Elevated base line as might be seen with faulty valves of a circle breathing system.

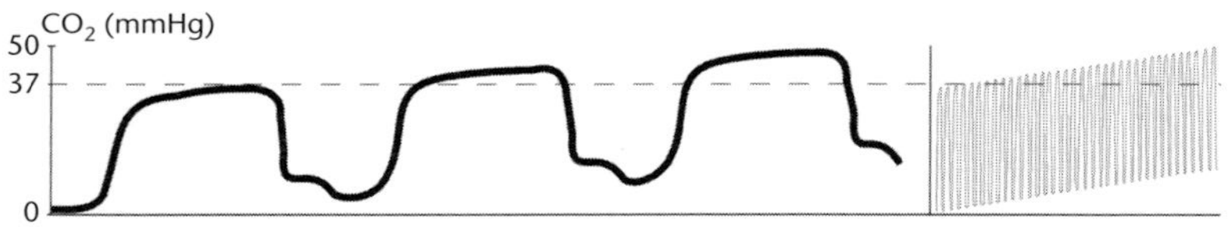

Additional waveform patterns

Asthma

Capnograms of data from a normal subject and a subject with asthma (note: short plateau phase: either shorter time base than normal or tachypnea).
(Adapted with permission from Yaron, M., Padyk, P., Hutsinpiller, M. & Cairns, C.B. (1996). Utility of the expiratory capnogram in the assessment of bronchospasm. *Ann. Emerg. Med.*, **28(4)**: 403–407).

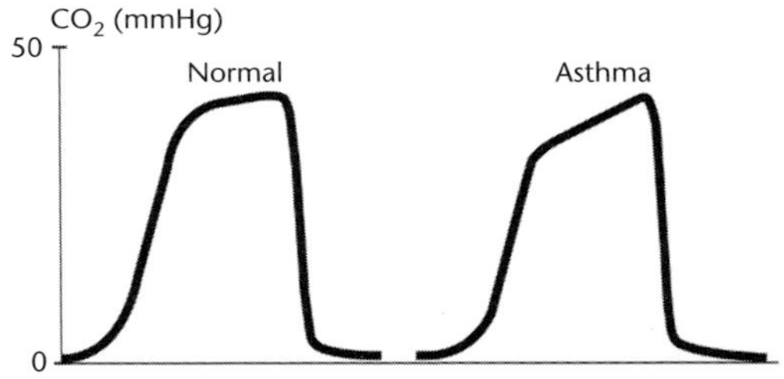

Cardiogenic oscillations

Cardiogenic oscillations as might be seen when the action of the heart cause small tidal volumes during prolonged breath-holding in patients with open glottis (or patent endotracheal tube).

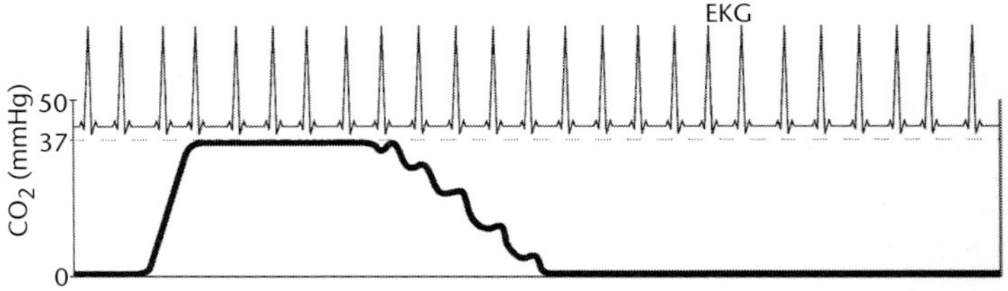

Cardiopulmonary resuscitation

Serial changes in the $P_{et}CO_2$ concentration in a representative patient before and immediately after cardiac arrest, during precordial compression and after defibrillation and resuscitation.
(Adapted with permission from Falk, J.L., Rackow, E.C. & Weil, M.H. (1988). End-tidal carbon dioxide concentration during cardiopulmonary resuscitation. *New Engl. J. Med.*, **318**: 607–611).

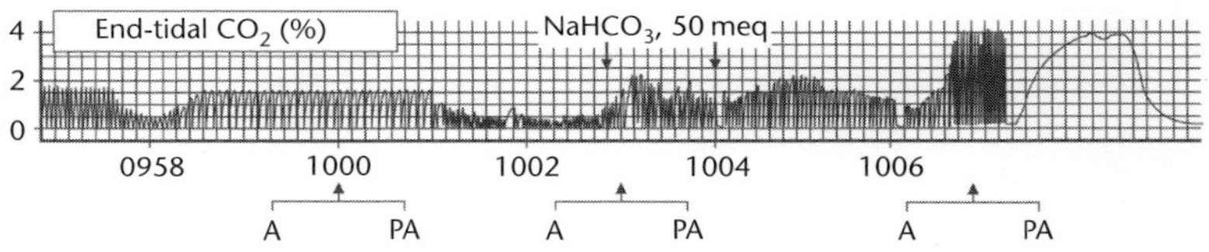

INDEX